Contents

Mosby's TEXTBOOK FOR MEDICATION ASSISTANTS

Adapted from Basic Pharmacology for Nurses, 14th Edition

SHEILA A. SORRENTINO, PhD, RN
Curriculum and Health Care Consultant
Anthem, Arizona

LEIGHANN N. REMMERT, BSN, RN
Staff Nurse, Memorial Medical Center
Springfield, Illinois

BRUCE D. CLAYTON, BS, PharmD, RPh
Professor of Pharmacy Practice
College of Pharmacy & Health Sciences
Butler University
Indianapolis, Indiana

YVONNE N. STOCK, MS, RN
Professor Emeritus, Nursing
Health Occupations Department
Iowa Western Community College
Council Bluffs, Iowa

RENAE D. HARROUN, MSN, RN
Assistant Professor
Trinity College of Nursing and Health Sciences
Rock Island, Illinois

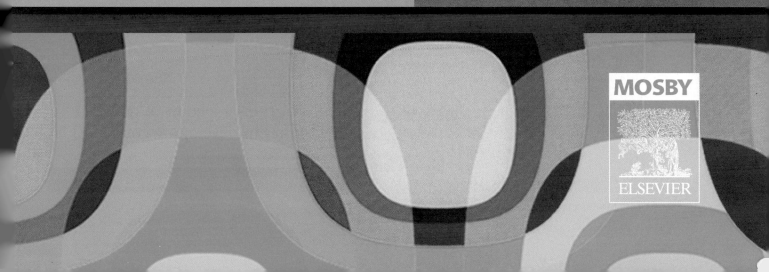

MOSBY

ELSEVIER

11830 Westline Industrial Drive
St. Louis, Missouri 63146

MOSBY'S TEXTBOOK FOR MEDICATION ASSISTANTS ISBN: 978-0-323-04687-9
Copyright © 2009 by Mosby, Inc., an affiliate of Elsevier Inc.

Notice

Knowledge and best practice in this field are constantly changing. As new research and experience broaden our knowledge, changes in practice, treatment, and drug therapy may become necessary or appropriate. Readers are advised to check the most current information provided (i) on procedures featured or (ii) by the manufacturer of each product to be administered, to verify the recommended dose or formula, the method and duration of administration, and contraindications. It is the responsibility of practitioners, relying on their own experience and knowledge of the patient, to make diagnoses, to determine dosages and the best treatment for each individual patient, and to take all appropriate safety precautions. To the fullest extent of the law, neither the Publisher nor the Authors assumes any liability for any injury and/or damage to persons or property arising out of or related to any use of the material contained in this book.

The Publisher

Library of Congress Control Number 2008031311

Library of Congress Cataloging-in-Publication Data

Sorrentino, Sheila A.
    Mosby's textbook for medication assistants / Sheila A. Sorrentino, Leighann Remmert. -- 1st ed.
      p. ; cm.
    Includes index.
    Adapted from: Basic pharmacology for nurses / Bruce D. Clayton, Yvonne N. Stock, Renae D. Harroun. 14th ed. 2007.
    ISBN 978-0-323-04687-9 (pbk. : alk. paper)
    1. Pharmacology. 2. Drugs--Administration. 3. Nurses' aides. I. Remmert, Leighann. II. Clayton, Bruce D., 1947-Basic pharmacology for nurses. III. Title. IV. Title: Textbook for medication assistants.
    [DNLM: 1. Pharmacology--Nurses' Instruction. 4. Education, Pharmacy--methods--Nurses' Instruction. QV 4 S714m 2009]
    RM300.S67 2009
615'.1071--dc22

                                        2008031311

Executive Editor: Susan R. Epstein
Senior Developmental Editor: Maria Broeker
Publishing Services Manager: John Rogers
Senior Project Manager: Cheryl A. Abbott
Text Designer: Renee Duenow

Printed in Canada
Last digit is the print number: 9 8 7 6

To
Carly, Tony, and Mike,
my niece and nephews.
You have grown up to be a fine young woman and fine young men.
I am very proud of you. May your lives be blessed with health, happiness, and success.

With much love,
Aunt Sheila

To my husband, Shane, for your unending love and support.
To my family for your constant encouragement.
And, to Sheila for an incredible opportunity and your exceptional mentoring.
Thank you all. I am truly grateful.

Leighann

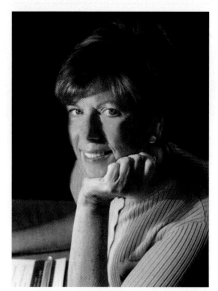

http://www.spindelvisions.com

Sheila A. Sorrentino is currently a curriculum and health care consultant focusing on effective delegation and partnering with assistive personnel in hospitals, long-term care centers, and home care agencies.

Dr. Sorrentino was instrumental in the development and approval of CNA-PN-ADN programs in the Illinois Community College System and has taught in nursing assistant, practical nursing, associate degree, and baccalaureate and higher degree programs. Her career includes experiences as a nursing assistant, staff nurse, charge nurse, head nurse, nursing educator, assistant dean, dean, and consultant.

A Mosby author since 1982, Dr. Sorrentino is the author of *Mosby's Textbook for Nursing Assistants (7e)* and several other textbooks for nursing assistive personnel. She was also involved in the development of *Mosby's Nursing Assistant Skills Videos* and *Mosby's Nursing Skills Videos,* winner of the 2003 AJN Book of the Year Award (electronic media). An earlier version of nursing assistant skills videos won the 1992 International Medical Films Award on caregiving.

Dr. Sorrentino has a bachelor of science degree in nursing, a master of arts in education, a master of science degree in community nursing, and a PhD in higher education administration. She is a member of the Anthem Rotary Club, Sigma Theta Tau International, the Honor Society of Nursing, and former member and chair of the Central Illinois Higher Education Health Care Task Force. She also served on the Iowa-Illinois Safety Council Board of Directors and the Board of Directors of Our Lady of Victory Nursing Center in Bourbonnais, Ill. In 1998 she received an alumni achievement award from Lewis University for outstanding leadership and dedication in nursing education. In 2005 she was inducted into the Illinois State University College of Education Hall of Fame. Her presentations at national and state conferences focus on delegation and other issues relating to nursing assistive personnel.

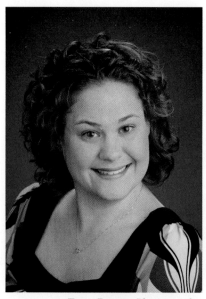

Terry Farmer Photography

Leighann N. Remmert received her bachelor of science degree in nursing from Bradley University in Peoria, Illinois. During her undergraduate study, she was inducted into Sigma Theta Tau International, the Honor Society of Nursing, and the Phi Kappa Phi Honor Society. Leighann was selected as the student representative to address the faculty, families, and classmates in attendance at the nursing department's pinning ceremony for her graduating class. She graduated summa cum laude, with highest honors, from Bradley University.

After receiving her baccalaureate degree, Leighann accepted a position as a registered nurse in the emergency department at Memorial Medical Center in Springfield, Illinois. Leighann has continued to function in this role and has earned her certification as a Trauma Nurse Specialist. She presently functions as a staff nurse, charge nurse, nurse preceptor, and trauma nurse at Memorial Medical Center, currently the Level I trauma center for its region.

Leighann is an active member of the High Reliability Team Steering Committee, which exists to enhance teamwork, accountability, and communication within the emergency department. She is a certified basic life support instructor, and she substitutes as a clinical and skills lab instructor at the Capital Area School of Practical Nursing in Springfield, Illinois. Leighann is pursuing a master's degree in nursing education at Southern Illinois University Edwardsville.

Leighann and her husband, Shane, volunteer as senior high youth sponsors at Elkhart Christian Church in Elkhart, Illinois. Leighann regularly participates in community blood drives and instructs CPR and First Aid training courses for the church and community.

Reviewers

Linda Castaldi, MNSc, RN
Division Chair
National Park Community College
Hot Springs, Arkansas

Ruth Ann Eckenstein, MEd, RN
Program Specialist
Oklahoma Department of Career and Technology
Education
Stillwater, Oklahoma

Stephen M. Setter, PharmD, CDE, CGP, FASCP
Associate Professor of Pharmacotherapy
Washington State University
Elder Services/Visiting Nurses Association
Spokane, Washington

Acknowledgments

Many individuals and agencies have contributed to this first edition of *Mosby's Textbook for Medication Assistants* by providing information, insights, and resources. We are especially grateful and appreciative of the contributions and efforts by:

- Bruce Clayton, Yvonne Stock, and Renae Harroun for graciously allowing their book, *Basic Pharmacology for Nurses* (14e), to be the foundation of *Mosby's Textbook for Medication Assistants*. (See "Instructor Preface.")
- Pamela Randolph, MSN, RN—Associate Director of Education and Evidenced Based Regulation at the Arizona State Board of Nursing (Phoenix, Arizona)—for having the insight that a book for medication assistants was very much needed. We had many discussions about the content and scope of such a book. She is a treasured friend and colleague.
- Diann Muzyka, PhD, RN, Clinical Associate Professor and Site Coordinator at Arizona State University in Tempe, Arizona (formerly Coordinator of Health Programs and Community Education and Workforce Development at Columbus State Community College in Columbus, Ohio) for writing the workbook and instructor ancillary materials. She, too, is a treasured friend and colleague.
- Doug McDermott, math instructor at Scottsdale Christian Academy (Scottsdale, AZ), for reviewing and proofreading the arithmetic appendix. Doug and his family are wonderful neighbors.
- Mary Beth Sorrentino Herron for promptly accommodating countless requests for documents, deliveries, research, and for many other favors and requests. What would we do without you?
- Tim and Linda Sorrentino, owners of the Inkwell (Peru, IL), for accommodating urgent photocopying needs. Their graciousness and generosity are appreciated.
- The artists at Graphic World in St. Louis, Missouri, for their talented work.
- Linda Castaldi, Ruth Ann Eckenstein, and Stephen M. Setter for reviewing the manuscript and for their candor and suggestions. They have contributed to the thoroughness and accuracy of this book.
- Gina Keckritz for serving as copy editor. It was a pleasure talking to her.
- And finally, especially because of all the challenges that surfaced during the development, manuscript, and production processes, to the talented and dedicated Elsevier/Mosby staff, especially:
  - Suzi Epstein (Executive Editor)—Suzi once again gave guidance and support and kept the project on track. She also stressed the importance of taking care of self and family. Suzi believes in us and supports us. Her vision, creativity, and resourcefulness are amazing. She is dedicated to her authors and titles and is a master at what she does.
  - Maria Broeker (Senior Developmental Editor)—Maria handled numerous details, manuscript needs, tasks, and issues. She always has an empathetic ear and time to listen to author wants, needs, and frustrations. Said many, many times, what would we do without Maria?
  - Mary Jo Adams and Sarah Graddy (Editorial Assistants)—they provided prompt clerical and secretarial assistance. They are simply pleasant and delights to work with.
  - John Rogers (Publishing Services Manager) and members of his team—Kathy Teal (Senior Project Manager) and Cheryl Abbott (Senior Project Manager). With all the features and design elements of this book, the book has a user friendly and attractive layout.
  - Renee Duenow (Senior Book Designer) took all of our ideas, some rather abstract, and created a unique, colorful, and up-lifting book and cover design. As always, the book is distinctive from the rest.
- And to all those who contributed to this effort in any way, we are sincerely grateful.

Sheila A. Sorrentino
Leighann N. Remmert

Instructor Preface

Mosby's Textbook for Medication Assistants, in great part, is an adaption of the 50th anniversary, 14th edition of *Basic Pharmacology for Nurses,** first established in 1957. That popular practical nursing/vocational nursing textbook, focused on safe medication administration, is authored by:

- Bruce D. Clayton, BS, PharmD, RPh—Professor of Pharmacy Practice in the College of Pharmacy and Health Sciences at Butler University in Indianapolis, Indiana.
- Yvonne N. Stock, MS, RN—Professor Emeritus of Nursing in the Health Occupations Department at Iowa Western Community College in Council Bluffs, Iowa.
- Renae D. Harron, MSN, RN—Assistant Professor at Trinity College of Nursing and Health Sciences in Rock Island, Illinois.

As more and more states sanctioned the medication assistant role or conducted feasibility studies focused on that role, the need for a textbook became evident. Information and curricula from those states were reviewed along with the curriculum by the National Council of State Boards of Nursing (NCSBN). Like the nursing assistant role, states vary regarding curricula, program length, range of functions, title, and so on. As the scope, content, and depth of the proposed book began to emerge, the possibility of adapting an existing textbook for the medication assistant role was explored because of the time-consuming and monumental task of researching countless drugs and reducing volumes of information into a user-friendly format for instructional and reference purposes. Requiring the cooperation and respect of all the authors and editorial teams involved, adapting *Basic Pharmacology for Nurses* by Clayton, Stock, and Harroun was ultimately viewed as a very feasible, beneficial, and expeditious avenue to meet the needs of the medication assistant market.

For purposes of standardization and to meet the needs of all states while maintaining neutrality and centrality, *Mosby's Textbook for Medication Assistants* follows the NCSBN's "Medication Assistant-Certified (MA-C) Model Curriculum." And with NCSBN approval, medication assistant-certified (MA-C) is used when referring to medication assistants and nursing assistive personnel with similar titles.

This textbook is designed to serve the teaching and learning needs of instructors and students focused on the MA-C role. It is a valuable resource for competency test review and a reference for the MA-C who seeks to learn or review additional information about drugs and giving them safely.

ORGANIZATIONAL STRATEGIES

Building on the nursing assistant role and assuming prior learning, *Mosby's Textbook for Medication Assistants* embraces the core values and principles in *Mosby's Textbook for Nursing Assistants (7e), Mosby's Textbook for Long-Term Care Assistants (5e), Essentials for Nursing Assistants (3e), Basic Skills for Nursing Assistants in Long-Term Care,* and *Assisting With Patient Care (2e).* Those values and principles, as they relate to this book, are:

- Patients and residents are persons who have inherent dignity and value. They have basic needs and protected rights.
- Federal and state laws—directly and indirectly—define the roles, range of functions, and limitations of the MA-C role.
- MA-C roles and functions vary among states and agencies.
- The MA-C role has legal and ethical aspects.
- MA-C functions and role limits depend on effective delegation by a licensed nurse. *Delegation Guidelines* are integrated throughout the book as appropriate.
- Safety is a critical need for the person and MA-C.
- Understanding body structure and function is an essential aspect of safety.
- The nursing process is the basis for safe medication administration. The MA-C assists the nurse with and has a valuable role in the nursing process.

Learning about medications and how to safely give them inherently present teaching and learning challenges. Therefore, additional strategies are employed to foster a user friendly format for teaching and learning.

---

*A complete listing of illustrations, boxes, and tables in this adaptation that originally appeared in *Basic Pharmacology for Nurses,* 14th edition, is on p. 465.

- An appropriate reading level is necessary to facilitate the learning process. Because of generic and trade names and the nature of pharmacology, the reading level is approximately that of the eighth grade.
- For readability and learning ease, some terms are purposefully hyphenated. Cortico-steroid, anti-cholinergic, vaso-dilator, vaso-constriction, broncho-dilator, and broncho-spasm are examples. And "drug," rather than "medication," is used for reading ease and simplification.
- With safety as an ultimate goal, the *Six Rights of Drug Administration* are stressed in text and in the procedures focused on various routes of drug administration.
- Parenteral dose forms—intradermal, subcutaneous, intramuscular, and intravenous—are NOT included in this book.
- Adult dosages are the focus. Pediatric dosages are not included. Even if a drug has no pediatric use, phrases such as "adult dosages" and "initial adult dosage" are used throughout the book for safety purposes.
- The MA-C is an assistant to the nurse. He or she, at all times, functions under the direction and supervision of a licensed nurse. The MA-C does not function independently and does not make patient or resident care decisions. The nursing process serves as the framework for presenting drug information.
- The person's safety and comfort are central to the MA-C role. *Promoting Safety and Comfort* boxes are integrated throughout the book as appropriate.
- Body structure and function and common health problems are integrated into the drug chapters.
- A template is used to present classes of drugs and specific drug information. That template includes a description of the drug's action, uses, and goals of therapy followed by "Assisting With the Nursing Process" for that drug class or drug:
  - Assessment—the observations to report and record
  - Planning—dose forms
  - Implementation—dosages and when and how to give the drug
  - Evaluation—side effects to report and record

FEATURES AND DESIGN

Besides content issues, attention also is given to the book's features and designs. The following features and design elements make the book readable and user friendly (see Student Preface, pp. xiii-xvi):
- **Illustrations**—the book contains numerous full-color photographs and line art.
- **Objectives**—list the learning objectives for the chapter.

- **Procedures**—a list of the procedures in the chapter follows the objectives.
- **Key Terms with definitions**—are at the beginning of each chapter.
- **Key Abbreviations**—for quick reference, the abbreviations used in the chapter are listed in the chapter opening section. Some are used, but not defined, in the chapter. Examples include mg, mL, g, mcg, MAR. Defined in earlier chapters, they are included for reference purposes in the "Key Abbreviations" lists.
- **Key terms in bold print**—are throughout the text. The definition is presented in narrative in the text.
- **Boxes and tables**—list principles, guidelines, signs and symptoms, nursing measures, and drug information. They are an efficient way for instructors to highlight content. And they are useful study guides for students.
- **Procedure icons**—in section headings alert the student to an associated procedure. Procedure boxes contain the same icon.
- **Delegation Guidelines**—are associated with procedures and drug classes. They focus on the information needed from the nurse and the care plan about critical aspects of the procedure and the observations to report and record. Step 1 in the procedures refers the student to the appropriate *Delegation Guidelines*.
- **Promoting Safety and Comfort boxes**—focus the student's attention on the need to be safe and cautious and promote comfort when giving drugs. "Safety" and "Comfort" subtitles are used. Step 1 in the procedures refers the student to the appropriate *Promoting Safety and Comfort* boxes.
- **Procedure boxes divided into Quality of Life, Pre-Procedure, Procedure, and Post-Procedure steps**—Each procedure section has a subtitle. *Quality of Life, Pre-Procedure,* and *Post-Procedure* steps are included to show the procedure as a whole and reinforce learning. The *Quality of Life* section in the procedure boxes reminds the student of six fundamental courtesies:
  - Knock before entering the room.
  - Address the person by name.
  - Introduce one's self by name and title.
  - Explain the procedure to the person before beginning and during the procedure.
  - Protect the person's rights during the procedure.
  - Handle the person gently during the procedure.
- **Focus on Older Persons boxes**—provide age-specific information about giving drugs to older persons.
- **Focus on Communication boxes**—suggest what to say and questions to ask when interacting with patients, residents, and the nursing team.

- **Review Questions**—are found at the end of each chapter. A page number is given for where to find the answers. The goal is to provide the student with a mechanism to review the chapter content. The questions are not intended to be test questions. They are structured to allow a thorough review of the content.

All textbook manuscripts are reviewed by instructors representing the various regions of the United States. Manuscripts are reviewed for accuracy, relevancy, and currency. Because of the ever changing pharmacology arena, the final manuscript for this textbook was reviewed by Bruce Clayton, co-author of *Basic Pharmacology for Nurses* (14e) and Stephen M. Setter, Associate Professor of Pharmacotherapy.

The manuscript and production processes for this book presented many challenges. At every turn the Food and Drug Administration approved new drugs, issued new warnings, and removed drugs from the market. Varying state requirements and curricula presented another set of challenges. What was projected to work in manuscript sometimes had to be modified, revised, or rejected. But finally, we are proud of the first edition of *Mosby's Textbook for Medication Assistants* and hope that Bruce Clayton, Yvonne Stock, and Renae Harroun are proud of it too.

**Sheila A. Sorrentino,
BSN, MA, MSN, PhD, RN
Leighann N. Remmert, BSN, RN**

Student Preface

This book was designed for you. It was designed to help you learn. The book is a useful resource as you gain experience and expand your knowledge.

This preface gives some study guidelines and helps you use the book. When given a reading assignment do you read from the first page to the last page without stopping? How much do you remember? You will learn more if you use a study system. A useful study system has these steps:

- Survey or preview
- Question
- Read and record
- Recite and review

PREVIEW

Before you start a reading assignment, preview or survey the assignment. This gives you an idea of what the assignment covers. It also helps you recall what you already know about the subject. Carefully look over the assignment. Preview the chapter title, headings, subheadings, and terms or ideas in bold print or italics. Also survey the objectives, key terms, boxes, and review questions at the end of the chapter. Previewing only takes a few minutes. Remember, previewing helps you become familiar with the material.

QUESTION

After previewing, you need to form questions to answer while you read. Questions should relate to what might be asked on a test or how the information applies to giving care. Use the title, headings, and subheadings to form questions. Avoid questions that have one word answers. Questions that begin with what, how, or why are helpful. While reading, you may find that a question does not help you study. If so, just change the question. Remember, questioning sets a purpose for reading. So changing a question only makes this step more useful.

READ AND RECORD

Reading is the next step. Reading is more productive after determining what you already know and what you need to learn. Read to find answers to your questions. The purpose of reading is to:

- Gain new information
- Connect new information to what you know already

Break the assignment into smaller parts. Then answer your questions as you read each part. Also, mark important information—underline, highlight, or make notes. Underlining and highlighting remind you of what you need to learn. Go back and review the marked parts later. Making notes results in more immediate learning. To make notes, write down important information in the margins or in a notebook. Use words and statements to jog your memory about the material.

You need to remember what you read. To do so, work with the information. Organize information into a study guide. Study guides have many forms. Diagrams or charts show relationships or steps in a process. Note taking in outline format is also very useful. The following is a sample outline.

1. Main heading
   a. Second level
   b. Second level
      i. Third level
      ii. Third level
2. Main heading

RECITE AND REVIEW

Finally, recite and review. Use your notes and study guides. Answer the questions you formed earlier. Also answer other questions that came up when reading and answering the "Review Questions" at the end of a chapter. Answer all questions out loud (recite).

Reviewing is more about when to study rather than what to study. You already determined what to study during the preview, question, and reading steps. The best times to review are right after the first study session, one week later, and before a quiz or test.

This book was also designed to help you study. Special design features are described on the next pages.

We hope you enjoy learning and your work. You and your work are important. You and the care you give make a difference in the person's life!

Sheila A. Sorrentino
Leighann N. Remmert

Procedures list identifies the procedures presented in the chapter.

Objectives tell what is presented in the chapter.

Key Terms are the important words and phrases in the chapter. Definitions are given for each term. The key terms introduce you to the chapter content. They are also a useful study guide.

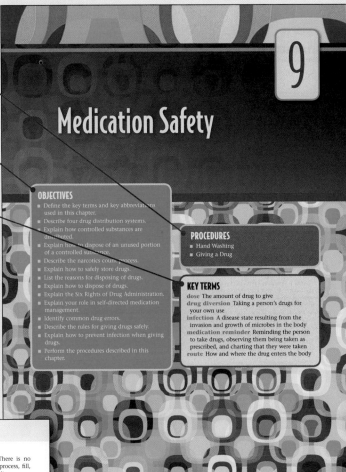

9

Medication Safety

OBJECTIVES
- Define the key terms and key abbreviations used in this chapter.
- Describe four drug distribution systems.
- Explain how controlled substances are distributed.
- Explain how to dispose of an unused portion of a controlled substance.
- Describe the narcotics count process.
- Explain how to safely store drugs.
- List the reasons for disposing of drugs.
- Explain how to dispose of drugs.
- Explain the Six Rights of Drug Administration.
- Explain your role in self-directed medication management.
- Identify common drug errors.
- Describe the rules for giving drugs safely.
- Explain how to prevent infection when giving drugs.
- Perform the procedures described in this chapter.

PROCEDURES
- Hand Washing
- Giving a Drug

KEY TERMS
dose The amount of drug to give
drug diversion Taking a person's drugs for your own use
infection A disease state resulting from the invasion and growth of microbes in the body
medication reminder Reminding the person to take drugs, observing them being taken as prescribed, and charting that they were taken
route How and where the drug enters the body

KEY ABBREVIATIONS
ADE Adverse drug event
ALR Assisted living residence
CDC Centers for Disease Control and Prevention
FDA Food and Drug Administration
HBV Hepatitis B virus
HIV Human immunodeficiency virus
ID Identification
IM Intramuscular
ISMP Institute for Safe Medication Practices
IV Intravenous
MAR Medication administration record
mg Milligram
NDC National Drug Code
OPIM Other potentially infectious materials
OSHA Occupational Safety and Health Administration
PPE Personal protective equipment
PRN When necessary; as needed
STAT At once; immediately
subcut Subcutaneous; subcutaneously

Medication safety involves the correct dispensing of the drug, correct storage, and correct disposal. Errors must be prevented. They must also be prevented when giving drugs to a person. To prevent drug errors and give drugs safely, you must follow the *Six Rights of Drug Administration*. The *right* drug must be given at the *right* time in the *right* dose to the *right* person using the *right* route. *Right* documentation follows giving a drug.

Safety involves protecting the person and yourself from infection. This chapter includes a review of medical asepsis, hand hygiene, and Standard Precautions.

DRUG DISTRIBUTION SYSTEMS

The pharmacy processes and fills drug orders. Then they are distributed (dispensed) to the nursing unit. Each agency has its own drug distribution system. The following systems are common.

See *Promoting Safety and Comfort: Drug Distribution Systems.*

Floor or Ward Stock System

With the *floor or ward stock system,* frequently used drugs are kept on the nursing unit (Fig. 9-1). Dangerous and rarely used drugs are kept in the pharmacy. Small hospitals and some nursing centers may use this system. Some government hospitals may use this system if drugs are not charged directly to the patient.

Ordered drugs are readily available. There is no waiting or lag time for the pharmacy to process, fill, and send the drug order to the nursing unit.

Safety issues for this system include:
- Many drugs are stocked on the nursing unit. This increases the risk for drug errors. For example, you must select the right drug and the right dose from all the drugs stocked.
- Monitoring drug expiration dates is hard. Over time, the chemical nature of a drug can change. In other words, the drug deteriorates. A once helpful drug can turn harmful.
- The nursing unit may not have enough space to store all drugs safely.
- Agency personnel have access to many drugs. Drug diversion is a risk.

Individual Prescription Order System

The *individual prescription order system* also involves storing drugs on the nursing unit. For a patient or resident, the pharmacy sends a 3- to 5-day supply of an ordered drug to the nursing unit. The drugs are stored in small bins in a cabinet on the nursing unit. Each person has a bin. Bins are arranged alphabetically by the person's name. Or bins are arranged by room and bed numbers.

This system is safer than the floor or ward stock system.
- A pharmacist and a nurse review the order before the drug is given.
- The pharmacy monitors drug expiration dates. This lessens the danger of drugs deteriorating.
- Fewer drugs are available for drug diversion.

Like the floor or ward stock system, drugs are available for STAT or PRN use. While fewer drugs are available, drug diversion remains a risk.

PROMOTING SAFETY AND COMFORT
Drug Distribution Systems

SAFETY
Always check drugs received from the pharmacy. Compare the pharmacy label against the drug order on the medication administration record (MAR). Also check that the number of doses is correct. If the number of doses is not correct, tell the nurse before continuing. It is possible that:
- The drug was discontinued.
- Another staff member gave the drug.
- The pharmacy omitted a dose.
- The drug was given to the wrong person.
- The drug was diverted by a staff member. **Drug diversion** is taking a person's drugs for your own use. This is illegal.

Follow agency policy for reporting a drug error (p. 118).

Key Abbreviations are a quick reference to the abbreviations used in the chapter. They are listed after the "Key Terms."

Promoting Safety and Comfort boxes focus your attention on the need to be safe and cautious and promote comfort when giving drugs. "Safety" and "Comfort" subtitles are used.

KEY ABBREVIATIONS

TDD Transdermal drug delivery

Topical refers to a surface of a part of the body. A **topical medication** is a drug applied to the skin. The absorption of a topical drug is affected by:

* The strength of the drug
* How long the drug is in contact with the skin
* The size of the area of application
* Skin thickness
* Amount of water in the tissues
* Amount of skin breakdown or irritation

Drugs are applied topically to:

* Clean and debride a wound. **Debride** means to remove. Wounds are debrided to remove dirt, damaged tissue, foreign objects, and drainage. This is done to prevent infection and to promote healing.
* Hydrate (add water) the skin.
* Reduce inflammation.
* Relieve itching or a rash.
* Provide a protective barrier to the skin.
* Reduce thickening of the skin. Callous formation is an example.

TOPICAL DOSE FORMS

Creams, lotions, ointments and powders are common topical dose forms.

* *Creams.* A **cream** is a semi-solid emulsion containing a drug. An *emulsion* contains small droplets of water-in-oil or oil-in-water. The cream base is usually non-greasy. Creams are removed with water.
* *Lotions.* A **lotion** is a watery preparation containing suspended particles. Shake all lotions before the application. Then gently but firmly pat the lotion onto the skin. Do not rub the lotion into the skin. Rubbing increases circulation and itching. Rubbing also causes friction, which can irritate the skin. Lotions are used to:
  * Soothe and protect the skin
  * Relieve rashes and itching
  * Cleanse the skin
* *Ointments.* An **ointment** is a semi-solid preparation containing a drug in an oily base. Ointments are not easily removed with water. Therefore the drug has longer contact with the skin.
* *Powders.* A **powder** is a finely ground drug in a talc base. Powders are used to absorb moisture. They also dry, cool, and protect the skin. Powder is applied to dry skin in a thin, even layer.

BOX 11-1   Rules for Applying Creams, Lotions, Ointments, and Powders

* Practice hand hygiene before and after the application.
* Follow Standard Precautions.
* Follow isolation precautions as ordered (Appendix B).
* Wear gloves.
* Do not let the dose form touch your skin.
* Provide for privacy.
* Position the person to expose the application site. Avoid unnecessary exposure.
* Clean and dry the skin as directed by the nurse before applying a dose form. Usually soap and water are used if the person's skin condition allows. Make sure previous applications are thoroughly removed.
* Observe the skin. Report and record your observations. See *Delegation Guidelines: Applying Creams, Lotions, Ointments, and Powders.*
* See *Promoting Safety and Comfort: Applying Creams, Lotions, Ointments, and Powders.*
* Shake lotions thoroughly. The lotion should have a uniform color throughout.
* Apply the dose form to clean, dry skin.
* Apply the correct amount. Use a sterile tongue blade or sterile cotton-tipped applicator to remove the dose from a jar. If applying the drug by hand or finger, use the tongue blade or cotton-tipped applicator to transfer the dose to your gloved hand or finger.
* Do not let the drug container touch the person's skin.
* Cover the site with gauze or other covering as directed by the nurse, care plan, and MAR. Ointments and creams may stain or soil garments and linens.
* See procedure: *Applying Nitroglycerin Ointment,* p. 145.

Text continued on p. 144.

Bold type is used to highlight the key terms in the text. You again see the key term and read its definition. This helps reinforce your learning.

FOCUS ON COMMUNICATION

The Self-Administration of Drugs

To remind a person to take his or her drugs, you can say:

* "Ms. Epstein, it's time to take your 8 o'clock pills."
* "Mr. Ladd, you'll need to take your pills in about 10 minutes."
* "Mrs. Young, are you ready to take your pills?"

To read a drug label to a person, read the following:

* The name of the person on the drug label
* The name of the drug
* How to take the drug (by mouth, with food, with a full glass of water; apply to the skin, rectally, and so on)
* The dosage
* When to take the drug (before meals, with meals, after meals, and so on)
* How often to take the drug
* Warnings and other information on the drug label

BOX 9-3   Examples of Drug Errors

PRESCRIBING ERRORS

* Prescribing the wrong drug for the person's diagnosis
* Prescribing a drug to which the person is allergic
* Prescribing the wrong dose for the person's diagnosis

TRANSCRIPTION ERRORS

* Misinterpreting or misunderstanding the drug ordered or the directions
* Interpreting hand-writing that is not legible
* Using unapproved abbreviations
* Omitting a drug order
* Using the wrong spelling
* Writing the wrong dates or times

DISPENSING

* Sending the wrong drug or dose to the nursing unit
* Using the wrong formulation
* Using the wrong dosage form

GIVING DRUGS

* Giving the wrong drug
* Giving the wrong dose
* Giving an extra dose
* Giving a drug not ordered for the person
* Missing or skipping a dose
* Giving a drug at the wrong time
* Giving the drug in the wrong way
* Not recording that a drug was given

Focus on Communication suggests what to say and questions to ask when interacting with patients, residents, and the nursing team.

BOX 9-4   Safety Rules for Giving Drugs

* Follow the *Six Rights of Drug Administration* p. 113.
* Store all drugs properly (p. 112).
* Make sure you have good lighting. You must be able to read the MAR and drug labels correctly.
* Stay focused. Do not allow yourself to become distracted. Ask other staff not to interrupt you unless the situation is critical.
* Keep your working area clean, neat, and orderly.
* Check the container label for the drug name, dose, and route.
* Check the person's chart, Kardex, MAR, and ID bracelet for allergies. Also ask the person before giving a drug if he or she has any allergies.
* Check the person's chart, Kardex, and MAR for rotation schedules for drugs applied to the skin (Chapter 11).
* Know why the drug was ordered. Also know its side effects and possible adverse reactions.
* Calculate drug dosages accurately (if allowed by your state and agency). Ask a nurse to check your calculation.
* Identify the person before giving any drug.
* Position the person for the route of administration. For example, for an oral drug the person should be in a sitting or Fowler's position to promote swallowing. Check the care plan and with the nurse for any position limits.
* Have correct fluids ready for the person to swallow oral drugs.
* Stay with the person to make sure that all drugs have been swallowed. If necessary, check the person's mouth—under the tongue and between teeth and the cheeks.
* Follow agency policy for self-administered drugs.
* Never leave a drug in the person's room for the person to take later (unless there is a doctor's order to do so). Always make sure the person takes the drug in your presence.
* Never leave a drug unattended.
* Refer any questions about the person's drug or treatment plan to the nurse.

Continued

Boxes and tables contain important rules, principles, guidelines, signs and symptoms, nursing measures, and drug information in a list format. They identify important information and are useful study guides.

Heading icons alert you to associated procedures. Procedure boxes contain the same icon.

Focus on Older Persons provides age-specific information about giving drugs to older persons.

Delegation Guidelines describe what information you need from the nurse and care plan before giving a drug. They also tell you what information to report and record.

Applying Creams, Lotions, Ointments, and Powders

Each topical dose form is applied differently. Lotions are dabbed on the skin with gauze or a cotton ball. A tongue blade, cotton-tipped applicator, or a gloved hand or finger is used to apply ointments and creams. Powders are applied in a thin, even layer. To safely apply a topical dose form, follow the rules in Box 11-1. Also practice medication safety (Chapter 9). To apply a nitroglycerin ointment, see p. 144.

See *Focus on Older Persons: Applying Creams, Lotions, Ointments, and Powders.*

See *Delegation Guidelines: Applying Creams, Lotions, Ointments, and Powders.*

See *Promoting Safety and Comfort: Applying Creams, Lotions, Ointments, and Powders.*

FOCUS ON OLDER PERSONS

Applying Creams, Lotions, Ointments, and Powders

Dry skin occurs with aging. Soap also dries the skin. Dry skin is easily damaged. Thorough rinsing is needed when using soap. The nurse and care plan may direct you to use a different cleansing agent.

DELEGATION GUIDELINES
Applying Creams, Lotions, Ointments, and Powders

Before applying a topical dose form, you need the following information from the nurse, care plan, and MAR:
* If isolation precautions are required. If yes:
  * What type of precaution
  * What personal protective equipment is needed
* Special measures for cleaning and drying the skin.
* What cleansing agent to use.
* The exact site of application.
* What to use to apply the drug—tongue blade, cotton-tipped applicator, or gloved hand or finger.
* If you need to cover the application. If yes, how to cover the application site—gauze, see-through dressing and tape, and so on.
* What observations to report and record:
  * The color of the skin
  * The location and description of rashes
  * Dry skin
  * Bruises or open skin areas
  * Pale or reddened areas, particularly over bony parts
  * Blisters
  * Drainage or bleeding from wounds or body openings
  * Skin temperature
  * Complaints of pain or discomfort
  * [ ]n to report observations.
* [ ]t specific patient or resident concerns to report [ ]ce.

PROMOTING SAFETY AND COMFORT
Applying Creams, Lotions, Ointments, and Powders

SAFETY

Use caution when applying powder. Inhaling powder can irritate the airway and lungs. Do not shake or sprinkle powder onto the person. To safely apply powder:
* Turn away from the person.
* Sprinkle a small amount of powder onto your hands or a cloth.
* Apply the powder in a thin layer.
* Make sure powder does not get on the floor. Powder is slippery and can cause falls.

COMFORT

A skin area is exposed to apply topical dose forms. Provide for privacy. Screen the person. Close doors and window coverings—drapes, shades, blinds, shutters, and so on. Avoid unnecessary exposure. Expose only the area needed.

The person may have a rash or skin lesion. A skin disorder may be contagious. The person knows the disease can be spread to others. Self-esteem may suffer. He or she may feel dirty and undesirable. Treat the person with dignity and respect.

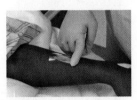

Fig. 11-1 A cream is applied with a gloved index finger. (Courtesy Rick Brady, from Lilley LL and others: *Pharmacology and the nursing process,* ed 5, St Louis, 2007, Mosby.)

APPLYING A CREAM, LOTION, OINTMENT, AND POWDER

QUALITY OF LIFE

Remember to:
* Knock before entering the person's room.
* Address the person by name.
* Introduce yourself by name and title.

* Explain the procedure to the person before beginning and during the procedure.
* Protect the person's rights during the procedure.
* Handle the person gently during the procedure.

PRE-PROCEDURE

1. Follow *Delegation Guidelines: Applying Creams, Lotions, Ointments, and Powders.* See *Promoting Safety and Comfort: Applying Creams, Lotions, Ointments, and Powders.*
2. Check the drug order. **(First safety check.)** Focus on:
   * Right drug
   * Right time
   * Right dose
   * Right person
   * Right route

3. Check with the nurse if you have any questions.
4. Practice hand hygiene.
5. Collect needed items:
   * Soap or other cleansing agent
   * Washcloth and towel
   * Wash basin with warm water
   * Gauze squares or cotton balls
   * Sterile tongue blade
   * Sterile cotton-tipped applicator
   * Gloves
   * MAR

PROCEDURE

6. Unlock the drug cart.
7. Read the order on the MAR.
8. Select the right drug from the person's drawer. Lock the drug cart.
9. Compare the drug order on the MAR against the pharmacy label on the drug container. **(Second safety check.)** Check for the:
   * Right drug
   * Right time
   * Right dose
   * Right person
   * Right route
10. Check the drug container for an expiration date.
11. Identify the person. Check the ID bracelet against the MAR. Make sure you use at least two identifiers according to agency policy. Also call the person by name. Follow agency policy if using a bar code scanner.
12. Provide for privacy.
13. Put on gloves.
14. Position the person to expose the application site. Expose the site.
15. Clean and dry the application site.
16. Observe the application site.
17. Remove and discard the gloves. Practice hand hygiene. Put on clean gloves.
18. Compare the drug order on the MAR against the pharmacy label on the drug container. **(Third safety check.)** Check for the:
    * Right drug
    * Right time
    * Right dose
    * Right person
    * Right route
19. Shake the lotion thoroughly.

20. Open the container. Place the lid or cap upside down on a clean surface. For an ointment or cream:
    a. *From a jar:* use a tongue blade to remove the ordered amount.
    b. *From a tube:* squeeze the ordered amount onto a tongue blade or cotton-tipped applicator.
21. Close the container. Compare the drug order on the MAR against the pharmacy label on the drug container. **(Fourth safety check.)** Check for the:
    * Right drug
    * Right time
    * Right dose
    * Right person
    * Right route
22. Apply the topical dose form.
    a. Lotion:
       (1) Hold the bottle in your non-dominant hand. The label is in the palm of your hand. This prevents the contents from running down and smearing the label during pouring.
       (2) Pour some lotion onto a cotton ball or gauze square. Do not let any part of the container touch the cotton ball.
       (3) Dab the lotion onto the skin. Do not rub.
       (4) Repeat steps 22 a (1)–(3) with a new cotton ball or gauze square until the area is covered.
    b. Cream or ointment:
       (1) Transfer the cream or ointment from the tongue blade or cotton-tipped applicator to your gloved hand or index finger (if necessary).
       (2) Apply the agent to the skin with the tongue blade, cotton-tipped applicator, or your gloved hand or finger (Fig. 11-1).
       (3) Apply the agent in a thin layer in the direction of hair growth. Use firm, gentle strokes.

Continued

Procedure icons in the title bar alert you to associated content areas. Heading icons and procedure icons are the same.

Procedures are written in a step-by-step format. They are divided into *Quality of Life, Pre-Procedure, Procedure,* and *Post-Procedure* sections for studying ease. The Quality of Life section lists six simple courtesies that show respect for the person.

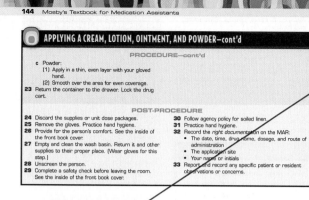

APPLYING A CREAM, LOTION, OINTMENT, AND POWDER—cont'd

PROCEDURE—cont'd

c Powder:
  (1) Apply in a thin, even layer with your gloved hand.
  (2) Smooth over the area for even coverage.
23 Return the container to the drawer. Lock the drug cart.

POST-PROCEDURE

24 Discard the supplies or unit dose packages.
25 Remove the gloves. Practice hand hygiene.
26 Provide for the person's comfort. See the inside of the front book cover.
27 Empty and clean the wash basin. Return it and other supplies to their proper place. (Wear gloves for this step.)
28 Unscreen the person.
29 Complete a safety check before leaving the room. See the inside of the front book cover.

30 Follow agency policy for soiled linen.
31 Practice hand hygiene.
32 Record the *right documentation* on the MAR:
  • The date, time, drug name, dosage, and route of administration
  • The application site
  • Your name or initials
33 Report and record any specific patient or resident observations or concerns.

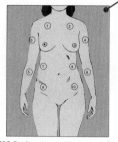

Fig. 11-2 Sites for applying nitroglycerin ointment. The sites also are used for a transdermal drug delivery system.

Applying Nitroglycerin Ointment. Nitroglycerin ointment is used to prevent angina (chest pain). It relaxes the heart's blood vessels and increases the blood and oxygen supply to the heart. See Chapter 21.

The dosage applied must be accurate. To properly apply nitroglycerin ointment, follow these rules:
• Apply the drug to clean, dry skin that has little or no hair (Fig. 11-2).
• Do not shave an area to apply the ointment. Shaving can cause skin irritation.
• Do not apply the ointment to irritated, scarred, open, broken, or calloused skin areas. Such areas can affect drug absorption.
• Wear gloves. Do not let any ointment touch any part of your skin.
• Check for an old application:
  • Check the MAR.
  • Ask the person the location of an existing application.
• Do not assume that there are no applications or that one has fallen off. Carefully check the person's skin. This is especially important if the person is confused, sedated, or non-responsive.
• Remove the old application before applying a new one. Check the person carefully to make sure there is only one old application. If you find more than one, tell the nurse at once. Remove all applications before applying a new one.

Color illustrations and photographs visually present key ideas, concepts, or procedure steps. They help you apply and remember the written material.

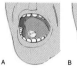 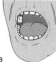

Fig. 10-18 A, A sublingual tablet is placed under the tongue. **B,** A buccal tablet is placed between the cheek and upper molar.

SUBLINGUAL AND BUCCAL DRUGS

Sublingual means under *(sub)* the tongue *(lingual)*. Sublingual tablets are placed under the tongue. They are dissolved and absorbed through the many blood vessels in that area.

Buccal means inside the cheek *(bucco)*. Buccal tablets are placed between the cheek and the molar teeth. A buccal tablet is absorbed by the blood vessels in the cheek.

Drugs are rapidly absorbed through the sublingual and buccal routes. Therefore the onset of action is rapid.

To give a sublingual or buccal tablet, follow the procedure, *Giving a Drug,* in Chapter 9. To give the drug, do the following:
1 Put on a glove.
2 For a sublingual drug: place the tablet under the tongue (Fig. 10-18, *A*).
3 For a buccal drug: place the tablet between the upper molar and the cheek (Fig. 10-18, *B*).
4 Do not give the person water to drink.
5 Encourage the person to:
  a Allow the drug to dissolve where placed. Remind the person not to move the drug to another part of the mouth.
  b Hold saliva in the mouth until the tablet is dissolved.
6 Remove and discard the glove.
7 Practice hand hygiene.

REVIEW QUESTIONS

Circle the BEST answer.

1 The wrong oral drug was given to a person. If necessary, how is the drug retrieved?
  a by giving an enema
  b by giving water to dilute the drug
  c by lavage
  d through surgery

2 Which person can receive oral drugs?
  a the person who is alert, oriented
  b the person who is vomiting
  c the person who is at risk for aspiration
  d the person who is comatose

3 To receive oral drugs, the person must be able to
  a state his or her name   c sit in Fowler's position
  b identify the drug   d swallow

4 Oral drug orders are written as follows. Which should you question?
  a 10 mL PO   c 10 mL orally
  b 10 mL per os   d 10 mL by mouth

5 Which dose form contains granules?
  a tablet
  b capsule
  c timed-release capsule
  d lozenge

6 Which dose form is held in the mouth to dissolve?
  a tablet
  b capsule
  c timed-release capsule
  d lozenge

Review Questions are useful study guides. They help you to review what you have learned. They can also be used when studying for a test or competency evaluation. Answers are given at the back of the book beginning on p. 443.

Contents

The Medication Assistant

OBJECTIVES

- Define the key terms and key abbreviations used in this chapter.
- Describe nurse practice acts.
- Identify the reasons for denying, revoking, or suspending a license or certification.
- Describe the standards for nursing assistive personnel.
- Describe how regulatory agencies are responsible for nursing assistive personnel.
- Explain how to maintain professional boundaries.
- Explain how to become a medication assistant-certified.
- Identify where medication assistants-certified can work.
- Explain the importance of a job description for medication assistants-certified.
- Explain the role and range of functions for medication assistants-certified.
- Identify what medication assistants-certified can and cannot do.

KEY TERMS

boundary crossing A brief act or behavior outside of the helpful zone

boundary signs Acts, behaviors, or thoughts that warn of a boundary crossing or violation

boundary violation An act or behavior that meets your needs, not the person's

drug A chemical substance that has an effect on a living organism

medication A drug used to prevent and treat disease; medicine

medication assistant-certified (MA-C) Nursing assistive personnel who are allowed by state law to give drugs

medicine See "medication"

nursing assistive personnel Individuals employed to give direct hands-on care and perform delegated nursing care tasks under the supervision of a licensed nurse

nurse practice act The law that regulates nursing practice in a state

professional boundaries That which separates helpful behaviors from behaviors that are not helpful

professional sexual misconduct An act, behavior, or comment that is sexual in nature and occurs within the scope of employment

standard of care Refers to the skills, care, and judgment required by nursing assistive personnel under similar conditions

KEY ABBREVIATIONS

CNA Certified nursing assistant
EMT Emergency medical technician
GED General education diploma
IM Intramuscular
IV Intravenous
LNA Licensed nursing assistant
LPN Licensed practical nurse
LVN Licensed vocational nurse
MA-C Medication assistant-certified
MAR Medication administration record
NCSBN National Council of State Boards of Nursing
PRN, prn As needed
RN Registered nurse
RNA Registered nurse aide

Nursing assistive personnel are individuals employed to give direct hands-on care and perform delegated nursing care tasks under the supervision of a licensed nurse. Licensed nurses are registered nurses (RNs) and licensed practical nurses (LPNs)/licensed vocational nurses (LVNs). Nursing assistive personnel assist nurses in giving care. State laws determine what nursing assistive personnel can do. In some states, they can give (administer) certain types of drugs. **Drugs** are chemical substances that have an effect on living organisms. **Medications** or **medicines** are those drugs used to prevent and treat disease.

Nursing assistive personnel who are allowed by state law to give drugs are called **medication assistants-certified (MA-C).** Some states use other titles. *Medication aide, certified medication aide,* and *certified medication technician* are examples. MA-C is used in this book. MA-Cs:

- Are certified nursing assistants (CNAs). Some states use the terms licensed nursing assistant (LNA) and registered nurse aide (RNA). CNA is used in this book.
- Have additional education and training as required by state law.
- Have passed the required certification tests.
- May give prescribed drugs within the limits defined by state law.
- Are supervised by licensed nurses.

STATE LAWS AND AGENCIES

Each state has a **nurse practice act.** The law regulates nursing practice in that state. It does so to protect the public's welfare and safety. A nurse practice act:

- Defines RN and LPN/LVN.
- Describes the scope of practice for RNs and LPNs/LVNs.
- Describes education and licensing requirements for RNs and LPNs/LVNs.
- Protects the public from persons practicing nursing without a license. Persons who do not meet the state's requirements cannot perform nursing functions.

The law allows for denying, revoking, and suspending licenses and certifications covered under the law. The purpose for doing so is to protect the public from unsafe nursing personnel. Reasons include:

- Being convicted of a crime in any state
- Selling or distributing drugs
- Using the person's drugs for oneself
- Placing a person in danger from the over-use of alcohol or drugs
- Demonstrating grossly negligent nursing practice
- Being convicted of abusing or neglecting children or older persons
- Violating a nurse practice act and its rules and regulations
- Demonstrating incompetent behaviors
- Aiding or assisting another person to violate a nurse practice act and its rules and regulations
- Making medical diagnoses
- Prescribing drugs and treatments

Nursing Assistive Personnel

A state's nurse practice act is used to decide what nursing assistive personnel can do. Some nurse practice acts also regulate CNA and MA-C roles, functions, education, and certification requirements. In other states, there are separate laws for nursing assistive personnel.

Legal and advisory opinions about nursing assistive personnel are based on the state's nurse practice act. So are any state laws about their roles and functions. If you do something beyond the legal limits of your role, you could be practicing nursing without a license. This creates serious legal problems for you and the nurse supervising your work.

In most states, nursing assistants are certified after passing the state's education and competency evaluation program for nursing assistants. They have the title of certified nursing assistant (CNA). Some states license or register nursing assistants. They are LNAs or RNAs.

Medication assistants are certified after passing the

state's education and competency evaluation program for medication assistants. Titles vary among states. The National Council of State Boards of Nursing (NCSBN) uses the title *medication assistant-certified (MA-C)*.

Nursing assistive personnel must be able to function with reasonable skill and safety. Like nurses, they can have their certification, license, or registration denied, revoked, or suspended. The NCSBN lists these reasons for doing so:

- Drug or substance abuse or dependency.
- Abandoning a patient or resident.
- Abusing a patient or resident.
- Fraud or deceit. Examples include:
  - Filing false personal information
  - Providing false information when applying for certification—initial, re-instatement, or renewal
- Neglecting a patient or resident.
- Violating professional boundaries (p. 4).
- Giving unsafe care.
- Performing acts beyond the CNA or MA-C role.
- Misappropriation (stealing, theft) or mis-using property.
- Obtaining money or property from a patient or resident. Doing so through fraud, falsely representing oneself, or through force are examples.
- Having been convicted of a crime. Examples include murder, assault, kidnapping, rape or sexual assault, robbery, sexual crimes involving children, criminal mistreatment of children or a vulnerable adult, drug trafficking, embezzlement (to take a person's property for one's own use), theft, and arson (starting fires).
- Failing to conform to the standards for nursing assistive personnel (Box 1-1).
- Putting patients and residents at risk for harm.
- Violating the privacy of a patient or resident.
- Failing to maintain the confidentiality of patient or resident information.

Regulatory Agencies

Each state has a *state board of nursing* or similar agency. The board is created and given powers by the state's nurse practice act. The board protects the public's health, safety, and welfare. It does so by regulating nursing education and nursing practice. In many states, the board of nursing also regulates the education and practice of nursing assistive personnel. In others, a different state agency has that responsibility. A Department of Public Health is an example.

The regulatory agency responsible for nursing assistive personnel:

- Makes sure that standards of care are met. **Standard of care** refers to the skills, care, and judgment required by nursing assistive personnel under similar conditions.

| BOX 1-1 | Nursing Assistive Personnel Standards |

- Performs nursing tasks within the range of functions allowed by the state's laws and rules regulating nursing assistive personnel.
- Is honest and shows integrity in performing nursing tasks.
- Bases nursing tasks on his or her education and training. Also bases them on the nurse's directions.
- Is accountable for his or her behavior and actions while assisting the nurse and helping patients and residents.
- Performs delegated aspects of the person's nursing care.
- Assists the nurse in observing patients and residents. Also assists in identifying their needs.
- Communicates:
  - Progress toward completing delegated nursing tasks
  - Problems in completing delegated nursing tasks
  - Changes in the person's status
- Asks the nurse to clarify what is expected when unsure.
- Uses educational and training opportunities as available.
- Practices safety measures to protect the person, others, and self.
- Respects the person's rights, concerns, decisions, and dignity.
- Functions as a member of the health team. Helps implement the care plan.
- Respects the person's property and the property of others.
- Protects confidential information unless required by law to share the information.

Modified from National Council of State Boards of Nursing, Inc., *Draft model language: nursing assistive personnel*, 2005, Chicago, Ill.

- Makes sure that they are competent.
- Approves individuals for initial certification, re-instatement, and certification renewal.
- Approves educational programs for nursing assistive personnel.
- Investigates complaints about a CNA or MA-C violating a law.
- Takes disciplinary action if a CNA or MA-C violated a law. Possible actions include:
  - Denying, suspending, or revoking certification.
  - Filing a letter of concern. This is done when the regulatory agency does not have enough evidence to take other action.
  - Noting on the certification and registry that there is a complaint against the CNA or MA-C.
  - Referring criminal violations to a law enforcement agency.
  - Imposing a fine.
- Maintains a state registry for nursing assistive personnel.

PROFESSIONAL BOUNDARIES

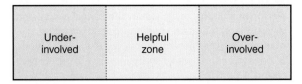

Under-involved	Helpful zone	Over-involved

Fig. 1-1 Professional boundaries. (Modified and redrawn from the National Council of State Boards of Nursing, Inc., *Professional boundaries: a nurse's guide to the importance of appropriate professional boundaries*, 1996, Chicago, Ill.)

PROFESSIONAL BOUNDARIES

A *boundary* limits or separates something. For example, a fence forms a boundary. It tells you to stay within or on the side of the fenced area. As a nursing assistant, you help patients, residents, and families. Therefore you enter into a helping relationship with them. The helping relationship has professional boundaries.

Professional boundaries separate helpful behaviors from behaviors that are not helpful (Fig. 1-1). The boundaries create a helpful zone. If your behaviors are outside of the helpful zone, you are over-involved with the person or under-involved. Boundary crossings, boundary violations, or professional sexual misconduct can occur.

A **boundary crossing** is a brief act or behavior outside of the helpful zone. The act or behavior may be thoughtless or something you did not mean to do. Or it could be on purpose if it meets the person's needs. For example, you give a crying patient a hug. The hug meets the person's needs at that time. If you give the hug to meet your needs, the act is wrong. Also, it is wrong to hug the person every time you see him or her.

A **boundary violation** is an act or behavior that meets your needs, not the person's. The act or behavior is unethical. It violates the standards in Box 1-1. The person could be harmed. Boundary violations include:
- Abuse.
- Giving a lot of personal information about yourself. You tell a person about your personal relationships or problems.
- Keeping secrets with the person.

Professional sexual misconduct is an act, behavior, or comment that is sexual in nature and occurs within the scope of employment. It is sexual misconduct even if the person consents or makes the first move.

Some boundary violations and some professional sexual misconduct also are crimes. To maintain professional boundaries, follow the rules in Box 1-2. Be alert to boundary signs. **Boundary signs** are acts, behaviors, or thoughts that warn of a boundary crossing or violation (Box 1-3).

Some patients, residents, and families want to thank the staff for the care given. Sometimes they send thank you cards and letters. Sometimes they offer gifts—candy, cookies, money, gift cards, flowers, and so on. Accepting gifts is a boundary violation. When offered a gift, you can say:
- "Thank you so much for thinking of me. It's very kind of you. However, it is against agency policy to accept gifts of any kind. I do appreciate your offer."
- "Thank you for wanting me to have the flowers your friend sent. They are lovely. However, staff cannot receive gifts because it is against agency policy. Let me help you find a way to take them home."

BECOMING AN MA-C

MA-C training involves classroom learning and clinical experiences. This includes practicing and demonstrating required skills. Giving oral drugs, applying ointments to the skin, and applying eye drops are examples. The training program length and number of hours vary by state.

Eligibility Requirements

To become an MA-C, you need to take a state-approved training program. But first you must meet program entrance requirements. Most states require that you:
- Be at least 18 years old.
- Have a high school diploma or general education diploma (GED).
- Read, write, spell, speak, and understand English
- Be a CNA.
- Have worked as a CNA. The length of time worked varies among states—90 days to 1 year. Six months is common.

Certification and Registry Requirements

MA-C certification and registry requirements vary by state. Generally they involve:
- Successfully completing a state-approved training program—classroom training, demonstrating required skills, and clinical experience
- Passing a competency evaluation—written test and skills test
- Completing an application form
- Paying required application fees
- Submitting fingerprint information

Certification can be denied for the reasons listed on p. 3.

BOX 1-2   Rules for Maintaining Professional Boundaries

- Follow the standards listed in Box 1-1.
- Talk to the nurse if you sense a boundary sign, crossing, or violation.
- Avoid caring for family, friends, and people with whom you do business. This may be hard to do in a small community. Always tell the nurse if you know the person. The nurse may need to change your assignment.
- Do not date, flirt with, kiss, or have a sexual relationship with current patients or residents. The same applies to family members of current patients or residents.
- Do not make sexual comments or jokes.
- Do not use offensive language.
- Do not discuss your sexual relationships with patients, residents, or their families.
- Do not say or write things that could suggest a romantic or sexual relationship with a patient, resident, or family member.
- Use touch correctly. Do not touch or handle sexual and genital areas except when necessary to give care. Such areas include the breasts, nipples, perineum, buttocks, and anus.
- Do not accept gifts, loans, money, credit cards, or other valuables from a patient, resident, or family member.
- Do not give gifts, loans, money, credit cards, or other valuables to a patient, resident, or family member.
- Do not borrow from a patient, resident, or family member. This includes money, personal items, and transportation.
- Maintain a professional relationship at all times. Do not develop any personal relationship or friendship with the person or family member.
- Do not visit or spend extra time with a person that is not part of your assignment.
- Do not share personal or financial information with a person or family member.
- Do not help a person or family member with his or her finances.
- Ask these questions before you date or marry a person whom you cared for. Be aware of the risk for sexual misconduct.
  - How long ago did you assist with the person's care?
  - Was the person's care short-term or long-term?
  - What kind and how much information do you have about the person? How will that information affect your relationship with the person?
  - Will the person need more care in the future?
  - Does dating or marrying the person place the person at risk for harm?

BOX 1-3   Boundary Signs

- You think about the person when you are not at work.
- You organize your work and provide other care around the person's needs.
- You spend free time with the person. You visit with the person during breaks, meal times, when off duty, and so on.
- You trade assignments with other staff so you can provide the person's care.
- You give more care or attention to the person at the expense of other patients and residents.
- You believe that you are the only person who understands the person and his or her needs.
- The person gives you gifts or money.
- You give the person gifts or money.
- You share information about yourself with the person.
- You talk about your work situation with the person.
- You flirt with the person.
- You make comments that have a sexual message.
- You tell the person "off-color" jokes.
- You notice more touch between you and the person.
- You use foul, vulgar, or offensive language when talking to the person.
- You and the person have secrets.
- You choose the person's side when he or she disagrees with other staff or the family.
- You select what you report and record. You do not give complete information.
- You do not like questions about the care you give or your relationship with the person.
- You change how you dress or your appearance when you will work with the person.
- You receive gifts from the person after he or she leaves the agency.
- You have contact with the person after he or she leaves the agency.

Certification Renewal

MA-Cs must renew their certification every year or every two years as required by state law. Each state has renewal requirements. Generally, an MA-C must provide the following to the regulatory agency:
- A completed renewal application.
- The required fee.
- A verified statement about any felony convictions:
  - Since initial certification
  - Since last certification renewal
- Evidence of continuing education. The number of required hours varies by state.
- Evidence of having worked as an MA-C or CNA during the renewal period. The number of required hours varies by state.
- Other state requirements.

WORK SETTINGS

Before accepting a job, you must know where MA-Cs are allowed to work in your state. MA-Cs usually work in agencies that employ licensed nurses. They include:
- Hospitals
- Long-term care facilities (nursing homes, nursing centers)
- Prisons and other correctional facilities
- Assisted living residences
- Centers for persons who are developmentally disabled
- Home health agencies
  States may allow MA-Cs to work in settings without a licensed nurse. Such settings include:
- Child day care centers
- Adult day care centers
- Private homes when supervised by the patient or his or her caregiver
- Schools
- Foster family homes
- Group homes

JOB DESCRIPTION

Your job description is a document describing what the agency expects you to do. It also states educational requirements.

Always obtain a written job description when you apply for a job. Ask questions about it during your job interview. Before accepting a job as an MA-C, make sure it includes giving drugs. Tell the employer about administration methods and routes that you did not learn. Also advise the employer of drugs that you cannot give for moral or religious reasons. Clearly understand what is expected before taking a job. Do not take a job that requires you to:
- Act beyond the legal limits of your role
- Function beyond your training limits
- Perform acts that are against your morals or religion

Your training prepares you to give drugs in certain ways. The agency may not let you do everything you learned. Other agencies want you to do things that you did not learn. Use your job description to discuss such issues with your supervisor.

No one can force you to do something beyond the legal limits of your role. Sometimes jobs are threatened for refusing to follow a nurse's orders. Often staff obey out of fear. That is why you must understand your role and functions.

ROLE AND RANGE OF FUNCTIONS

To protect persons from harm, you must understand what you can do, what you cannot do, and the legal limits of your role. In some states, this is called *scope of practice*. The NCSBN calls it *range of functions*.

Your role as an MA-C is to give drugs. When working in an agency—hospital, nursing center, or other health care facility—*you should not have a patient care or resident care assignment*. You should not be assisting persons with hygiene, elimination, moving and transfers, comfort, or other nursing care measures. You must not be distracted or taken away from your role of giving drugs. If you are assisting one person in a private home, you can assist the person with his or her other needs.

MA-C functions and responsibilities vary among states and agencies. Before giving a drug, make sure that:
- Your state allows MA-Cs to do so.
- It is in your job description.
- You have the necessary education and training.
- A nurse is available to answer questions and to supervise you.

Box 1-4 describes the MA-C role. State laws differ. You must know what you can do in the state in which you are working. For example, you move from Oregon to Texas. You must learn the laws and rules in Texas. Or you might work in two states. For example, you work in agencies in Kansas and Oklahoma. You must know the laws and rules of both states.

Some MA-Cs are also emergency medical technicians (EMTs). EMTs give emergency care outside of health care settings ("in the field"). EMTs work under the direction of doctors in hospital emergency departments. State laws and rules for EMTs and

BOX 1-4	Functions and Role Limits of the MA-C

FUNCTIONS

- Gives drugs under the supervision of a licensed nurse unless otherwise allowed by state law.
- Uses the medication administration record (MAR) to give drugs and to record the drugs given.
- Gives drugs following the Six Rights of Drug Administration (Chapter 9):
  - Right person
  - Right drug
  - Right time
  - Right route
  - Right dose
  - Right documentation
- Gives "as needed" (PRN, prn) drugs to a person as specified by the nurse.
- Prevents drug errors.
- Reports signs and symptoms, side effects, and adverse reactions.
- Reports the following to the nurse at once:
  - Signs and symptoms that appear life-threatening
  - Events that appear life-threatening
  - Drugs that have no results as observed by you or as reported by the person
  - Drugs that have undesirable effects as observed by you or as reported by the person
- Measures, reports, and records measurements as they relate to ordered drugs. Such measurements include:
  - Vital signs—temperature, pulse, respirations, blood pressure, and pain
  - Weight and height
  - Intake and output
  - Blood glucose
- Records the drugs given following agency policy and procedures.
- Follows agency policies and procedures for reporting and recording drug errors or suspected drugs errors.

ROLE LIMITS

- Does not give a drug, unless allowed by state law, if:
  - The person's need for the drug must be assessed. Only licensed nurses assess.
  - The drug requires a dosage calculation (Chapter 9 and Appendix A).
  - The dosage of the drug must be converted from one measurement system to another (Chapter 9 and Appendix A).
  - The nurse is not available to monitor the person's progress.
  - The nurse is not available to monitor how the drug affects the person.
  - The person is not stable.
  - The person's nursing needs are changing.
- Does not give the first dose of a newly ordered drug.
- Does not make decisions about as needed (PRN, prn) drugs.
- Does not make decisions about with-holding (not giving) a drug.
- Does not call doctors.
- Does not accept verbal or telephone orders from doctors or other health professionals authorized by state law to prescribe drugs.
- Does not give drugs that must be injected into the person's body by needle or other means: intramuscular (IM), subcutaneous, intradermal, intravenous (IV), and so on.
- Does not regulate IV fluids.
- Does not program insulin pumps.

Modified from National Council of State Boards of Nursing, Inc. *Draft model language: nursing assistive personnel*, 2005, Chicago, Ill.

MA-Cs differ. For example, Joan Woods is an EMT for a fire department. When off duty, she is an MA-C at Deer Valley Nursing Center. Her state allows EMTs to start IVs and give IV drugs in the field. However, MA-Cs do not start IVs or give IV drugs. Ms. Woods cannot start IVs or give IV drugs when working as an MA-C.

The situation is similar for persons who were medics or corpsmen in military service. When working as MA-Cs, medics and corpsmen must follow their state laws and rules for MA-Cs. As with EMTs, the ability to do something does not give the right to do so in all settings.

State laws and rules limit MA-C functions. Your job description reflects those laws and rules. An agency can further limit what you can do. So can a nurse based on the person's needs. However, no agency or nurse can expand your range of functions beyond what is allowed by your state's laws and rules.

REVIEW QUESTIONS

Circle the BEST answer.

1 Nursing assistive personnel can give drugs only if
a the person's condition is stable
b a licensed nurse is in the agency
c it is part of the CNA job description
d allowed by state law

2 You are an MA-C working in a nursing center. You are supervised by
a a licensed nurse
b a CNA
c the person needing the drug
d the doctor who ordered the drug

3 The purpose of a nurse practice act is to
a protect the public's welfare and safety
b deny, suspend, or revoke nursing licenses
c regulate nursing education
d determine what nursing assistive personnel can do

4 Medication assistants are certified after
a becoming a CNA
b passing the state-required education and competency evaluation
c meeting the requirements of the National Council of State Boards of Nursing
d working 1 year as a CNA

5 You are an MA-C. You can have your certification revoked for the following reasons *except*
a drug abuse
b deciding to give a drug without the nurse's consent
c taking telephone orders from a doctor
d refusing to give the first dose of a newly ordered drug

6 You are an MA-C. You can have your certification revoked for the following reasons *except*
a taking a person's drugs for your own use
b assessing a person's need for a drug
c violating a person's privacy
d refusing to accept a verbal order from a doctor

7 You are not sure if you should give a certain drug. What should you do?
a Ask the patient or resident.
b Ask the nurse.
c Give the drug.
d Report the error.

8 Which agency can deny, revoke, or suspend an MA-C's certification?
a the state board of nursing
b the state regulatory agency responsible for MA-Cs
c the National Council of State Boards of Nursing
d the agency in which the MA-C is employed

9 On your days off, you call the agency to check on a patient. This is a
a professional boundary
b boundary crossing
c boundary violation
d boundary sign

10 To maintain professional boundaries, your behaviors must
a help the person
b meet your needs
c be biased
d show that you care

11 A patient asks you out to dinner. You accept. This is a
a professional boundary
b boundary crossing
c boundary violation
d boundary sign

12 A friend's mother is a resident where you work. You helped with her care. This is a
a professional boundary
b boundary crossing
c boundary violation
d boundary sign

13 To renew your MA-C certification, you will likely need
a proof of continuing education hours
b to take another written exam
c to take another skills test
d a physical examination

14 You give a person a drug for pain relief. Later the person continues to complain of pain. What should you do?
a Give the same drug again.
b Tell the nurse at once.
c Offer other comfort measures.
d Tell the person to give the drug more time to take effect.

15 MA-Cs can
a give oral drugs
b give IV drugs
c give IM drugs
d program insulin pumps

Circle T if the statement is true. Circle F if the statement is false.

16 T F   Some states allow MA-Cs to work in settings that do not employ a licensed nurse.

17 T F   You are a CNA and an MA-C. Your agency's job description for nursing assistive personnel does not include giving drugs. Because you are an MA-C, you can still give drugs as directed by the nurse.

18 T F   You are an MA-C. A nurse tells you to give a drug that requires using a needle. You can give the drug.

19 T F   State law allows you to give a certain drug. A nurse or an agency can make you give the drug.

20 T F   You are assigned to give drugs and the personal care for 8 residents. Resident care is part of your role as an MA-C.

Answers to these questions are on p. 443.

Delegation

OBJECTIVES

- Define the key terms and key abbreviations used in this chapter.
- Describe the delegation process.
- Explain your role in the delegation process.
- Explain how to accept or refuse a delegated task.
- Describe the MA-C's role in the medication administration process.
- Explain what nurses can and cannot delegate to MA-Cs.

KEY TERMS

accountable Being responsible for one's actions and the actions of others who performed the delegated tasks; answering questions about and explaining one's actions and the actions of others

delegate To authorize another person to perform a nursing task in a certain situation

nursing task Nursing care or a nursing function, procedure, activity, or work that does not require an RN's professional knowledge or judgment

KEY ABBREVIATIONS

CNA Certified nursing assistant
LPN Licensed practical nurse
LVN Licensed vocational nurse
MA-C Medication assistant-certified
mg Milligram
NCSBN National Council of State Boards of Nursing
PRN As needed
RN Registered nurse

Licensed nurses supervise your work. You perform nursing tasks related to the person's care. A **nursing task** is the nursing care or a nursing function, procedure, activity, or work that does not require an RN's professional knowledge or judgment. If allowed by state law, giving certain drugs is a nursing task that can be delegated to MA-Cs.

MA-C functions and responsibilities vary among states and agencies. Before you give any drug, make sure that:
* Your state allows you to do so
* The task is in your job description
* You have the necessary education and training
* A nurse is available to answer questions and to supervise you

DELEGATION PRINCIPLES

Delegate means to authorize another person to perform a nursing task in a certain situation. The person must be competent to perform a task in the given situation. For example, you know how to give oral drugs. However, Mr. Jones has developed a swallowing problem. The nurse wants to assess if he has a problem swallowing drugs. You do not assess. Therefore the nurse gives the oral drugs.

Who Can Delegate

RNs can delegate nursing tasks to LPNs/LVNs and CNAs and MA-Cs. In some states, LPNs/LVNs can delegate tasks to CNAs and MA-Cs. RNs and LPNs/LVNs can only delegate tasks within their scope of practice. And they can only delegate tasks that are in the CNA's or MA-C's job description.

Delegation decisions must protect the person's health and safety. The delegating nurse is legally accountable for the nursing task. **Accountable** means to be responsible for one's actions and the actions of others who performed the delegated tasks. It also involves answering questions about and explaining one's actions and the actions of others.

The delegating nurse must make sure that the task was completed safely and correctly. If the RN delegates, the RN is responsible for the delegated task. If the LPN/LVN delegates, the LPN/LVN is responsible for the delegated task. The RN also supervises LPNs/LVNs. Therefore the RN is legally accountable for the tasks that LPNs/LVNs delegate to CNAs and MA-Cs. The RN is accountable for all nursing care.

CNAs and MA-Cs cannot delegate. You cannot delegate any task to other nursing assistive personnel or to any other worker. You can ask someone to help you. But you cannot ask or tell someone to do your work.

Delegation Process

To make delegation decisions, the nurse follows a process. The person's needs, the nursing task, and the staff member doing the task must fit. The nurse can decide *to delegate* the task to you. Or the nurse can decide *not to delegate* the task. The person's needs and the task may require a nurse's knowledge, judgment, and skill. You may be asked to assist.

Do not get offended or angry if you cannot perform a task that is usually delegated to you. The nurse decides what is best for the person at the time. That decision is also best for you at that time. You should not do something that requires a nurse's judgment. For example, you always give Mrs. Doyle her oral drugs. Now she is weak and refusing her drugs. The nurse wants to assess her behaviors while she is refusing her drugs. The nurse decides to give the drugs. At this time Mrs. Doyle needs the nurse's judgment and knowledge.

The person's circumstances are central factors in delegation decisions. Delegation decisions must result in the best care for the person. A nurse risks a person's health and safety with poor delegation decisions. Also, the nurse may face serious legal problems. If you perform a task that places the person at risk, you can also face serious legal problems.

The National Council of State Boards of Nursing (NCSBN) describes the delegation process in four steps.

Step 1—Assess and Plan. Step 1 is done by the nurse. To safely delegate, the nurse needs to understand the person's needs. And the nurse needs to know your knowledge, skills, and job description.

When assessing the person's needs, the nurse answers these questions.
* What is the nature of the person's needs? How complex are the needs? How can they vary? How urgent are the care needs?

- What are the most important long-term needs? What are the most important short-term needs?
- How much judgment is needed to meet the person's needs and give care?
- How predictable is the person's health status? How does the person respond to health care?
- What kind of problems might arise from the needed nursing task? How severe might the problems be?
- What actions are needed if a problem arises? How complex are those actions?
- What kind of emergencies or incidents might arise? How likely might they occur?
- How involved is the person in health care decisions? How involved is the family?
- How will delegating the nursing task help the person? What are the risks to the person?

To assess your knowledge and skills, the nurse answers these questions.

- What knowledge and skills are needed to safely perform the nursing task?
- What is your role in the agency? What is in your job description?
- What are the conditions under which the nursing task will be performed?
- What is expected after the nursing task is performed?
- What problems can arise from the nursing task? What problems might the person develop during the nursing task?

The nurse then decides if it is safe to delegate the nursing task. It must be safe for the person and safe for you. If unsafe, the nurse stops the delegation process. If it is safe for the person and you, the nurse moves to step 2.

Step 2—Communication. This step involves the nurse and you. The nurse must provide clear and complete directions about:

- How to perform and complete the task
- What observations to report and record
- When to report observations
- What specific patient and resident concerns to report at once
- Priorities for nursing tasks
- What to do if the person's condition or needs change

The nurse needs to make sure that you understand the directions. The nurse asks you questions to make sure you understand. He or she may ask you to explain what you are going to do. You should not be annoyed or insulted by the nurse's questions. He or she must make sure that safe care is given. This protects the person and you.

Before performing a delegated nursing task, you must have the opportunity to discuss the task with the nurse. Make sure that you:

- Ask questions about the delegated task.
- Ask questions about what you are expected to do.
- Tell the nurse if you have not done the task before. Also tell the nurse if you have not done it often.
- Ask for needed training or supervision.
- Re-state what is expected of you.
- Re-state what specific patient or resident concerns to report to the nurse and when.
- Explain how and when you will report your progress in completing the task.
- Know how to contact the nurse if there is an emergency.
- Know what the nurse wants you to do if there is an emergency.

After completing a delegated task, you must report and record the care given. You also report and record your observations. See Chapter 4.

Step 3—Surveillance and Supervision. *Surveillance* means to keep a close watch over someone or something. *Supervise* means to oversee, direct, or manage. In this step, the nurse observes the care you give. The nurse has to make sure that you complete the task correctly. The nurse also observes the person's condition and response to your care. How often the nurse makes observations depends on:

- The person's health status and needs.
- If the person's condition is stable or unstable.
- If the nurse can predict the person's responses and risk to care.
- The setting where the nursing task occurs.
- The resources and support available.
- If the nursing task is simple or complex.

The nurse must follow-up on any problems or concerns. For example, the nurse must take action if you did not complete the nursing task in a timely manner. The nurse also must take action if the nursing task did not meet expectations. An unexpected change in the person's condition is also cause for the nurse to act.

The nurse must be alert for signs and symptoms that signal a possible change in the person's condition. This way the nurse, with your help, can take action before the person's condition changes in a major way.

Sometimes problems arise in completing a nursing task. By supervising you, the nurse can detect and solve problems early. This helps you complete the task safely and on time.

After you complete the task, the nurse may review and discuss what happened with you. This helps you learn. If a similar situation happens in the future, you have ideas about how to adjust.

Step 4—Evaluation and Feedback.

This step is done by the nurse. *Evaluate* means to judge. The nurse decides if the delegation was successful. The nurse answers these questions:

- Was the nursing task done correctly?
- Did the person respond to the nursing task as expected?
- Was the outcome (the result) as desired? Was it satisfactory or not satisfactory?
- Was communication between you and the nurse timely and effective?
- What went well? What were the problems?
- Does the care plan need to change (Chapter 4)? Or can the plan stay the same?
- Did the nursing task present ways for the nurse or you to learn?
- Did the nurse give you the right feedback? *Feedback* means to respond. The nurse tells you what you did correctly. If you did something wrong, the nurse tells you that too. Feedback is another way in which you can learn and improve the care you give.
- Did the nurse thank you for completing the nursing task?

The Five Rights of Delegation

The NCSBN's *The Five Rights of Delegation* is another way to view the delegation process. In using the "five rights," the nurse answers the questions listed in the four steps described above. *The Five Rights of Delegation* are:

- *The right task.* Can the task be delegated? Is the nurse allowed to delegate the task? Is the task in your job description?
- *The right circumstances.* What are the person's physical, mental, emotional, and spiritual needs at this time?
- *The right person.* Do you have the training and experience to safely perform the task for this person?
- *The right directions and communication.* The nurse must give clear directions. The nurse tells you what to do and when to do it. The nurse tells you what observations to make and when to report back. The nurse allows questions and helps you set priorities.
- *The right supervision.* The nurse guides, directs, and evaluates the care you give. The nurse demonstrates tasks as necessary and is available to answer questions. The less experience you have with a task, the more supervision you need. Complex tasks require more supervision than do basic tasks. Also, the

person's circumstances affect how much supervision you need. The nurse assesses how the task affected the person and how well you performed the task. The nurse tells you what you did well and how to improve your work. This helps you learn and give better care.

Your Role in Delegation

You perform delegated nursing tasks for or on *a person.* You must protect the person from harm. You have two choices when a task is delegated to you. You either *agree* or *refuse* to do the task. Use *The Five Rights of Delegation* in Box 2-1.

BOX 2-1 | **The Five Rights of Delegation for Nursing Assistive Personnel**

THE RIGHT TASK
- Does your state allow you to perform the task?
- Were you trained to do the task?
- Do you have experience performing the task?
- Is the task in your job description?

THE RIGHT CIRCUMSTANCES
- Do you have experience performing the task given the person's condition and needs?
- Do you understand the purposes of the task for the person?
- Can you perform the task safely under the current circumstances?
- Do you have the equipment and supplies to safely complete the task?
- Do you know how to use the equipment and supplies?

THE RIGHT PERSON
- Are you comfortable performing the task?
- Do you have concerns about performing the task?

THE RIGHT DIRECTIONS AND COMMUNICATION
- Did the nurse give clear directions and instructions?
- Did you review the task with the nurse?
- Do you understand what the nurse expects?

THE RIGHT SUPERVISION
- Is a nurse available to answer questions?
- Is a nurse available if the person's condition changes or if problems occur?

Modified from the National Council of State Boards of Nursing, Inc., *The five rights of delegation,* 1997, Chicago, Ill.

Accepting a Task. When you agree to perform a task, you are responsible for your own actions. What you do or fail to do can harm the person. *You must complete the task safely.* Ask for help when you are unsure or have questions about a task. Report to the nurse what you did and the observations you made.

Refusing a Task. You have the right to say "no." Sometimes refusing to follow the nurse's directions is your right and duty. You should refuse to perform a task when:

- The task is beyond the legal limits of your role.
- The task is not in your job description.
- You were not prepared to perform the task.
- The task could harm the person.
- The person's condition has changed.
- You do not know how to use the supplies or equipment.
- Directions are not ethical or legal.
- Directions are against agency policies.
- Directions are unclear or incomplete.
- A nurse is not available for supervision.

Use common sense. This protects you and the person. Ask yourself if what you are doing is safe for the person.

Never ignore an order or a request to do something. Tell the nurse about your concerns. If the task is within the legal limits of your role and in your job description, the nurse can help increase your comfort with the task. The nurse can:

- Answer your questions
- Demonstrate the task
- Show you how to use supplies and equipment
- Help you as needed
- Observe you performing the task
- Check on you often
- Arrange for needed training

Do not refuse a task because you do not like it or do not want to do it. You must have sound reasons. Otherwise, you place the person at risk for harm. You also could lose your job.

DELEGATING TO MA-Cs

The actual task of giving certain drugs may not require a nurse's judgment. Therefore nurses can delegate to MA-Cs the task of giving such drugs. However, *the nurse cannot delegate the nursing actions and judgments needed before and after a drug is given.*

Figure 2-1 shows the MA-C's place and role in the entire process of medication administration. The

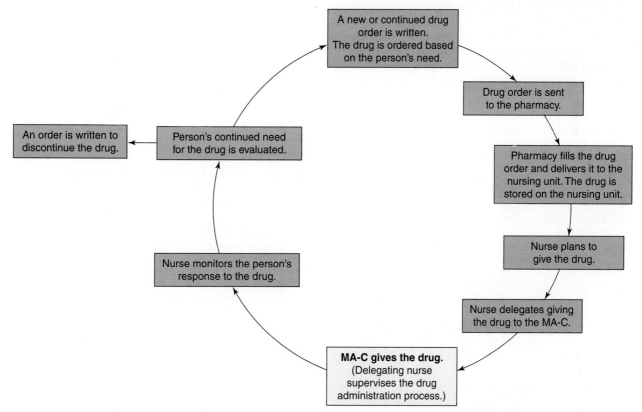

Fig. 2-1 The MA-C's place and role in the medication administration process. (Adapted and redrawn from The Interface of the Licensed Nurse with the Medication Aide: A Position Statement. North Carolina Board of Nursing, Board Approved Statement May 15, 2003, North Carolina Board of Nursing.)

MA-C's role is to give the drug. It is one step in the process. The nurse cannot delegate any other step in the process shown in Figure 2-1. Those steps involve:
- Assessing the person's need for a drug
- Determining the need for PRN drugs
- Assessing and evaluating side effects
- Recognizing allergic reactions
- Assessing and evaluating immediate desired effects
- Assessing and evaluating effects that are unusual and not expected
- Recognizing when continued use of the drug may be harmful
- Recognizing when the person no longer needs the drug
- Anticipating effects which may rapidly affect the person's life or well-being
- Making judgments and decisions about what actions to take if the person's life or well-being is threatened

Sometimes a drug dosage needs to be converted or calculated before the drug is given. For example, the doctor orders 500 mg (milligrams) of a drug. Each tablet contains 250 mg. A calculation shows to give 2 tablets. Some states do not allow MA-Cs to convert or calculate drug dosages. Therefore the nurse cannot delegate the task. Other states allow MA-Cs to do simple conversions and calculations. Converting and calculating dosages is described in Appendix A.

REVIEW QUESTIONS

Circle the **BEST** answer.

1 You are responsible for
 a supervising other nursing assistants
 b delegation decisions
 c completing delegated tasks safely
 d nursing tasks

2 You are asked to give a drug. Your state does not allow MA-Cs to give that drug. Which is *true*?
 a If a nurse delegated the task, there is no legal problem.
 b You could be practicing nursing without a license.
 c You can give the drug if giving drugs is in your job description.
 d If you give the drug safely, there is no legal problem.

3 A nurse delegates giving drugs to you. Which is *false*?
 a Nurses can delegate to you the responsibility of giving drugs.
 b The delegation decision must be safe for the person.
 c The delegated task must be in your job description.
 d The delegating nurse is responsible for making sure the drugs were given safely.

4 Giving certain drugs is in your job description. Which is *false*?
 a The nurse must delegate the task to you.
 b The nurse can delegate the task if the person's circumstances are right.
 c You must have the necessary education and training to complete the task.
 d You must have clear directions before you perform the task.

5 The nurse decided that Mr. Monroe needs a drug for pain relief. The nurse delegates the task of giving the drug to you. You must
 a complete the task
 b decide to accept or refuse the task
 c delegate the task if you are busy
 d ignore the request if you do not know what to do

6 The nurse asks you to give a drug. You can refuse to perform a task for these reasons *except*
 a the task is beyond the legal limits of your role
 b the task is not in your job description
 c you do not like the task
 d a nurse is not available to supervise you

7 You decide to refuse the task of giving a certain drug. What should you do?
 a Delegate the task to a CNA.
 b Communicate your concerns to the nurse.
 c Ignore the request.
 d Talk to the director of nursing.

8 Mr. Monroe complains of pain. He asks for a pain-relief drug. What should you do?
 a Assess his complaint of pain.
 b Tell the nurse.
 c Call the doctor.
 d Give the drug.

9 As an MA-C, what is your role in the medication administration process?
 a sending drug orders to the pharmacy
 b receiving filled drug orders from the pharmacy
 c giving drugs as delegated by the nurse
 d monitoring the person's response to the drug

10 Which of the following can the nurse delegate to you?
 a determining if a person needs a PRN drug
 b evaluating side effects and allergic reactions
 c deciding when a drug is no longer needed
 d making and reporting observations

Answers to these questions are on p. 443.

3

Ethics and Laws

OBJECTIVES

- Define the key terms and key abbreviations used in this chapter.
- Describe ethical conduct.
- Describe the rules of conduct for MA-Cs.
- Explain the rights of hospital patients and nursing center residents.
- Identify two types of advance directives.
- Explain the Federal Food, Drug, and Cosmetic Act.
- Explain the Comprehensive Drug Abuse Prevention and Control Act.
- Explain how unintentional torts, intentional torts, and crimes differ.
- Explain why possessing a controlled substance is a crime.
- Describe elder, child, and domestic abuse.

KEY TERMS

abuse The intentional mistreatment or harm of another person

advance directive A document stating a person's wishes about health care when that person cannot make his or her own decisions

assault Intentionally attempting or threatening to touch a person's body without the person's consent

battery Touching a person's body without his or her consent

civil law Laws concerned with relationships between people

crime An act that violates a criminal law

criminal law Laws concerned with offenses against the public and society in general

defamation Injuring a person's name and reputation by making false statements to a third person

ethics Knowledge of what is right conduct and wrong conduct

false imprisonment Unlawful restraint or restriction of a person's freedom of movement

fraud Saying or doing something to trick, fool, or deceive a person

invasion of privacy Violating a person's right not to have his or her name, photo, or private affairs exposed or made public without giving consent

Continued

KEY TERMS—cont'd

law A rule of conduct made by a government body

libel Making false statements in print, writing, or through pictures or drawings

malpractice Negligence by a professional person

neglect Failure to provide the person with the goods or services needed to avoid physical harm, mental anguish, or mental illness

negligence An unintentional wrong in which a person did not act in a reasonable and careful manner and a person or the person's property was harmed

protected health information Identifying information and information about the person's health care that is maintained or sent in any form (paper, electronic, oral)

slander Making false statements orally

tort A wrong committed against a person or the person's property

vulnerable adult A person 18 years old or older who has a disability or condition that makes him or her at risk to be wounded, attacked, or damaged

KEY ABBREVIATIONS

AHA American Hospital Association

DEA Drug Enforcement Administration

DNR Do not resuscitate

FDA Food and Drug Administration

HIPAA Health Insurance Portability and Accountability Act of 1996

MA-C Medication assistant-certified

OBRA Omnibus Budget Reconciliation Act of 1987

Nurse practice acts, your training and job description, and safe delegation serve to protect patients and residents from harm (Chapter 2). Protecting them from harm also involves a complex set of rules and standards of conduct. They form the ethical and legal aspects of care.

ETHICAL ASPECTS

Ethics is knowledge of what is right conduct and wrong conduct. Morals are involved. It also deals with choices or judgments about what should or should not be done. An ethical person behaves and acts in the right way. He or she does not cause a person harm.

Ethical behavior also involves not being *prejudiced* or *biased*. To be prejudiced or biased means to make judgments and have views before knowing the facts. Judgments and views usually are based on one's values

| BOX 3-1 | Code of Conduct for Nursing Assistive Personnel |

- Respect each person as an individual.
- Know the limits of your role and knowledge.
- Perform only those tasks that are within the legal limits of your role.
- Perform only those tasks that you have been prepared to do.
- Perform no act that will cause the person harm.
- Take a drug only when prescribed and ordered by a doctor.
- Carry out the directions and instructions of the nurse to your best possible ability.
- Follow the agency's policies and procedures.
- Complete each task safely.
- Be loyal to your employer and co-workers.
- Act as a responsible citizen at all times.
- Keep the person's information confidential.
- Protect the person's privacy.
- Protect the person's property.
- Consider the person's needs to be more important than your own.
- Report errors and incidents at once.
- Be accountable for your actions.

and standards. They are based on the person's culture, religion, education, and experiences. Do not judge the person by your values and standards. Do not avoid persons whose standards and values differ from your own.

Ethical problems involve making choices. You must decide what is the right thing to do. The rules of conduct for nursing assistive personnel can guide your thinking and behavior (Box 3-1). Also see "Professional Boundaries" in Chapter 1.

THE PERSON'S RIGHTS

In April, 2003, the American Hospital Association (AHA) adopted *The Patient Care Partnership: Understanding Expectations, Rights, and Responsibilities* (Box 3-2). The document explains the person's rights and expectations during hospital stays. The relationship between the doctor, the health team, and the patient is stressed.

Nursing center residents have rights as United States citizens. They also have rights under the Omnibus Budget and Reconciliation Act of 1987 (OBRA). OBRA is a federal law. It applies to all 50 states. Nursing centers must provide care in a manner and in a setting that maintains or improves each person's quality of life, health, and safety. Resident rights are a major part of OBRA (Box 3-3, pp. 18-19).

BOX 3-2 The Patient Care Partnership: Understanding Expectations, Rights, and Responsibilities

When you need hospital care, your doctor and the nurses and other professionals at our hospital are committed to working with you and your family to meet your health care needs. Our dedicated doctors and staff serve the community in all its ethnic, religious, and economic diversity. Our goal is for you and your family to have the same care and attention we would want for our families and ourselves.

The sections below explain some of the basics about how you can expect to be treated during your hospital stay. They also cover what we will need from you to care for you better. If you have questions at any time, please ask them. Unasked or unanswered questions can add to the stress of being in the hospital. Your comfort and confidence in your care are very important to us.

WHAT TO EXPECT DURING YOUR HOSPITAL STAY

- **High quality hospital care.** Our first priority is to provide you the care you need, when you need it, with skill, compassion, and respect. Tell your caregivers if you have concerns about your care or if you have pain. You have the right to know the identity of doctors, nurses, and others involved in your care, and you have the right to know when they are students, residents, or other trainees.
- **A clean and safe environment.** Our hospital works hard to keep you safe. We use special policies and procedures to avoid mistakes in your care and keep you free from abuse or neglect. If anything unexpected and significant happens during your hospital stay, you will be told what happened, and any resulting changes in your care will be discussed with you.
- **Involvement in your care.** You and your doctor often make decisions about your care before you go to the hospital. Other times, especially in emergencies, those decisions are made during your hospital stay. When decision-making takes place, it should include:
  - *Discussing your medical condition and information about medically appropriate treatment choices.* To make informed decisions with your doctor, you need to understand:
    - The benefits and risks of each treatment.
    - Whether your treatment is experimental or part of a research study.
    - What you can reasonably expect from your treatment and any long-term effects it might have on your quality of life.
    - What you and your family will need to do after you leave the hospital.
    - The financial consequences of using uncovered services or out of network providers.

    Please tell your caregivers if you need more information about treatment choices.
  - *Discussing your treatment plan.* When you enter the hospital, you sign a general consent to treatment. In some cases, such as surgery or experimental treatment, you may be asked to confirm in writing that you understand what is planned and agree to it.

This process protects your right to consent to or refuse a treatment. Your doctor will explain the medical consequences of refusing recommended treatment. It also protects your right to decide if you want to participate in a research study.

- *Getting information from you.* Your caregivers need complete and correct information about your health and coverage so that they can make good decisions about your care. That includes:
  - Past illnesses, surgeries, or hospital stays.
  - Past allergic reactions.
  - Any medicines or dietary supplements (such as vitamins and herbs) that you are taking.
  - Any network or admission requirements under your health plan.
- *Understanding your health care goals and values.* You may have health care goals and values or spiritual beliefs that are important to your well-being. They will be taken into account as much as possible throughout your hospital stay. Make sure your doctor, your family, and your care team know your wishes.
- *Understanding who should make decisions when you cannot.* If you have signed a health care power of attorney stating who should speak for you if you become unable to make health care decisions for yourself, or a "living will" or "advance directive" that states your wishes about end-of-life care, give copies to your doctor, your family, and your care team. If you or your family need help making difficult decisions, counselors, chaplains, and others are available to help.
- **Protection of your privacy.** We respect the confidentiality of your relationship with your doctor and other caregivers and the sensitive information about your health and health care that are part of that relationship. State and federal laws and hospital operating policies protect the privacy of your medical information. You will receive a Notice of Privacy Practices that describes the ways that we use, disclose, and safeguard patient information and that explains how you can obtain a copy of information from our records about your care.
- **Preparing you and your family for when you leave the hospital.** Your doctor works with hospital staff and professionals in your community. You and your family also play an important role in your care. The success of your treatment often depends on your efforts to follow medication, diet, and therapy plans. Your family may need to help care for you at home. You can expect us to help you identify sources of follow-up care and let you know if our hospital has a financial interest in any referrals. As long as you agree we can share information about your care with them, we will coordinate our activities with your caregivers outside the hospital. You can also expect to receive information and, where possible, training about the self-care you will need when you go home.

Courtesy American Hospital Association. Copyright 2003.

Continued

BOX 3-2 **The Patient Care Partnership: Understanding Expectations, Rights, and Responsibilities—cont'd**

- **Help with your bill and filing insurance claims.** Our staff will file claims for you with health care insurers or other programs such as Medicare and Medicaid. They also will help your doctor with needed documentation. Hospital bills and insurance coverage are often confusing. If you have questions about your bill, contact our business office. If you need help understanding your insurance coverage or health plan, start with your insurance company or health benefits manager. If you do not have health coverage, we will try to help you and your family find financial help or make other arrangements. We need your help with collecting needed information and other requirements to obtain coverage or assistance.

  While you are here, you will receive more detailed notices about some of the rights you have as a hospital patient and how to exercise them. We are always interested in improving. If you have questions, comments, or concerns, please contact _____.

Reprinted with permission of the American Hospital Association, copyright 2003.

BOX 3-3 **Resident's Rights**

THE RIGHT TO INFORMATION
- The person has access to all of his or her records—medical record, contracts, incident reports, and financial records.
- The person receives information about his or her total health condition. Information is given in language the person can understand. Interpreters are used as needed. Sign language or other aids are used for those with hearing losses.
- The person receives information about his or her doctor. This includes the doctor's name, specialty, and how to contact the doctor.

THE RIGHT TO REFUSE TREATMENT
- The person must consent to treatment or to take part in research. If a person does not give consent or refuses treatment, it cannot be given. This includes refusing drugs. If a person refuses a certain treatment, the center must provide all other services.
- Advance directives are part of the right to refuse treatment. They include living wills or instructions about life support.

THE RIGHT TO PRIVACY AND CONFIDENTIALITY
- The person's body is not exposed unnecessarily.
- Only staff directly involved in care and treatments are present. The person must give consent for others to be present.
- The bathroom is used in private.
- Privacy is maintained for personal care measures.
- Privacy is maintained when visiting with others and for phone calls.
- Mail is sent, received, and opened without others interfering. No one can open mail the person sends or receives without his or her consent.
- Information about the person's care, treatment, and condition is kept confidential. So are medical and financial records.

THE RIGHT TO PERSONAL CHOICE
- Residents can choose their own doctors.
- Residents take part in planning and deciding about their care and treatment. They can choose activities, schedules, and care based on their preferences.
- Residents can choose friends and visitors inside and outside the center.

THE RIGHT TO DISPUTES AND GRIEVANCES
- Residents can voice concerns, questions, and complaints about treatment or care.
- The person cannot be punished in any way for voicing the dispute or grievance.

THE RIGHT TO WORK OR NOT TO WORK
- The person does not work for care, care items, or other things or privileges.
- The person is not required to perform services for the center.
- The person *can* work or perform services if he or she wants to. A person may want to garden, repair or build things, sew, mend, or cook. Other persons need work for rehabilitation or activity reasons. The desire or need for work is part of the person's care plan.

THE RIGHT TO PARTICIPATION IN RESIDENT AND FAMILY GROUPS
- Residents can form and take part in resident and family groups. Groups can discuss concerns and suggest center improvements. They also can plan activities.
- Residents can take part in social, cultural, religious, and community events. They have the right to help in getting to and from events of their choice.

BOX 3-3   Resident's Rights—cont'd

THE RIGHT TO CARE AND SECURITY OF PERSONAL POSSESSIONS

- Residents can keep and use personal items. This includes clothing and some furnishings.
- The center must protect the person's property. Items are labeled with the person's name.
- The center must investigate reports of lost, stolen, or damaged items. Police help is sometimes needed.

THE RIGHT TO FREEDOM FROM ABUSE, MISTREATMENT, AND NEGLECT

- Residents must be free from verbal, sexual, physical, or mental abuse (p. 22) and involuntary seclusion. Involuntary seclusion is:
  - Separating a person from others against his or her will
  - Keeping the person confined to a certain area
  - Keeping the person away from his or her room without consent
- Nursing centers must investigate suspected or reported cases of abuse.
- Nursing centers cannot employ persons who were convicted of abusing, neglecting, or mistreating others.

THE RIGHT TO FREEDOM FROM RESTRAINT

- Residents have the right not to have body movements restricted.
- Restraints and certain drugs restrict body movements. Some drugs can restrain the person because they affect mood, behavior, and mental function.
- Sometimes residents are restrained to protect them from harming themselves or others. A doctor's order is needed for restraint use.
- Restraints are not used for staff convenience or to discipline a person.

THE RIGHT TO QUALITY OF LIFE

- Nursing centers must care for residents in a manner that promotes dignity and self-esteem. It must also promote physical, psychological, and mental well-being.
- The person is spoken to in a polite and courteous manner.
- The person is given good, honest, and thoughtful care.
- Nursing centers provide activity programs that allow personal choice. They must promote physical, intellectual, social, spiritual, and emotional well-being. Many centers provide religious services for spiritual health.
- The center's environment must promote quality of life. It must be clean, safe, and as home-like as possible.

ADVANCE DIRECTIVES

The Patient Self-Determination Act and OBRA give persons the right to accept or refuse medical treatment. They also give the right to make advance directives. An **advance directive** is a document stating a person's wishes about health care when that person cannot make his or her own decisions. Advance directives usually forbid certain care if there is no hope of recovery. Living wills and durable power of attorney are common advance directives.

A *living will* is a document about measures that support or maintain life when death is likely. Tube feedings, ventilators, and cardio-pulmonary resuscitation are examples. A living will may instruct doctors:

- Not to start measures that prolong dying
- To remove measures that prolong dying

Durable power of attorney for health care also is an advance directive. It gives the power to make health care decisions to another person. Usually this is a family member, friend, or lawyer. When a person cannot make health care decisions, the person with durable power of attorney can do so.

Doctors often write *do not resuscitate (DNR)* or *no code* orders for terminally ill persons. This means that the person will not be resuscitated. The person is allowed to die with peace and dignity. The orders are written after consulting with the person and family. The family and doctor make the decision if the person is not mentally able to. Some advance directives address resuscitation.

You may not agree with care and resuscitation decisions. However, you must follow the person's or family's wishes and the doctor's orders. These may be against your personal, religious, and cultural values. If so, discuss the matter with the nurse. An assignment change may be needed.

Quality of care cannot be less because of the person's advance directives. Health care agencies must inform all persons of the right to advance directives on admission. This information is in writing. The medical record must document whether the person has made them.

FEDERAL DRUG LAWS

A **law** is a rule of conduct made by a government body. The U.S. Congress and state legislatures make laws. Enforced by the government, laws protect the public welfare. The intent of federal drug laws is to protect patients, residents, and anyone who uses drugs. The goal is safe and effective drug use.

Federal Food, Drug, and Cosmetic Act of 1938

The Federal Food, Drug, and Cosmetic Act of 1938 gives the Food and Drug Administration (FDA) the power to:

- Determine the safety and effectiveness of drugs before marketing
- Ensure that manufacturers meet labeling requirements
- Ensure advertising standards are met when manufacturers market drugs

Manufacturers must submit new drug applications to the FDA. The FDA reviews safety studies before approving a drug for sale.

The law was strengthened in 1952 by the *Durham-Humphrey Amendment*. It restricted the re-filling of prescriptions. To be re-filled, certain drugs need a new prescription from a doctor.

The Kefauver-Harris Amendment was passed in 1962. It requires that a drug be proven both safe and effective before it is approved for sale.

Comprehensive Drug Abuse Prevention and Control Act of 1970

The Comprehensive Drug Abuse Prevention and Control Act of 1970 serves to control the manufacturing, distributing, and dispensing of certain drugs. It is commonly called the *Controlled Substance Act*. The Drug Enforcement Administration (DEA) enforces this law. The DEA gathers intelligence, trains, and conducts research about dangerous drugs and drug abuse.

The Act has five classifications or *schedules* of controlled substances (Box 3-4). How a drug is scheduled depends on:

- The degree of control
- Required record-keeping
- Required order forms
- Other regulations

All drugs in Schedules II, III, and IV require a prescription. So do some drugs in Schedule V. The pharmacist must have the prescriber's approval before re-filling a prescription.

Prescriptions must contain:

- The prescriber's name, address, and DEA registration number
- The prescriber's signature
- The name and address of the patient or resident
- The date of issue

When a Schedule II drug is given, the person giving the drug must record the following information:

- The name of the person receiving the drug
- The date and time the drug was given
- The drug given
- The dosage given

BOX 3-4 Schedules of Controlled Substances

SCHEDULE I C DRUGS
- High potential for abuse.
- No currently accepted medical use in the United States.
- Lack accepted safety for use under medical supervision.
- Examples—lysergic acid diethylamide (LSD), marijuana, peyote, heroin, hashish.

SCHEDULE II C DRUGS
- High potential for abuse.
- Have an accepted medical use in the United States.
- May lead to severe psychological or physical dependence.
- Examples—secobarbital, pentobarbital, amphetamines, morphine, meperidine, methadone, Percodan, methylphenidate.

SCHEDULE III C DRUGS
- High potential for abuse. Less potential than schedule I and II drugs.
- Have an accepted medical use in the United States.
- May lead to moderate or low physical dependence. May lead to high psychological dependence.
- Examples—Lortab, Fiorinal, Tylenol with codeine.

SCHEDULE IV C DRUGS
- Low potential for abuse. Less potential than those in Schedule III.
- Have an accepted medical use in the United States.
- May lead to limited physical or psychological dependence.
- Examples—phenobarbital, Darvon, chloral hydrate, Librium, Valium, Dalmane, temazepam.

SCHEDULE V C DRUGS
- Low potential for abuse. Less potential than those in Schedule IV.
- Have an accepted medical use in the United States.
- Have limited potential for physical or psychological dependence.
- A prescription may not be required.
- Examples—Lomotil, Robitussin A-C.

TORTS AND CRIMES

Civil laws are concerned with relationships between people. Examples of civil laws are those that involve contracts and nursing practice. A person found guilty of breaking a civil law usually has to pay a sum of money to the injured person.

Criminal laws are concerned with offenses against the public and society in general. An act that violates a criminal law is called a **crime.** A person found guilty of a crime is fined or sent to prison.

You are legally responsible *(liable)* for your own actions. The nurse is liable as your supervisor. However, you are not relieved of personal liability. Remember, sometimes refusing to follow the nurse's directions is your right and duty (Chapter 2).

Torts

Tort comes from the French word meaning *wrong.* Torts are part of civil law. A **tort** is a wrong committed against a person or the person's property. Torts may be unintentional. Harm was not intended. Some torts are intentional. Harm was intended.

Unintentional Torts. Negligence is an unintentional wrong. The negligent person did not act in a reasonable and careful manner. As a result, a person or the person's property was harmed. The person causing the harm did not intend or mean to cause harm. The person failed to do what a reasonable and careful person would have done. Or he or she did what a reasonable and careful person would not have done. The negligent person may have to pay damages (a sum of money) to the one injured.

Malpractice is negligence by a professional person. A person has professional status because of training and the service provided. Nurses, doctors, and pharmacists are examples.

What you do or do not do can lead to a lawsuit if harm results to the person or property of another. *Standard of care* refers to skills, care, and judgments required by a health team member under similar conditions (Chapter 1). Standards of care come from:
- Laws, including nurse practice acts
- Textbooks
- Agency policies and procedures
- Manufacturer instructions for equipment and supplies
- Job descriptions
- Approval and accrediting agency standards
- Standards and guidelines issued by government agencies

As an MA-C, the following actions could lead to charges of negligence:
- You give a drug to the wrong person.
- You give the wrong drug.
- You give the wrong dosage.
- You give a drug the wrong way.
- You give a drug at the wrong time.
- You do not give an ordered drug.

BOX 3-5 Protecting the Right to Privacy

- Keep all information about the person confidential.
- Cover the person when he or she is being moved in hallways.
- Screen the person. Close the privacy curtain and the door when giving care. Also close window coverings.
- Expose only the body part involved in care or a procedure.
- Do not discuss the person or the person's treatment with anyone except the nurse supervising your work. "Shop talk" is a common cause of invasion of privacy. ("Shop talk" is jargon or subject matter related to your work.)
- Ask visitors to leave the room when care is given.
- Do not open the person's mail.
- Allow the person to visit with others in private.
- Allow the person to use the phone in private.
- Follow agency policies and procedures required to protect privacy. This includes those related to computer use.

Intentional Torts. Intentional torts are acts meant to be harmful. The act is done knowingly.
- **Defamation** is injuring a person's name and reputation by making false statements to a third person. **Libel** is making false statements in print, writing, or through pictures or drawings. **Slander** is making false statements orally.
- **False imprisonment** is the unlawful restraint or restriction of a person's freedom of movement.
- **Invasion of privacy** is violating a person's right not to have his or her name, photo, or private affairs exposed or made public without giving consent. The Health Insurance Portability and Accountability Act of 1996 (HIPAA) protects the privacy and security of a person's health information. **Protected health information** refers to identifying information and information about the person's health care that is maintained or sent in any form (paper, electronic, oral). Failure to comply with HIPAA rules can result in fines, penalties, and criminal action including jail time. Follow agency policies and procedures. Direct any questions about the person or the person's care to the nurse. Box 3-5 lists ways to protect the person's privacy.
- **Fraud** is saying or doing something to trick, fool, or deceive a person. The act is fraud if it does or could cause harm to a person or the person's property.

Crimes

Murder, robbery, rape, kidnapping, and abuse (p. 22) are crimes. So is possession of a controlled substance. Assault and battery may result in both civil and criminal charges.

Assault and Battery. Assault is intentionally attempting or threatening to touch a person's body without the person's consent. The person fears bodily harm.

Battery is touching a person's body without his or her consent. Consent is the important factor in assault and battery. The person must consent to any procedure, treatment, or other act that involves touching the body. The person has the right to withdraw consent at any time.

Protect yourself from being accused of assault and battery. Explain to the person what is to be done and get the person's consent. Consent may be verbal—"yes" or "okay." Or it can be a gesture—a nod, turning over for a back rub, or holding out an arm so you can take a pulse.

Possession of Controlled Substances. Federal and state laws make the possession of controlled substances a crime. Nurses give controlled substances only under the direction of a licensed doctor or dentist.

Nurses can have controlled substances in their possession if:
* The nurse is giving a controlled substance to a person under a doctor's order.
* The nurse is a patient for whom a doctor has prescribed a controlled substance.
* The nurse is the official custodian of a limited supply of controlled substances on a nursing unit in an agency.

A controlled substance may be ordered for a person but not used. The drug must be returned to where it was obtained—doctor or pharmacy.

Violating or failing to comply with the Controlled Substance Act can result in a fine, a prison term, or both. State laws vary about MA-Cs giving Schedule II drugs. So do MA-C job descriptions. You must know what your state and agency allow you to do.

REPORTING ABUSE

Abuse is the intentional mistreatment or harm of another person. Abuse is a crime. It can occur at home or in a health care agency. Abuse has one or more of these elements:
* Willful causing of injury
* Unreasonable confinement
* Intimidation (to make afraid with threats of force or violence)
* Punishment
* Depriving the person of the goods or services needed for physical, mental, or psychosocial well-being

Abuse causes physical harm, pain, or mental anguish. Protection against abuse extends to persons in a coma. The abuser is usually a family member or caregiver—spouse, partner, adult child, and others. The abuser can be a friend, neighbor, landlord, or other person. Both men and women are abusers. Both men and women are abused.

Accrediting agencies and OBRA do not allow agencies to employ persons who were convicted of abuse, neglect, or mistreatment. Before hiring, the agency must thoroughly check the applicant's work history. All references are checked. Efforts must be made to find out about any criminal records.

The agency also checks nursing assistive personnel registries for findings of abuse, neglect, or mistreatment. It also is checked for mis-using or stealing a person's property.

Vulnerable Adults

Vulnerable comes from the Latin word *vulnerare,* which means *to wound.* Vulnerable adults are persons 18 years old or older who have disabilities or conditions that make them at risk to be wounded, attacked, or damaged. They have problems caring for or protecting themselves due to:
* A mental, emotional, physical, or developmental disability
* Brain damage
* Changes from aging

Patients and residents, regardless of age, are considered vulnerable. Older persons and children are at risk for abuse.

Elder Abuse

Elder abuse is any knowing, intentional, or negligent act by a caregiver or any other person to an older adult. The act causes harm or serious risk of harm. Nursing assistive personnel have lost their certification, license, or registration because of elder abuse. Elder abuse can take these forms:
* *Physical abuse.* This involves inflicting, or threatening to inflict, pain or injury. Grabbing, hitting, slapping, kicking, pinching, hair-pulling, or beating are examples. It also includes *corporal punishment*—punishment inflicted directly on the body. Beatings, lashings, and whippings are examples. Depriving the person of a basic need also is physical abuse.
* *Neglect.* Failure to provide the person with the goods or services needed to avoid physical harm, mental anguish, or mental illness is called neglect. This includes failure to provide health care, food, clothing, hygiene, shelter, or other needs.
* *Verbal abuse.* Using oral or written words or statements that speak badly of, sneer at, criticize, or condemn the person is called verbal abuse. It includes unkind gestures.
* *Involuntary seclusion.* This involves confining the person to a certain area. People have been locked in closets, basements, attics, and other spaces.

- *Financial exploitation.* To *exploit* means to use unjustly. Financial exploitation means that the older person's resources (money, property, assets) are misused by another person. Or the resources are used for the other person's profit or benefit. The person's money is stolen or used by another person. It is also mis-using a person's property.
- *Emotional abuse.* This involves inflicting mental pain, anguish, or distress through verbal or nonverbal acts. Humiliation, harassment, ridicule, and threats of punishment are examples. It includes being deprived of needs such as food, clothing, care, a home, or a place to sleep.
- *Sexual abuse.* The person is harassed about sex or is attacked sexually. The person may be forced to perform sexual acts out of fear of punishment or physical harm.
- *Abandonment. Abandon* means to leave or desert someone. The person is deserted by someone who is responsible for his or her care.

There are many signs of elder abuse. The abused person may show only some of the signs in Box 3-6.

Federal and state laws require the reporting of elder abuse. If abuse is suspected, it must be reported. Where and how to report abuse vary among states. You may suspect abuse. If so, discuss the matter and your observations with the nurse. Give as many details as possible. The nurse contacts health team members as needed.

The nurse also contacts community agencies that investigate elder abuse. They act at once if the problem is life-threatening. Sometimes the help of police or the courts is necessary.

Child Abuse and Neglect

Child abuse and neglect involve the following:
- A child 18 years old or younger.
- Any recent act or failure to act on the part of a parent or caregiver.
- The act or failure to act results in death, serious physical or emotional harm, sexual abuse, or exploitation.
- The act or failure to act presents a likely or immediate risk for harm.

The abuser usually is a household member—parent, a parent's partner, brother or sister, nanny. Usually an abuser is someone the family knows.

Types of Child Abuse and Neglect. Child abuse and neglect can take different forms. Often more than one type is present.
- *Physical abuse* is injuring the child on purpose. It can cause death. Forms of physical abuse include striking, kicking, burning, or biting the child. Any action that causes physical impairment of the child is physical abuse.
- *Neglect* can be physical or emotional. *Physical neglect* means to deprive the child of food, clothing, shelter, and medical care. *Emotional neglect* is not meeting the child's need for affection and attention.

BOX 3-6 **Signs of Elder Abuse**

- Living conditions are unsafe, unclean, or inadequate.
- Personal hygiene is lacking. The person is not clean. Clothes are dirty.
- Weight loss—there are signs of poor nutrition and inadequate fluid intake.
- Assistive devices are missing or broken—eyeglasses, hearing aids, dentures, cane, walker.
- Medical needs are not met.
- Frequent injuries—conditions behind the injuries are strange or seem impossible.
- Old and new injuries—bruises, pressure marks, welts, scars, fractures, and punctures.
- Complaints of pain or itching in the genital area.
- Bleeding and bruising around the breasts or in the genital area.
- Burns on the feet, hands, buttocks, or other parts of the body. Cigarettes and cigars cause small circle-like burns.
- Pressure ulcers or contractures.
- The person seems very quiet or withdrawn.
- Unexplained withdrawal from normal activities.
- The person seems fearful, anxious, or agitated.
- Sudden change in alertness.
- Depression.
- Sudden changes in finances.
- The person does not seem to want to talk or answer questions.
- The person is restrained. Or the person is locked in a certain area for long periods.
- The person cannot reach toilet facilities, food, water, and other needed items.
- Private conversations are not allowed. The caregiver is present during all conversations.
- Strained or tense relationships with a caregiver.
- Frequent arguments with a caregiver.
- The person seems anxious to please the caregiver.
- Drugs are not taken properly. Drugs are not bought. Or too much or too little of the drug is taken.
- Visits to the emergency room may be frequent.
- The person may change doctors often. Some people do not have a doctor.

- *Sexual abuse* is using, persuading, or forcing a child to engage in sexual conduct. It can take many forms:
  - *Rape or sexual assault*—forced sexual acts with a person against his or her will.
  - *Molestation*—sexual advances toward a child. It includes kissing, touching, or fondling sexual areas. The abuser may kiss, touch, or fondle the child. Or the child is forced to kiss, touch, or fondle the abuser.
  - *Incest*—sexual activity between family members. The abuser may be a parent, step-parent, brother or sister, step-brother or step-sister, aunt or uncle, cousin, or grandparent.
  - *Child pornography*—taking pictures or video-taping a child involved in sexual acts.
  - *Child prostitution*—forcing a child to engage in sexual activity for money. Usually the child is forced to have many sexual partners.
- *Emotional abuse* is injuring the child mentally. The child has changes in behavior, emotional responses, thinking, reasoning, learning, and so on. The child may show anxiety, depression, withdrawal, or aggressive behaviors.
- *Substance abuse* is part of child abuse and neglect in some states. A *controlled substance* is a drug or chemical substance whose possession and use are controlled by law. Substance abuse involves:
  - Making a controlled substance in the presence of a child
  - Making a controlled substance on the premises occupied by a child
  - Allowing a child to be present where there are chemicals or equipment used to make or store a controlled substance
  - Selling, distributing, or giving drugs or alcohol to a child
  - Using a controlled substance that impairs a care-giver's ability to adequately care for a child
  - Exposing a child to equipment and supplies for using, selling, or distributing drugs
  - Exposing a child to other drug-related activities
- *Abandonment* is when a parent's identity or where-abouts are unknown. The child was left by the parent in circumstances where the child suffers serious harm. Or the parent fails to maintain contact with the child or provide support for the child.

Box 3-7 lists the signs of child abuse and neglect. You must be alert for any unexplained changes in the child's body or behavior. Child and parent behaviors may signal that something is wrong. The child may be quiet and withdrawn. He or she may fear adults. Sometimes children are afraid to go home. Sudden behavior changes are common in sexual abuse. Bed-wetting, thumb-sucking, loss of appetite, poor grades, and running away from home are examples. Some children attempt suicide.

Parents give different stories about what happened. Injuries are blamed on play accidents or other children. Frequent emergency room visits are common.

Child abuse is complex. Many more behaviors, signs, and symptoms are present than discussed here. The health team must be alert for signs and symptoms of child abuse. All states require the reporting of suspected child abuse. However, someone should not be falsely accused.

If you suspect child abuse, share your concerns with the nurse. Give as much detail as you can. The nurse contacts health team members and child protection agencies as needed.

Domestic Abuse

Domestic abuse—also called domestic violence, intimate partner abuse, partner abuse, and spousal abuse—occurs in relationships. One partner has power and control over the other. Such power and control occur through abuse. Fear and harm occur. Abuse may be physical, sexual, verbal, economic, or social. Usually more than one type of abuse is present.

- *Physical abuse*—unwanted punching, slapping, grabbing, choking, poking, biting, pulling hair, twisting arms, or kicking. It may involve burns and weapons. Physical injuries occur. Death is a constant threat.
- *Sexual abuse*—unwanted sexual contact.
- *Verbal abuse*—unkind and hurtful remarks. They make the person feel unwhole, unattractive, and without value.
- *Economic abuse*—controlling money. Having or not having a job is controlled by the abuser. So are paychecks, money gifts from family and friends, and money for household expenses (food, clothing).
- *Social abuse*—controlling friendships and other relationships. The abuser controls phone calls, car use, leaving the home, and visits with family and friends.

Patients and residents can suffer from domestic abuse. For example, a husband slaps his wife during a visit. Or a wife uses her husband's money for her own benefit rather than buying her husband's drugs.

Domestic abuse is a safety issue. Like child and elder abuse, domestic abuse is complex. The victim often hides the abuse. He or she may protect the abusive partner. State laws vary about reporting domestic abuse. However, the health team has an ethical duty to give information about safety and community resources. If you suspect domestic abuse, share your concerns with the nurse. The nurse gathers information to help the person.

BOX 3-7 **Signs and Symptoms of Child Abuse and Neglect**

PHYSICAL ABUSE
- Bruises on the face (eyes, lips, mouth, cheeks), back, buttocks, abdomen, chest, and inner thighs.
- Welts on the face (lips, mouth, cheeks), back, buttocks, abdomen, chest, and inner thighs.
  - The shape of the object causing the welt may be seen. The shape may be of a belt, belt buckle, wooden spoon, chain, clothes hanger, rope, or other object.
- Burns and scalds on the feet, hands, back, buttocks, or other body parts.
  - Intentional burns leave a pattern from the item causing the burn: cigarettes, irons, curling irons, ropes, stove burners, and radiators are examples.
  - In scalds, the area put in hot liquid is clearly marked. For example, a scald to the hand looks like a glove. A scald to the foot looks like a sock.
- Fractures of the nose, skull, arms, or legs.
- Bite marks.

NEGLECT
- Fails to gain weight
- Shows great affection to others
- Wants to eat large amounts of food
- Steals food
- Is dirty or has a severe body odor
- Lacks the correct clothing for the weather
- Abuses alcohol or drugs
- States that no one is home

SEXUAL ABUSE
- Bleeding, cuts, and bruises of the genitalia, anus, breasts, or mouth
- Stains or blood on underclothing
- Painful urination
- Signs and symptoms of urinary tract infection
- Vaginal discharge
- Genital odor
- Genital pain
- Difficulty walking or sitting
- Pregnancy
- Fearful behaviors—nightmares, depression, unusual fears, attempts to run away
- Sexual behavior that does not fit with one's age

EMOTIONAL ABUSE
- Sudden changes in self-confidence
- Headaches
- Stomach aches
- Abnormal fears
- Nightmares
- Attempts to run away

REVIEW QUESTIONS

Circle the BEST answer.

1 Ethics is
   a making judgments before you have the facts
   b knowledge of what is right and wrong conduct
   c a behavior that meets your needs, not the person's
   d skills, care, and judgments required of a health team member

2 Which of the following is ethical behavior?
   a sharing information about a patient with your family
   b accepting gifts from a resident's family
   c reporting errors
   d calling your family before answering a signal light

3 A person has made an advance directive. The person wants measures removed that prolong dying. What should you do about the drugs ordered?
   a Discuss the drug orders with the nurse.
   b With-hold the drugs.
   c Give the drugs as needed.
   d Return the drugs to the pharmacy.

4 The Federal Food, Drug, and Cosmetic Act requires the following *except*
   a that a drug is safe before it is marketed
   b that manufacturers meet labeling requirements
   c that advertising standards are met
   d that drugs fit into one of the 5 drug classifications

Continued

REVIEW QUESTIONS—cont'd

5 What is another name for the Comprehensive Drug Abuse Prevention and Control Act?
   a the Federal Food, Drug, and Cosmetic Act
   b the Patient Self-Determination Act
   c the Controlled Substance Act
   d the Omnibus Budget Reconciliation Act

6 A prescription must contain the following *except*
   a the cost of the drug
   b the prescriber's DEA registration number
   c the name of the patient or resident
   d the date the prescription was issued

7 All Schedule V drugs require a prescription.
   a True
   b False

8 Which has no medical use in the United States?
   a Schedule I drugs   c Schedule III drugs
   b Schedule II drugs   d Schedule IV drugs

9 Which is *not* a crime?
   a abuse   c negligence
   b murder   d robbery

10 These statements are about negligence. Which is *true*?
   a It is an intentional tort.
   b The negligent person acted in a reasonable manner.
   c Harm was caused to a person or a person's property.
   d A prison term is likely.

11 Threatening to touch the person's body without the person's consent is
   a assault   c defamation
   b battery   d false imprisonment

12 Restraining a person's freedom of movement is
   a assault   c defamation
   b battery   d false imprisonment

13 Photos of Mr. Blue are shown to others without his consent. This is
   a battery   c invasion of privacy
   b fraud   d malpractice

14 A person asks if you are a nurse. You answer "yes." This is
   a negligence   c libel
   b fraud   d slander

15 Possessing a controlled substance is a crime.
   a True
   b False

16 Who is at risk for being wounded, attacked, or damaged?
   a children
   b older adults
   c persons with disabilities
   d all patients and residents

17 You scold an older person for refusing to take ordered drugs. This is
   a physical abuse
   b neglect
   c emotional abuse
   d verbal abuse

18 Which is *not* a sign of elder abuse?
   a stiff joints and joint pain
   b old and new bruises
   c poor personal hygiene
   d frequent injuries

19 A child is deprived of food, clothing, and shelter. This is
   a physical abuse   c abandonment
   b neglect   d emotional abuse

20 A child has a black eye, bruises on her face, and bite marks on her arms. These are signs of
   a physical abuse   c neglect
   b sexual abuse   d substance abuse

21 A child is dirty and has a body odor. These are signs of
   a physical abuse   c neglect
   b sexual abuse   d substance abuse

22 You find blood stains on a child's underpants. This is a sign of
   a physical abuse   c neglect
   b sexual abuse   d substance abuse

23 These statements are about domestic abuse. Which is *true*?
   a It always involves physical harm.
   b It always involves violence.
   c One partner has control over the other partner.
   d Only one type of abuse is usually present.

24 You suspect a person was abused. What should you do?
   a Tell the family.
   b Call the police.
   c Tell the nurse.
   d Ask the person about the abuse.

Answers to these questions are on p. 443.

4

Assisting With the Nursing Process

OBJECTIVES

- Define the key terms and key abbreviations used in this chapter.
- Explain the purpose of the nursing process.
- Explain your role in each step of the nursing process.
- Explain the difference between objective data and subjective data.
- Identify the observations that you need to report to the nurse.
- Explain how to measure vital signs, weight and height, and blood glucose.
- Explain how to communicate with the nursing team.
- Explain how to accurately report and record.
- Perform the procedures described in this chapter.

PROCEDURES

- Taking a Temperature
- Taking a Pulse
- Counting Respirations
- Measuring Blood Pressure
- Measuring Weight and Height
- Measuring Blood Glucose

KEY TERMS

assessment Collecting information about the person; a step in the nursing process

evaluation To measure if goals in the planning step were met; a step in the nursing process

implementation To perform or carry out nursing measures in the care plan; a step in the nursing process

nursing care plan A written guide about the person's care; care plan

nursing diagnosis Describes a health problem that can be treated by nursing measures; a step in the nursing process

Continued

KEY TERMS—cont'd

nursing intervention An action or measure taken by the nursing team to help the person reach a goal

nursing process The method nurses use to plan and deliver nursing care; its five steps are assessment, nursing diagnosis, planning, implementation, and evaluation

objective data Information that is seen, heard, felt, or smelled by an observer; signs

observation Using the senses of sight, hearing, touch, and smell to collect information

planning Setting priorities and goals; a step in the nursing process

signs See "objective data"

subjective data Things a person tells you about that you cannot observe through your senses; symptoms

symptoms See "subjective data"

vital signs Temperature, pulse, respirations, blood pressure, and pain

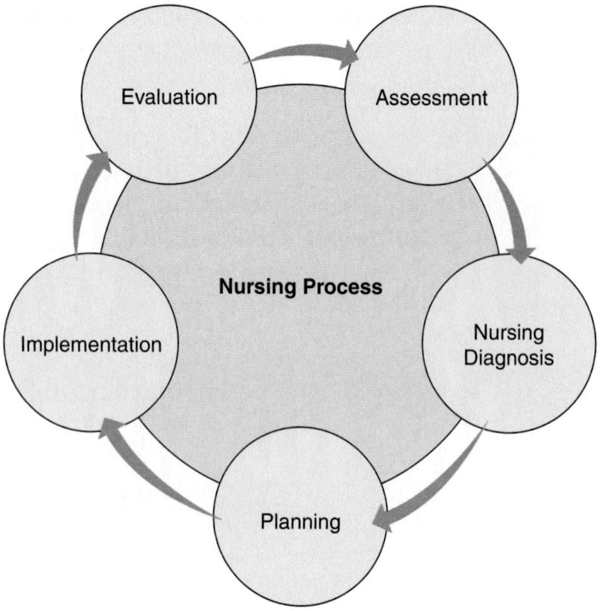

KEY ABBREVIATIONS

C Celsius; centigrade
F Fahrenheit
Hg Mercury
IV Intravenous
MDS Minimum Data Set
mm Millimeter
mm Hg Millimeters of mercury
NANDA-I North American Nursing Diagnosis Association International
OBRA Omnibus Budget Reconciliation Act of 1987
OSHA Occupational Safety and Health Administration

Nurses communicate with each other about the person's strengths, problems, needs, and care. This information is shared through the nursing process. The **nursing process** is the method nurses use to plan and deliver nursing care. It has five steps:

- Assessment
- Nursing diagnosis
- Planning
- Implementation
- Evaluation

THE NURSING PROCESS

The nursing process focuses on the person's nursing needs. Good communication is needed between the person and the nursing team.

Each step is important. If done in order with good communication, nursing care is organized and has

Fig. 4-1 The nursing process is continuous.

purpose. All nursing team members do the same things for the person. They have the same goals. The person feels safe and secure with consistent care.

The nursing process is ongoing. New information is gathered, and the person's needs may change. However, the steps remain the same. You will see the continuous nature of the nursing process as each step is explained (Fig. 4-1).

Assessment

Assessment involves collecting information about the person. Nurses use many sources. Health and drug histories are taken. The drug history includes drugs used currently—prescription drugs, over-the-counter drugs, herbal products, and street drugs. Drug allergies also are part of the drug history. The health and drug histories tell about current and past health problems.

The family's health history is important. Many diseases are genetic. That is, the risk for certain diseases is inherited from parents. For example, a mother had breast cancer. Her daughters are at risk.

Information from the doctor is reviewed. So are test results and past medical records.

An RN assesses the person's body systems and mental status. You assist the nurse with assessment by reporting and recording what you observe about the person.

Observation is using the senses of sight, hearing, touch, and smell to collect information:

- You *see* how the person lies, sits, or walks. You see flushed or pale skin. You see red and swollen body areas.

- You *listen* to the person breathe, talk, and cough. You use a stethoscope to listen to the heartbeat and to measure blood pressure.
- Through *touch,* you feel if the skin is hot or cold, or moist or dry. You use touch to take the person's pulse.
- *Smell* is used to detect body, wound, and breath odors. You also smell odors from urine and bowel movements.

Objective data (signs) are seen heard, felt, or smelled by an observer. You can feel a pulse. You can see urine. You cannot feel or see the person's pain, fear, or nausea. **Subjective data (symptoms)** are things a person tells you about that you cannot observe through your senses. For example, the person says: "Whenever I take this drug, I feel sick to my stomach."

Box 4-1 lists the basic observations you need to make and report to the nurse. Box 4-2, p. 30 lists the observations that you must report at once. You also measure vital signs, height, and weight. In some states and agencies, you measure blood glucose (p. 46). Make notes of your observations and measurements. Use them when reporting and recording (pp. 50-51).

BOX 4-1   Basic Observations

ABILITY TO RESPOND
- Is the person easy or hard to wake up?
- Can the person give his or her name, the time, and location when asked?
- Does the person identify others correctly?
- Does the person answer questions correctly?
- Does the person speak clearly?
- Are instructions followed correctly?
- Is the person calm, restless, or excited?
- Is the person conversing, quiet, or talking a lot?

MOVEMENT
- Can the person squeeze your fingers with each hand?
- Can the person move arms and legs?
- Are the person's movements shaky or jerky?
- Does the person complain of stiff or painful joints?

PAIN OR DISCOMFORT
- Where is the pain located? (Ask the person to point to the pain.)
- Does the pain go anywhere else?
- How does the person rate the severity of the pain—mild, moderate, severe?
- How does the person rate the pain on a scale of 1 to 10 (Chapter 17)?
- When did the pain begin?
- What was the person doing when the pain began?
- How long does the pain last?
- How does the person describe the pain?
  - Sharp
  - Severe
  - Knife-like
  - Dull
  - Burning
  - Aching
  - Comes and goes
  - Depends on position
- Was a pain-relief drug given?
- Did the pain-relief drug relieve the pain? Is the pain still present?
- Is the person able to sleep and rest?
- What is the position of comfort?

SKIN
- Is the skin pale or flushed?
- Is the skin cool, warm, or hot?
- Is the skin moist or dry?
- What color are the lips and nail beds?
- Is the skin intact? Are there broken areas? If so, where?
- Are sores or reddened areas present?
- Are bruises present? Where are they located?
- Does the person complain of itching? If yes, where?

EYES, EARS, NOSE, AND MOUTH
- Is there drainage from the eyes? What color is the drainage?
- Are the eyelids closed? Do they stay open?
- Are the eyes reddened?
- Does the person complain of spots, flashes, or blurring?
- Is the person sensitive to bright lights?
- Is there drainage from the ears? What color is the drainage?
- Can the person hear? Is repeating necessary? Are questions answered appropriately?
- Is there drainage from the nose? What color is the drainage?
- Can the person breathe through the nose?
- Is there breath odor?
- Does the person complain of a bad taste in the mouth?
- Does the person complain of painful gums or teeth?

RESPIRATIONS
- Do both sides of the person's chest rise and fall with respirations?
- Is breathing noisy?
- Does the person complain of pain or difficulty breathing?
- What is the amount and color of sputum?
- What is the frequency of the person's cough? Is it dry or productive?

Continued

BOX 4-1   Basic Observations—cont'd

BOWELS AND BLADDER
- Is the abdomen firm or soft?
- Does the person complain of gas?
- What are the amount, color, and consistency of bowel movements?
- What is the frequency of bowel movements?
- Can the person control bowel movements?
- Does the person have pain or difficulty urinating?
- What is the amount of urine?
- What is the color of urine?
- Is urine clear? Are there particles in the urine?
- Does urine have a foul smell?
- Can the person control the passage of urine?
- What is the frequency of urination?

APPETITE
- Does the person like the food served?
- How much of the meal is eaten?
- What foods does the person like?
- Can the person chew food?
- What is the amount of fluid taken?
- What fluids does the person like?
- How often does the person drink fluids?

APPETITE—cont'd
- Can the person swallow food and fluids?
- Does the person complain of nausea?
- What is the amount and color of material vomited?
- Does the person have hiccups?
- Is the person belching?
- Does the person cough when swallowing?

ACTIVITIES OF DAILY LIVING
- Can the person perform personal care without help?
  - Bathing?
  - Brushing teeth?
  - Combing and brushing hair?
  - Shaving?
- Which does the person use: toilet, commode, bedpan, or urinal?
- Does the person feed himself or herself?
- Can the person walk?
- What amount and kind of help is needed?

OTHER
- Is the person bleeding from any body part? If yes, where and how much?

BOX 4-2   Observations to Report at Once

- A change in the person's ability to respond
  - A responsive person is no longer responding.
  - A non-responsive person is now responding.
- A change in the person's mobility
  - The person cannot move a body part.
  - The person is now able to move a body part.
- Complaints of sudden, severe pain
- A sore or reddened area on the person's skin
- Complaints of a sudden change in vision
- Complaints of pain or difficulty breathing
- Abnormal respirations
- Complaints of or signs of difficulty swallowing
- Vomiting
- Bleeding
- Vital signs outside their normal ranges

FOCUS ON OLDER PERSONS

Assessment

The Omnibus Budget Reconciliation Act of 1987 (OBRA) requires the Minimum Data Set (MDS) for nursing center residents. The MDS is an assessment and screening tool. The form is completed when the person is admitted to the center. It provides extensive information about the person. Examples include memory, communication, hearing and vision, physical function, and activities.

The nurse uses your observations to complete the MDS. The RN responsible for the person's care makes sure the MDS is complete. The MDS is updated before each care conference. A new MDS is completed once a year and whenever a significant change occurs in the person's health status. An RN signs the MDS. A signed MDS means that it is complete and accurate.

The assessment step never ends. New information is collected with every patient or resident contact. New observations are made. The person shares more information. Often the family adds more information.

See *Focus on Older Persons: Assessment.*

Nursing Diagnosis

The RN uses assessment information to make a nursing diagnosis. A **nursing diagnosis** describes a health problem that can be treated by nursing measures. Some nursing diagnoses associated with drug therapy are listed in Box 4-3. The problem may exist or develop. Nursing diagnoses can relate to the desired (therapeutic) effects of drugs. They also can relate to the side effects of drugs. For example: *Injury, Risk for: related to side effects of confusion, disorientation, dizziness, and light-headedness.*

BOX 4-3	Nursing Diagnoses Approved by the North American Nursing Diagnosis Association International (NANDA-I)

- Activity Intolerance
- Airway Clearance, Ineffective
- Anxiety
- Aspiration, Risk for
- Body Temperature, Risk for Imbalanced
- Breathing Pattern, Ineffective
- Cardiac Output, Decreased
- Communication, Impaired Verbal
- Confusion, Acute
- Confusion, Risk for Acute
- Confusion, Chronic
- Constipation
- Constipation, Perceived
- Constipation, Risk for
- Coping, Ineffective
- Diarrhea
- Dressing/Grooming Self-Care Deficit
- Falls, Risk for
- Fatigue
- Fluid Volume, Deficient
- Fluid Volume, Excess
- Fluid Volume, Risk for Deficient
- Fluid Volume, Risk for Imbalanced
- Gas Exchange, Impaired
- Glucose Level, Blood, Risk for Unstable
- Grieving
- Grieving, Complicated
- Incontinence, Urinary, Functional
- Incontinence, Urinary, Overflow
- Incontinence, Urinary, Reflex

- Incontinence, Urinary, Stress
- Incontinence, Urinary, Total
- Incontinence, Urinary, Urge
- Incontinence, Urinary, Urge, Risk for
- Infection, Risk for
- Injury, Risk for
- Insomnia
- Knowledge, Deficient (Specify)
- Lifestyle, Sedentary
- Memory, Impaired
- Mobility, Impaired Physical
- Nausea
- Noncompliance
- Nutrition, Imbalanced: Less Than Body Requirements
- Pain, Acute
- Pain, Chronic
- Post-Trauma Syndrome
- Sensory Perception, Disturbed (Specify type: visual, auditory, kinesthetic, gustatory, tactile, olfactory)
- Sexual Dysfunction
- Suicide, Risk for
- Swallowing, Impaired
- Thought Processes, Disturbed
- Tissue Integrity, Impaired
- Tissue Perfusion, Ineffective (Specify type: renal, cerebral, cardio-pulmonary, gastro-intestinal, peripheral)
- Urinary Retention
- Violence, Risk for Other-Directed
- Violence, Risk for Self-Directed

Modified from NANDA International: *Nursing diagnoses: definitions and classification 2007-2008*, Philadelphia, 2007, NANDA-I.

Nursing diagnoses and medical diagnoses are not the same. A *medical diagnosis* is the identification of a disease or condition by a doctor. Cancer, stroke, heart attack, infection, and diabetes are examples. Doctors order drugs, therapies, and surgery to cure or heal.

A person can have many nursing diagnoses. They deal with the total person—physical, emotional, social, and spiritual needs. They may change as assessment information changes. Or new nursing diagnoses are added.

Planning

The person, family, and health team help the RN plan care. **Planning** involves setting priorities and goals. Priorities relate to what is most important for the person. Goals are aimed at the person's highest level of well-being and function—physical, emotional, social, spiritual. Goals promote health and prevent health problems. They also promote rehabilitation.

Nursing interventions are chosen after goals are set.

An *intervention* is an action or measure. A **nursing intervention** is an action or measure taken by the nursing team to help the person reach a goal. *Nursing intervention, nursing action,* and *nursing measure* mean the same thing. A nursing intervention does not need a doctor's order. Nursing interventions related to drug therapy include:

- Actions to minimize expected side effects. For example, a drug causes dry mouth. The care plan includes frequent oral hygiene.
- The side effects to report at once. See Box 4-2.

Some nursing measures come from a doctor's order. For example, a doctor orders a pain-relief drug for Mrs. Lange. The nurse includes this order in the care plan.

The **nursing care plan** (care plan) is a written guide about the person's care. It has the person's nursing diagnoses and goals. It also has the measures or actions for each goal. The care plan is a communication tool. Nursing staff use it to see what care to give. The care plan helps ensure that the nursing team members give the same care.

Each agency has a care plan form. It is found in the medical record, on the Kardex, or on a computer.

The RN may conduct a care conference to share information and ideas about the person's care. The purpose is to develop or revise the person's nursing care plan. Effective care is the goal. Nursing assistants usually take part in the conference.

The plan is carried out. It may change as the person's nursing diagnoses change.

Implementation

To *implement* means to perform or carry out. The implementation step is performing or carrying out nursing measures in the care plan. Care is given in this step.

Nursing care ranges from simple to complex. The nurse delegates nursing tasks that are within your legal limits and job description. The nurse may ask you to assist with complex measures.

You report the care given to the nurse. You record the care given in the person's medical record. Reporting and recording are done *after* giving care, not before. Also report and record your observations. Observing is part of assessment. New observations may change the nursing diagnoses. If so, care plan changes are made. To give correct care, you need to know about any changes in the care plan.

Evaluation

Evaluation means to measure. The evaluation step involves measuring if the goals in the planning step were met. Progress is evaluated. Goals may be met totally, in part, or not at all. Assessment information is used for this step. Changes in nursing diagnoses, goals, and the care plan may result.

To evaluate the goals related to drug therapy, the RN:
- Assesses the person's response to the drug prescribed
- Observes for signs and symptoms of recurring illness
- Observes for signs and symptoms of adverse drug effects
- Determines the person's ability to receive information about his or her drugs
- Determines the person's ability to self-administer drugs
- Assesses if the person will comply with ordered drug therapies—take drugs as ordered, at the right time, in the right way

The nursing process never ends. Nurses constantly collect information about the person. Nursing diagnoses, goals, and the care plan may change as the person's needs change.

ASSISTING WITH ASSESSMENT

Vital signs, weight, and blood glucose are measurements used to assess and evaluate the person's response to drug therapy. Often a specific measurement is needed before giving a drug. For example, a person is to receive a drug that lowers the heart rate. Before giving the drug, you take the person's pulse. If the pulse is too low, the nurse tells you not to give the drug.

Accurate measurements are essential. So is accurate reporting and recording.

Vital Signs

The vital signs of body function are:
- Temperature
- Pulse
- Respirations
- Blood pressure
- Pain (Chapter 17)

A person's vital signs vary within certain limits. They are affected by such factors as sleep, activity, eating, weather, noise, exercise, drugs, anger, fear, anxiety, pain, and illness.

Vital signs are measured to detect changes in normal body function. They tell about responses to treatment. They often signal life-threatening events.

Unless otherwise ordered, measure temperature, pulse, respirations, and blood pressure with the person lying or sitting. The person is at rest when vital signs are measured. Report the following at once:
- Any vital sign that is changed from a prior measurement
- Vital signs above the normal range
- Vital signs below the normal range

You learned how to measure vital signs in your CNA training program. A basic review is provided here.

Body Temperature. *Body temperature* is the amount of heat in the body. It is a balance between the amount of heat produced and the amount lost by the body.

Thermometers are used to measure temperature. It is measured using the Fahrenheit (F) and centigrade or Celsius (C) scales. See Box 4-4 for temperature sites. See Table 4-1 for the normal ranges for each site.

Glass Thermometers. The glass thermometer is filled with a mercury-free mixture. When heated, the substance expands and rises in the tube. When cooled, the substance contracts and moves down the tube.

BOX 4-4 Temperature Sites

ORAL SITE

Oral temperatures are *not* taken if the person:
- Is an infant or child under 6 years of age
- Is unconscious
- Has had surgery or an injury to the face, neck, nose, or mouth
- Is receiving oxygen
- Breathes through the mouth
- Has a naso-gastric tube
- Is delirious, restless, confused, or disoriented
- Is paralyzed on one side of the body
- Has a sore mouth
- Has a convulsive (seizure) disorder

RECTAL SITE

Rectal temperatures are taken when the oral site cannot be used. Rectal temperatures are *not* taken if the person:
- Has diarrhea
- Has a rectal disorder or injury
- Has heart disease
- Had rectal surgery
- Is confused or agitated

TYMPANIC MEMBRANE SITE

The site has fewer microbes than the mouth or rectum. Therefore the risk of spreading infection is reduced. This site is *not* used if the person has:
- An ear disorder
- Ear drainage

TEMPORAL ARTERY SITE

Measures body temperature at the temporal artery in the forehead. The site is non-invasive.

AXILLARY (UNDERARM) SITE

Less reliable than the other sites. It is used when the other sites cannot be used.

TABLE 4-1 Normal Body Temperatures

SITE	BASELINE	NORMAL RANGE
Oral	98.6° F (37° C)	97.6° to 99.6° F (36.5° to 37.5° C)
Rectal	99.6° F (37.5° C)	98.6° to 100.6° F (37.0° to 38.1° C)
Tympanic membrane	98.6° F (37° C)	98.6° F (37° C)
Temporal artery	99.6° F (37.5° C)	99.6° F (37.5° C)
Axillary	97.6° F (36.5° C)	96.6° to 98.6° F (35.9° to 37.0° C)

PROMOTING SAFETY AND COMFORT
Glass Thermometers

SAFETY

Glass thermometers break easily. Broken rectal thermometers can injure the rectum and colon. The person may bite down and break an oral thermometer. Cuts in the mouth are risks.

Older glass thermometers contain mercury. Swallowed mercury can cause mercury poisoning. Therefore, the Occupational Safety and Health Administration (OSHA) recommends using mercury-free devices. Some patients in home settings may still have mercury thermometers.

If a mercury-glass thermometer breaks, tell the nurse at once. Mercury is a hazardous substance. Do not touch the mercury. Do not let the person do so. Follow agency procedures for handling hazardous materials.

Do the following to prevent infection, promote safety, and obtain an accurate measurement:
- Use the person's thermometer.
- Use a rectal thermometer only for rectal temperatures.
- Follow Standard Precautions (Chapter 9) and the Bloodborne Pathogen Standard (Appendix C).

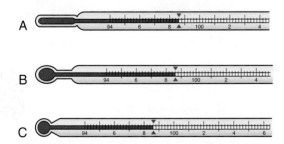

Fig. 4-2 Types of glass thermometers. **A,** The long or slender tip. **B,** The pear-shaped tip. **C,** The stubby tip (rectal thermometer).

Long- or slender-tip thermometers are used for oral and axillary temperatures (Fig. 4-2, *A*). So are thermometers with stubby and pear-shaped tips (Fig. 4-2, *B*). Rectal thermometers have stubby tips (Fig. 4-2, *C*). Thermometers are color-coded:
- Blue—oral and axillary thermometers
- Red—rectal thermometers
  See *Promoting Safety and Comfort: Glass Thermometers.*

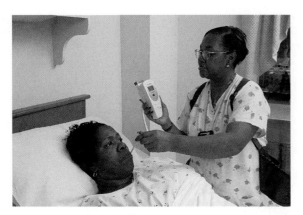

Fig. 4-3 The covered probe of the electronic thermometer is inserted under the tongue.

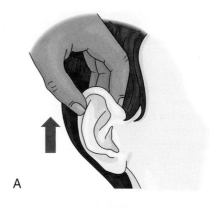

A

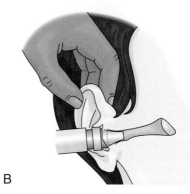

B

Fig. 4-4 Using a tympanic membrane thermometer. **A,** The ear is pulled up and back. **B,** The probe is inserted into the ear canal.

Electronic Thermometers. Electronic thermometers are used for oral, rectal, and axillary temperatures (Fig. 4-3). The temperature is measured in a few seconds and is shown on the front of the device.

A disposable cover (sheath) protects the probe. The probe cover is discarded after use. This helps prevent the spread of infection.

Tympanic Membrane Thermometers. Tympanic membrane thermometers measure temperature at the tympanic membrane in the ear (Fig. 4-4). The temperature is measured in 1 to 3 seconds.

These thermometers are comfortable. They are not invasive like rectal thermometers. The ear has fewer microbes than the mouth or rectum. There is less risk of spreading infection.

Temporal Artery Thermometers. Body temperature is measured at the temporal artery (Fig. 4-5). The device is gently stroked across the forehead and temporal artery. The temperature of the blood in the temporal artery is measured—the same temperature as the blood from the heart.

Body temperature is measured in 3 to 4 seconds. Follow the manufacturer's instructions for using, cleaning, and storing the device. Some devices have probe covers. To measure temperature:
- Choose the side of the head that is exposed. Do not use the side covered by hair, a dressing, hat, or other covering. If the person was in the side-lying position, do not use the side that was on a pillow.
- Place the thermometer at the side of forehead between the hairline and eyebrows.
- Slide the thermometer across the forehead.
- Read the temperature display.

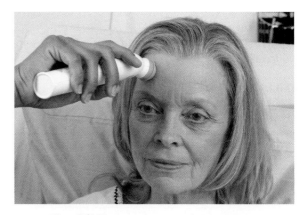

Fig. 4-5 Temporal artery thermometer.

Taking Temperatures. The site used to measure body temperature depends on the person's condition. The equipment used depends on the person's condition and what is used in your agency.

See *Delegation Guidelines: Taking Temperatures.*
See *Promoting Safety and Comfort: Taking Temperatures.*

DELEGATION GUIDELINES
Taking Temperatures

Before taking a person's temperature, you need this information from the nurse and the care plan:
- What site to use for each person—oral, rectal, axillary, tympanic membrane, or temporal artery
- What thermometer to use for each person—glass, electronic, or other type
- How long to leave a glass thermometer in place
- When to take temperatures
- Which persons are at risk for elevated temperatures
- What observations to report and record:
  - A temperature that is changed from a prior measurement
  - A temperature above or below the normal range for the site used
- When to report observations
- What specific patient or resident concerns to report at once

PROMOTING SAFETY AND COMFORT
Taking Temperatures

SAFETY
Thermometers are inserted into the mouth, rectum, axilla, and ear. Each area has many microbes. The area may contain blood. Therefore each person has his or her own glass thermometer. This prevents the spread of microbes and infection.

When taking a rectal temperature, your gloved hands may come in contact with feces. If so, remove the gloves and practice hand hygiene. Then note the temperature on your notepad or assignment sheet. Put on clean gloves to complete the procedure.

Follow Standard Precautions (Chapter 9) and the Bloodborne Pathogen Standard (Appendix C) when taking temperatures.

COMFORT
Remove the thermometer in a timely manner. Do not leave it place longer than needed. This affects the person's comfort. For example, an oral (glass) thermometer is left in place for 2 to 3 minutes. Do not leave it in place longer than that.

TAKING A TEMPERATURE

QUALITY OF LIFE

Remember to:
- Knock before entering the person's room.
- Address the person by name.
- Introduce yourself by name and title.

- Explain the procedure to the person before beginning and during the procedure.
- Protect the person's rights during the procedure.
- Handle the person gently during the procedure.

PRE-PROCEDURE

1 Follow *Delegation Guidelines: Taking Temperatures.* See *Promoting Safety and Comfort:*
   - *Glass Thermometers,* p. 33
   - *Taking Temperatures*
2 For an *oral temperature,* ask the person not to eat, drink, smoke, or chew gum for at least 15 to 20 minutes or as required by agency policy.
3 Practice hand hygiene.
4 Collect the following:
   - Thermometer—glass, electronic, tympanic membrane, temporal artery
   - Probe and probe covers (if needed)

- Tissues
- Plastic covers if used (glass thermometers)
- Gloves
- Toilet tissue (rectal temperature)
- Water-soluble lubricant (rectal temperature)
- Towel (axillary temperature)
5 Plug the oral or rectal probe into the electronic thermometer.
6 Decontaminate your hands.
7 Identify the person. Check the ID bracelet against the assignment sheet. Also call the person by name.
8 Provide for privacy.

PROCEDURE

9 Position the person for an oral, rectal (Sims' position), axillary, or tympanic membrane temperature.
10 Put on gloves if contact with blood, body fluids, secretions, or excretions is likely.
11 Insert the probe into a probe cover.

12 For a *glass thermometer:*
   a Rinse the glass thermometer in cold water if it was soaking in a disinfectant. Dry it with tissues.
   b Check for breaks, cracks, or chips.
   c Shake down the thermometer below the lowest number. Hold the thermometer by the stem.
   d Insert it into a plastic cover if used.

Continued

PROCEDURE—cont'd

13 For an *oral temperature*:
  a Ask the person to moisten his or her lips.
  b Place the covered probe at the base of the tongue and to one side. If using a glass thermometer, place the bulb end under the tongue and to one side (Fig. 4-6).
  c Ask the person to close the lips around the thermometer to hold it in place.
  d Ask the person not to talk. Remind the person not to bite down on a glass thermometer.
  e Leave a glass thermometer in place for 2 to 3 minutes or as required by agency policy.

14 For a *rectal temperature*:
  a Put a small amount of lubricant on a tissue.
  b Lubricate the bulb end of the thermometer.
  c Expose the anal area.
  d Raise the upper buttock to expose the anus (Fig. 4-7).
  e Insert the glass thermometer 1 inch into the rectum. Insert an electronic thermometer $1/2$ inch into the rectum. Do not force the thermometer.
  f Hold the probe or thermometer. Hold a glass thermometer in place for 2 minutes or as required by agency policy. Do not let go of it while it is in the rectum.

15 For an *axillary temperature*:
  a Help the person remove an arm from the gown. Do not expose the person.
  b Dry the axilla with the towel.
  c Place the covered probe in the axilla. For a glass thermometer, place the bulb end of the thermometer in the center of the axilla.
  d Ask the person to place the arm over the chest to hold the thermometer in place (Fig. 4-8). Hold it and the arm in place if he or she cannot help.
  e Hold the probe in place. Leave a glass thermometer in place for 5 to 10 minutes or as required by agency policy.

16 For a *tympanic membrane temperature*:
  a Ask the person to turn his or her head so the ear is in front of you.
  b Pull up and back on the ear to straighten the ear canal.
  c Insert the covered probe gently.

17 For an *electronic or tympanic membrane thermometer*:
  a Start the thermometer.
  b Hold the probe in place until you hear a tone or see a flashing or steady light.
  c Read the temperature on the display.
  d Remove the probe. Press the eject button to discard the cover.

18 For a *glass thermometer*:
  a Remove the glass thermometer.
  b Use tissues to remove the plastic cover. Discard the cover and tissues. Wipe the thermometer with a tissue if no cover was used. Wipe from the stem to the bulb end. Discard the tissue.
  c Read the thermometer.
    (1) Hold it at the stem. Bring it to eye level.
    (2) Turn it until you can see the numbers and the long and short lines.
    (3) Turn it back and forth slowly until you can see the silver or red line (Fig. 4-9).
    (4) Read the nearest degree (long line). For a Fahrenheit (F) thermometer, every other long line is an even degree from 94° to 108° F. For a centigrade thermometer, each long line means 1 degree.
    (5) Read the nearest tenth of a degree (short line). For a Fahrenheit thermometer, the short lines mean 0.2 (two-tenths) of a degree. For a centigrade thermometer, each short line means 0.1 (one-tenth) of a degree.

19 Note the person's name, temperature, and temperature site on your notepad or assignment sheet.

20 Return the probe to the holder.

21 For a *rectal temperature*:
  a Place used toilet tissue on several thicknesses of toilet tissue to avoid soiling linen.
  b Place the glass thermometer on clean toilet tissue.
  c Wipe the anal area to remove excess lubricant and any feces.
  d Cover the person.

22 For an *axillary temperature*: Help the person put the gown back on.

23 Shake down the glass thermometer.

24 Clean the glass thermometer according to agency policy. Return it to the holder.

25 Discard tissues, and dispose of toilet tissue.

26 Remove the gloves. Decontaminate your hands.

POST-PROCEDURE

27 Provide for comfort. See the inside of the front book cover.

28 Place the signal light within reach.

29 Unscreen the person.

30 Complete a safety check of the room. See the inside of the front book cover.

31 Return the electronic or tympanic membrane thermometer to the charging unit.

32 Decontaminate your hands.

33 Report and record the temperature. Note the temperature site when reporting and recording. Report any abnormal temperature at once.

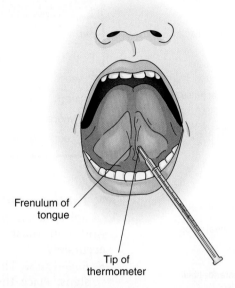

Frenulum of
tongue

Tip of
thermometer

Fig. 4-6 The thermometer is placed at the base of the tongue and to one side.

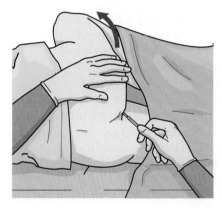

Fig. 4-7 The rectal temperature is taken with the person in Sims' position. The buttock is raised to expose the anus.

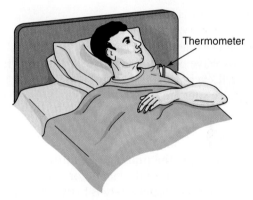

Thermometer

Fig. 4-8 The thermometer is held in place in the axilla by bringing the person's arm over the chest.

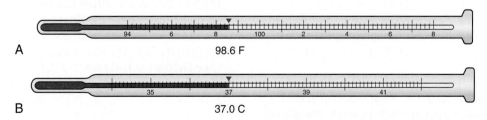

A   98.6 F

B   37.0 C

Fig. 4-9 A, A Fahrenheit thermometer. The temperature measurement is 98.6° F. **B,** Centigrade thermometer. The temperature measurement is 37.0° C.

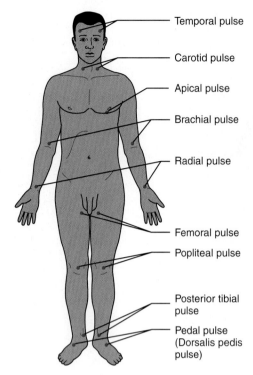

Temporal pulse
Carotid pulse
Apical pulse
Brachial pulse
Radial pulse
Femoral pulse
Popliteal pulse
Posterior tibial pulse
Pedal pulse (Dorsalis pedis pulse)

Fig. 4-10 The pulse sites.

TABLE 4-2	Pulse Ranges By Age	
AGE	**PULSE RATE PER MINUTE**
Birth to 1 year	80—190
2 years	80—160
6 years	75—120
10 years	70—110
12 years and older	60—100

Pulse. The *pulse* is the beat of the heart felt at an artery as a wave of blood passes through the artery. A pulse is felt every time the heart beats.

The pulse sites are shown in Figure 4-10. The radial pulse is used most often. It is easy to reach and find. You can take a radial pulse without disturbing or exposing the person.

The *pulse rate* is the number of heartbeats or pulses felt in 1 minute. The rate varies for each age group (Table 4-2). The adult pulse rate is between 60 and 100 beats per minute. A rate of less than 60 or more than 100 is considered abnormal. Report abnormal pulses to the nurse at once.

- *Tachycardia* is a rapid *(tachy)* heart rate *(cardia)*. The heart rate is more than 100 beats per minute.
- *Bradycardia* is a slow *(brady)* heart rate *(cardia)*. The heart rate is less than 60 beats per minute.

The *rhythm* of the pulse should be regular. That is, pulses are felt in a pattern. The same time interval occurs between beats. An irregular pulse occurs when the beats are not evenly spaced or beats are skipped.

Force relates to pulse strength. A forceful pulse is easy to feel. It is described as *strong, full,* or *bounding.* Hard-to-feel pulses are described as *weak, thready,* or *feeble.*

Taking a Pulse. You will take radial, apical, and apical-radial pulses. You must count accurately. And you must report and record the pulse rate accurately.

- *Radial pulse.* The *radial pulse* is used for routine vital signs. Place the first 2 or 3 fingers of one hand against the radial artery. The radial artery is on the thumb side of the wrist (Fig. 4-11). Count the pulse for 30 seconds. Then multiply the number by 2. This gives the number of beats per minute. If the pulse is irregular, count it for 1 minute. In some agencies, all radial pulses are taken for 1 minute. Follow agency policy.
- *Apical pulse.* The *apical pulse* is on the left side of the chest slightly below the nipple (Fig. 4-12). Apical pulses are taken on persons who:
  - Have heart disease
  - Have irregular heart rhythms
  - Take drugs that affect the heart

  Count the apical pulse for 1 minute. The heartbeat normally sounds like a *lub-dub.* Count each *lub-dub* as one beat. Do not count the *lub* as one beat and the *dub* as another. The apical pulse is taken with a stethoscope.
- *Apical-radial pulse.* The apical and radial pulse rates should be equal. Sometimes heart contractions are not strong enough to create pulses in the radial artery. Then the radial pulse rate is less than the apical pulse rate. This may occur in people with heart disease. To see if the apical and radial pulses are equal, two staff members are needed. One takes the radial pulse; the other takes the apical pulse. The *pulse deficit* is the difference between the apical and radial pulse rates. To obtain the pulse deficit, subtract the radial rate from the apical rate. (The apical pulse rate is never less than the radial pulse rate.)

See *Delegation Guidelines: Taking a Pulse.*
See *Promoting Safety and Comfort: Taking a Pulse.*

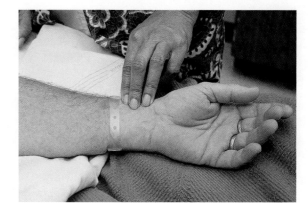

Fig. 4-11 The middle three fingers are used to take the radial pulse.

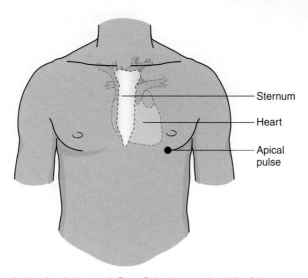

Sternum

Heart

Apical pulse

Fig. 4-12 The apical pulse is located 2 to 3 inches to the left of the sternum (breastbone) and below the left nipple.

DELEGATION GUIDELINES
Taking a Pulse

Before taking a pulse, you need this information from the nurse and the care plan:
- What pulse to take for each person—radial, apical, or apical-radial
- When to take the pulse
- What other vital signs to measure
- How long to count the pulse—30 seconds or 1 minute
- If the nurse has concerns about certain patients or residents
- What observations to report and record:
  - The pulse site
  - The pulse rate—report a pulse rate less than 60 (bradycardia) or more than 100 beats (tachycardia) per minute at once
  - Pulse deficit for an apical-radial pulse
  - If the pulse is regular or irregular
  - Pulse force—strong, full, bounding, weak, thready, or feeble
- When to report the pulse measurement
- What specific patient or resident concerns to report at once

PROMOTING SAFETY AND COMFORT
Taking a Pulse

SAFETY
Do not use your thumb to take a pulse. The thumb has a pulse. You could mistake the pulse in your thumb for the person's pulse. Reporting and recording the wrong pulse rate can harm the person.

Stethoscopes are in contact with many persons and staff. Therefore you must prevent infection. Wipe the earpieces and diaphragm with antiseptic wipes before and after use.

COMFORT
Stethoscope diaphragms tend to be cold. Warm the diaphragm in your hand before applying it to the person. Cold diaphragms can startle the person.

TAKING A PULSE

QUALITY OF LIFE

Remember to:
- Knock before entering the person's room.
- Address the person by name.
- Introduce yourself by name and title.

- Explain the procedure to the person before beginning and during the procedure.
- Protect the person's rights during the procedure.
- Handle the person gently during the procedure.

PRE-PROCEDURE

1 Follow *Delegation Guidelines: Taking a Pulse*, p. 39. See *Promoting Safety and Comfort: Taking a Pulse*, p. 39.
2 Ask a nursing team member to help you take an apical-radial pulse.
3 Practice hand hygiene.

4 Collect a stethoscope and antiseptic wipes for an apical pulse or an apical-radial pulse.
5 Decontaminate your hands.
6 Identify the person. Check the ID bracelet against the assignment sheet. Also call the person by name.
7 Provide for privacy.

PROCEDURE

8 Clean the earpieces and diaphragm with the wipes.
9 Have the person sit or lie down.
10 For a *radial pulse:*
   a Locate the radial pulse. Use your first 2 or 3 middle fingers.
   b Note if the pulse is strong or weak, and regular or irregular.
   c Count the pulse for 30 seconds. Multiply the number of beats by 2. Or count the pulse for 1 minute if:
      - Directed by the nurse and care plan.
      - Required by agency policy.
      - The pulse was irregular.
      - Required for your state competency test.
11 For an *apical pulse:*
   a Expose the nipple area of the left chest. Do not expose a woman's breasts.
   b Warm the diaphragm in your palm.
   c Place the earpieces in your ears.
   d Find the apical pulse. Place the diaphragm 2 to 3 inches to the left of the breastbone and below the left nipple.

   e Count the pulse for 1 minute. Note if it was regular or irregular.
   f Cover the person. Remove the earpieces.
12 For an *apical-radial pulse:*
   a Follow steps 11 a–c.
   b Find the apical pulse. Your helper finds the radial pulse (Fig. 4-13).
   c Give the signal to begin counting.
   d Count the pulse for 1 minute.
   e Give the signal to stop counting.
   f Subtract the radial pulse from the apical pulse for the pulse deficit. Note whether the pulse was regular or irregular.
13 Note the person's name and pulse on your notepad or assignment sheet. For an apical-radial pulse, note the apical and radial pulse rates and the pulse deficit. Note the strength of the pulse. Note if it was regular or irregular.

POST-PROCEDURE

14 Provide for comfort. See the inside of the front book cover.
15 Place the signal light within reach.
16 Unscreen the person.
17 Complete a safety check of the room. See the inside of the front book cover.
18 Clean the earpieces and diaphragm with the wipes.

19 Return the stethoscope to its proper place.
20 Decontaminate your hands.
21 Report and record your observations. Record the pulse rate and note the site. Report an abnormal pulse rate at once. For an apical-radial pulse, note:
   - The apical and radial pulse rates
   - The pulse deficit

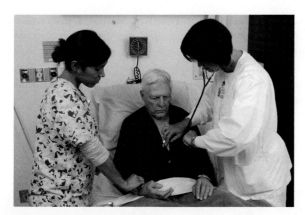

Fig. 4-13 Taking an apical-radial pulse. One worker takes the apical pulse. The other takes the radial pulse.

 Respirations. *Respiration* means breathing air into (inhalation) and out of (exhalation) the lungs. Each respiration involves one inhalation and one exhalation. The chest rises during inhalation. It falls during exhalation.

The healthy adult has 12 to 20 respirations per minute. Respirations are normally quiet, effortless, and regular. Both sides of the chest rise and fall equally.

Count respirations when the person is at rest. Position the person so you can see the chest rise and fall. People tend to change their breathing patterns when they know their respirations are being counted. Therefore the person should not know that you are counting them.

DELEGATION GUIDELINES
Respirations

Before counting respirations, you need this information from the nurse and the care plan:
* How long to count respirations for each person—30 seconds or 1 minute
* When to count respirations
* If the nurse has concerns about certain patients or residents
* What other vital signs to measure
* What observations to report and record:
  * The respiratory rate
  * Equality and depth of respirations
  * If the respirations were regular or irregular
  * If the person has pain or difficulty breathing
  * Any respiratory noises
  * An abnormal respiratory pattern
* When to report observations
* What specific patient or resident concerns to report at once

Count respirations right after taking a pulse. Keep your fingers or stethoscope over the pulse site. (The person assumes you are taking the pulse). To count respirations, watch the chest rise and fall. Count them for 30 seconds. Multiply the number by 2 for the number of respirations in 1 minute. If an abnormal pattern is noted, count the respirations for 1 minute.

In some agencies, respirations are counted for 1 minute. Follow agency policy.

See *Delegation Guidelines: Respirations.*

COUNTING RESPIRATIONS

PROCEDURE

1 Follow *Delegation Guidelines: Respirations.*
2 Keep your fingers or stethoscope over the pulse site.
3 Do not tell the person you are counting respirations.
4 Begin counting when the chest rises. Count each rise and fall of the chest as 1 respiration.
5 Note the following:
  * If respirations are regular
  * If both sides of the chest rise equally
  * The depth of respirations
  * If the person has any pain or difficulty breathing
  * An abnormal respiratory pattern

6 Count respirations for 30 seconds. Multiply the number by 2. Count respirations for 1 minute if:
  * Directed by the nurse and care plan.
  * Required by agency policy.
  * They are abnormal or irregular.
  * Required for your state competency test.
7 Note the person's name, respiratory rate, and other observations on your notepad or assignment sheet.

POST-PROCEDURE

8 Provide for comfort. See the inside of the front book cover.
9 Place the signal light within reach.
10 Unscreen the person.
11 Complete a safety check of the room. See the inside of the front book cover.
12 Decontaminate your hands.
13 Report and record the respiratory rate and your observations. Report abnormal respirations at once.

Blood Pressure. *Blood pressure* is the amount of force exerted against the walls of an artery by the blood. The period of heart muscle contraction is called *systole*. The heart is pumping blood. The period of heart muscle relaxation is called *diastole*. The heart is at rest.

Systolic and diastolic pressures are measured. The *systolic pressure* is the amount of force needed to pump blood out of the heart into the arterial circulation. It is the higher pressure. The *diastolic pressure* is the pressure in the arteries when the heart is at rest. It is the lower pressure.

Blood pressure is measured in millimeters (mm) of mercury (Hg). The systolic pressure is recorded over the diastolic pressure. A systolic pressure of 120 mm Hg (millimeters of mercury) and a diastolic pressure of 80 mm Hg is written as 120/80 mm Hg.

Because it can vary so easily, blood pressure has normal ranges:
- *Systolic pressure*—less than 120 mm Hg
- *Diastolic pressure*—less than 80 mm Hg

A stethoscope and a sphygmomanometer are used to measure blood pressure. The sphygmomanometer has a cuff and a measuring device. The cuff is wrapped around the upper arm. Tubing connects the cuff to the manometer. Another tube connects the cuff to a small, hand-held bulb. A valve on the bulb is turned so the cuff inflates as the bulb is squeezed. The inflated cuff causes pressure over the brachial artery. The valve is turned the other way to deflate the cuff. Blood pressure is measured as the cuff is deflated.

Blood pressure is normally measured in the brachial artery. Box 4-5 lists the guidelines for measuring blood pressure. The stethoscope is used to listen to the sounds in the brachial artery as the cuff is deflated. Stethoscopes are not needed with electronic manometers.

See *Delegation Guidelines: Blood Pressure.*
See *Promoting Safety and Comfort: Blood Pressure.*

DELEGATION GUIDELINES
Blood Pressure

Before measuring blood pressure, you need this information from the nurse and the care plan:
- When to measure blood pressure
- If the person has an arm injury, IV infusion, cast, or dialysis access site
- If the person had breast surgery, on what side was the surgery done
- The person's normal blood pressure range
- If the nurse has concerns about certain patients or residents
- If the person needs to be lying down, sitting, or standing
- What size cuff to use—regular, child-size, or extra large
- What observations to report and record:
  - When to report the blood pressure measurement
  - What specific patient or resident concerns to report at once

---

BOX 4-5   **Guidelines for Measuring Blood Pressure**

- Do not take blood pressure on an arm with an IV (intravenous) infusion, a cast, or a dialysis access site. If a person had breast surgery, do not take blood pressure on that side. Avoid taking blood pressure on an injured arm.
- Let the person rest for 10 to 20 minutes before measuring blood pressure.
- Measure blood pressure with the person sitting or lying. Sometimes the doctor orders blood pressure measured in the standing position.
- Apply the cuff to the bare upper arm. Clothing can affect the measurement.
- Make sure the cuff is snug. Loose cuffs can cause inaccurate readings.
- Use a larger cuff if the person is obese or has a large arm. Use a small cuff if the person has a very small arm. Ask the nurse what size to use.
- Place the diaphragm of the stethoscope firmly over the brachial artery. The entire diaphragm must have contact with the skin.

- Make sure the room is quiet. Talking, TV, radio, and sounds from the hallway can affect an accurate measurement.
- Have the sphygmomanometer where you can clearly see it.
- Measure the systolic and diastolic pressures.
  - Expect to hear the first blood pressure sound at the point where you last felt the radial or brachial pulse. The first sound is the systolic pressure.
  - The point where the sound disappears is the diastolic pressure.
- Take the blood pressure again if you are not sure of an accurate measurement. Wait 30 to 60 seconds before repeating the measurement.
- Tell the nurse at once if you cannot hear the blood pressure.

PROMOTING SAFETY AND COMFORT
Blood Pressure

SAFETY

Some sphygmomanometers contain mercury. Mercury is a hazardous substance. OSHA recommends that health care agencies replace out-dated sphygmomanometers with mercury-free devices. If using a mercury sphygmomanometer, handle the device carefully. If one breaks, call for the nurse at once. Do not touch the mercury. Do not let the person touch it. The agency must follow special procedures for handling all hazardous substances.

COMFORT

Inflate the cuff only to the extent necessary (see procedure: *Measuring Blood Pressure*). The inflated cuff causes discomfort. The higher the inflation, the greater the discomfort.

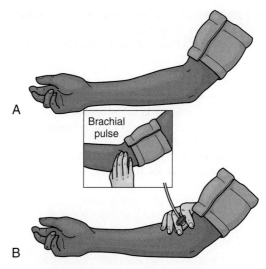

Fig. 4-14 Measuring blood pressure. **A,** The cuff is over the brachial artery. **B,** The diaphragm of the stethoscope is over the brachial artery.

 # MEASURING BLOOD PRESSURE

QUALITY OF LIFE

Remember to:
- Knock before entering the person's room.
- Address the person by name.
- Introduce yourself by name and title.

- Explain the procedure to the person before beginning and during the procedure.
- Protect the person's rights during the procedure.
- Handle the person gently during the procedure.

PRE-PROCEDURE

1 Follow *Delegation Guidelines: Blood Pressure*. See *Promoting Safety and Comfort*:
- *Taking a Pulse*, p. 39
- *Blood Pressure*
2 Practice hand hygiene.
3 Collect the following:
- Sphygmomanometer
- Stethoscope
- Antiseptic wipes

4 Decontaminate your hands.
5 Identify the person. Check the ID bracelet against the assignment sheet. Also call the person by name.
6 Provide for privacy.

PROCEDURE

7 Wipe the stethoscope earpieces and diaphragm with the wipes. Warm the diaphragm in your palm.
8 Have the person sit or lie down.
9 Position the person's arm level with the heart. The palm is up.
10 Stand no more than 3 feet away from the manometer.
11 Expose the upper arm.

12 Squeeze the cuff to expel any remaining air. Close the valve on the bulb.
13 Find the brachial artery at the inner aspect of the elbow. (The brachial artery is on the little finger side of the arm.) Use your fingertips.
14 Place the arrow on the cuff over the brachial artery (Fig. 4-14, *A*). Wrap the cuff around the upper arm at least 1 inch above the elbow. It is even and snug.

Continued

MEASURING BLOOD PRESSURE—cont'd

PROCEDURE—cont'd

15 *One-step method:*
- **a** Place the stethoscope earpieces in your ears.
- **b** Find the radial or brachial artery.
- **c** Inflate the cuff until you can no longer feel the pulse. Note this point.
- **d** Inflate the cuff 30 mm Hg beyond the point where you last felt the pulse.

16 *Two-step method:*
- **a** Find the radial or brachial artery.
- **b** Inflate the cuff until you can no longer feel the pulse. Note this point.
- **c** Inflate the cuff 30 mm Hg beyond the point where you last felt the pulse.
- **d** Deflate the cuff slowly. Note the point when you feel the pulse.
- **e** Wait 30 seconds.
- **f** Place the stethoscope earpieces in your ears.
- **g** Inflate the cuff 30 mm Hg beyond the point where you felt the pulse return.

17 Place the diaphragm of the stethoscope over the brachial artery (Fig. 4-14, *B*, p. 43). Do not place it under the cuff.

18 Deflate the cuff at an even rate of 2 to 4 millimeters per second. Turn the valve counter-clockwise to deflate the cuff.

19 Note the point where you hear the first sound. This is the systolic reading. It is near the point where the radial pulse disappeared.

20 Continue to deflate the cuff. Note the point where the sound disappears. This is the diastolic reading.

21 Deflate the cuff completely. Remove it from the person's arm. Remove the stethoscope earpieces from your ears.

22 Note the person's name and blood pressure on your notepad or assignment sheet.

23 Return the cuff to the case or wall holder.

POST-PROCEDURE

24 Provide for comfort. See the inside of the front book cover.

25 Place the signal light within reach.

26 Unscreen the person.

27 Complete a safety check of the room. See the inside of the front book cover.

28 Clean the earpieces and diaphragm with the wipes.

29 Return the equipment to its proper place.

30 Decontaminate your hands.

31 Report and record the blood pressure. Report an abnormal blood pressure at once.

Measuring Weight and Height

Weight and height are measured on admission to the agency. The doctor uses the measurements to determine the dosages of some drugs. Then the person is weighed daily, weekly, or monthly. This is done to measure weight gain or loss.

When measuring weight and height, follow these guidelines:

- The person only wears a gown or pajamas. Clothes add weight. No footwear is worn. Footwear adds to the weight and height measurements.
- The person voids before being weighed. A full bladder adds weight.
- Weigh the person at the same time of day. Before breakfast is the best time. Food and fluids add weight.
- Use the same scale for daily, weekly, and monthly weights. Scales weigh differently.
- Balance the scale at zero (0) before weighing the person. For balance scales, move the weights to zero. A digital scale should read at zero.

See *Delegation Guidelines: Measuring Weight and Height.*

See *Promoting Safety and Comfort: Measuring Weight and Height.*

DELEGATION GUIDELINES
Measuring Weight and Height

Before measuring weight and height, you need this information from the nurse and the care plan:
- When to measure weight and height
- What scale to use
- When to report the measurements
- What specific patient or resident concerns to report at once

PROMOTING SAFETY AND COMFORT
Measuring Weight and Height

SAFETY
Follow the manufacturer's instructions when using chair, bed, or lift scales. Also follow the agency's procedures. Practice safety measures to prevent falls.

COMFORT
The person wears only a gown or pajamas for the weight measurement. Prevent chilling and drafts.

MEASURING WEIGHT AND HEIGHT

QUALITY OF LIFE

Remember to:
- Knock before entering the person's room.
- Address the person by name.
- Introduce yourself by name and title.

- Explain the procedure to the person before beginning and during the procedure.
- Protect the person's rights during the procedure.
- Handle the person gently during the procedure.

PRE-PROCEDURE

1 Follow *Delegation Guidelines: Measuring Weight and Height.* See *Promoting Safety and Comfort: Measuring Weight and Height.*
2 Ask the person to void.
3 Practice hand hygiene.
4 Bring the scale and paper towels (for a standing scale) to the person's room.

5 Decontaminate your hands.
6 Identify the person. Check the ID bracelet against the assignment sheet. Also call the person by name.
7 Provide for privacy.

PROCEDURE

8 Place the paper towels on the scale platform.
9 Raise the height rod.
10 Move the weights to zero (0). The pointer is in the middle.
11 Have the person remove the robe and footwear. Assist as needed.
12 Help the person stand on the scale. The person stands in the center of the scale. Arms are at the sides.
13 Move the weights until the balance pointer is in the middle (Fig. 4-15, p. 46).
14 Note the weight on your notepad or assignment sheet.

15 Ask the person to stand very straight.
16 Lower the height rod until it rests on the person's head (Fig. 4-16, p. 46).
17 Note the height on your notepad or assignment sheet.
18 Raise the height rod. Help the person step off of the scale.
19 Help the person put on a robe and non-skid footwear if he or she will be up. Or help the person back to bed.
20 Lower the height rod. Adjust the weights to zero (0) if this is your agency's policy.

POST-PROCEDURE

21 Provide for comfort. See the inside of the front book cover.
22 Place the signal light within reach.
23 Raise or lower bed rails. Follow the care plan.
24 Unscreen the person.
25 Complete a safety check of the room. See the inside of the front book cover.

26 Discard the paper towels.
27 Return the scale to its proper place.
28 Decontaminate your hands.
29 Report and record the measurements.

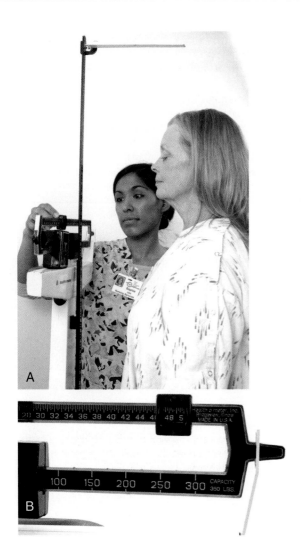

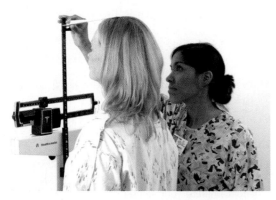

Fig. 4-15 A, The person is weighed. **B,** The weight is read when the balance pointer is in the middle.

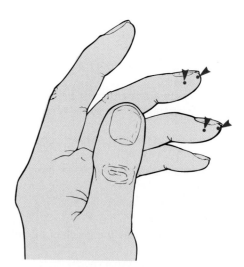

Fig. 4-16 Height is measured.

Blood Glucose Testing

Blood glucose testing is used for persons with diabetes. The doctor uses the results to regulate the person's drugs and diet. For the test, capillary blood is obtained through a skin puncture.

With skin punctures, a few drops of capillary blood are obtained. A fingertip is the most common site for skin punctures. The earlobe also is a site. These sites provide easy access and do not require clothing removal. The person feels a sharp pinch. Discomfort is brief.

Inspect the site carefully. Look for signs of trauma and skin breaks. Avoid sites that are swollen, bruised, cyanotic (bluish color), scarred, or calloused. Blood flow to these areas is poor. A *callus* is a thick, hardened area on the skin. Calluses often form over frequently used areas, such as the tips of the thumbs and index fingers. Therefore the thumbs and index fingers are not good sites for skin punctures.

Do not use the center, fleshy part of the fingertip. The site has many nerve endings. A puncture at the site is painful. Use the side toward the tip of the fingertip on the middle or ring finger (Fig. 4-17).

A sterile lancet is used to puncture the skin (Fig. 4-18). A *lancet* is a short, pointed blade. The short blade punctures but does not cut the skin. The lancet is inside a protective cover. You do not touch the actual blade. All types of lancets are disposable. A lancet is discarded into the sharps container after use.

Fig. 4-17 Site for skin punctures. (From Bonewit-West, K: *Clinical procedures for medical assistants,* ed 5, Philadelphia, 2000, Saunders.)

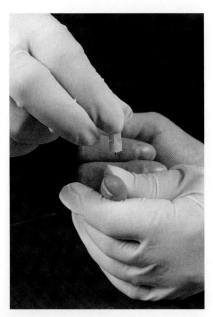

Fig. 4-18 A lancet. (From Bonewit-West, K: *Clinical procedures for medical assistants,* ed 6, St. Louis, 2004, Saunders.)

A glucose meter (glucometer) is used to measure blood glucose. The blood glucose level is shown on the monitor. Many different glucose meters are available. The speed with which results are displayed varies with the manufacturer. Some take 1 minute. Others take 15 seconds or less.

Before inserting the reagent strip into the device, follow the manufacturer's instructions. One of the following is usually required:

* *Dry-wipe.* Blood is wiped off the reagent strip with a cotton ball.
* *Wet-wash.* The reagent strip is flushed with water to rinse blood off.
* *No-wipe.* No wiping or rinsing. The reagent strip is inserted directly into the device.

In agencies, glucose meters are tested daily for accuracy. The manufacturer has instructions for testing the device.

There are many different kinds of glucometers. You will learn to use the device used in your agency. Always follow the manufacturer's instructions.

See *Delegation Guidelines: Blood Glucose Testing.*

See *Promoting Safety and Comfort: Blood Glucose Testing.*

DELEGATION GUIDELINES
Blood Glucose Testing

Many states and agencies allow nursing assistive personnel to test blood glucose. If the task is delegated to you, make sure that:

* Your state allows nursing assistive personnel to perform the procedure
* The procedure is in your job description
* You have the necessary training
* You know how to use the agency's equipment
* You review the procedure with a nurse
* The nurse is available to answer questions and to supervise you

If the above conditions are met, you need the following information from the nurse:

* What sites you can use for the skin puncture
* What sites to avoid for the skin puncture
* What to report and record:
  * The time the specimen was collected
  * The blood glucose test results
  * The site used for the skin puncture
  * The amount of bleeding at the skin puncture site
  * Any signs of a *hematoma* (a swelling [*oma*] that contains blood [*hemat*])
  * How the person tolerated the procedure
  * Complaints of pain at the skin puncture site
  * Other observations or patient or resident complaints
* When to report observations and the blood glucose measurement
* What specific patient or resident concerns to report at once

---

PROMOTING SAFETY AND COMFORT
Blood Glucose Testing

SAFETY
Accurate results are important. Inaccurate results can harm the person. Follow the rules in Box 4-6 (p. 48) when testing blood specimens for glucose.

Make sure you know how to use the equipment before testing blood. Also check the manufacturer's instructions for the reagent strip to use. Use only the type of reagent strip specified by the manufacturer. Otherwise you will get inaccurate results.

Contact with blood is likely. Follow Standard Precautions (Chapter 9) and the Bloodborne Pathogen Standard (Appendix C).

COMFORT
The heel is used for skin punctures in infants who are not yet walking. The third finger (ring finger) is used for children. See Figure 4-19 (p. 48).

Older persons often have poor circulation in their fingers. To increase blood flow, apply a warm washcloth or wash the hands in warm water.

BOX 4-6 Rules for Blood Glucose Testing

- Follow the manufacturer's instructions for the glucose meter.
- Know how to use the equipment. Request any necessary training.
- Make sure the glucose meter was tested for accuracy. Check the testing log.
- Check the color of reagent strips. Do not use discolored strips.
- Check the expiration date of the reagent strips. Do not use them if the date has passed.
- Use a watch with a sweep hand to time the test (if necessary). Follow the manufacturer's instructions for test times.
- Report the results to the nurse at once.
- Record the result following agency policy.

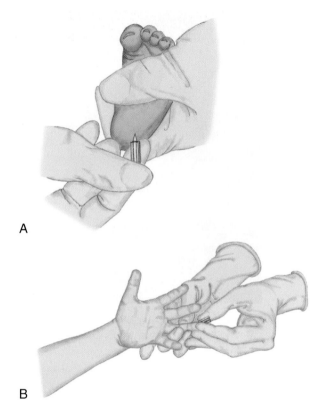

A

B

Fig. 4-19 A, Heel site is used for skin punctures in infants. **B,** The third finger (ring finger) is used for skin punctures in children. (From James SR, Ashwill JW, Droske SC: *Nursing care of children: principles and practice,* ed 3, St. Louis, 2007, Saunders.)

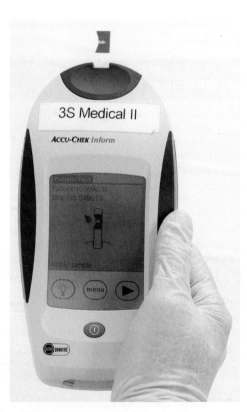

Fig. 4-20 A reagent strip is in the glucose meter.

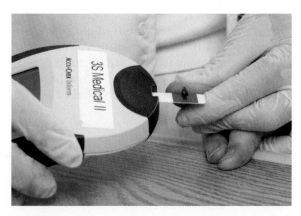

Fig. 4-21 A drop of blood is applied to the reagent strip.

MEASURING BLOOD GLUCOSE

QUALITY OF LIFE

Remember to:
- Knock before entering the person's room.
- Address the person by name.
- Introduce yourself by name and title.

- Explain the procedure to the person before beginning and during the procedure.
- Protect the person's rights during the procedure.
- Handle the person gently during the procedure.

PRE-PROCEDURE

1 Follow *Delegation Guidelines: Blood Glucose Testing,* p. 47. See *Promoting Safety and Comfort: Blood Glucose Testing,* p. 47.
2 Practice hand hygiene.
3 Collect the following:
- Sterile lancet
- Antiseptic wipes
- Gloves
- Cotton balls
- Glucose meter
- Reagent strips (Use the correct ones for the meter. Check the expiration date.)
- Paper towels
- Washcloth
- Soap, towel, and wash basin

4 Read the manufacturer's instructions for the lancet and glucose meter.
5 Arrange your work area.
6 Identify the person. Check the ID bracelet against the assignment sheet. Also call the person by name.
7 Provide for privacy.
8 Raise the bed for body mechanics. The far bed rail is up if used.

PROCEDURE

9 Help the person to a comfortable position.
10 Assist with hand washing.
11 Put on the gloves.
12 Prepare the supplies:
   a Open the antiseptic wipes.
   b Remove a reagent strip from the bottle. Place it on the paper towel. Place the cap securely on the bottle.
   c Prepare the lancet.
   d Turn on the glucose meter.
   e Insert a reagent strip into the glucose meter (Fig. 4-20).
13 Perform a skin puncture to obtain a drop of blood:
   a Inspect the person's fingers. Select a skin puncture site.
   b Warm the finger. Rub it gently or apply a warm washcloth.
   c Massage the hand and finger toward the puncture site. This brings more blood to the site.
   d Lower the finger below the person's waist. This increases blood flow to the site.
   e Hold the finger with your thumb and forefinger. Use your non-dominant hand. Hold the finger until step 13-k.
   f Clean the site with an antiseptic wipe. *Do not touch the site after cleaning.*
   g Let the site dry.
   h Pick up the sterile lancet.
   i Place the lancet against the side of the finger or the top of the fingertip.

   j Push the button on the lancet to puncture the skin. (Follow the manufacturer's instructions.)
   k Wipe away the first blood drop. Use a cotton ball.
   l Apply gentle pressure below the puncture site.
   m Let a large drop of blood form.
14 Collect and test the specimen. Follow the manufacturer's instructions and agency procedures for the glucose meter used.
   a Hold the test area of the reagent strip close to the drop of blood.
   b Lightly touch the reagent strip to the blood drop (Fig. 4-21). Do not smear the blood.
   c Set the timer on the glucose meter (if necessary). NOTE: Some glucose meters start timing automatically when the blood is applied.
   d Wait the length of time required by the manufacturer.
   e Apply pressure to the puncture site until bleeding stops. Use a cotton ball. If able, let the person apply pressure to the site.
   f Read the result on the display (Fig. 4-22, p. 50). Note the result, and tell the person the result.
   g Turn off the glucose meter.
15 Discard the lancet into the sharps container.
16 Discard the cotton balls following agency policy.
17 Remove and discard the gloves. Decontaminate your hands.

Continued

MEASURING BLOOD GLUCOSE—cont'd

POST-PROCEDURE

18 Provide for comfort. See the inside of the front book cover.
19 Place the signal light within reach.
20 Lower the bed to its lowest position.
21 Raise or lower bed rails. Follow the care plan.
22 Unscreen the person.
23 Discard used supplies. Clean and return the bath basin to its proper place.

24 Complete a safety check of the room. See the inside of the front book cover.
25 Follow agency policy for soiled linen.
26 Decontaminate your hands.
27 Return the glucose meter to its proper place.
28 Report and record the test result and your observations.

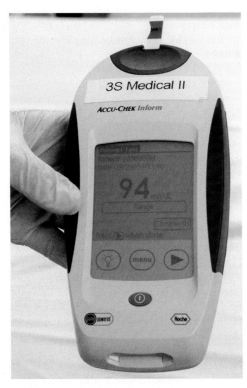

Fig. 4-22 The result is displayed on the glucose meter.

COMMUNICATION

Communication is essential for successful use of the nursing process. Nursing team members must communicate effectively with one another. For good communication:

- Use words that mean the same thing to you and the receiver of the message. "Small," "moderate," and "large" mean different things to different people. Is small the size of a dime? Or is it the size of a quarter? In health care, different meanings can cause serious problems. Avoid words with more than one meaning.
- Use familiar words. If you do not know what a word means, ask the nurse. Or use a medical dictionary.
- Be brief and concise. Do not add unrelated or unnecessary information. Stay on the subject. Avoid wandering in thought. Do not get wordy.
- Give information in a logical and orderly manner. Organize your thoughts. Present them step-by-step.
- Give facts and be specific. The receiver should have a clear picture of what you are saying. You report a pulse rate of 110. It is more specific and factual than saying the "pulse is fast."

Reporting and Recording

The nursing team communicates by reporting and recording. *Reporting* is the oral account of care and observations. *Recording (charting)* is the written account of care and observations.

Reporting. You report care and observations to the nurse. Follow these rules:

- Be prompt, thorough, and accurate.
- Give the person's name and room and bed number.
- Give the time your observations were made or the care was given.
- Report only what you observed or did yourself.
- Give reports as often as the person's condition requires. Or give them when the nurse asks you to do so.
- Report any changes from normal or changes in the person's condition. Report these changes at once.
- Use your written notes to give a specific, concise, and clear report.

Recording. When recording on the person's chart, you must communicate clearly and thoroughly. Follow the rules in Box 4-7. Anyone who reads your charting should know:

- What you observed
- What you did
- The person's response

The medication administration record is used to record what drugs were given and when. See Chapter 8.

Recording Time. The 24-hour clock (military time or international time) has four digits (Fig. 4-23). The first two digits are for the hours: 0100 = 1:00 AM; 1300 = 1:00 PM. The last two digits are for minutes: 0110 = 1:10 AM. The AM and PM abbreviations are not used.

The hour is the same for morning times, but AM is not used. For PM times add 12 to the clock time. If it is 2:00 PM, add 12 and 2 for 1400. For 8:35 PM, add 12 and 835 for 2035.

Communication is better with the 24-hour clock. You must use AM and PM with conventional clock time. Someone may forget to use AM or PM. Or writing may be unclear. This means that the correct time is not communicated. Harm to the person could result.

Communication Barriers

Communication barriers prevent the sending and receiving of messages. Communication fails. You must avoid these barriers when communicating with the nurse:

- Using unfamiliar language
- Cultural differences
- Changing the subject
- Giving your opinion
- Failing to listen

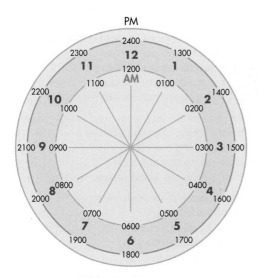

Fig. 4-23 The 24-hour clock.

BOX 4-7 Rules for Recording

- Always use ink. Use the ink color required by the agency.
- Include the date and time for every recording. Use conventional time (AM or PM) or 24-hour clock time according to agency policy.
- Make sure writing is readable and neat.
- Use only agency-approved medical abbreviations.
- Use correct spelling, grammar, and punctuation.
- Do not use ditto marks.
- Never erase or use correction fluid. Draw a line through the incorrect part. Date and initial the line. Write "mistaken entry" over it if this is agency policy. Then rewrite the part. Follow agency policy for correcting errors.
- Sign all entries with your name and title as required by agency policy.
- Do not skip lines. Draw a line through the blank space of a partially completed line or to the end of the page. This prevents others from recording in a space with your signature.
- Make sure each form has the person's name and other identifying information.
- Record only what you observed and did yourself. Do not record for another person.
- Never chart a procedure, treatment, or care measure until after it is completed.
- Be accurate, concise, and factual. Do not record judgments or interpretations.
- Record in a logical and sequential manner.
- Be descriptive. Avoid terms with more than one meaning.
- Use the person's exact words whenever possible. Use quotation marks to show that the statement is a direct quote.
- Chart any changes from normal or changes in the person's condition. Also chart that you informed the nurse (include the nurse's name), what you told the nurse, and the time you made the report.
- Do not omit information.
- Record safety measures. Examples include placing the signal light within reach, assisting a person when up, or reminding a person not to get out of bed.

REVIEW QUESTIONS

Circle the BEST answer.

1 Which is *not* a step in the nursing process?
a observation
b assessment
c planning
d implementation

2 The nursing process
a involves guidelines for care plans
b is a care conference
c involves a health history and a drug history
d is the method nurses use to plan and deliver nursing care

3 What happens during assessment?
a Goals are set.
b Information is collected.
c Nursing measures are carried out.
d Progress is evaluated.

4 Which is a symptom?
a redness
b vomiting
c pain
d pulse rate of 78

5 Which is a sign?
a nausea
b headache
c dizziness
d dry skin

6 You gave a drug to a person. Which observation should you report at once?
a The person had a bowel movement.
b The person is not responding to you.
c The person's pulse is 80 beats per minute.
d The person complains of stiff, painful joints.

7 You gave a drug to a person. Which observation should you report at once?
a The person can no longer move a body part.
b The person answers questions correctly.
c The person has a breath odor.
d The person walked to the dining room.

8 Measures in the nursing care plan are carried out. This is
a a nursing diagnosis
b planning
c implementation
d evaluation

9 Which statement is *true?*
a The nursing process is done without the person's input.
b You are responsible for the nursing process.
c The nursing process is used to communicate the person's care.
d Nursing process steps can be done in any order.

10 The nursing care plan is
a written by the doctor
b a guide with measures to help the person
c the same for all persons
d the drugs ordered for the person

11 Which is a nursing diagnosis?
a cancer
b heart attack
c kidney failure
d acute pain

12 The nurse uses the following to evaluate the person's response to drug therapy *except*
a vital signs
b weight
c Minimum Data Set
d blood glucose

13 Which temperature is *not* normal?
a an oral temperature of 99.8° F
b a rectal temperature of 99.6° F
c a tympanic membrane temperature of 98.6° F
d a temporal artery temperature of 99.6° F

14 A person has heart disease. You can measure temperature at the following sites *except*
a the oral site
b the rectal site
c the tympanic membrane site
d the temporal artery site

15 You take a person's pulse. Before giving a drug, which should you report to the nurse?
a a rate of 82
b a strong pulse
c an irregular pulse
d a pulse deficit of 0

16 Which respiratory rate is *not* normal for an adult?
a 12 respirations per minute
b 16 respirations per minute
c 20 respirations per minute
d 24 respirations per minute

17 When measuring vital signs, you count respirations
a before taking the temperature
b before taking the pulse
c after taking the pulse
d after taking the blood pressure

18 Blood pressure is usually measured
a in the radial artery
b in the brachial artery
c in the carotid artery
d at the apical pulse

19 Which blood pressure is *not* normal?
a 118/80 mm Hg
b 128/72 mm Hg
c 114/68 mm Hg
d 110/74 mm Hg

20 The diastolic blood pressure is
a 30 mm Hg above where the pulse was last felt
b 30 mm Hg below where the pulse was last felt
c where the first sound is heard
d where the last sound is heard

21 Which is the best site for a skin puncture?
a the thumb
b the index finger
c the ring finger
d the little finger

22 Which is used to measure blood glucose?
a glucose meter
b lancet
c reagent strip
d sphygmomanometer

23 You are measuring blood glucose. How long should you time the test?
a 30 seconds
b 1 minute
c 2 minutes
d as stated in the manufacturer's instructions

24 When should you record that you gave a person a drug?
a before giving the drug
b after giving the drug
c at the end of the shift
d when reporting to the nurse

Circle T if the statement is true. Circle F if the statement is false.

25 T F Drugs can affect a person's vital signs.

26 T F A person receives drugs for heart disease. When taking the pulse, you use the apical site.

27 T F A person has an IV in the left arm. You should measure blood pressure in the left arm.

28 T F Reagent strips for blood glucose are discolored. You should use the reagent strips.

29 T F A drug is ordered for 1630. You should give the drug at 4:30 PM.

30 T F You make a mistake when recording a drug. You can erase the error.

Answers to these questions are on p. 443.

5

Body Structure and Function

OBJECTIVES

- Define the key terms and key abbreviations used in this chapter.
- Identify the basic structures of the cell.
- Explain how cells divide.
- Describe four types of tissue.
- Identify the structures of each body system.
- Identify the functions of each body system.

KEY TERMS

artery A blood vessel that carries blood away from the heart

capillary A tiny blood vessel; food, oxygen, and other substances pass from the capillaries into the cells

cell The basic unit of body structure

digestion The process of physically and chemically breaking down food so that it can be absorbed for use by the cells

hemoglobin The substance in red blood cells that carries oxygen and gives blood its color

hormone A chemical substance secreted by the endocrine glands into the bloodstream

immunity Protection against a disease or condition; the person will not get or be affected by the disease

menstruation The process in which the lining of the uterus breaks up and is discharged from the body through the vagina

metabolism The burning of food for heat and energy by the cells

organ Groups of tissues with the same function

peristalsis Involuntary muscle contractions in the digestive system that move food down the esophagus through the alimentary canal

respiration The process of supplying the cells with oxygen and removing carbon dioxide from them

Continued

system Organs that work together to perform special functions

tissue A group of cells with similar functions

vein A blood vessel that returns blood back to the heart

KEY ABBREVIATIONS

ACTH Adrenocorticotropic hormone
ADH Antidiuretic hormone
CNS Central nervous system
GH Growth hormone
GI Gastro-intestinal
mL Milliliter
RBC Red blood cell
TH Thyroid hormone; thyroxine
TSH Thyroid-stimulating hormone
WBC White blood cell

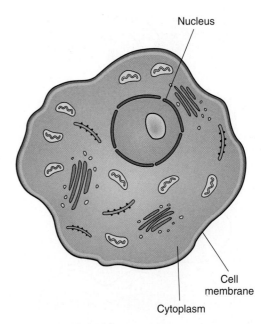

Fig. 5-1 Parts of a cell.

You help patients and residents meet basic needs. Their bodies do not work at peak levels because of illness, disease, or injury. Your care promotes comfort, healing, and recovery. You need to know the body's normal structure and function. It will help you understand signs, symptoms, and the reasons for drug therapy.

CELLS, TISSUES, AND ORGANS

The basic unit of body structure is the **cell.** Cells have the same basic structure. Function, size, and shape may differ. Cells are very small. You need a microscope to see them. Cells need food, water, and oxygen to live and function.

Figure 5-1 shows the cell and its structures. The *cell membrane* is the outer covering. It encloses the cell and helps it hold its shape. The *nucleus* is the control center of the cell. It directs the cell's activities. The nucleus is in the center of the cell. The *cytoplasm* surrounds the nucleus. Cytoplasm contains smaller structures that perform cell functions. *Protoplasm* means *living substance*. It refers to all structures, substances, and water within the cell. Protoplasm is a semi-liquid substance much like an egg white.

Chromosomes are thread-like structures in the nucleus. Each cell has 46 chromosomes. Chromosomes contain *genes*. Genes control the traits children inherit from their parents. Height, eye color, and skin color are examples.

The nucleus controls cell reproduction. Cells reproduce by dividing in half. The process of cell division is called *mitosis*. It is needed for tissue growth and repair. During mitosis, the 46 chromosomes arrange themselves in 23 pairs. As the cell divides, the 23 pairs are pulled in half. The two new cells are identical. Each has 46 chromosomes (Fig. 5-2, p. 56).

Cells are the body's building blocks. Groups of cells with similar functions combine to form **tissues:**
- *Epithelial tissue* covers internal and external body surfaces. Tissue lining the nose, mouth, respiratory tract, stomach, and intestines is epithelial tissue. So are the skin, hair, nails, and glands.
- *Connective tissue* anchors, connects, and supports other tissues. It is in every part of the body. Bones, tendons, ligaments, and cartilage are connective tissue. Blood is a form of connective tissue.
- *Muscle tissue* stretches and contracts to let the body move.
- *Nerve tissue* receives and carries impulses to the brain and back to body parts.

Groups of tissue with the same function form **organs.** An organ has one or more functions. Examples of organs are the heart, brain, liver, lungs, and kidneys. **Systems** are formed by organs that work together to perform special functions (Fig. 5-3, p. 56).

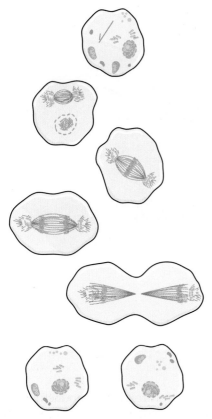

Fig. 5-2 Cell division.

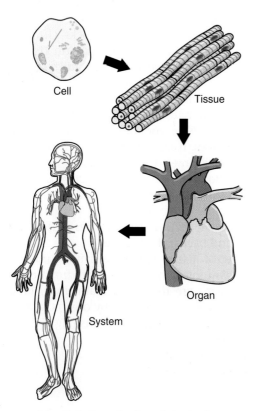

Fig. 5-3 Organization of the body.

THE INTEGUMENTARY SYSTEM

The *integumentary system,* or *skin,* is the largest system. *Integument* means *covering.* The skin covers the body. It has epithelial, connective, and nerve tissue. It also has oil glands and sweat glands. There are two skin layers (Fig. 5-4):

- The *epidermis* is the outer layer. It has living cells and dead cells. The dead cells were once deeper in the epidermis. They were pushed upward as the cells divided. Dead cells constantly flake off. They are replaced by living cells. Living cells also die and flake off. Living cells of the epidermis contain *pigment.* Pigment gives skin its color. The epidermis has no blood vessels and few nerve endings.
- The *dermis* is the inner layer. It is made up of connective tissue. Blood vessels, nerves, sweat glands, and oil glands are in the dermis. So are hair roots.

The epidermis and dermis are supported by *subcutaneous tissue.* The subcutaneous tissue is a thick layer of fat and connective tissue.

Oil glands, sweat glands, hair, and *nails* are skin appendages:

- Hair—covers the entire body, except the palms of the hands and the soles of the feet. Hair in the nose and ears and around the eyes protects these organs from dust, insects, and other foreign objects.
- Nails—protect the tips of the fingers and toes. Nails help fingers pick up and handle small objects.
- Sweat glands—help the body regulate temperature. Sweat consists of water, salt, and a small amount of wastes. Sweat is secreted through pores in the skin. The body is cooled as sweat evaporates.
- Oil glands—lie near the hair shafts. They secrete an oily substance into the space near the hair shaft. Oil travels to the skin surface. This helps keep the hair and skin soft and shiny.

The skin has many functions:

- It is the body's protective covering.
- It prevents microorganisms and other substances from entering the body.
- It prevents excess amounts of water from leaving the body.
- It protects organs from injury.
- Nerve endings in the skin sense both pleasant and unpleasant stimulation. Nerve endings are over the entire body. They sense cold, pain, touch, and pressure to protect the body from injury.
- It helps regulate body temperature. Blood vessels dilate (widen) when temperature outside the body is high. More blood is brought to the body surface for cooling during evaporation. When blood vessels constrict (narrow), the body retains heat. This is because less blood reaches the skin.

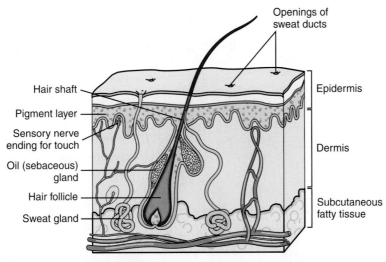

Fig. 5-4 Layers of the skin.

THE MUSCULOSKELETAL SYSTEM

The musculoskeletal system provides the framework for the body. It lets the body move. This system also protects and gives the body shape.

Bones

The human body has *206 bones* (Fig. 5-5, p. 58). There are four types of bones:

* *Long bones* bear the body's weight. Leg bones are long bones.
* *Short bones* allow skill and ease in movement. Bones in the wrists, fingers, ankles, and toes are short bones.
* *Flat bones* protect the organs. They include the ribs, skull, pelvic bones, and shoulder blades.
* *Irregular bones* are the vertebrae in the spinal column. They allow various degrees of movement and flexibility.

Bones are hard, rigid structures. They are made up of living cells. They are covered by a membrane called *periosteum.* Periosteum contains blood vessels that supply bone cells with oxygen and food. Inside the hollow centers of the bones is a substance called *bone marrow.* Blood cells are formed in the bone marrow.

Joints

A *joint* is the point at which two or more bones meet. Joints allow movement. *Cartilage* is the connective tissue at the end of the long bones. It cushions the joint so that the bone ends do not rub together. The *synovial membrane* lines the joints. It secretes *synovial fluid.* Synovial fluid acts as a lubricant so the joint can move smoothly. Bones are held together at the joint by strong bands of connective tissue called *ligaments.*

There are three major types of joints (Fig. 5-6, p. 58):

* *Ball-and-socket joint* allows movement in all directions. It is made up of the rounded end of one bone and the hollow end of another bone. The rounded end of one fits into the hollow end of the other. The joints of the hips and shoulders are ball-and-socket joints.
* *Hinge joint* allows movement in one direction. The elbow is a hinge joint.
* *Pivot joint* allows turning from side to side. A pivot joint connects the skull to the spine.

Muscles

The human body has more than *500 muscles* (Figs. 5-7 and 5-8, p. 59). Some are voluntary. Others are involuntary.

* *Voluntary muscles* can be consciously controlled. Muscles attached to bones *(skeletal muscles)* are voluntary. Arm muscles do not work unless you move your arm; likewise for leg muscles. Skeletal muscles are *striated.* That is, they look striped or streaked.
* *Involuntary muscles* work automatically. You cannot control them. They control the action of the stomach, intestines, blood vessels, and other body organs. Involuntary muscles also are called *smooth muscles.* They look smooth, not streaked or striped.
* *Cardiac muscle* is in the heart. It is an involuntary muscle. However, it appears striated like skeletal muscle.

Muscles have three functions:

* Movement of body parts
* Maintenance of posture
* Production of body heat

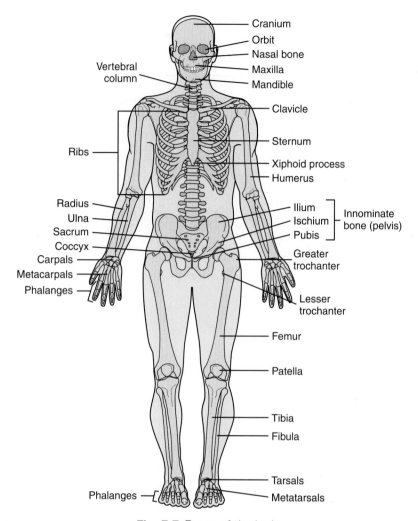

Fig. 5-5 Bones of the body.

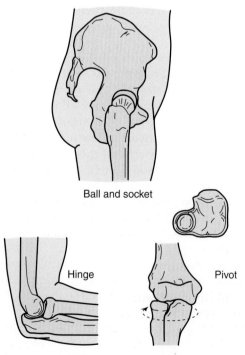

Ball and socket

Hinge   Pivot

Fig. 5-6 Types of joints.

Strong, tough connective tissues called *tendons* connect muscles to bones. When muscles contract (shorten), tendons at each end of the muscle cause the bone to move. The body has many tendons. See the Achilles tendon in Figure 5-8. Some muscles constantly contract to maintain the body's posture. When muscles contract, they burn food for energy. Heat is produced. The more muscle activity, the greater the amount of heat produced. Shivering is how the body produces heat when exposed to cold. Shivering is from rapid, general muscle contractions.

THE NERVOUS SYSTEM

The nervous system controls, directs, and coordinates body functions. Its two main divisions are:

- The *central nervous system* (CNS). It consists of the brain and spinal cord (Fig. 5-9, p. 60).
- The *peripheral nervous system*. It involves the *nerves* throughout the body (Fig. 5-10, p. 60).

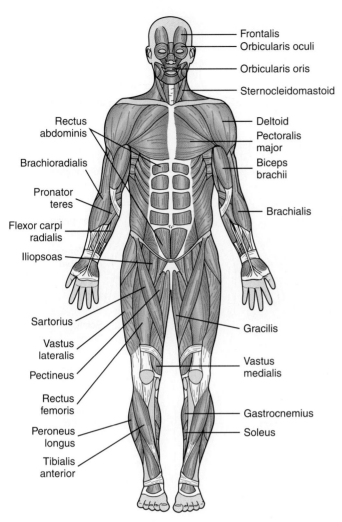

Fig. 5-7 Anterior view of the muscles of the body.

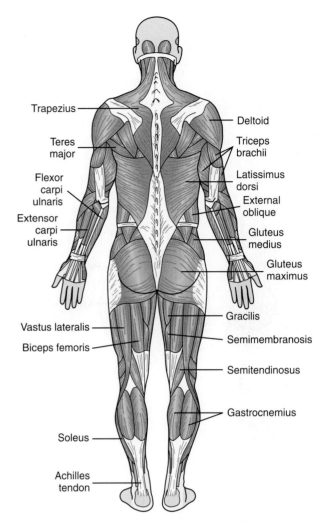

Fig. 5-8 Posterior view of the muscles of the body.

Nerves carry messages or impulses to and from the brain. Nerves connect to the spinal cord. They are easily damaged and take a long time to heal. Some nerve fibers have a protective covering called a *myelin sheath*. The myelin sheath also insulates the nerve fiber. Nerve fibers covered with myelin conduct impulses faster than those fibers without it.

The Central Nervous System

The *brain* and *spinal cord* make up the central nervous system. The brain is covered by the skull. The three main parts of the brain are the *cerebrum*, the *cerebellum*, and the *brainstem* (Fig. 5-11, p. 60).

The cerebrum is the largest part of the brain. It is the center of thought and intelligence. The cerebrum is divided into two halves called the *right* and *left hemispheres*. The right hemisphere controls movement and activities on the body's left side. The left hemisphere controls the right side.

The outside of the cerebrum is called the *cerebral cortex*. It controls the highest functions of the brain. These include reasoning, memory, consciousness, speech, voluntary muscle movement, vision, hearing, sensation, and other activities.

The cerebellum regulates and coordinates body movements. It controls balance and the smooth movements of voluntary muscles. Injury to the cerebellum results in jerky movements, loss of coordination, and muscle weakness.

The brainstem connects the cerebrum to the spinal cord. The brainstem contains the *midbrain, pons,* and *medulla.* The midbrain and pons relay messages between the medulla and the cerebrum. The medulla is below the pons. The medulla controls heart rate, breathing, blood vessel size, swallowing, coughing, and vomiting. The brain connects to the spinal cord at the lower end of the medulla.

The spinal cord lies within the spinal column. The cord is 17 to 18 inches long. It contains pathways that conduct messages to and from the brain.

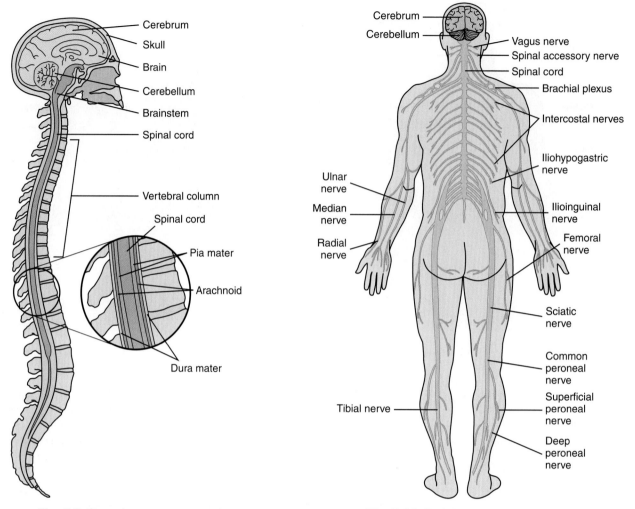

Fig. 5-9 Central nervous system.

Fig. 5-10 Peripheral nervous system.

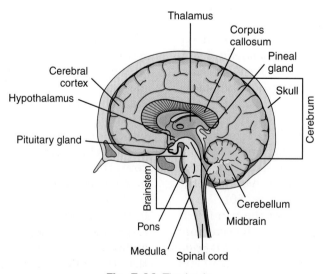

Fig. 5-11 The brain.

The brain and spinal cord are covered and protected by three layers of connective tissue called meninges:
- The outer layer lies next to the skull. It is a tough covering call the *dura mater.*
- The middle layer is the *arachnoid.*
- The inner layer is the *pia mater.*

The space between the middle layer (arachnoid) and inner layer (pia mater) is the *arachnoid space.* The space is filled with *cerebrospinal fluid.* It circulates around the brain and spinal cord. Cerebrospinal fluid protects the central nervous system. It cushions shocks that could easily injure brain and spinal cord structures.

The Peripheral Nervous System

The peripheral nervous system has 12 pairs of *cranial nerves* and 31 pairs of *spinal nerves.* Cranial nerves conduct impulses between the brain and the head, neck, chest, and abdomen. They conduct impulses for smell, vision, hearing, pain, touch, temperature, and pressure. They also conduct impulses for voluntary and involuntary muscles. Spinal nerves carry impulses from the skin, extremities, and the internal structures not supplied by cranial nerves.

Some peripheral nerves form the *autonomic nervous system.* This system controls involuntary muscles and certain body functions. The functions include the heartbeat, blood pressure, intestinal contractions, and glandular secretions. These functions occur automatically.

The autonomic nervous system is divided into the *sympathetic nervous system* and the *parasympathetic nervous system.* They balance each other. The sympathetic nervous system speeds up functions. The parasympathetic nervous system slows functions. When you are angry, scared, excited, or exercising, the sympathetic nervous system is stimulated. The parasympathetic nervous system is activated when you relax. It also is activated when the sympathetic system is stimulated for too long.

The Sense Organs

The five senses are *sight, hearing, taste, smell,* and *touch.* Receptors for taste are in the tongue. They are called *taste buds.* Receptors for smell are in the nose. Touch receptors are in the dermis, especially in the toes and fingertips.

The Eye. Receptors for vision are in the *eyes* (Fig. 5-12). The eye is easily injured. Bones of the skull, eyelids and eyelashes, and tears protect the eyes from injury. The eye has three layers:
- The *sclera,* the white of the eye, is the outer layer. It is made of tough connective tissue.

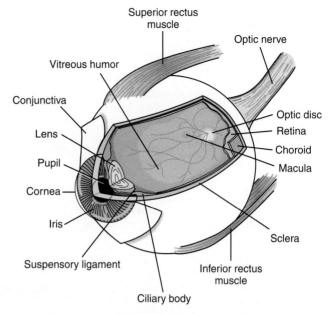

Fig. 5-12 The eye.

- The *choroid* is the second layer. Blood vessels, the *ciliary muscle,* and the *iris* make up the choroid. The iris gives the eye its color. The opening in the middle of the iris is the *pupil.* Pupil size varies with the amount of light entering the eye. The pupil constricts (narrows) in bright light. It dilates (widens) in dim or dark places.
- The *retina* is the inner layer. It has receptors for vision and the nerve fibers of the *optic nerve.*

Light enters the eye through the *cornea.* It is the transparent part of the outer layer that lies over the eye. Light rays pass to the *lens,* which lies behind the pupil. The light is then reflected to the retina. Light is carried to the brain by the optic nerve.

The *aqueous chamber* separates the cornea from the lens. The chamber is filled with a fluid called *aqueous humor.* The fluid helps the cornea keep its shape and position. The *vitreous humor* is behind the lens. It is a gelatin-like substance that supports the retina and maintains the eye's shape.

The Ear. The *ear* is a sense organ (Fig. 5-13, p. 62). It functions in hearing and balance. It has three parts: the *external ear, middle ear,* and *inner ear.*

The external ear (outer part) is called the *pinna* or *auricle.* Sound waves are guided through the external ear into the *auditory canal.* Glands in the auditory canal secrete a waxy substance called *cerumen.* The auditory canal extends about 1 inch to the *eardrum.* The eardrum *(tympanic membrane)* separates the external and middle ear.

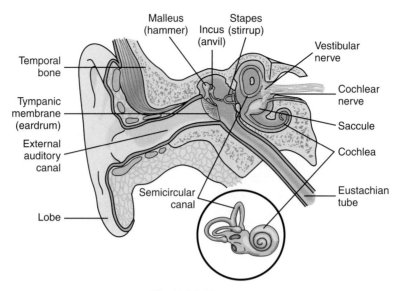

Fig. 5-13 The ear.

The middle ear is a small space. It contains the *eustachian tube* and three small bones called *ossicles*. The eustachian tube connects the middle ear and the throat. Air enters the eustachian tube so that there is equal pressure on both sides of the eardrum. The ossicles amplify sound received from the eardrum and transmit the sound to the inner ear. The three ossicles are:

- The *malleus*. It looks like a hammer.
- The *incus*. It looks like an anvil.
- The *stapes*. It is shaped like a stirrup.

The inner ear consists of *semicircular canals* and the *cochlea*. The cochlea looks like a snail shell. It contains fluid. The fluid carries sound waves from the middle ear to the *auditory nerve*. The auditory nerve then carries the message to the brain.

The three semicircular canals are involved with balance. They sense the head's position and changes in position. They send messages to the brain.

THE CIRCULATORY SYSTEM

The circulatory system is made up of the *blood, heart,* and *blood vessels*. The heart pumps blood through the blood vessels. The circulatory system has many functions:

- Blood carries food, oxygen, and other substances to the cells.
- Blood removes waste products from cells.
- Blood and blood vessels help regulate body temperature. The blood carries heat from muscle activity to other body parts. Blood vessels in the skin dilate to cool the body. They constrict to retain heat.
- The system produces and carries cells that defend the body from microbes that cause disease.

The Blood

The blood consists of blood cells and *plasma*. Plasma is mostly water. It carries blood cells to other body cells. Plasma also carries substances that cells need to function. This includes food (proteins, fats, and carbohydrates), hormones (p. 69), and chemicals.

Red blood cells (RBCs) are called *erythrocytes*. They give blood its red color because of a substance in the cell called **hemoglobin.** As RBCs circulate through the lungs, hemoglobin picks up oxygen. Hemoglobin carries oxygen to the cells. When blood is bright red, hemoglobin in the RBCs is saturated (filled) with oxygen. As blood circulates through the body, oxygen is given to the cells. Cells release carbon dioxide (a waste product). It is picked up by the hemoglobin. RBCs saturated with carbon dioxide make the blood look dark red.

The body has about 25 trillion (25,000,000,000,000) RBCs. About 4½ to 5 million cells are in a cubic millimeter of blood (the size of a tiny drop). RBCs live for 3 or 4 months. They are destroyed by the liver and spleen as they wear out. New RBCs are formed in the bone marrow. About 1 million RBCs are produced every second.

White blood cells (WBCs) are called *leukocytes*. They have no color. They protect the body against infection. There are about 5,000 to 10,000 WBCs in a cubic millimeter of blood. At the first sign of infection, WBCs rush to the infection site. There they multiply rapidly. The number of WBCs increases when there is an infection. WBCs are formed by the bone marrow. They live about 9 days.

Platelets (thrombocytes) are needed for blood clotting. They are formed by the bone marrow. There are about 200,000 to 400,000 platelets in a cubic millimeter of blood. A platelet lives about 4 days.

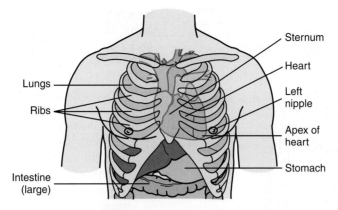

Fig. 5-14 Location of the heart in the chest cavity.

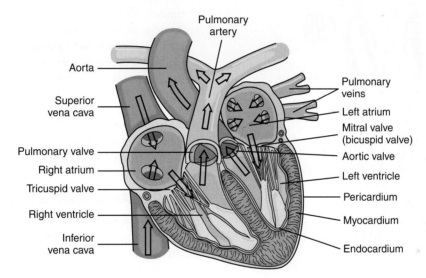

Fig. 5-15 Structures of the heart.

The Heart

The heart is a muscle. It pumps blood through the blood vessels to the tissues and cells. The heart lies in the middle to lower part of the chest cavity toward the left side (Fig. 5-14). The heart is hollow and has three layers (Fig. 5-15):

* The *pericardium* is the outer layer. It is a thin sac covering the heart.
* The *myocardium* is the second layer. It is the thick, muscular part of the heart.
* The *endocardium* is the inner layer. A membrane, it lines the inner surface of the heart.

The heart has four chambers (see Fig. 5-15). Upper chambers receive blood and are called *atria*. The *right atrium* receives blood from body tissues. The *left atrium* receives blood from the lungs. Lower chambers are called *ventricles*. Ventricles pump blood. The *right ventricle* pumps blood to the lungs for oxygen. The *left ventricle* pumps blood to all parts of the body.

Valves are between the atria and ventricles. The valves allow blood flow in one direction. They prevent blood from flowing back into the atria from the ventricles. The *tricuspid valve* is between the right atrium and the right ventricle. The *mitral valve (bicuspid valve)* is between the left atrium and left ventricle.

Heart action has two phases:

* *Diastole.* It is the resting phase. Heart chambers fill with blood.
* *Systole.* It is the working phase. The heart contracts. Blood is pumped through the blood vessels when the heart contracts.

The Blood Vessels

Blood flows to body tissues and cells through the blood vessels. There are three groups of blood vessels: arteries, capillaries, and veins.

Arteries carry blood away from the heart. Arterial blood is rich in oxygen. The *aorta* is the largest artery.

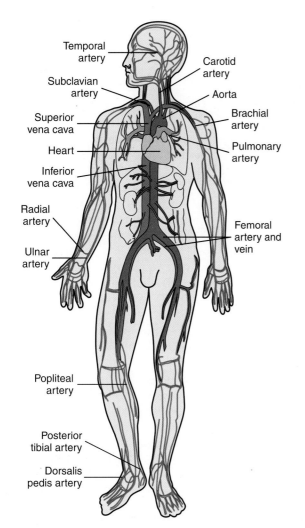

Fig. 5-16 Arterial and venous systems. Arterial system is *red.* Venous system is *blue.*

It receives blood directly from the left ventricle. The aorta branches into other arteries that carry blood to all parts of the body (Fig. 5-16). These arteries branch into smaller parts within the tissues. The smallest branch of an artery is an *arteriole.*

Arterioles connect to **capillaries.** Capillaries are very tiny blood vessels. Food, oxygen, and other substances pass from capillaries into the cells. The capillaries pick up waste products (including carbon dioxide) from the cells. Veins carry waste products back to the heart.

Veins return blood back to the heart. They connect to the capillaries by *venules.* Venules are small veins. Venules branch together to form veins. The many veins also branch together as they near the heart to form two main veins (see Fig. 5-16). The two main veins are the *inferior vena cava* and the *superior vena cava.* Both empty into the right atrium. The inferior vena cava carries blood from the legs and trunk. The

superior vena cava carries blood from the head and arms. Venous blood is dark red. It has little oxygen and a lot of carbon dioxide.

Blood flow through the circulatory system is shown in Fig. 5-15. The path of blood flow is as follows:
- Venous blood, poor in oxygen, empties into the right atrium.
- Blood flows through the tricuspid valve into the right ventricle.
- The right ventricle pumps blood into the lungs to pick up oxygen.
- Oxygen-rich blood from the lungs enters the left atrium.
- Blood from the left atrium passes through the mitral valve into the left ventricle.
- The left ventricle pumps the blood to the aorta. It branches off to form other arteries.
- Arterial blood is carried to the tissues by arterioles and to the cells by capillaries.
- Cells and capillaries exchange oxygen and nutrients for carbon dioxide and waste products.
- Capillaries connect with venules.
- Venules carry blood that has carbon dioxide and waste products.
- Venules form veins.
- Veins return blood to the heart.

THE RESPIRATORY SYSTEM

Oxygen is needed to live. Every cell needs oxygen. Air contains about 21% oxygen. This meets the body's needs under normal conditions. The respiratory system (Fig. 5-17) brings oxygen into the lungs and removes carbon dioxide. **Respiration** is the process of supplying the cells with oxygen and removing carbon dioxide from them. Respiration involves *inhalation* (breathing in) and *exhalation* (breathing out). The terms *inspiration* (breathing in) and *expiration* (breathing out) also are used.

Air enters the body through the *nose.* The air then passes into the *pharynx* (throat). It is a tube-shaped passageway for air and food. Air passes from the pharynx into the *larynx* (voice box). A piece of cartilage, the *epiglottis,* acts like a lid over the larynx. The epiglottis prevents food from entering the airway during swallowing. During inhalation the epiglottis lifts up to let air pass over the larynx. Air passes from the larynx into the *trachea* (windpipe).

The trachea divides at its lower end into the *right bronchus* and the *left bronchus.* Each bronchus enters a lung. Upon entering the lungs, the bronchi divide many times into smaller branches. The smaller branches are called *bronchioles.* Eventually the bronchioles subdivide. They end up in tiny one-celled air sacs called *alveoli.*

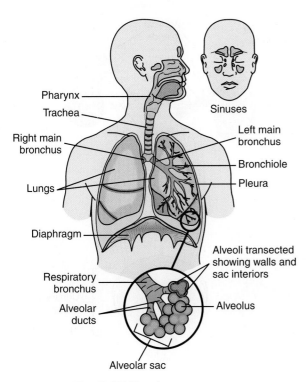

Fig. 5-17 Respiratory system.

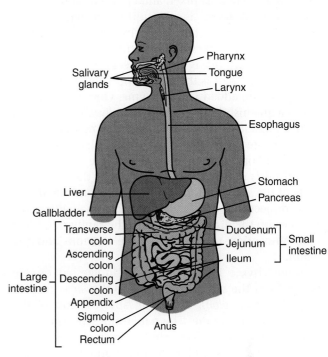

Fig. 5-18 Digestive system.

Alveoli look like small clusters of grapes. They are supplied by capillaries. Oxygen and carbon dioxide are exchanged between the alveoli and capillaries. Blood in the capillaries picks up oxygen from the alveoli. Then the blood is returned to the left side of the heart and pumped to the rest of the body. Alveoli pick up carbon dioxide from the capillaries for exhalation.

The lungs are spongy tissues. They are filled with alveoli, blood vessels, and nerves. Each lung is divided into lobes. The right lung has three lobes; the left lung has two. The lungs are separated from the abdominal cavity by a muscle called the *diaphragm.*

Each lung is covered by a two-layered sac called the *pleura.* One layer is attached to the lung and the other to the chest wall. The pleura secretes a very thin fluid that fills the space between the layers. The fluid prevents the layers from rubbing together during inhalation and exhalation. A bony framework made up of the ribs, sternum, and vertebrae protects the lungs.

THE DIGESTIVE SYSTEM

The digestive system breaks down food physically and chemically so it can be absorbed for use by the cells. This process is called **digestion.** The digestive system is also called the *gastro-intestinal (GI) system.* The system also removes solid wastes from the body.

The digestive system involves the *alimentary canal (GI tract)* and the accessory organs of digestion

(Fig. 5-18). The alimentary canal is a long tube. It extends from the mouth to the anus. Its major parts are the mouth, pharynx, esophagus, stomach, small intestine, and large intestine. Accessory organs are the teeth, tongue, salivary glands, liver, gallbladder, and pancreas.

Digestion begins in the *mouth.* The mouth also is called the *oral cavity.* It receives food and prepares it for digestion. Using chewing motions, the *teeth* cut, chop, and grind food into small particles for digestion and swallowing. The *tongue* aids in chewing and swallowing. Taste buds on the tongue's surface contain nerve endings. Taste buds allow sweet, sour, bitter, and salty tastes to be sensed. *Salivary glands* in the mouth secrete *saliva.* Saliva moistens food particles to ease swallowing and begin digestion. During swallowing, the tongue pushes food into the *pharynx.*

The pharynx (throat) is a muscular tube. Swallowing continues as the pharynx contracts. Contraction of the pharynx pushes food into the *esophagus.* The esophagus is a muscular tube about 10 inches long. It extends from the pharynx to the *stomach.* Involuntary muscle contractions called **peristalsis** move food down the esophagus through the alimentary canal.

The stomach is a muscular, pouch-like sac. It is in the upper left part of the abdominal cavity. Strong stomach muscles stir and churn food to break it up into even smaller particles. A mucous membrane lines the stomach. It contains glands that secrete *gastric juices.* Food is mixed and churned with the gastric juices to form a semi-liquid substance called *chyme.* Through peristalsis, the chyme is pushed from the stomach into the small intestine.

The *small intestine* is about 20 feet long. It has three parts. The first part is the *duodenum.* There more digestive juices are added to the chyme. One is called *bile.* Bile is a greenish liquid made in the *liver.* Bile is stored in the *gallbladder.* Juices from the *pancreas* and small intestine are added to the chyme. Digestive juices chemically break down food so it can be absorbed.

Peristalsis moves the chyme through the two other parts of the small intestine: the *jejunum* and the *ileum.* Tiny projections called *villi* line the small intestine. Villi absorb the digested food into the capillaries. Most food absorption takes place in the jejunum and the ileum.

Some chyme is not digested. Undigested chyme passes from the small intestine into the *large intestine (large bowel* or *colon).* The colon absorbs most of the water from the chyme. The remaining semi-solid material is called *feces.* Feces contain a small amount of water, solid wastes, and some mucus and germs. These are the waste products of digestion. Feces pass through the colon into the *rectum* by peristalsis. Feces pass out of the body through the *anus.*

THE URINARY SYSTEM

The digestive system rids the body of solid wastes. The lungs rid the body of carbon dioxide. Water and other substances leave the body through sweat. There are other waste products in the blood from cells burning food for energy. The urinary system (Fig. 5-19):

- Removes waste products from the blood
- Maintains water balance within the body

The *kidneys* are two bean-shaped organs in the upper abdomen. They lie against the back muscles on each side of the spine. They are protected by the lower edge of the rib cage.

Each kidney has over a million tiny *nephrons* (Fig. 5-20). Each nephron is the basic working unit of the kidney. Each nephron has a *convoluted tubule,* which is a tiny coiled tubule. Each convoluted tubule has a *Bowman's capsule* at one end. The capsule partly surrounds a cluster of capillaries called a *glomerulus.* Blood passes through the glomerulus and is filtered by the capillaries. The fluid part of the blood is squeezed into the Bowman's capsule. The fluid then passes into the tubule. Most of the water and other needed substances are re-absorbed by the blood. The rest of the fluid and the waste products form *urine* in the tubule. Urine flows through the tubule to a *collecting tubule.* All collecting tubules drain into the *renal pelvis* in the kidney.

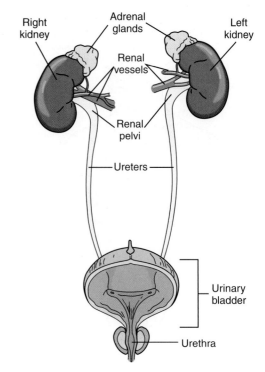

Fig. 5-19 Urinary system.

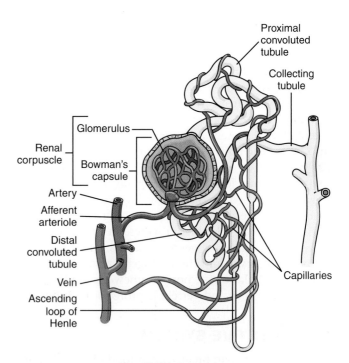

Fig. 5-20 A nephron.

A tube, called the *ureter,* is attached to the renal pelvis of the kidney. Each ureter is about 10 to 12 inches long. The ureters carry urine from the kidneys to the *bladder.* The bladder is a hollow, muscular sac. It lies toward the front in the lower part of the abdominal cavity.

Urine is stored in the bladder until the need to urinate is felt. This usually occurs when there is about a half pint (250 mL) of urine in the bladder. Urine passes from the bladder through the *urethra.* The opening at the end of the urethra is the *meatus.* Urine passes from the body through the meatus. Urine is a clear, yellowish fluid.

THE REPRODUCTIVE SYSTEM

Human reproduction results from the union of a male sex cell and a female sex cell. The male and female reproductive systems are different. This allows for the process of reproduction.

The Male Reproductive System

The male reproductive system is shown in Figure 5-21. The *testes (testicles)* are the male sex glands. Sex glands also are called *gonads.* The two testes are oval or almond-shaped glands. Male sex cells are produced in the testes. Male sex cells are called *sperm* cells.

Testosterone, the male hormone, is produced in the testes. This hormone is needed for reproductive organ function. It also is needed for the development of the male secondary sex characteristics. These include facial hair; pubic and axillary (underarm) hair; and hair on the arms, chest, and legs. Neck and shoulder sizes increase.

The testes are suspended between the thighs in a sac called the *scrotum.* The scrotum is made of skin and muscle.

Sperm travel from the testis to the *epididymis.* The epididymis is a coiled tube on top and to the side of the testis. From the epididymis, sperm travel through a tube called the *vas deferens.* Each vas deferens joins a *seminal vesicle.* The two seminal vesicles store sperm and produce *semen.* Semen is a fluid that carries sperm from the male reproductive tract. The ducts of the seminal vesicles unite to form the *ejaculatory duct.* It passes through the *prostate gland.*

The prostate gland lies just below the bladder. It is shaped like a donut. The gland secretes fluid into the semen. As the ejaculatory ducts leave the prostate, they join the *urethra.* The urethra runs through the prostate gland. The urethra is the outlet for urine and semen. The urethra is contained within the *penis.*

The penis is outside of the body and has *erectile* tissue. When a man is sexually excited, blood fills the erectile tissue. The penis enlarges and becomes hard and erect. The erect penis can enter a female's vagina. The semen, which contains sperm, is released into the vagina.

The Female Reproductive System

Figure 5-22 shows the female reproductive system. The female gonads are two almond-shaped glands called *ovaries.* An ovary is on each side of the uterus in the abdominal cavity.

The ovaries contain *ova* or eggs. Ova are the female sex cells. One ovum (egg) is released monthly during the woman's reproductive years. Release of an ovum is called *ovulation.*

The ovaries secrete the female hormones *estrogen* and *progesterone.* These hormones are needed for reproductive system function. They also are needed for the development of secondary sex characteristics in

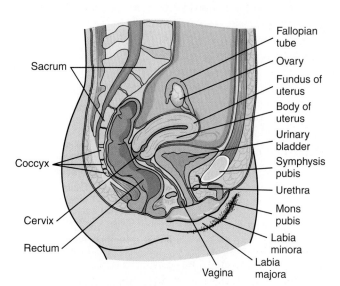

Fig. 5-21 Male reproductive system.

Fig. 5-22 Female reproductive system.

the female. These include increased breast size, pubic and axillary (underarm) hair, slight deepening of the voice, and widening and rounding of the hips.

When an ovum is released from an ovary, it travels through a *fallopian tube*. There are two fallopian tubes, one on each side. The tubes are attached at one end to the uterus. The ovum travels through the fallopian tube to the *uterus*.

The *uterus* is a hollow, muscular organ shaped like a pear. It is in the center of the pelvic cavity behind the bladder and in front of the rectum. The main part of the uterus is the *fundus*. The neck or narrow section of the uterus is the *cervix*. Tissue lining the uterus is called the *endometrium*. The endometrium has many blood vessels. If sex cells from the male and female unite into one cell, that cell implants into the endometrium. There the cell grows into a baby. The uterus serves as a place for the *fetus* (unborn baby) to grow and receive nourishment.

The cervix of the uterus projects into a muscular canal called the *vagina*. The vagina opens to the outside of the body. It is just behind the urethra. The vagina receives the penis during intercourse. It also is part of the birth canal. Glands in the vaginal wall keep it moistened with secretions. In young girls, the external vaginal opening is partially closed by a membrane called the *hymen*. The hymen ruptures when the female has intercourse for the first time.

The external female genitalia are called the *vulva* (Fig. 5-23):

- The *mons pubis* is a rounded, fatty pad over a bone called the *symphysis pubis*. The mons pubis is covered with hair in the adult female.
- The *labia majora* and *labia minora* are two folds of tissue on each side of the vaginal opening.
- The *clitoris* is a small organ composed of erectile tissue. It becomes hard when sexually stimulated.

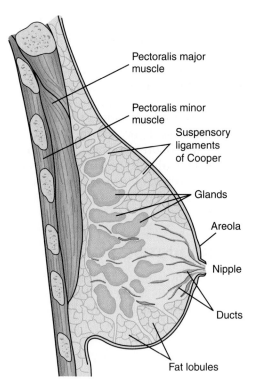

Pectoralis major muscle
Pectoralis minor muscle
Suspensory ligaments of Cooper
Glands
Areola
Nipple
Ducts
Fat lobules

Fig. 5-24 The female breast.

The *mammary glands (breasts)* secrete milk after childbirth. The glands are on the outside of the chest. They are made up of glandular tissue and fat (Fig. 5-24). The milk drains into ducts that open onto the *nipple*.

Menstruation. The endometrium is rich in blood to nourish the cell that grows into a fetus. If pregnancy does not occur, the endometrium breaks up. It is discharged from the body through the vagina. This process is called **menstruation.** Menstruation occurs about every 28 days. Therefore it is called the *menstrual cycle.*

The first day of the menstrual cycle begins with menstruation. Blood flows from the uterus through the vaginal opening. Menstrual flow usually lasts 3 to 7 days. Ovulation occurs during the next phase. An ovum matures in an ovary and is released. Ovulation usually occurs on or about day 14 of the cycle.

Meanwhile, estrogen and progesterone (the female hormones) are secreted by the ovaries. These hormones cause the endometrium to thicken for pregnancy. If pregnancy does not occur, the hormones decrease in amount. This causes the blood supply to the endometrium to decrease. The endometrium breaks up. It is discharged through the vagina. Another menstrual cycle begins.

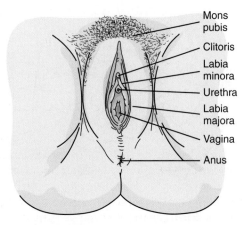

Mons pubis
Clitoris
Labia minora
Urethra
Labia majora
Vagina
Anus

Fig. 5-23 External female genitalia.

Fertilization

To reproduce, a male sex cell (sperm) must unite with a female sex cell (ovum). The uniting of the sperm and ovum into one cell is called *fertilization*. A sperm has 23 chromosomes. An ovum has 23 chromosomes. When the two cells unite, the fertilized cell has 46 chromosomes.

During intercourse, millions of sperm are deposited into the vagina. Sperm travel up the cervix, through the uterus, and into the fallopian tubes. If a sperm and an ovum unite in a fallopian tube, fertilization results. Pregnancy occurs. The fertilized cell travels down the fallopian tube to the uterus. After a short time, the fertilized cell implants in the thick endometrium and grows during pregnancy.

THE ENDOCRINE SYSTEM

The endocrine system is made up of glands called the *endocrine glands* (Fig. 5-25). The endocrine glands secrete chemical substances called **hormones** into the bloodstream. Hormones regulate the activities of other organs and glands in the body.

The *pituitary gland* is called the *master gland*. About the size of a cherry, it is at the base of the brain behind the eyes. The pituitary gland is divided into the *anterior pituitary lobe* and the *posterior pituitary lobe*. The anterior pituitary lobe secretes:
* *Growth hormone (GH)*—needed for growth of muscles, bones, and other organs. It is needed throughout life to maintain normal-size bones and muscles. Growth is stunted if a baby is born with deficient amounts of growth hormone. Too much of the hormone causes excessive growth.
* *Thyroid-stimulating hormone (TSH)*—needed for thyroid gland function.
* *Adrenocorticotropic hormone (ACTH)*—stimulates the adrenal gland.

The anterior lobe also secretes hormones that regulate growth, development, and function of the male and female reproductive systems.

The posterior pituitary lobe secretes *antidiuretic hormone (ADH)* and *oxytocin*. ADH prevents the kidneys from excreting excessive amounts of water. Oxytocin causes uterine muscles to contract during childbirth.

The *thyroid gland,* shaped like a butterfly, is in the neck in front of the larynx. *Thyroid hormone (TH, thyroxine)* is secreted by the thyroid gland. It regulates **metabolism.** Metabolism is the burning of food for heat and energy by the cells. Too little TH results in slowed body processes, slowed movements, and weight gain. Too much TH causes increased metabolism, excess energy, and weight loss. Some babies are born with deficient amounts of TH. Their physical growth and mental growth are stunted.

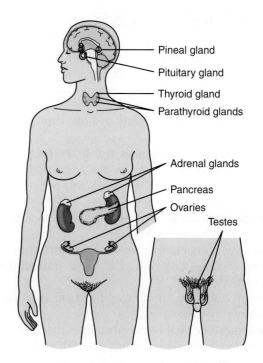

Fig. 5-25 Endocrine system.

The four *parathyroid glands* secrete *parathormone.* Two lie on each side of the thyroid gland. Parathormone regulates calcium use. Calcium is needed for nerve and muscle function. Insufficient amounts of calcium cause *tetany.* Tetany is a state of severe muscle contraction and spasm. If untreated, tetany can cause death.

There are two *adrenal glands.* An adrenal gland is on the top of each kidney. The adrenal gland has two parts: the *adrenal medulla* and the *adrenal cortex.* The adrenal medulla secretes *epinephrine* and *norepinephrine.* These hormones stimulate the body to quickly produce energy during emergencies. Heart rate, blood pressure, muscle power, and energy all increase.

The adrenal cortex secretes three groups of hormones needed for life:
* *Gluco-corticoids*—regulate the metabolism of carbohydrates. They also control the body's response to stress and inflammation.
* *Mineralo-corticoids*—regulate the amount of salt and water that is absorbed and lost by the kidneys.
* Small amounts of male and female sex hormones— p. 67.

The *pancreas* secretes *insulin.* Insulin regulates the amount of sugar in the blood available for use by the cells. Insulin is needed for sugar to enter the cells. If there is too little insulin, sugar cannot enter the cells. If sugar cannot enter the cells, excess amounts of sugar build up in the blood. This condition is called *diabetes.*

The *gonads* are the glands of human reproduction. Male sex glands (testes) secrete *testosterone.* Female sex glands (ovaries) secrete *estrogen* and *progesterone.*

THE IMMUNE SYSTEM

The immune system protects the body from disease and infection. Abnormal body cells can grow into tumors. Sometimes the body produces substances that cause the body to attack itself. Microorganisms (bacteria, viruses, and other germs) can cause an infection. The immune system defends against threats inside and outside the body.

The immune system gives the body **immunity.** Immunity means that a person has protection against a disease or condition. The person will not get or be affected by the disease:

- *Specific immunity* is the body's reaction to a certain threat.
- *Non-specific immunity* is the body's reaction to anything it does not recognize as a normal body substance.

Special cells and substances function to produce immunity:

- *Antibodies*—normal body substances that recognize abnormal or unwanted substances. They attack and destroy such substances.

- *Antigens*—abnormal or unwanted substances. An antigen causes the body to produce antibodies. The antibodies attack and destroy the antigens.
- *Phagocytes*—white blood cells that digest and destroy microorganisms and other unwanted substances (Fig. 5-26).
- *Lymphocytes*—white blood cells that produce antibodies. Lymphocyte production increases as the body responds to an infection.
- *B lymphocytes (B cells)*—cause the production of antibodies that circulate in the plasma. The antibodies react to specific antigens.
- *T lymphocytes (T cells)*—cells that destroy invading cells. *Killer T cells* produce poisons near the invading cells. Some T cells attract other cells. The other cells destroy the invaders.

When the body senses an antigen (an unwanted substance), the immune system acts. Phagocyte and lymphocyte production increases. Phagocytes destroy the invaders through digestion. The lymphocytes produce antibodies that attack and destroy the unwanted substances.

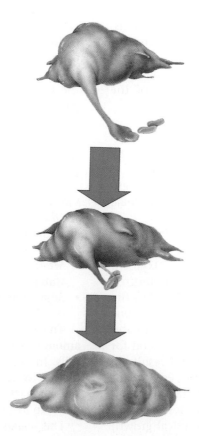

Fig. 5-26 A phagocyte digests and destroys a microorganism. (From Thibodeau GA, Patton KT: *Structure and function of the body,* ed 11, St Louis, 2000, Mosby.)

REVIEW QUESTIONS

Circle the BEST answer.

1 The basic unit of body structure is the
a cell
b neuron
c nephron
d ovum

2 The outer layer of the skin is called the
a dermis
b epidermis
c integument
d myelin

3 Which is *not* a function of the skin?
a provides the protective covering for the body
b regulates body temperature
c senses cold, pain, touch, and pressure
d provides the shape and framework for the body

4 Which allows movement?
a bone marrow
b synovial membrane
c joints
d ligaments

5 Skeletal muscles
a are under involuntary control
b appear smooth
c are under voluntary control
d appear striped and smooth

6 The highest functions in the brain take place in the
a cerebral cortex
b medulla
c brainstem
d spinal nerves

7 The ear is involved with
a regulating body movements
b balance
c smoothness of body movements
d controlling involuntary muscles

8 The liquid part of the blood is the
a hemoglobin
b red blood cell
c plasma
d white blood cell

9 Which part of the heart pumps blood to the body?
a right atrium
b left atrium
c right ventricle
d left ventricle

10 Which carry blood away from the heart?
a capillaries
b veins
c venules
d arteries

11 Oxygen and carbon dioxide are exchanged
a in the bronchi
b between the alveoli and capillaries
c between the lungs and pleura
d in the trachea

12 Digestion begins in the
a mouth
b stomach
c small intestine
d colon

13 Most food absorption takes place in the
a stomach
b small intestine
c colon
d large intestine

14 Urine is formed by the
a jejunum
b kidneys
c bladder
d liver

15 Urine passes from the body through the
a ureters
b urethra
c anus
d nephrons

16 The male sex gland is called the
a penis
b semen
c testis
d scrotum

17 The male sex cell is the
a semen
b ovum
c gonad
d sperm

18 The female sex gland is the
a ovary
b cervix
c uterus
d vagina

19 The discharge of the lining of the uterus is called
a the endometrium
b ovulation
c fertilization
d menstruation

20 The endocrine glands secrete
a hormones
b mucus
c semen
d insulin

21 The immune system protects the body from
a low blood sugar
b disease and infection
c loss of fluid
d stunted growth

Answers to these questions are on p. 443.

6

Basic Pharmacology

OBJECTIVES

- Define the key terms and key abbreviations used in this chapter.
- Explain how drugs are classified.
- Explain how drugs act in the human body.
- Explain how drugs are absorbed, distributed, metabolized, and excreted.
- Explain the difference between side effects, adverse drug reactions, idiosyncratic reactions, and allergic reactions.
- Describe the factors influencing a drug's action.
- Explain how drugs can interact with each other.
- Identify common resources of drug information.

KEY TERMS

adverse drug reaction (ADR) An unintended effect on the body from using a legal drug, illegal drug, or two or more drugs; drug reaction

allergic reaction An unfavorable response to a substance that causes a hyper-sensitivity reaction

anaphylactic reaction See "anaphylaxis"

anaphylaxis A severe, life-threatening sensitivity to an antigen; anaphylactic reaction

desired action Expected response

dilute To add the correct amount of water or other liquid

drug blood level The amount of a drug present in the blood

drug interaction When the action of one drug is altered by the action of another drug

drug reaction See "adverse drug reaction"

enteral route Drugs are given directly into the gastro-intestinal (GI) tract; *enteral* means *bowel*

generic name The drug's common name

hives See "urticaria"

idiosyncratic reaction Something unusual or abnormal that happens when a drug is first given

Continued

KEY TERMS—cont'd

intramuscular (IM) Within (*intra*) a muscle (*muscular*)

intravenous (IV) Within (*intra*) a vein (*venous*)

parenteral route Drugs bypass the GI tract (*para* means *beyond*; *enteral* means *bowel*)

percutaneous route Drugs are given through (*per*) the skin (*cutaneous*) or a mucous membrane

pharmacology The study of drugs and their actions on living organisms

placebo A drug dosage form that has no active ingredients

reconstitute To add water or other liquid to a powder or solid form of a drug

side effect An unintended reaction to a drug given in a normal dosage

subcutaneous Beneath (*sub*) the skin (*cutaneous*)

toxicity Exposure to large amounts of a substance that should not cause problems in smaller amounts; the reaction when side effects are severe

trademark The brand name or trade name of the drug

urticaria Raised, irregularly shaped patches on the skin and severe itching; hives

KEY ABBREVIATIONS

ADME Absorption, distribution, metabolism, excretion

ADR Adverse drug reaction

CNS Central nervous system

FDA Food and Drug Administration

GI Gastro-intestinal

IM Intramuscular

IV Intravenous

OTC Over-the-counter

PDR Physicians' Desk Reference

Pharmacology is the study of drugs and their actions on living organisms. There are thousands of drugs. New ones are developed every year.

Chemical name: 4-Thia-1-azabicyclo[3.2.0]heptane-2-carboxylic acid, 6-[(aminophenylacetyl)amino]-3,3-dimethyl-7-oxo-, [2S-[2α,-5α,6β(S*)]]-

Generic name: ampicillin

Official name: ampicillin, USP

Brand names: Principen, Polycillin

Fig. 6-1 Different names of the same drug.

DRUG NAMES

Drugs have different names. Many have similar spellings. The exact name and spelling are important. You must give the right drug to the right person.

Drugs have the following names (Fig. 6-1):

- *Chemical name*—the exact chemical structure of a drug.
- *Generic name*—the drug's common name. A generic drug is a copy of a brand name drug. The generic drug is the same in dosage, safety, strength, how it is taken, quality, performance, and intended use. All manufacturers of the drug use the generic name. The first letter is not capitalized.
- *Official name*—the name under which the drug is listed by the Food and Drug Administration (FDA).
- *Trademark*—the *brand name* or *trade name* of the drug. Only the manufacturer who owns the drug can use the brand or trade name. Brand or trade names are easier to spell, pronounce, and remember. The first letter is capitalized.

DRUG CLASSIFICATIONS

Classification means a group or category. Things in a group or category are similar and have common attributes and qualities. Drugs are classified by:

- *Body system.* Drugs are classified according to the body system they affect. Examples are drugs affecting the central nervous system (CNS) and drugs affecting the cardiovascular system.
- *Therapeutic use or clinical indications.* Therapeutic relates to treating or curing a disease or disorder. Clinical indications relate to the signs or reasons for using a drug. For example, a person has an infection. The doctor orders an antibiotic. An antibiotic is a drug that kills microbes and cures infections. (*Anti* means *against. Biotic* means *life.*)
- *Physiologic or chemical action.* The action relates to what the drug does in the body. Calcium channel blockers reduce calcium flow across the cell membranes in smooth muscles. They are used to prevent coronary artery spasms. This promotes blood flow through the coronary arteries to the heart muscle.
- *Prescription or non-prescription.* Prescription drugs require an order from a health professional licensed to prescribe—doctors, dentists, nurse practitioners, physician assistants, and pharmacists. The manufacturer's label contains the phrase "Rx only" or "Caution: Federal Law Prohibits Dispensing Without a Prescription." Non-prescription drugs also are called *over-the-counter (OTC) drugs.* These drugs are sold without a prescription. They are sold in drug stores, grocery stores, and other stores.

- *Illegal drugs.* These are drugs or chemical substances used for non-therapeutic reasons. They are obtained illegally. They are not approved for use by the FDA. They also are called *recreational drugs.*

BASIC PRINCIPLES

Drugs act in the human body in the following ways:

- Drugs change a physiologic activity within the body. They do not create new responses. Drug response is stated in relation to the physiologic activity before drug therapy. For example, a drug is given to lower blood pressure. The therapy is successful if blood pressure is lower during therapy than before therapy. The person's blood pressure is measured before and during drug therapy. The doctor and nurse use the measurements to evaluate if drug therapy was effective in lowering the person's blood pressure.
- Usually a drug forms chemical bonds within specific sites *(receptors)* within the body. The relationship between a drug and a receptor is like a key and lock (Fig. 6-2, *A*).
- Drugs that interact with a receptor to cause a response are *agonists* (Fig. 6-2, *B*). Drugs that attach to a receptor but do not cause a response are *antagonists* (Fig. 6-2, *C*). Drugs that interact with a receptor to cause a response but prevent other responses are *partial agonists* (Fig. 6-2, *D*).
- Once given, all drugs go through four stages: *a*bsorption, *d*istribution, *m*etabolism, and *e*xcretion (ADME).

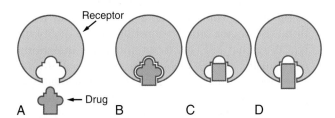

Fig. 6-2 A, Drugs act by forming a chemical bond with a specific receptor site. This is like a key and a lock. **B,** The better the fit of the key into the lock, the better the response. Those drugs with complete attachment are called *agonists.* **C,** *Antagonists* are drugs that attach but do not cause a response. **D,** *Partial agonists* attach and cause a small response. They also block other responses.

Absorption

Absorption is the process by which a drug is transferred from its site of body entry to circulating body fluids (blood, lymph) for distribution. The rate of absorption depends on:

- The route of administration
- Blood flow through the tissue where the drug was given
- How well the drug can dissolve (solubility)

To promote absorption, it is important to:

- Give oral drugs with enough fluid, usually 8 ounces of water.
- Reconstitute and dilute drugs as recommended by the manufacturer. **Reconstitute** means to add water or other liquid to a powder or solid form of a drug. **Dilute** means to add the correct amount of water or other liquid.
- Give drugs into the correct tissue.

Drugs are given in these ways:

- **Enteral route**—drugs are given directly into the gastro-intestinal (GI) tract. *Enteral* means *bowel.* Enteral drugs are given through the oral, rectal, and naso-gastric routes.
- **Parenteral route**—drugs bypass the GI tract. *(Para* means *beyond. Enteral* means *bowel.)* Parenteral routes include:
  - **Subcutaneous**—beneath *(sub)* the skin *(cutaneous).*
  - **Intramuscular (IM)**—within *(intra)* a muscle *(muscular).*
  - **Intravenous (IV)**—within *(intra)* a vein *(venous).*
- **Percutaneous route**—drugs are given through *(per)* the skin *(cutaneous)* or a mucous membrane. Inhalation, sublingual (under the tongue), and topical (on the skin) are examples.

A drug must dissolve in body fluids before it can be absorbed into body tissues. For example, a solid drug is taken orally. It must be absorbed into the bloodstream for transport to the site of action. First it must dissolve in the GI fluids. Then it must be transported across the stomach or intestinal lining into the blood.

The rate of absorption for parenteral drugs depends on the blood flow through the tissues. Circulatory problems and respiratory distress may lead to vasoconstriction. *(Vaso* means *blood vessel. Constriction* means *to narrow.)* Therefore the nurse does not give an injection in a site where circulation is impaired. Subcutaneous injections have the slowest absorption rate. IM injections are more rapidly absorbed. Blood flow to muscle is greater than to subcutaneous tissue. Drugs are dispersed throughout the body most rapidly when given by IV injection.

Absorption of drugs applied to the skin (topical route) is influenced by:
* The amount and strength of the drug
* Length of contact time
* Size of the affected area
* Thickness of the skin surface
* Tissue hydration (amount of water in the tissues)
* Skin condition—intact or non-intact

Distribution

Distribution refers to the ways drugs are transported by circulating body fluids to the sites of action (receptors) and to the sites of metabolism and excretion. Organs with the greatest blood supply (heart, liver, kidneys, and brain) receive the drug most rapidly. Areas with lesser blood supplies (muscle, skin, and fat) receive the drug more slowly.

Once absorbed into the blood, a drug's distribution is determined by:
* Its chemical properties
* How it is affected by the blood and tissues it contacts

A blood sample may be studied to determine the amount of a drug present in the blood. This is known as a **drug blood level.** If the drug blood level is low, the dosage is increased or the drug is given more often. If the drug blood level is too high, the person may show signs of toxicity. (*Toxin* means *poison.* **Toxicity** means exposure to large amounts of a substance that should not cause problems in smaller amounts.) The dosage is reduced or the drug is given less often.

The amount of drug that actually gets to the receptor sites determines the extent of the response. If little drug actually reaches and binds to the receptor sites, the response is minimal.

Metabolism

Metabolism is the process by which the body in-activates drugs. The liver is the primary site for drug metabolism. Other tissues and organs metabolize drugs to a minor extent—white blood cells, GI tract, lungs. Genetic, environmental, and physiologic factors help regulate drug metabolism. Use of other drugs, illnesses, and age are some other factors affecting metabolism.

Excretion

Excretion is the elimination of a drug from the body. Urine and feces are the primary routes of excretion. Others include evaporation from the skin, exhalation from the lungs, and secretion into saliva and breast milk.

DRUG ACTION

No drug has a single action. When a drug is absorbed and distributed, the **desired action** (expected response) usually occurs. All drugs can affect more than one body system. Therefore, side effects and adverse drug reactions can occur.
* **Side effects**—an unintended reaction to a drug given in a normal dosage. Usually the effect is not desired. Nausea, dry mouth, dizziness, blurred vision, and ringing in the ears *(tinnitus)* are common side effects. When side effects are severe, the reaction is sometimes called **toxicity.**
* **Drug reaction** or **adverse drug reaction (ADR)**—an unintended effect on the body from using a legal drug, illegal drug, or two or more drugs. Rash, itching, high blood sugar *(hyperglycemia)* and a reduced number of platelets *(thrombocytopenia)* are common ADRs. ADRs are a leading cause of death in the United States. Most can be prevented.

Each drug has parameters (measures)—therapeutic actions to expect, side effects to expect, ADRs to report, and probable drug interactions. The health team monitors the parameters. Dosages are adjusted for the best therapeutic effect and to reduce side effects and ADRs. Follow agency policy for reporting ADRs.

Idiosyncratic reactions and allergic reactions can occur. An **idiosyncratic reaction** is something unusual or abnormal that happens when a drug is first given. (*Idio* means *own. Syncratic* means *mixing together.*) The person has an over-response to the drug's action. The uncommon response is usually because the person cannot metabolize the drug.

An **allergic reaction** is an unfavorable response to a substance that causes a hyper-sensitivity reaction. *Hyper-sensitivity* means an exaggerated *(hyper)* response *(sensitivity)*. Allergic reactions occur in persons previously exposed to a drug. The person has developed antibodies to the drug. On re-exposure, the antibodies cause a reaction.

The most common allergic reaction is **urticaria (hives)**—raised, irregularly shaped patches on the skin and severe itching (Fig. 6-3, p. 76). Some persons have **anaphylaxis (anaphylactic reaction)**—a severe, life-threatening sensitivity to an antigen (an unwanted substance). (*Ana* means *without. Phylaxis* means *protection.*) A medical emergency, signs and symptoms can occur within seconds:
* Sweating
* Shortness of breath
* Low blood pressure
* Irregular pulse
* Respiratory congestion
* Swelling of the larynx (laryngeal edema)
* Hoarseness
* Dyspnea

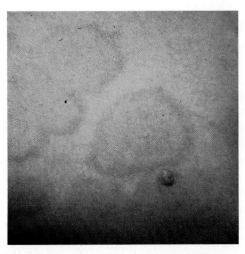

Fig. 6-3 Urticaria (hives). (Courtesy Dr. Donald W. Kress, Children's Hospital of Pittsburgh. From Zitelli BJ, Davis HW: *Atlas of pediatric physical diagnosis*, ed 4, St Louis, 2002, Mosby.)

A mild allergic reaction is a warning not to take the drug again. The person is at risk for anaphylaxis from the next exposure to the drug. The person must:
- Never use the drug again.
- Receive information about the drug.
- Tell health professionals about the reaction.
- Wear a medical alert bracelet or necklace that explains the allergy.
  See *Focus on Older Persons: Drug Action*.

Factors Influencing Drug Action

Exact responses to drug therapy are hard to predict. Drugs have strong effects in some people. Others show little response to the same dosage. Some people react differently to the same dosage given at different times. The following factors affect a person's response to drugs.
- *Age.* Infants and older persons are the most sensitive to drugs. The ADME of drugs differs in premature infants, full-term newborns, and children. Changes from aging affect the older person's response to drug therapy.
- *Body weight.* Very heavy persons may need higher dosages to attain the desired response. Persons who are underweight may need lower dosages for the desired response. Weight and height measurements are needed (Chapter 4). The doctor uses them to determine drug dosages.

FOCUS ON OLDER PERSONS

Drug Action

Older persons may not tolerate drug side effects well. For example, dizziness may cause an older person to decrease activity because he or she has fears of falling. Or a dry mouth can cause problems with dentures, taste, and chewing. Nutrition can suffer.

Many drugs cause depression, confusion, and delirium in older persons. Often confusion is the first and only sign of a drug-induced problem.

Always report signs, symptoms, and behavior changes to the nurse. The doctor may need to adjust the person's drug therapy.

- *Metabolic rate. Metabolism* is the burning of food for heat and energy by the cells. *Metabolic rate* is the amount of energy used in a given amount of time. People with a high metabolic rate tend to metabolize drugs faster. They need larger doses or drugs more often. The opposite is true for those with a low metabolic rate.
- *Illness.* Illness may affect ADME. For example, persons in shock have reduced circulation. They absorb IM or subcutaneous drugs slowly. With vomiting, drugs may not stay in the stomach long enough for absorption. Some persons do not have enough proteins in the blood to adequately distribute drugs. Many drugs are excreted by the kidneys. Persons with kidney failure need lower dosages.
- *Willingness to take drugs.* Some diseases have rapid effects if therapy is ignored. Diabetes is an example. Persons with diabetes usually take drugs as prescribed. Persons with high blood pressure may not have signs and symptoms. They may not take drugs as prescribed.
- *Placebo effect.* A **placebo** is a drug dosage form that has no active ingredients. A placebo is commonly called a "sugar pill." When taken, the person may report the desired response. Positive expectations about treatment and care can affect good therapy outcomes. This is called the *placebo effect.* In Latin, *placebo* means *shall please.* The American Pain Society recommends avoiding the deceitful (not honest) use of placebos to manage pain. This is because it violates the person's right to the highest quality of care possible.

- *Tolerance.* Tolerance occurs when a person begins to need higher dosages to produce the same effects that lower dosages once gave. For example, a person is addicted to heroin. Over time, larger and larger dosages are needed to give the same "high." Tolerance can be caused by psychologic dependence. Or the body may metabolize a drug faster than before. The effects of drugs diminish faster.
- *Dependence.* Drug dependence (addiction or habituation) occurs when a person cannot control the ingestion of drugs. Dependence may be physical. The person develops withdrawal symptoms if the drug is not taken for a certain period. Psychologic dependence is when the person is emotionally attached to the drug. Drug dependence is most common with scheduled or controlled drugs (Chapter 3). Many people worry about becoming addicted to pain-relief drugs. They may not take them even when needed. However, the risk of addiction is low. For the person's well-being, he or she should be as pain-free as possible.
- *Cumulative effect.* A drug may accumulate in the body if the next dose is given before the previous one is metabolized or excreted. Toxicity may result. For example, a person is drinking alcohol. The person becomes "drunk" when he or she drinks faster than the rate of alcohol metabolism and excretion.

DRUG INTERACTIONS

A **drug interaction** occurs when the action of one drug is altered by the action of another drug. This happens in two ways:

- Drugs, when combined, *increase* the actions of one or both drugs.
- Drugs, when combined, *decrease* the effectiveness of one or both drugs.

Some drug interactions are beneficial. For example, caffeine is a CNS stimulant. An antihistamine is a CNS depressant. When combined, the caffeine counter-acts the drowsiness from the antihistamine. The desired antihistamine effects are allowed.

DRUG INFORMATION

There are thousands of drugs. You cannot memorize information about all of them. Many drug resources are available in print, on CD-ROM, on-line, and in other electronic forms.

You must use accurate and current resources. Check for a current date on the resource. Also check other current resources to make sure the information is correct.

The following resources are helpful. Know where to find them on your nursing unit.

- *American Hospital Formulary Service Drug Information.* This resource has information about every drug available in the United States.
- *Drug Interaction Facts.* This book is about drug interactions.
- *Drug Facts and Comparisons.* The book is arranged by body systems. All drugs within each chapter are grouped by therapeutic use.
- *Handbook of Nonprescription Drugs.* The book is organized by body systems. Disorders are described. Non-prescription drugs, non-drug therapies, and prevention therapies follow.
- *Natural Medicines Comprehensive Database.* The book has five major sections: herbal monographs, references, brand name listing, charts section, and general index. More than 1000 herbal medicines are arranged alphabetically by the most common name.
- *Physicians' Desk Reference (PDR).* More than 4000 drugs are presented. Divided into sections, each section has a different page color. For example, Section 4 (gray) is the Product Identification Guide. It contains actual-size color photos of tablets and capsules provided by the manufacturers. Section 5 (white) is the Product Information Section. It contains reprints of package inserts. The insert describes the drug's action, uses, administration, dosages, contraindications, and other information.
- *Package inserts.* These are the inserts developed by the manufacturer and approved by the FDA.

REVIEW QUESTIONS

Circle the **BEST** answer.

1　The brand name of a drug is
   a　its trade name
   b　its chemical structure
   c　its common name
   d　the name listed by the FDA

2　A prescription drug
   a　affects one body system
   b　has one use
   c　needs a doctor's order
   d　is not approved for use by the FDA

3　Over-the-counter drugs
   a　are called recreational drugs
   b　are sold without a prescription
   c　have no therapeutic use
   d　require the phrase "Rx only" on the label

4　Drugs act in the human body by
   a　forming a chemical bond within specific sites
   b　creating new body responses
   c　reconstituting a body fluid
   d　diluting a body fluid

5　The process by which the body in-activates a drug is called
   a　absorption
   b　distribution
   c　metabolism
   d　excretion

6　A drug is given by the enteral route. You know that the drug is given
   a　into a vein
   b　into a muscle
   c　beneath the skin
   d　into the GI tract

7　The nurse tells you that the blood level of a drug is too high. You know that the
   a　person is taking illegal drugs
   b　person is at risk for toxicity
   c　the rate of absorption is low
   d　the rate of excretion is high

8　Most drugs are metabolized
   a　in the kidneys
   b　by white blood cells
   c　by the GI tract
   d　in the liver

9　Most drugs leave the body through
   a　the skin
   b　the lungs
   c　saliva
   d　urine and feces

10　Which is life-threatening?
   a　an allergic reaction
   b　an adverse drug reaction
   c　an idiosyncratic drug reaction
   d　an anaphylactic reaction

11　A person complains of severe itching. You observe raised, irregular patches on the person's skin. This is called
   a　a side effect
   b　an adverse drug reaction
   c　anaphylaxis
   d　hives

12　A hyper-sensitivity to a drug is called
   a　an allergic reaction
   b　an adverse effect
   c　a side effect
   d　an anaphylactic reaction

13　Which has no active ingredients?
   a　IM
   b　IV
   c　subcutaneous
   d　placebo

14　A person needs higher dosages of a drug to produce the same effects that lower dosages once gave. This is called
   a　tolerance
   b　dependence
   c　cumulative effect
   d　a drug interaction

15　When checking drug information, you must use
   a　the *PDR*
   b　package inserts
   c　the most current resource
   d　on-line resources

Answers to these questions are on p. 444.

7

Life Span Considerations

OBJECTIVES

- Define the key terms and key abbreviations used in this chapter.
- Know the age ranges for each age group.
- Identify the factors that affect drug absorption in children and older persons.
- Identify the factors that affect drug distribution in children and older persons.
- Identify the factors that affect drug metabolism in children and older persons.
- Identify the factors that affect drug excretion in children and older persons.
- Explain the purpose of therapeutic drug monitoring.
- Explain how to assist the nurse with therapeutic drug monitoring.
- Explain the factors and guidelines related to giving drugs to children.
- Identify the causes of drug toxicity in older persons.
- Explain how to help older persons with drug therapy.
- Explain how to help pregnant women and breast-feeding mothers with drug therapy.

KEY TERMS

absorption The process by which a drug is transferred from its site of body entry to circulating body fluids (blood, lymph) for distribution

distribution The ways drugs are transported by circulating body fluids to the sites of action (receptors) and to the sites of metabolism and excretion

enzymes Substances produced by body cells; using oxygen, enzymes break down glucose and other nutrients to release energy for cellular work

excretion The elimination of a drug from the body

metabolism The process by which the body in-activates drugs

metabolite A product of drug metabolism

therapeutic drug monitoring The measurement of a drug's concentration in body fluids

KEY ABBREVIATIONS

FDA Food and Drug Administration
GI Gastro-intestinal

Gender (male; female) affects drug therapy. Men and women respond to drugs differently. They also react to and experience disease differently.

The person's age can greatly affect drug therapy. See the different age groups in Box 7-1. Children and older persons require special considerations when giving drugs.

DRUG ABSORPTION

Absorption is the process by which a drug is transferred from its site of body entry to circulating body fluids (blood, lymph) for distribution.

Drugs Applied to the Skin

Absorption of drugs applied to the skin (topical drugs) is usually effective in infants. The outer skin layer is not fully developed. The skin is more fully hydrated (has more water) at this age. Skin absorption is enhanced when infants wear plastic-coated diapers. The plastic increases hydration of the skin. Inflammation of the skin also increases the amount of drug absorbed. Diaper rash is an example of skin inflammation.

Skin absorption in older persons is often hard to predict. Skin thickness decreases with aging and may enhance absorption. However, some factors lessen absorption. They include:

- Drier skin.
- Wrinkled skin.
- Decreased number of hair follicles.
- Decreased cardiac output. This decreases the amount of blood flow to tissues.

Drugs Given Orally

Most drugs are given orally. Some tablet and capsule forms are too large for children and older persons to swallow. With the nurse's permission, some tablets are crushed to mix with food. Or a liquid form is ordered. Taste is a factor when giving oral liquids. The liquid has contact with the taste buds.

Certain oral drug forms must not be crushed. Doing so affects the absorption rate. Toxicity also is a risk. Such oral drug forms are:

- Timed-release tablets (Chapter 10)
- Enteric-coated tablets (Chapter 10)
- Sublingual tablets (Chapter 10)

Infants and some older persons may not have enough teeth for chewable drugs. Do not give chewable tablets to anyone with loose teeth. Loose teeth are common in children and older persons. Always ask about loose teeth.

Saliva flow is often less in older persons. Chewing and swallowing are harder for them.

Gastro-intestinal (GI) absorption of drugs is influenced by disease processes and many factors. They include:

- *Gastric pH*—how much acid is in the stomach. Older persons have fewer acid-secreting cells. This means that they have a higher gastric pH. (The lower the pH, the more acid in the stomach.) Some drugs are destroyed by gastric acid. Older persons have less acid to destroy such drugs. Therefore drugs destroyed by gastric acid are absorbed faster in older persons. Blood levels also are higher. Penicillin is an example. Other drugs depend on gastric acid for absorption. They are poorly absorbed and have lower blood levels in older adults. Aspirin is an example.
- *Gastric emptying*—how fast the stomach empties. The stomach empties more slowly in older persons than in younger people. Drugs may have a longer time of tissue contact. This allows increased absorption. Increased absorption leads to a higher blood level. Toxicity is a risk from the extended contact time in the stomach. The risk of ulcers increases with some drugs.
- *Motility of the GI tract*—how fast digested food and fluids move through the GI tract. GI motility is decreased in older persons. This can alter the absorption of drugs. Constipation or diarrhea can occur.
- *Blood flow*—the amount of blood that reaches the stomach and intestines. Blood flow decreases in older persons. This can alter the absorption of drugs. Constipation or diarrhea can occur.

BOX 7-1 Age Groups	
Less than 38 weeks gestation	Premature
0 to 1 month	Newborn; neonate
1 to 24 months	Infant; baby
1 to 5 years	Young child
6 to 12 years	Older child
13 to 18 years	Adolescent
19 to 54 years	Adult
55 to 64 years	Older adult
65 to 74 years	Elderly; young old
75 to 84 years	The aged; old
85 years and older	The very old; old old

DRUG DISTRIBUTION

Distribution refers to the ways drugs are transported by circulating body fluids to the sites of action (receptors) and to the sites of metabolism and excretion. Most drugs are transported:

- Dissolved in the circulating body water (in blood). The amount of body water changes with age. About 74% of an infant's body is composed of water. About 60% of an adult man's body is composed of body water.
- Bound to plasma proteins within the blood. Albumin and globulins are plasma proteins. After age 40, protein composition begins to change. Albumin concentrations gradually decrease. The globulins increase. As albumin levels decrease, the amount of unbound, active drug increases. Some liver and kidney diseases lower albumin levels. If the albumin level is low, the person needs lower doses of some drugs. The doctor may slowly increase the dosage. The drug effect may be greater at first—there is more active drug available. However, the duration of action may be reduced. When the drug is not bound to protein, there is more drug available for metabolism and excretion.

DRUG METABOLISM

Metabolism is the process by which the body inactivates drugs. Enzymes are a factor in drug metabolism. **Enzymes** are substances produced by body cells. Using oxygen, enzymes break down glucose and other nutrients to release energy for cellular work. Enzyme systems in the liver provide the major pathway for drug metabolism. All enzyme systems are present at birth. However, they mature at different rates. They can take many weeks to 1 year to fully develop.

Liver weight, the number of functioning liver cells, and liver blood flow decrease with age. Therefore drug metabolism is slower in older adults. Reduced metabolism is made more serious by liver disease and heart failure. Drugs metabolized by the liver can have longer action if liver blood flow is reduced. Usually dosages are reduced or the time between doses is extended. This prevents the accumulation of active drugs. It also reduces the risk of toxicity.

Drug metabolism is also affected at all ages by genetics, smoking, diet, gender, liver disease, and other drugs. The doctor orders liver function tests. Dosages are adjusted as needed.

DRUG EXCRETION

Excretion is the elimination of a drug from the body. Metabolites of drugs, and sometimes the drug itself, are eventually excreted from the body. (A **metabolite** is a product of drug metabolism.) They are excreted mainly through the urine and feces. Minor routes of excretion are through the skin, lungs, saliva, and breast milk.

At birth, a full-term newborn has about 35% of the kidney capacity of an adult. Full adult function is achieved at 9 to 12 months. Some drugs are excreted mainly by the kidneys. As the child grows, dosages of such drugs are increased or given more often to maintain therapeutic blood levels.

Changes in the kidneys occur with aging. Kidney blood flow decreases. So does cardiac output. Kidney function decreases. The doctor orders kidney function tests as needed. Drug dosages are decreased or given less often to maintain therapeutic blood levels.

THERAPEUTIC DRUG MONITORING

Therapeutic drug monitoring is the measurement of a drug's concentration in body fluids. It is done to determine the drug dosage and the blood level of the drug in relation to the body's response. Blood testing is commonly used. Saliva tests are used for some drugs.

Therapeutic drug monitoring is essential in newborns, infants, and children and for persons with certain health problems. Heart failure and abnormal heart rhythms are examples. The doctor adjusts the dosage and how often the drug is given to maintain desired drug levels.

Blood levels are measured if drug toxicity is suspected. The doctor uses the blood level to decide how to treat the toxicity.

Blood and urine samples can be obtained for legal purposes if drug abuse is suspected.

Assisting With the Nursing Process

Vital signs and urinary output are used to plan dosages and monitor the effects of drug therapy in all persons. Accurate measurements are essential. You must know the normal ranges for the person. Report abnormal measurements at once.

For all drugs, health teaching is important. As needed, the nurse involves family members and caregivers in the health teaching plan. Patients and residents need to understand the purpose of the drugs they are taking. They also need to know the complications that could occur if they stop taking the drug.

Children. Infants and children are at great risk for complications from drug therapy. Their bodies and organ functions are developing. Remember the following when giving drugs to children:

- They are at risk for dehydration from fever, vomiting, and diarrhea.
- They grow rapidly and have growth spurts. The doctor may need to adjust dosages according to the child's weight. Accurate height and weight measurements are important.
- Report your observations to the nurse. Vital signs, intake and output measurements, appetite, appearance, and responsiveness are examples.
- Use appropriate devices when giving liquid drugs. Use a medicine cup, oral dropper, or oral syringe (Fig. 7-1).
- Children 5 years or older can usually swallow tablets and capsules. Many tablets that are not timed-release or enteric-coated can be crushed. Most capsules can be opened and the contents sprinkled on small amounts of food. Applesauce, jelly, and pudding are examples.
- Dilute oral drugs in powder form according to the manufacturer's instructions.
- Many drugs are not approved by the Food and Drug Administration (FDA) for use in children. Doctors may legally prescribe some drugs for what is called *off-label use.* The nurse must question a specific dose if it is not readily available for cross-checking in drug information resources. Before giving the drug, the nurse documents in the child's medical record that the drug order was verified. Follow agency policy. The nurse may need to give the drug.

- In general, salicylates (aspirin) should not be given to children from infancy through the teenage years. Taking aspirin puts children at risk for Reye's syndrome. It is a life-threatening illness. Reye's syndrome is a risk when a child takes aspirin at the time or shortly after chickenpox or influenza. Drugs routinely used to relieve pain or reduce fever in children are ibuprofen (Advil) and acetaminophen (Tylenol).
- Allergic reactions can occur rapidly in children. Reactions are most common from antibiotics, especially penicillins. Observe the child's response to the drug. Report adverse signs and symptoms to the nurse at once. Intense anxiety, weakness, sweating, and shortness of breath are common at first. Hypotension, shock, abnormal heart rhythms, respiratory congestion, laryngeal edema, nausea, and defecation may occur. Call for the nurse at once. Start cardio-pulmonary resuscitation if necessary.

See Box 7-2 for guidelines when giving oral drugs to children.

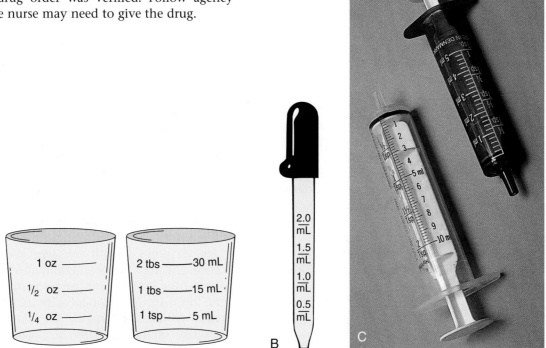

Fig. 7-1 Devices for giving oral drugs to children. **A,** Medicine cup. **B,** Oral dropper. **C,** Oral syringe.

BOX 7-2 Guidelines for Giving Oral Drugs to Children

INFANTS

- Use a calibrated dropper or oral syringe (see Fig. 7-1).
- Support the infant's head while holding him or her in your lap (Fig. 7-2).
- Give small amounts of the drug at a time. This helps prevent choking.
- Crush non-enteric coated or slow-release tablets to a powder. Sprinkle on small amounts of food that the child likes and is able to eat.

TODDLERS

- Let the toddler choose a position in which to take the drug.
- Disguise the drug's taste with a small amount of food or flavored drink. Let the child rinse with water or a flavored drink to help remove an unpleasant after-taste.
- Use simple commands in the toddler's jargon to obtain cooperation. For example, "This will make you feel better. Open up. Yummy, yummy."
- Let the toddler choose which drugs to take first. The child may need to take more than one drug.
- Use verbal and touch responses to promote the child's cooperation.
- Let the child become familiar with the oral dosing device. Let the child inspect the device.

PRE-SCHOOL CHILDREN

- Place a tablet or capsule near the back of the tongue. Then provide water or a flavored drink to help the child swallow the drug.
- Tell the nurse if the child has loose teeth. Chewable tablets are avoided if the child has loose teeth.
- Use a straw to give drugs that could stain teeth. The nurse tells you when straws are needed.
- Let the child rinse with water or a flavored drink to remove an unpleasant after-taste.
- Let the child help decide:
  - Where to take drugs
  - What to take first
  - If he or she will swallow and rinse with water or a flavored drink

Information from Isetts BJ, Brown LM: Patient assessment and consultation, *Handbook of Non-Prescription Drugs*, ed 14, Washington, DC, 2004, American Pharmaceutical Association.

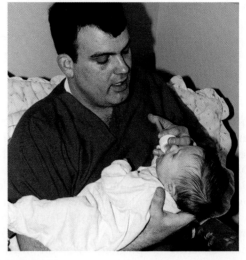

Fig. 7-2 The infant's head is supported when giving an oral drug.

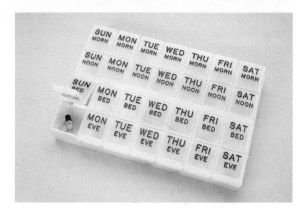

Fig. 7-3 Drug organizer.

Older Persons. Older persons are at great risk for drug interactions or drug toxicity. Causes include:

- Reduced liver function
- Reduced kidney function
- Chronic illnesses that require many drugs
- Poor nutrition

Remember the following when assisting older persons with drug therapy:

- Drug organizers (Fig. 7-3) and calendars are reminders for when to take drugs. They are useful for persons who can take their own drugs.
- Help the person destroy old prescriptions. This helps prevent confusion with current drug therapy.
- Older persons may have problems swallowing large tablets or capsules. You can crush them with the nurse's approval. Or you can break them in half if there is a "score" mark on the tablet (Fig. 7-4, p. 84). A *score* is a groove or indentation used to divide the tablet. A scored tablet is easily broken in half. Remember, timed-release tablets, enteric-coated tablets, and sublingual tablets are never crushed. Crushing affects the absorption rate and increases the risk of toxicity. Give crushed drugs with applesauce, ice cream, or jelly as the person's diet allows.

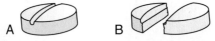

Fig. 7-4 A, A scored tablet. **B,** The scored tablet is broken in half.

Pregnant Women. Many drugs can injure the developing fetus. Drug therapy during pregnancy is avoided when possible. However many women take at least one drug while pregnant. Most of those drugs are non-prescription, self-care remedies. Pain-relief drugs, antacids, and cold and allergy products are commonly taken. Some drugs cause birth defects. They are contra-indicated during pregnancy.

When assisting a pregnant woman with drug therapy, remind her to:

- Take only drugs ordered by the doctor.
- Avoid drinking alcohol. Excessive use may cause the child to be born with fetal alcohol syndrome. It is a life-long condition with psychological, behavioral, and physical effects. It is avoided by not drinking alcohol during pregnancy. Women planning to become pregnant should stop drinking alcohol 2 to 3 months before conception.
- Not use tobacco. Mothers who smoke have a higher frequency of miscarriage, stillbirths, premature births, and low-birth-weight infants.

- Try non-drug treatments first. The following may help "morning sickness":
  - Lying down when feeling nauseated
  - Eating crackers or sipping small amounts of liquids before arising
  - Eating small, frequent meals high in carbohydrates
  - Lowering the fat content of meals
  - Avoiding spicy foods, dairy products, and smells or situations that may cause vomiting
- Avoid herbal medicines. They have not been scientifically tested on humans during pregnancy.

Breast-Feeding Women. Many drugs enter the breast milk of nursing mothers. Such drugs may harm the infant. If the breast-feeding mother is taking drugs, the best times to take them are:

- Right after the infant finishes breast-feeding
- Just before the infant's longer sleep period

Remind the mother about adverse effects that might occur in the infant.

REVIEW QUESTIONS

Circle the **BEST** answer.

1 Skin absorption of drugs is enhanced in infants. This is because their skin
   a   is thinner
   b   has more water
   c   is dry
   d   has few hair follicles

2 You are giving drugs to an older person. Which of the following may enhance skin absorption?
   a   thin skin
   b   dry skin
   c   wrinkled skin
   d   decreased blood flow to the skin

3 A tablet is too large for a person to swallow. With the nurse's permission you can
   a   crush the tablet and mix it with food
   b   give a liquid form of the same drug
   c   ask the person to chew the tablet
   d   dissolve the drug in water

4 Before giving a chewable tablet, you should
   a   taste the drug
   b   ask about the person's saliva flow
   c   mix the drug with food
   d   ask about loose teeth

5 These statements are about gastro-intestinal absorption of drugs in older persons. Which is *false?*
   a   Gastric acid secretion increases.
   b   Stomach emptying is slower.
   c   GI motility is slower.
   d   Blood flow to the stomach and intestines is decreased.

6 Drugs are given orally to an older person. The person is at risk for the following *except*
   a   enzymes
   b   ulcers
   c   constipation
   d   diarrhea

7 Drug distribution is likely to be greater in
   a   infants
   b   persons with liver disease
   c   persons with kidney disease
   d   older persons

8 In persons with liver or kidney disease, you should expect drug dosages to be
   a   increased
   b   decreased
   c   within the normal range
   d   half the normal range

9 Therapeutic drug monitoring is done to measure
   a   metabolites
   b   enzymes
   c   a drug's concentration in body fluids
   d   drug toxicity

10 You assist the nurse with therapeutic drug monitoring by measuring
   a   vital signs and urinary output
   b   gastric pH
   c   blood pH
   d   drug blood levels

11 The following are used to give oral drugs to children *except*
   a   medicine cups   c   oral syringes
   b   oral droppers   d   pacifiers

12 A child cannot swallow a capsule. With the nurse's permission you can
   a   sprinkle the contents onto small amounts of applesauce, jelly, or pudding
   b   sprinkle the contents into a flavored drink
   c   dilute the capsule following the manufacturer's instructions
   d   have the child chew the drug

13 From birth through the teenage years, children should *not* be given
   a   Tylenol   c   penicillin
   b   Advil   d   aspirin

14 When giving drugs to an infant, you should
   a   support the child's head
   b   let the child choose which drug to take first
   c   place a tablet near the back of the child's tongue
   d   use a straw if the drug can stain teeth

15 To remove an unpleasant after-taste, you should let the child
   a   have candy
   b   rinse with a flavored drink
   c   choose which drug form to take
   d   choose where to take the drug

16 Which is a useful reminder for when to take drugs?
   a   medicine cup   c   oral syringe
   b   oral dropper   d   drug organizer

17 A tablet is "scored." What does "scored" mean?
   a   You keep track of the number of tablets given to the person.
   b   The tablet can be broken in half.
   c   A "score" means 20. There are 20 doses in the tablet.
   d   The tablet is timed-release.

18 A pregnant woman should do the following *except*
   a   try non-drug treatments before trying drugs
   b   take only drugs ordered by the doctor
   c   have one alcoholic drink a day
   d   take prescribed drugs after the infant is done breast-feeding

Answers to these questions are on p. 444.

8

Drug Orders and Prescriptions

OBJECTIVES

- Define the key terms and key abbreviations used in this chapter.
- Identify the members of the health team who can give drug orders.
- List the parts of a drug order.
- Explain four types of drug orders.
- Identify the abbreviations commonly used in drug orders and prescriptions.
- Know the weights and measures used in drug orders and prescriptions.
- Identify common drug administration times.
- Describe the information on a prescription label.
- Describe the information contained in a person's medical record.
- Identify the information to include when recording a PRN drug in a person's medical record.
- Describe the parts of the medication administration record.
- Describe the parts of a PRN or unscheduled medication record.
- Explain the purpose of a Kardex.
- Explain how the nurse verifies and transcribes a drug order.
- Explain how to accurately transcribe a drug order.

KEY TERMS

chart See "medical record"

clinical record See "medical record"

drug order An order for a drug written on the agency's (hospital, nursing center) physician's order form for a patient or resident; medication order

medical record The written account of a person's condition and response to treatment and care; chart or clinical record

medication order See "drug order"

prescription A drug order written for a person leaving the hospital or nursing center or for a person seen in a clinic or doctor's office; it is written on a prescription pad or it is called in, faxed, or emailed to the pharmacy by the doctor

PRN order The nurse decides when to give the drug based on the person's needs

single order A drug is to be given at a certain time and only one time

standing order A drug is to be given for a certain number of doses or for a certain number of days

STAT order The drug is to be given at once and only one time

KEY ABBREVIATIONS

ISMP Institute for Safe Medication Practices
IV Intravenous; intravenously
MAR Medication administration record
PRN When necessary; as needed
STAT Immediately; at once
TO Telephone order
VO Verbal order

Licensed doctors and dentists order needed drugs for patients and residents. In some states nurse practitioners, nurse-midwives, nurse anesthetists, and physician assistants can order drugs. However, for purposes of this book, "doctor" is used when referring to drug orders.

- A **drug order (medication order)** is an order for a drug written on the agency's (hospital, nursing center) physician's order form for a patient or resident (Fig. 8-1, p. 88). Called the "doctor's order form" in this book, the order form is part of the person's medical record. In agencies with computerized charting systems, the order is entered into the system. The order is filled in the agency's pharmacy. Then it is sent to the nursing unit.
- A **prescription** is a drug order written for a person leaving the hospital or nursing center. Or it is written for a person seen in a clinic or doctor's office. It is written on a prescription pad (Fig. 8-2, p. 89). The prescription is taken to a local pharmacy (drug store) to be filled. Sometimes prescriptions are called in, faxed, or emailed to the pharmacy by the doctor.

Drug orders and prescriptions are essentially the same. They differ for:
- Where they are used—hospital, nursing center, home setting
- Where they are filled—within or outside the agency

PARTS OF A DRUG ORDER

All drug orders and prescriptions must contain:
- The person's full name
- The date
- Drug name
- Route of administration (Chapters 10, 11, 12, and 13)
- Dose
- Frequency of use
- Duration of the order
- The doctor's (or prescriber's) signature

TYPES OF DRUG ORDERS

There are four types of drug orders.
- **STAT order.** *STAT* come from the Latin word *statim*. It means *immediately* or *at once*. The drug is to be given at once and only one time. For example, a person is having a seizure. The ordered drug is given at once to stop the seizure. STAT orders are usually given for emergency or urgent situations.
- **Single order.** A drug is to be given at a certain time and only one time. For example, a drug to reduce fluid retention is ordered to be given at 0700.
- **Standing order.** A drug is to be given for a certain number of doses or for a certain number of days. For example, an antibiotic is ordered to be given daily for 10 days. The doctor must renew the order if he or she wants the drug to be given longer.
- **PRN order.** *PRN* comes from the Latin term *pro re nata*. It means *when necessary* or *as needed*. The nurse decides when to give the drug based on the person's needs.

ORDERING METHODS

The doctor can give drug orders in several ways.
- *Written order.* The doctor writes the order on the doctor's order form or prescription pad. The doctor then signs the order with his or her name. A copy of the order form is sent to the pharmacy. Some written orders are hard to read. If unsure of what is written, the nurse checks with the doctor before transcribing the order (p. 101). The pharmacist contacts the doctor if he or she has questions.
- *Verbal order (VO).* The doctor gives the order orally to a nurse. The nurse writes the order on the physician's order form or enters it into the computer system. VO is written on the order to show that it was given orally. The doctor signs the order later.
- *Telephone order (TO).* The doctor gives the order to a nurse over the phone. The nurse writes the order on the physician's order form or enters it into the computer system. TO is written on the order to show that it was given orally. The doctor signs the order later.
- *Faxed orders.* An order is faxed from a doctor's office to the nursing unit on which the person is a patient or resident. The doctor signs the orders at the agency within 24 hours of sending the fax.
- *Electronic orders.* The doctor enters the order into a computer. It is sent by email or computer network to the pharmacy.
  See *Focus on Older Persons: Ordering Methods*, p. 89.
  See *Promoting Safety and Comfort: Ordering Methods*, p. 89.

PHYSICIAN'S ORDER FORM

Addressograph here:

016-28-3978
Joseph Lorenzo
18 Bush Ave.
Hometown, USA

Dr. M. Martin
Unit-6W, Rm. 621

Martindale Hometown Hospital
Hometown, USA

Please Indicate Allergies

None	Codeine	Penicillin	Sulfa	Aspirin	Others

Date	Time	Prob. No.	Physician's Orders	Physician	Progress Record
1/6	1500	6	Erythromycin 250 mg, PO		
			q6h $\times$ 8 days	M. Martin	

Fig. 8-1 Physician's order form.

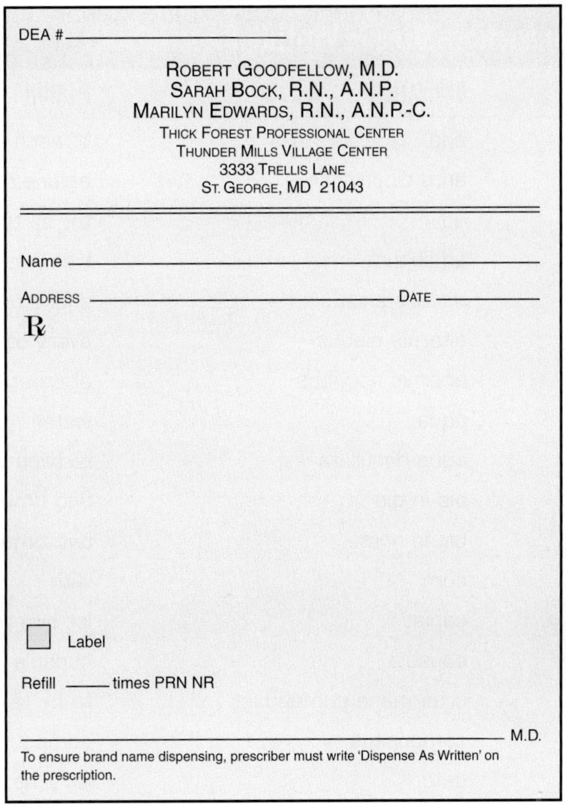

```
DEA #_____

              ROBERT GOODFELLOW, M.D.
               SARAH BOCK, R.N., A.N.P.
           MARILYN EDWARDS, R.N., A.N.P.-C.
             THICK FOREST PROFESSIONAL CENTER
             THUNDER MILLS VILLAGE CENTER
                     3333 TRELLIS LANE
                  ST. GEORGE, MD  21043


Name _____

ADDRESS _____ DATE _____

R



□  Label

Refill _____ times PRN NR

_____ M.D.
To ensure brand name dispensing, prescriber must write 'Dispense As Written' on
the prescription.
```

Fig. 8-2 Prescription pad. (From Edmunds MW: *Introduction to clinical pharmacology,* ed 5, St Louis, 2006, Mosby.)

FOCUS ON OLDER PERSONS

Ordering Methods

Some hospital patients are transferred to nursing centers. Faxed orders are often sent to nursing centers before the residents arrive there. This allows the center to prepare for the person's arrival. The person brings the original signed order to the nursing center.

PROMOTING SAFETY AND COMFORT
Ordering Methods

SAFETY
As an MA-C, you do not accept verbal or telephone orders from doctors. The nurse is responsible. Politely give your name and title, and ask the doctor to wait for a nurse. Promptly find a nurse to speak with the doctor.

ABBREVIATIONS

Abbreviations are commonly used in writing drug orders and prescriptions (Table 8-1, p. 90). The Joint Commission and the Institute for Safe Medication Practices (ISMP) recommend using only agency-approved abbreviations. If other abbreviations are used, they can lead to confusion and drug errors. Each agency is required to have a "Do Not Use" list (Table 8-2, p. 92).

Text continued on p. 92

TABLE 8-1	Common Abbreviations Used in Writing Prescriptions	
ABBREVIATION	**DERIVATION**	**MEANING**
$\overline{aa}$	ana	of each
a.c.; AC	ante cibum	before meals
ad	ad	to, up to
ad lib.	ad libitum	freely as desired
agit. ante sum.	agitare ante	shake before taking
alt. dieb.	alternis diebus	every other day
alt. noct.	alternis noctibus	alternate nights
aq.	aqua	water
aq. dest.	aqua destillata	distilled water
b.i.d.; bid	bis in die	two times a day
b.i.n.	bis in nocte	two times a night
c., $\overline{c}$	cum	with
Cap.	capiat	let him take
caps.	capsula	capsule
c.m.s.	cras mane sumendus	to be taken tomorrow morning
comp.	compositus	compound
Det.	detur	let it be given
Dieb. tert.	diebus tertiis	every third day
dil.	dilutus	dilute
elix.	elixir	elixir
ext.	extractum	extract
fld.	fluidus	fluid
Ft.	fiat	make
g	gramme	gram
gt	gutta	a drop
gtt; gtts	guttae	drops
h.; h	hora	hour
M.	misce	mix
mist.	mistura	mixture
non rep.	non repetatur	not to be repeated
noct.	nocte	in the night
ol.	oleum	oil
o.h.	omni hora	every hour
o.n.	omni nocte	every night
oz	uncia	ounce
p.c.; PC	post cibum	after meals
per	per	through or by
pil.	pilula	pill
p.o.; PO	per os	orally
p.r.n.; PRN	pro re nata	when required
q	quaque	every

Modified from *Mosby's dictionary of medicine, nursing, and health professions*, ed 7, St Louis, 2006, Mosby.

TABLE 8-1	Common Abbreviations Used in Writing Prescriptions—cont'd	
ABBREVIATION	**DERIVATION**	**MEANING**
q.h.; qh	quaque hora	every hour
q.2h.; q2h		every two hours
q.3h.; q3h		every three hours
q.4h.; q4h		every four hours
q.6h.; q6h		every six hours
q.8h.; q8h		every eight hours
q.12h.; q12h		every twelve hours
q.i.d.; qid	quater in die	four times a day
q.l.	quantum libet	as much as desired
q.p.	quantum placeat	as much as desired
q.v.	quantum vis	as much as you please
q.s.	quantum sufficit	as much as is required
℞	recipe	take
Rep.	repetatur	let it be repeated
s, s̄	sine	without
seq. luce.	sequenti luce	the following day
Sig. or S.	signa	write on label
s.o.s.	si opus sit	if necessary
sp.	spiritus	spirits
stat.; STAT	statim	immediately
syr.	syrupus	syrup
t.i.d.; tid	ter in die	three times a day
t.i.n.	ter in nocte	three times a night
tr. or tinct.	tinctura	tincture
ung.	unguentum	ointment
ut. dict.	ut dictum	as directed

TABLE 8-2	The Joint Commission "Do Not Use" List of Abbreviations

OFFICIAL "DO NOT USE" LIST[1]

DO NOT USE	POTENTIAL PROBLEM	USE INSTEAD
U (unit)	Mistaken for "O" (zero), the number "4" (four) or "cc"	Write "unit"
IU (International Unit)	Mistaken for IV (intravenous) or the number 10 (ten)	Write "International Unit"
Q.D., QD, q.d., qd (daily)	Mistaken for each other	Write "daily"
Q.O.D., QOD, q.o.d., qod (every other day)	Period after the Q mistaken for "I" and the "O" mistaken for "I"	Write "every other day"
Trailing zero (X.0 mg)*	Decimal point is missed	Write X mg
Lack of leading zero (.X mg)		Write 0.X mg
MS	Can mean morphine sulfate or magnesium sulfate	Write "morphine sulfate"
MSO_4 and $MgSO_4$	Confused for one another	Write "magnesium sulfate"

[1]Applies to all orders and all medication-related documentation that is handwritten (including free-text computer entry) or on pre-printed forms.

*Exception: A "trailing zero" may be used only where required to demonstrate the level of precision of the value being reported, such as for laboratory results, imaging studies that report size of lesions, or catheter/tube sizes. It may not be used in medication orders or other medication-related documentation.

ADDITIONAL ABBREVIATIONS, ACRONYMS AND SYMBOLS (FOR POSSIBLE FUTURE INCLUSION IN THE OFFICIAL "DO NOT USE" LIST)

DO NOT USE	POTENTIAL PROBLEM	USE INSTEAD
> (greater than)	Misinterpreted as the number "7" (seven) or the letter "L"	Write "greater than"
< (less than)	Confused for one another	Write "less than"
Abbreviations for drug names	Misinterpreted due to similar abbreviations for multiple drugs	Write drug names in full
Apothecary units	Unfamiliar to many practitioners Confused with metric units	Use metric units
@	Mistaken for the number "2" (two)	Write "at"
cc	Mistaken for U (units) when poorly written	Write "mL" or "milliliters"
μg	Mistaken for mg (milligrams) resulting in one thousand-fold overdose	Write "mcg" or "micrograms"

From The Joint Commission, 2005. Reprinted with permission.

ROMAN NUMERALS, WEIGHTS, AND MEASURES

Roman numerals are sometimes used by doctors when prescribing drugs. Key numerals are listed in Box 8-1. See Appendix A for how to use Roman numerals.

The household and metric systems of measurement are used to calculate, prepare, and give drugs (Box 8-1). See Appendix A for how to calculate dosages using these systems.

The *unit* and *milli-equivalent (mEq)* are other measures used in drug orders. These quantities are stated with a number and "units" or "mEq" following. The following are examples:

- 300,000 units of penicillin
- 40 mEq of potassium chloride

BOX 8-1 Roman Numerals, Weights, and Measures

ROMAN NUMERALS
 I = 1
 V = 5
 X = 10
 L = 50
 C = 100
 D = 500
 M = 1000

HOUSEHOLD MEASUREMENTS
 1 quart = 4 cups
 1 pint = 2 cups
 1 cup = 8 ounces
 1 teacup = 6 ounces
 1 tablespoon = 3 teaspoons
 1 teaspoon = about 5 mL

METRIC SYSTEM
Units of Length (Meter)
 1 millimeter = 0.001 (meaning 1/1000)
 1 centimeter = 0.01 (meaning 1/100)
 1 decimeter = 0.1 (meaning 1/10)
 1 meter = 1 (meter)

Units of Volume (Liter)
 1 milliliter = 0.001 (meaning 1/1000)
 1 centiliter = 0.01 (meaning 1/100)
 1 deciliter = 0.1 (meaning 1/10)
 1 liter = 1 (liter)

Units of Weight (Gram)
 1 microgram = 0.000001 (meaning 1/1,000,000)
 1 milligram = 0.001 (meaning 1/1000)
 1 centigram = 0.01 (meaning 1/100)
 1 gram = 1 (gram)
 1 kilogram = 1000 grams

TABLE 8-3 Examples of Standard Drug Administration Times

ORDER	TIMES
Daily; once daily	0900 (9:00 AM)
Bedtime; nightly, at bedtime	2100 (9:00 PM)
Twice a day	0900 (9:00 AM) and 1700 (5:00 PM)
Three times a day	0900 (9:00 AM), 1300 (1:00 PM), and 1700 (5:00 PM)
Four times a day	0900 (9:00 AM), 1300 (1:00 PM), 1700 (5:00 PM), and 2100 (9:00 PM)
Every 6 hours	0600 (6:00 AM); 1200 (12:00 PM, noon), 1800 (6:00 PM), and 2400 (12:00 AM; midnight):
Every 8 hours	0800 (8:00 AM); 1600 (4:00 PM); 2400 (12:00 AM; midnight)
Every 12 hours	0900 (9:00 AM) and 2100 (9:00 PM)
Before meals	0700 (7:00 AM), 1100 (11:00 AM); 1600 (4:00 PM)
After meals	0800 (8:00 AM), 1200 (12:00 PM, noon); 1800 (6:00 PM)

ADMINISTRATION TIMES

Agencies have standard drug administration times. This helps prevent drug errors. And they help make sure that drugs are given safely and on time. Examples of administration times are listed in Table 8-3. The times may vary among agencies. Always use the standard times used in your agency.

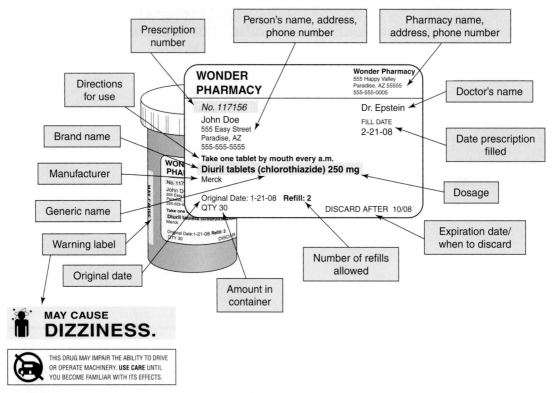

Fig. 8-3 Drug label.

PRESCRIPTION LABELS

Health care agencies have drug distribution systems (Chapter 9). Prescriptions filled in local pharmacies are labeled with the following information (Fig. 8-3):

- The person's name, address, and phone number
- The pharmacy's name, address, and phone number
- The prescription number
- The date the prescription was filled
- Original date of the prescription
- Doctor's name
- Brand name of the drug
- Generic name of the drug
- Manufacturer's name
- Drug dosage
- Amount in the container
- How often to take the drug
- Directions for use
- Warnings
- Number of refills allowed
- Expiration date or when to discard

Always read the label carefully. Make sure it is complete before giving the drug. If it is not complete, tell the nurse at once. Read and follow warnings and directions on the label. Also check the expiration date. If the date has passed, do not give the drug.

MEDICAL RECORD FORMS

The **medical record (chart; clinical record)** is the written account of a person's condition and response to treatment and care. It is a way for the health team to share information about the person. The record is permanent. It can be used years later if the person's health history is needed. The record is a legal document. It can be used as evidence in a court of law of the person's problems, treatment, and care.

The record has many forms. They are organized into sections for easy use. Each form has the person's name, room and bed number, and other identifying information. This helps prevent errors and improper placement of records. The record includes the person's:

- Admission form
- Health history
- Physical examination results
- Doctor's order form
- Doctor's progress notes
- Progress notes (nursing team and health team)
- Graphic sheet
- Flow sheets
- Laboratory and x-ray reports
- IV (intravenous) therapy record
- Respiratory therapy record
- Consultation reports
- Surgery and anesthesia reports
- Assessments and reports from social services, dietary services, and physical, occupational, speech, and recreational therapies
- Consent forms
- Medication administration record (MAR) or medication profile
- PRN or unscheduled medication record

Health team members record information on the forms for their departments. Other health team members read the information. It tells the care provided and the person's response.

Agencies have policies about medical records and who can see them. Policies address:

- Who records
- When to record
- Abbreviations
- Correcting errors
- Ink color
- Signing entries

You have an ethical and legal duty to keep the person's information confidential. You may know someone in the agency. If you do not give care to that person, you have no right to review the person's chart. To do so is an invasion of privacy.

Patients and residents have the right to the information in their medical records. The person or the person's legal representative may ask you for the chart. Report the request to the nurse. The nurse deals with the request.

The following parts of the medical record relate to your work as an MA-C.

The Graphic Sheet

The *graphic sheet* is used to record measurements and observations made daily, every shift, or 3 to 4 times a day (Fig. 8-4, p. 96). Information includes vital signs—temperature, pulse, respirations, blood pressure. It also includes daily weight, intake and output, bowel movements (feces), and doctor's visits.

You may have to check the graphic sheet before giving a drug. For example, you may need to check the person's intake and output, daily weight, or when the person last had a bowel movement.

Med-Forms, Inc.
FORM #MF37079 (Rev 9/95)

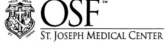

OSF℠
ST. JOSEPH MEDICAL CENTER
Bloomington, Illinois 61701

DAILY SUMMARY AND GRAPHIC

TEMPERATURE
Write in 105° or over

	2400	0400	0800	1200	1600	2000	2400	0400	0800	1200	1600	2000	2400	0400	0800	1200	1600	2000	2400	0400	0800	1200	1600	2000
DATE																								
HOSPITAL DAY																								
POST OP DAY																								
HOUR	2400	0400	0800	1200	1600	2000	2400	0400	0800	1200	1600	2000	2400	0400	0800	1200	1600	2000	2400	0400	0800	1200	1600	2000
B/P																								

TEMPERATURE

104 40
102.2 39
100.4 38
98.6 37
96.6 36

PULSE																								
RESPIRATION																								
WEIGHT																								
DR. VISIT																								

INTAKE	2300-0700	0700-1500	1500-2300	TOTAL	2300-0700	0700-1500	1500-2300	TOTAL	2300-0700	0700-1500	1500-2300	TOTAL	2300-0700	0700-1500	1500-2300	TOTAL
Oral																
IV																
Tube Feedings																
PPN/TPN/Lipids																
Blood/Blood Products																
IV Meds																
Chemotherapy																
Unreturned irr. sol.																
TOTAL INTAKE																
OUTPUT	2300-0700	0700-1500	1500-2300	TOTAL	2300-0700	0700-1500	1500-2300	TOTAL	2300-0700	0700-1500	1500-2300	TOTAL	2300-0700	0700-1500	1500-2300	TOTAL
Urine																
GI																
Emesis																
Drains																
TOTAL OUTPUT																
Feces																

Fig. 8-4 Graphic sheet. (Courtesy OSF St. Joseph Medical Center, Bloomington, Ill.)

Progress Notes

The *progress notes* describe the care given and the person's response and progress (Fig. 8-5). In some agencies they are called the *nurses' notes*. The nursing team uses this form to record:

- The person's signs and symptoms
- Information about treatments
- Information about all PRN drugs
- Information about patient or resident teaching and counseling
- Procedures performed by the doctor
- Visits by other health team members

PRN drugs are recorded right *after* they are given. Depending on the drug, the person's vital signs are taken before giving the drug. The person's condition is monitored after the drug is given. Observations about the person's condition are then recorded in the progress notes. This includes vital signs if indicated.

The Medication Administration Record

The *medication administration record (MAR)* is called the *medication profile* in some agencies. Depending on the agency, it is a computerized form or hand written. The MAR lists all drugs to be given to a person (Fig. 8-6, pp. 98-100). The drug order written by the doctor is transferred to the MAR.

The drugs are sometimes grouped as follows:

- *Scheduled medications.* These drugs are scheduled on a regular basis. Daily, every 6 hours, twice a day, and at bedtime are examples.
- *Parenteral medications. Parenteral* involves piercing the skin or mucous membranes through a needle stick. Injections ("shots") and drugs given intravenously (IV) are in this group.
- *STAT medications.* These drugs are given at once after receiving the order.
- *Pre-operative medications.* These drugs are given before surgery.
- *PRN medications.* These drugs are given as needed. They are usually listed at the bottom of the MAR or on a separate page.

Date	Time	Nursing Margin / Other Depts Margin
3-19	1700	Out with family for dinner. Jane Doe, LPN
	1930	Returned from outing accompanied by her son. States she had a pleasant time Mary Smith, CNA
3-20	0900	In bed. Complains of headache. T 98.4 orally, radial pulse 72 and regular, respirations 18 and unlabored. BP 134/84 left arm lying down. Alice Jones, RN notified of resident complaint and vital signs. Ann Adams, CNA
	0910	In bed resting. States she has had a headache for about 1/2 hour. Denies nausea and dizziness. No other complaints. PRN Tylenol given. Instructed resident to use signal light if headache worsens or other symptoms occur. Alice Jones, RN
	0945	Resting quietly. Denies headache at this time. T 98.4 orally, radial pulse 70 and regular, respirations 18 and unlabored. BP 132/84 left arm lying down. Alice Jones, RN

Fig. 8-5 Progress notes. Note that other members of the health team also can record on this form.

MARTINDALE HOMETOWN HOSPITAL

MEDICATION ADMINISTRATION RECORD

				Init	Signature	Title
NAME:	Joseph Lorenzo	RM-BD: 621-2				
ID NO.	016-28-3978	AGE: 62				
DIAGNOSIS	Myocardial Infarction	SEX: M				
PHYSICIAN	M. Martin, M.D.	Ht: 6' Wt: 200				

	SCHEDULED MEDICATIONS			
DATES:	MEDICATION—STRENGTH—FORM—ROUTE	0030-0729	0730-1529	1530-0029

1/25	RANITIDINE
	  ZANTAC
	  150 MG TABLET ORAL
	    TWICE A DAY
			0900	1800

1/25	DILTIAZEM HYDROCHLORIDE
	  CARDIZEM
	  90 MG TABLET ORAL
	  4 TIMES DAILY
			0900
			1300
				1800
				2100

1/25	WARFARIN SODIUM
	  COUMADIN
	  1 MG TABLET ORAL
	    EVERY OTHER DAY
		NOT GIVEN	TODAY	

	IV AND PIGGYBACK ORDERS			

1/25	CEFTAZIDIME (FORTAZ) 1 G IV
	  SODIUM CHLORIDE 0.9% 50 ML
	  EVERY 8 HOURS INFUSE: 20 MIN
		0200	1000	1800

1/25	GENTAMICIN PREMIX 80 MG IV
	  ISO-OSMOTIC SOLN 100 ML
	  BY IV PUMP
	  EVERY 12 HOURS INFUSE: 30 MIN
		0200	1400	

1/25	BY IV PUMP 1 IV
	  D5W 1000 ML
	          RATE: 100 ML/HR			

	PRN MEDICATIONS			

1/25	ACETAMINOPHEN
	  TYLENOL
	  650 MG TABLET ORAL
	  EVERY 4 HOURS AS NEEDED PRN			

1/25	MAGNESIUM HYDROXIDE
	  MILK OF MAGNESIA
	  60 ML (CONC) ORAL CONC
	    AS NEEDED PRN			

1/25	ALBUTEROL
	  PROVENTIL INHALER
	  90 MCG/INH AEROSOL INH
	  AS NEEDED PRN
	  SEE RESPIRATORY THERAPY NOTES
	    AT BEDSIDE			

Age/Sex	HT	WT	Date	ALLERGIES CODEINE
62/ M	6'0"	200 lbs	1/25	
Room-Bd	Name			
621 2	Joseph Lorenzo			

A

Fig. 8-6 Medication administration records. **A,** A computer generated MAR. Recordings are hand written.

The MAR provides a space for recording the time the drug was given and who gave it. This recording is done at once after giving the drug. Depending on the system used, you will:

- Initial the time when the drug was given. You will write your initials, your signature, and title in the space provided. See Figure 8-6, *A* and *C*.
- Follow agency policy if using a computerized charting system. See Figure 8-6, *B*.

MARs are kept in a notebook or clipboard file on the medication cart. Or they are accessed on the computer following agency policy. MARs may be for a shift (8, 10, or 12 hours), 24 hours, or for as long as 1 month.

See *Promoting Safety and Comfort: The Medication Administration Record.*

**PROMOTING SAFETY AND COMFORT
The Medication Administration
Record**

SAFETY

The MAR includes a place to note the person's allergies (see Fig. 8-6. *A* and *C*). Before giving a drug, always compare it to the allergies listed. Tell the nurse at once if the person is allergic to a drug ordered. If unsure, check with the nurse before giving the drug.

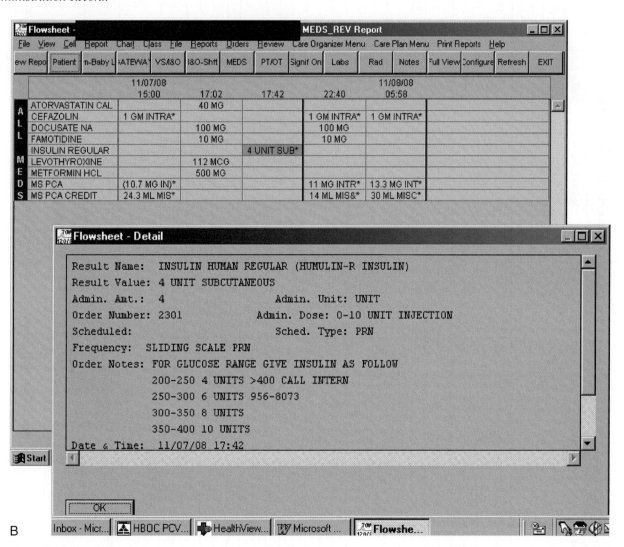

Fig. 8-6, cont'd Medication administration records. **B,** A computer generated MAR. Recordings are computerized. (**B,** Courtesy of Creighton University Medical Center, Omaha, Nebraska.) *Continued*

MEDICATION ADMINISTRATION RECORD

Nursing Home Name	PHARMACY PROVIDER	INIT.=GIVEN R=REFUSED V=VOMITED H=HELD O=HOME	INIT.	SIGNATURE	INIT.	SIGNATURE	INIT.	SIGNATURE	INIT.	SIGNATURE
Mo. ___ Yr. ___										

RX#—DATE ORDERED MEDICATION—DOSE—ROUTE	TIME	1	2	3	4	5	6	7	8	9	10	11	12	13	14	15	16	17	18	19	20	21	22	23	24	25	26	27	28	29	30	31

ALLERGIES   **DIAGNOSIS**

LAST NAME	FIRST	INIT.	LEVEL OF CARE	ROOM-BED	SEX	BIRTHDATE	DIET	IDENTIFICATION #	PHYSICIAN

DATE OF MED. REVIEW _____   REVIEWED BY _____ (RPh)
_____ (RN)

C

Fig. 8-6, cont'd Medication administration records. **C,** An MAR used in a nursing center.

Medication Records in Assisted Living Residences. Residents manage and take their own drugs if able. Some residents need help. A medication record is kept for each person needing help with drugs. The record includes:

- The person's name
- Drug name, dose, directions, and route of administration
- Date and time to take the drug
- Date and time help was given
- Signature or initials of the person assisting

PRN or Unscheduled Medication Record

Some agencies use a PRN or unscheduled medication record (Fig. 8-7, p. 102). The following information is recorded:

- The date and time
- The drug given
- The dose given
- The route
- Reason for giving the PRN drug
- The person's response

The Kardex

The *Kardex* is a type of card file. It summarizes information found in the medical record—drugs, treatments, diagnoses, routine care measures, equipment, and special needs. The Kardex is a quick, easy source of information about the person (Fig. 8-8, p. 103).

Often completed in pencil, it is updated regularly. Old information or orders are erased, new ones are added. The Kardex is not a formal, legal part of the medical record. It is destroyed when the person is discharged from the agency.

THE NURSE'S ROLE

A nurse verifies and transcribes the drug order. To *verify* an order means to make sure the drug order is safe for the person. The nurse makes professional judgments about:

- The type of drug
- The drug's therapeutic intent
- The usual dosage of the drug
- The person's ability to tolerate the dosage form ordered
- If the person has any allergies to the drug

The nurse decides if the drug is safe to give. If the drug order is deemed safe, the nurse sends the drug order to the pharmacy. If it is not deemed safe, the doctor is contacted. The nurse explains why the nursing team cannot give the drug. Usually the doctor will re-write the order. If not, the nurse follows agency policy for refusing to give a drug.

After verifying the order, it is transcribed. To *transcribe* means *to copy.* Transcribing is necessary to put the order into action. The process involves:

- Copying the order onto the Kardex and MAR or entering it into the computer. This may be done by the nurse or unit secretary. In some states and agencies, you may be allowed to transcribe orders, p. 104.
- Signing the order. In some agencies this is called *noting the order* or *posting the order.* The nurse reviews the transcription to make sure it is correct. Then the nurse signs, dates, and times the transcription on the original order. This means that the order was received and verified.
- Sending the order to the pharmacy following agency policy. This involves sending a copy of the doctor's order form or sending the order by computer. For nursing centers, the order is faxed or emailed to a local pharmacy.

Text continued on p. 104

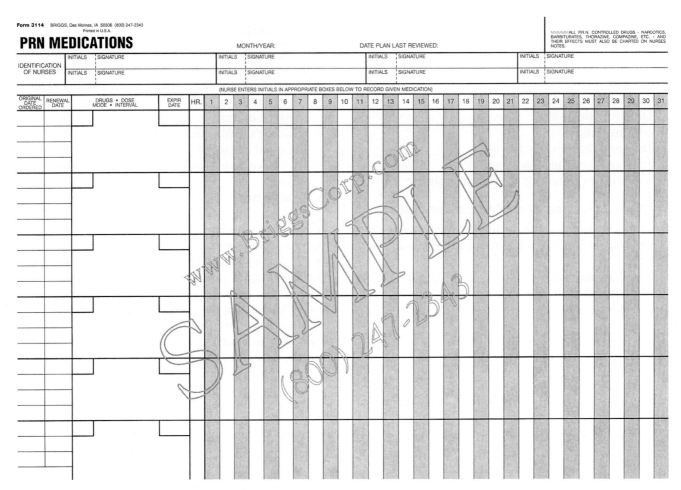

Fig. 8-7 PRN or unscheduled medication record. (Reprinted with permission of Briggs Corporation, Des Moines, Iowa, [800] 247-2343.)

DIET	NOURISHMENT/SPECIAL FEEDING	INTAKE/OUTPUT

DIET _Regular_

Hold:

NOURISHMENT/SPECIAL FEEDING _Health shake at Bedtime_

INTAKE/OUTPUT
Encourage/(Restrict) Fluids _2000_ mL/24 Hr.
7-3 _1000_   3-11 _800_   11-7 _200_

FUNCTIONAL STATUS

	SELF	ASSIST	TOTAL	OTHER	SPECIFY
Feeding	☐	☒	☐	☐	
Bathing	☐	☒	☐	☐	
Toileting	☐	☒	☐	☐	
Oral Care	☐	☒	☐	☐	
Positioning	☒	☐	☐	☐	
Transferring	☒	☐	☐	☐	
Wheeling	☐	☐	☐	☐	
Walking	☒	☐	☐	☐	
	☐	☐	☐	☐	

ACTIVITIES
Bedrest & BRP ____
Bedside Commode ____
Up ad Lib _X_
Chair ____
Ambulatory _X_
Ambulate & Assist ____
Turn ____
Dangle ____
Mode of Travel ____

ELIMINATION
Bladder - Cont. (Incont.)
Catheter ____
Date Changed ____
Irrigations ____
Bowel - (Cont.)/ Incont.
Ostomy ____
Irrigations ____

VITALS
Temp. _qid_
Pulse _qid_
Resp. _qid_
BP _qid_
Weight _daily_
Other:
Pulse OX
daily

COMMUNICATION DEFICITS ☐ None
Hearing _Hard-of-hearing_
Vision _Impaired_
Speech ____
Language _Impaired_

SPECIAL CONDITIONS (Paralysis, Pressure Ulcers, Etc.)

SAFETY/SUPPORTIVE MEASURES
Bed rails: ☐ Nights Only ☐ Constant ☐ No Need
Restraints: ☐ PRN ☐ Constant
Support Devices: ☐ PRN ☐ Constant

RESPIRATORY THERAPY
Aerosol
IPPB
Ultrasonic
Rx Med ____

OXYGEN
_2_ Liter/Minute
☒ PRN ☐ Constant
___ Tent ___ Catheter
___ Mask _X_ Cannula

PROSTHESIS ☐ None
Glasses _X_   Dentures _X_
Contacts ____   Limb ____
Hearing Aid _L ear_

DATE	TREATMENTS/MISCELLANEOUS

SPECIAL EQUIPMENT/PROCEDURES/ANCILLARY SERVICES/ETC.
Speech therapy 3 times/wk.

ORDERED	SCHEDULED	COMPLETED	X-RAY AND SPECIAL DIAGNOSTIC EXAMS
10-20	10-20	10-20	Chest x-ray

START DATE	SCHEDULED MEDICATIONS	STOP DATE	RENEW	START DATE	STOP OR RENEW	SITE	IV FLUID & RATE	DATE & TIME CHANGED TUBING	DRESS.	SITE
10-19	Lasix 40 mg PO daily									
10-19	Lanoxin 0.25 mg PO daily									

DATE	ONE TIME ORDERS

DATE	DAILY/REPEATING ORDERS
10-20	Serum potassium daily

DATE	TIME	PRN MEDICATIONS
10-19	2100	Ativan 0.25 mg PO q4h PRN anxiety

MISCELLANEOUS

ALLERGIES:
☒ None Known

NURSING ALERTS:

EMERGENCY CONTACT:
Name: _Parker, Marie_   Telephone No. Home: _555-1212_
Relationship: _Wife_   Bus: ____

ROOM	NAME	PHYSICIAN	ADMITTING DIAGNOSIS/PROBLEM	HOSP. NO.
310	Parker, Edwin	Dr. S Epstein	1. CHF 2. Dementia	1035B

Fig. 8-8 A sample Kardex. (Reprinted with permission of Briggs Corporation, Des Moines, Iowa [800] 247-2343.)

Assisting With Transcription

Some states and agencies may allow you to transcribe drug orders from the doctor's order form to the Kardex and MAR or computer. *Accuracy* is a must. When transcribing, follow the guidelines in Box 8-2. Also follow agency policies and procedures.

BOX 8-2 Guidelines for Transcribing

GENERAL RULES

- Make sure your state and agency allow you to transcribe drug orders.
- Make sure you have received the necessary education and training.
- Make sure that a nurse will review and complete the transcription process.
- Follow agency policy whenever transcribing. Agency policies may vary from the rules listed in this box.
- Make sure the form has the person's identifying information.
- Make sure the form has the person's current diagnoses.
- Make sure the form lists any known allergies.
- Follow the rules for reporting and recording. See Chapter 4.
- Use only the abbreviations allowed in your agency. Tell the nurse if an abbreviation on the "Do Not Use" list is used.
- Use only the drug times approved for use in your agency.
- Tell the nurse at once of any STAT order.
- Use the ink color required by your agency. Never use pencil on a doctor's order form or MAR.
- Press hard enough that your writing goes through all copy layers.
- Write clearly and neatly. Your writing must be legible.
- Ask a nurse to clarify if you cannot read or are not sure of something on the order.
- Place a check-mark next to each order transcribed. Do this *after* transcribing each order. The check-mark shows that the order was transcribed.
- Write "noted" or "posted," and sign, date, and time the doctor's order form after transcribing all orders. This tells the nurse that:
  - You have transcribed all orders.
  - The orders are ready for the nurse to review and sign. After checking for accuracy, the nurse will write "verified" and sign, date, and time when this was done.

ADDING A NEW DRUG

- Transfer the following information from the drug order to the MAR:
  - The name of the drug. Some agencies require both the brand and generic names.
  - The strength of the drug. This is the amount of drug in each tablet, capsule, and so on.
  - The dose and amount of the drug to give.
  - How to give the drug (the route to use).
  - What time or times to give the drug. Or how many times a day to give the drug.
  - When the order was written.
  - When to start the drug (if written). This is usually the day the drug was ordered.
  - When to stop the drug (if written).
  - Special instructions or precautions. For example: "Do not give if apical pulse is less than 60 per minute."
- Note the times to give the drug. Use the agency's standard set of times (p. 93). For example, a drug is ordered 4 times a day. An agency may give drugs ordered 4 times a day at 0900 (9:00 AM), 1300 (1:00 PM), 1700 (5:00 PM), and 2100 (9:00 PM).
- Put an X through every date and time not included in the order.

DISCONTINUING A DRUG

- Draw a diagonal line or straight line through the drug order and all dates affected on the MAR.
- Write "discontinued" and the date above or next to the diagonal line or straight line.
- Sign your name next to or under "discontinued" and the date.
- Use a highlighter to mark out the line and the dates affected according to agency policy.

CHANGING AN ORDER

- Discontinue the current order.
- Transcribe the new order on a new line or in a new box on the MAR.
- Put an X through every date and time not included in the order.

STAT OR "ONE-TIME-ONLY" ORDERS

- Transfer all information from the drug order to the MAR.
- Put an X through every date and time not included in the order.

REVIEW QUESTIONS

Circle the BEST answer.

1 Drug orders written on a prescription pad are usually filled
  a on the nursing unit
  b in the hospital pharmacy
  c at a local pharmacy
  d at the doctor's office

2 A STAT drug order is to be given
  a at once
  b as needed
  c at a certain time
  d at bedtime

3 A PRN order means that a drug is given
  a at once
  b as needed
  c at a certain time
  d at bedtime

4 A single drug order is given
  a at once
  b as needed
  c at a certain time
  d at bedtime

5 Which abbreviation is on the "Do Not Use" list?
  a QD
  b PO
  c AC
  d q6h

6 Which abbreviation is safe to use?
  a cc
  b U
  c QOD
  d mL

7 A prescription label is not complete. What should you do?
  a Check the expiration date.
  b Call the pharmacy.
  c Tell the nurse.
  d Give the drug.

8 A drug order states to give the drug if the person has not had a bowel movement for 3 days. Where will you find information about the drug order?
  a the Kardex
  b the graphic sheet
  c the progress notes
  d the care plan

9 You gave a PRN drug as directed by the nurse. Besides the MAR, where should you record giving the drug?
  a the Kardex
  b the graphic sheet
  c the progress notes
  d the care plan

10 Where do you record giving a drug?
  a the Kardex
  b the MAR
  c the graphic sheet
  d a flow sheet

11 When do you record giving a drug?
  a before giving the drug
  b after giving the drug
  c at the end of your shift
  d when you have time

12 Before giving a drug, you must
  a check the person's allergies
  b take the person's pulse
  c measure the person's blood pressure
  d check the care plan

13 When is a copy of the order sent to the pharmacy?
  a as soon as it is written
  b after it is transcribed
  c at the end of the shift
  d at the time noted by the doctor

14 A drug order contains an abbreviation on the agency's "Do Not Use" list. What should you do?
  a Transcribe the order as written.
  b Tell the nurse.
  c Call the pharmacist.
  d Call the doctor.

15 You are not sure of something on a drug order. What should you do?
  a Transcribe the order as written.
  b Tell the nurse.
  c Call the pharmacist.
  d Call the doctor.

16 After transcribing a drug order, you should do the following *except*
  a place a check mark by the order
  b write "noted" or "posted" on the order
  c sign, date, and time the order
  d give the drug

17 A drug is to be given daily. What time should you put on the MAR?
  a 0900
  b the agency's standard time for a drug given daily
  c the time the drug was ordered
  d the time preferred by the person

18 A drug order was changed from daily to twice a day. When transcribing the new order to the MAR, you should do the following *except*
  a erase the first order
  b discontinue the first order
  c put an X through every date and time not included in the order
  d transcribe the new order on a new line

Continued

REVIEW QUESTIONS—cont'd

Circle T if the statement is true. Circle F if the statement is false.

19 T F Only doctors can order or prescribe drugs.

20 T F The doctor's order form is a permanent part of the person's medical record.

21 T F All drug orders must contain the prescriber's signature.

22 T F All drug orders must include the route of administration.

23 T F You can accept telephone orders from doctors.

24 T F You can accept verbal orders from doctors.

25 T F Standard drug administration times help prevent drug errors.

26 T F You can discuss the person's drug orders with anyone in the agency.

27 T F The Kardex is a permanent part of the person's medical record.

28 T F You can verify drug orders.

29 T F You can use a pencil to transcribe a drug order to the MAR.

30 T F A drug order was discontinued. It is erased from the Kardex.

Answers to these questions are on p. 444.

Medication Safety

OBJECTIVES

- Define the key terms and key abbreviations used in this chapter.
- Describe four drug distribution systems.
- Explain how controlled substances are distributed.
- Explain how to dispose of an unused portion of a controlled substance.
- Describe the narcotics count process.
- Explain how to safely store drugs.
- List the reasons for disposing of drugs.
- Explain how to dispose of drugs.
- Explain the Six Rights of Drug Administration.
- Explain your role in self-directed medication management.
- Identify common drug errors.
- Describe the rules for giving drugs safely.
- Explain how to prevent infection when giving drugs.
- Perform the procedures described in this chapter.

PROCEDURES

- Hand Washing
- Giving a Drug

KEY TERMS

dose The amount of drug to give

drug diversion Taking a person's drugs for your own use

infection A disease state resulting from the invasion and growth of microbes in the body

medication reminder Reminding the person to take drugs, observing them being taken as prescribed, and charting that they were taken

route How and where the drug enters the body

KEY ABBREVIATIONS

ADE Adverse drug event
ALR Assisted living residence
CDC Centers for Disease Control and Prevention
FDA Food and Drug Administration
HBV Hepatitis B virus
HIV Human immunodeficiency virus
ID Identification
IM Intramuscular
ISMP Institute for Safe Medication Practices
IV Intravenous
MAR Medication administration record
mg Milligram
NDC National Drug Code
OPIM Other potentially infectious materials
OSHA Occupational Safety and Health Administration
PPE Personal protective equipment
PRN When necessary; as needed
STAT At once; immediately
subcut Subcutaneous; subcutaneously

Medication safety involves the correct dispensing of the drug, correct storage, and correct disposal. Errors must be prevented. They must also be prevented when giving drugs to a person. To prevent drug errors and give drugs safely, you must follow the *Six Rights of Drug Administration*. The *right* drug must be given at the *right* time in the *right* dose to the *right* person using the *right* route. *Right* documentation follows giving a drug.

Safety involves protecting the person and yourself from infection. This chapter includes a review of medical asepsis, hand hygiene, and Standard Precautions.

DRUG DISTRIBUTION SYSTEMS

The pharmacy processes and fills drug orders. Then they are distributed (dispensed) to the nursing unit. Each agency has its own drug distribution system. The following systems are common.

See *Promoting Safety and Comfort: Drug Distribution Systems.*

Floor or Ward Stock System

With the *floor or ward stock system*, frequently used drugs are kept on the nursing unit (Fig. 9-1). Dangerous and rarely used drugs are kept in the pharmacy. Small hospitals and some nursing centers may use this system. Some government hospitals may use this system if drugs are not charged directly to the patient.

Ordered drugs are readily available. There is no waiting or lag time for the pharmacy to process, fill, and send the drug order to the nursing unit.

Safety issues for this system include:

- Many drugs are stocked on the nursing unit. This increases the risk for drug errors. For example, you must select the right drug and the right dose from all the drugs stocked.
- Monitoring drug expiration dates is hard. Over time, the chemical nature of a drug can change. In other words, the drug deteriorates. A once helpful drug can turn harmful.
- The nursing unit may not have enough space to store all drugs safely.
- Agency personnel have access to many drugs. Drug diversion is a risk.

Individual Prescription Order System

The *individual prescription order system* also involves storing drugs on the nursing unit. For a patient or resident, the pharmacy sends a 3- to 5-day supply of an ordered drug to the nursing unit. The drugs are stored in small bins in a cabinet on the nursing unit. Each person has a bin. Bins are arranged alphabetically by the person's name. Or bins are arranged by room and bed numbers.

This system is safer than the floor or ward stock system.

- A pharmacist and a nurse review the order before the drug is given.
- The pharmacy monitors drug expiration dates. This lessens the danger of drugs deteriorating.
- Fewer drugs are available for drug diversion.

Like the floor or ward stock system, drugs are available for STAT or PRN use. While fewer drugs are available, drug diversion remains a risk.

PROMOTING SAFETY AND COMFORT
Drug Distribution Systems

SAFETY

Always check drugs received from the pharmacy. Compare the pharmacy label against the drug order on the medication administration record (MAR). Also check that the number of doses is correct. If the number of doses is not correct, tell the nurse before continuing. It is possible that:

- The drug was discontinued.
- Another staff member gave the drug.
- The pharmacy omitted a dose.
- The drug was given to the wrong person.
- The drug was diverted by a staff member. *Drug diversion* is taking a person's drugs for your own use. This is illegal.

Follow agency policy for reporting a drug error (p. 118).

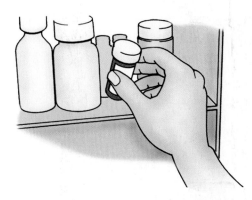

Fig. 9-1 Floor or ward stock system. (From Edmunds MW: *Introduction to clinical pharmacology*, ed 5, St Louis, 2006, Mosby.)

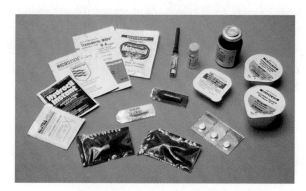

Fig. 9-2 Unit dose packages.

Unit Dose System

With the *unit dose system*, a single-unit dose package of a drug is dispensed for each dose ordered (Fig. 9-2). Placed in a packet, each packet is labeled according to agency policy. A 24-hour supply is provided in hospitals. For example, a person receives a drug 4 times a day. Four doses are included in the packet. The pharmacist refills the drawers every 24 hours.

A drawer in a drug cart is labeled with the person's name and room and bed number (Fig. 9-3). The cart is kept at the nurses' station. It is wheeled to each person's room to give the drugs.

The unit dose system is very common. It is safe and cost and time efficient.

* The nursing team spends less time preparing to give drugs.
* The pharmacy has a list of all drugs ordered for a person. The pharmacist can check for drug interactions or contraindications.
* The pharmacist determines the correct dosage. For example, 100 mg (milligrams) of a drug was ordered. The drug is supplied in 50 mg tablets. The pharmacist determines that 2 tablets are needed.
* Every dose must be accounted for on the MAR. This reduces the risk of drug diversion.
* Fewer drugs are available for drug diversion.

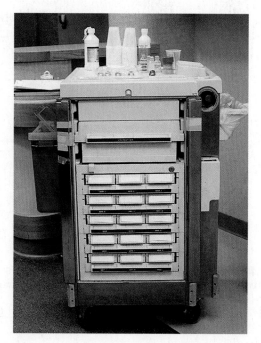

Fig. 9-3 Unit dose cart. Each drawer is labeled with a person's name and room and bed number.

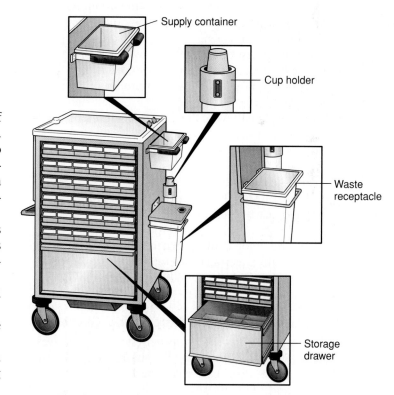

Fig. 9-4 Storage areas on a unit dose drug cart.

Unit dose carts have compartments for medicine bottles too large to fit in the person's drawer. There also are storage areas for supplies—medicine cups, drinking cups, straws, and so on (Fig. 9-4).

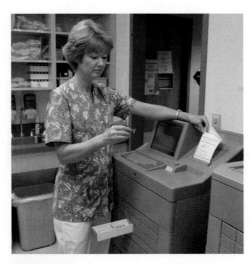

Fig. 9-5 Using a computer-controlled dispensing system. (Courtesy Rick Brady, from Lilley LL and others: *Pharmacology and the nursing process*, ed 5, St Louis, 2007, Mosby.)

The Unit Dose System in Nursing Centers.
Each drawer in the drug cart is large enough to hold drug containers for a 1 week or 1 month supply. Each drawer is labeled with a person's name, room and bed number, pharmacy name and phone number, and the center's name.

The pharmacist fills a container with the prescribed drug. Each container has sections for each day of the week. Each section contains the number of doses for that day.

Some systems have color codes for different times of day. For example:
- Purple—0600 (6:00 AM)
- Pink—0800 (8:00 AM)
- Yellow—1200 (12:00 PM; noon)
- Green—1400 (2:00 PM) or 1600 (4:00 PM)
- Orange—early evening
- Red—PRN

With the color coding, you can remove the drug containers for a certain time of day. For example, a person receives 4 drugs at 0800. You can remove the 4 pink containers for 0800.

Computer-Controlled Dispensing System

The *computer-controlled dispensing system* is the newest system (Fig. 9-5). Each day the pharmacy stocks the nursing unit's drug cart with the drugs ordered for patients and residents on that unit. You use a security code and password to access the system. In some agencies, you use a thumbprint or fingerprint.

In 2004, the Food and Drug Administration (FDA) issued a rule titled *Bar Code Label Requirements for Human Drug Products and Biological Products*. The rule is intended to improve safety by reducing drug errors. This FDA rule requires bar codes on most prescription drugs and on over-the-counter drugs commonly used in hospitals. The bar codes must contain the drug's National Drug Code (NDC).

With a computer-controlled dispensing system, bar codes work as follows:
- The person receives a bar-coded identification (ID) bracelet when admitted to the agency. The bar code on the ID bracelet is linked to the person's computerized medical record.
- The agency has bar code scanners (bar code readers) linked to the computer system.
- You log onto the system. Then you bring up the person's computerized medical record.
- The drug orders appear on the screen. You select the drugs to be given at that time. A section of the cart opens for you to take the person's drugs out of the cart.
- At the bedside, you use a hand-held bar code scanner to read the bar code on your ID badge, the person's ID bracelet, and the unit-dose packet. All information is linked to the person's database.
  - *If there is an error*—An alarm sounds and an error message appears. The wrong drug, wrong dose, wrong time, or wrong person are examples. Or the person's drug orders have changed since the cart was filled.
  - *If the process is correct*—There is automatic documentation in the person's MAR.

Computer-controlled systems are safe and time efficient. However, the systems are costly.

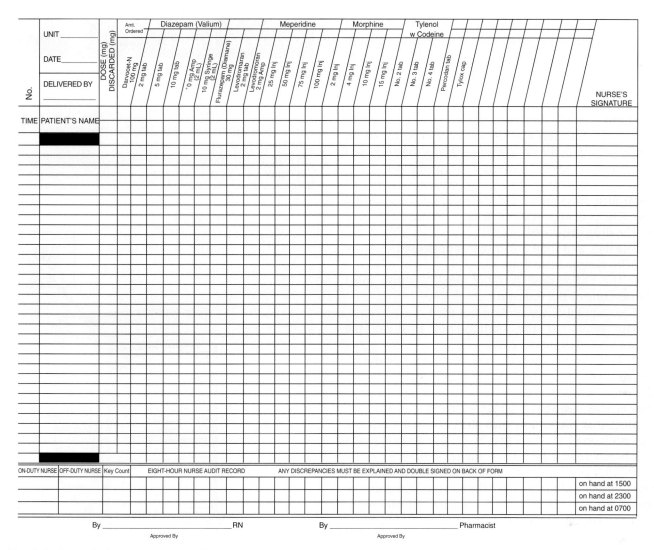

Fig. 9-6 Controlled substances inventory control sheet. (Courtesy The Nebraska Medical Center.)

Narcotic Control Systems

As explained in Chapter 3, federal laws regulate the use of controlled substances. These laws are strictly enforced.

In hospitals and nursing centers, controlled substances are issued in single-unit packages. The packages are kept in a locked cabinet in the medicine room or in a locked drawer in the drug cart. If a computer-controlled dispensing system is not used, the nurse manager or charge nurse is responsible for the key to the cabinet or drawer. The key is commonly called the "narcotics key." The cabinet or drawer is locked and the key returned to the nurse after the dose is obtained and the paperwork is complete.

An inventory control sheet lists each type of controlled substance and the number of doses issued (Fig. 9-6). The nurse receiving the drug supply:

- Counts and verifies the number and types of drugs received
- Signs a form indicating that the count is accurate
- Locks the controlled substances in a cabinet or drug cart drawer

The inventory control sheet is used to account for each drug and dose given. When a drug is removed from the locked storage area to give to a patient or resident, the following are documented on the inventory control sheet:

- The time
- The person's name
- The drug
- The dose
- The signature of the nurse or MA-C removing the drug

Sometimes the prescribed dose is smaller than that supplied. Disposal procedures are followed for the unused portion. When a nurse gives the drug, another nurse must check:

- The dose
- How the drug is prepared
- Disposal of the unused portion

Both nurses then sign the inventory control sheet. If you are giving the drug, a nurse checks the drug. You and the nurse sign the inventory control sheet.

With computer-controlled dispensing systems, all controlled drugs are kept in the automated dispensing cart. The system provides a detailed record of:

- The drug dispensed
- The date and time the drug was dispensed
- Who accessed the drug

If the entire dose was not used, a nurse must witness one of the following:

- The disposal of the portion not used
- The return of the portion not used to the automated dispensing cart

The inventory control sheet is a legal document. Follow the rules for recording (Chapter 4).

Narcotics Count. Controlled substances are inventoried at the end of each shift. A nurse from the on-coming shift counts the drugs with a nurse going off-duty. Each container and the remaining doses are counted. For each, the number remaining is added to the number used. The total should equal the number issued by the pharmacy. For example, the pharmacy issued 10 doses of a drug. Four were used during the shift. Six should remain in the container. With a computer-controlled dispensing system, the computer generates an end-of-shift report.

If the count is not correct, an investigation is started. The nurse manager or charge nurse will:

- Check with the nursing team to see if all controlled substances were charted
- Check all medical records to see if all controlled substances recorded are consistent with the inventory control sheet
- Contact the pharmacy and the nursing service office

During the narcotics count, unopened boxes and containers are inspected for tampering. Suspected tampering is reported to the pharmacy and the nursing service office.

See *Promoting Safety and Comfort: Narcotics Count.*

STORING DRUGS

All drugs must be safely stored. If the nursing unit has a medicine room, only authorized staff can enter the room. The room is locked when not in use.

Drug carts are locked when not in use. If you need to leave the drug cart to go into a person's room, lock

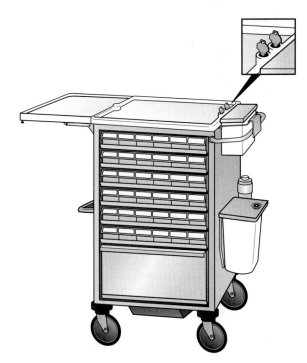

Fig. 9-7 Drug cart left unattended with keys (including the narcotics key) in the lock. This is a most unsafe practice.

the cart first. Always keep the keys with you. Do not leave keys in the lock or on the cart (Fig. 9-7).

Also follow these rules to properly store drugs:

- Open only one bin or drawer at a time. This prevents you from taking the wrong drugs or putting drugs back in the wrong bin or drawer.
- Store drugs in their original containers or unit dose packets.
- Store drugs as noted on the label or unit dose packet. Some drugs are stored in a refrigerator. The refrigerator is for drugs only, not food or fluids.
- Keep drug containers closed tightly. Moisture and heat can destroy some drugs.

Assisted Living Residences

In assisted living residences (ALRs), many residents use drug organizers (Chapter 7). They have sections for days and times. Some are for a week. Others are for a month. The person takes the right drugs on the right day and at the right time.

Drugs are kept in a secure place. This prevents others from taking them. If the ALR stores the drugs, they are kept in a locked container, cabinet, or area.

Some persons manage and store their own drugs. If the room is shared, each person's ability to safely have drugs is assessed. If safety is a factor, drugs are kept in a locked container.

Drugs must have the original pharmacy label. They are stored as directed on the label. For example, some drugs are refrigerated. Others are kept away from light. The label also has an expiration date. To dispose of expired or discontinued drugs, follow the ALR's procedures.

Storing Narcotics

Narcotics are double locked. If kept in a medicine room, there is a locked cabinet for narcotics. If a drug cart is used, the cart has a second lock for the narcotics drawer. The narcotics drawer is kept locked with the key removed. Only open the narcotics drawer when you need to give an ordered drug. Do not leave the key in the lock.

DISPOSING OF DRUGS

Drugs are disposed of for many reasons. They include:
* A person refuses to take a drug after it is ready to give.
* A drug is dropped on the floor or bed.
* You are to give only part of a drug dispensed.
* The drug's expiration date has passed.
* A drug became contaminated.
* The person was discharged.
* The person died.
* The doctor discontinued the drug.

To dispose of a drug, follow agency policy. Do not return an unused dose or an unused portion to a stock supply bottle. Also follow agency policy for recording drug disposal.

See *Promoting Safety and Comfort: Disposing of Drugs.*

PROMOTING SAFETY AND COMFORT
Disposing of Drugs

SAFETY

Drug diversion is a crime. To protect yourself from being suspected or accused of drug diversion, have someone watch you dispose of a drug. When recording, include the full name and title of the person who witnessed the disposal.

THE SIX RIGHTS

When giving drugs, always protect the person's safety. This involves the *Six Rights of Drug Administration:*
* Right drug
* Right time
* Right dose
* Right person
* Right route
* Right documentation

Right Drug

Many drugs have similar names and spellings. And some drugs have look-alike packaging. Serious harm or even death can occur if the wrong drug is given.

Do not assume that the pharmacist provided the right drug. Before giving any drug, compare the exact spelling of the drug prescribed against the MAR. Always read the drug label:
* Before removing the drug from the unit dose cart or from the shelf.
* Before preparing or measuring the prescribed dose.
* Before returning the drug to the shelf. Or before opening a unit dose packet. (Open the unit dose right before giving the drug to the person.)

Right Time

Many factors are involved in giving a drug at the right time. They include the drug order, standard administration times (Chapter 8), blood levels, drug absorption, and diagnostic tests.
* The drug order states how often to give the drug. Often standard abbreviations are used (Chapter 8).
* Each agency has standard drug administration times. The standard times help prevent drug errors. They also help the nursing and health teams plan care activities. For example, all drugs ordered 4 times a day are given at 0900, 1300, 1700, and 2100 (9:00 AM, 1:00 PM, 5:00 PM, and 9:00 PM).
* Some drugs are given at certain times. This allows laboratory and diagnostic tests to be done and the results reported before the drug is given. For example, a drug affects the time it takes for blood to clot. If another dose is given when the blood level is too high, the person is at risk for severe bleeding or hemorrhage. Therefore the drug is given only if the person's clotting time is within a certain range. Laboratory staff obtain a blood specimen and report the results before the nurse lets you give the drug. Sometimes laboratory or diagnostic tests are done before starting a drug or before continuing the drug therapy.

- Some drugs require a consistent blood level to be effective. Such drugs are given on a regular basis. Every 6 hours is an example. If the drug is not given on time, the blood level lowers. The drug is less effective.
- Drugs must be properly absorbed by the body. Some drugs are absorbed better when the stomach is empty. They are given 1 to 2 hours after meals. Drugs that irritate the stomach are given with food. Still other drugs are not given with dairy products or antacids.

See *Promoting Safety and Comfort: Right Time.*

PRN, One-Time-Only, and STAT Orders. Before giving a drug ordered PRN (when necessary; as needed), one-time-only, or STAT (at once; immediately), make sure no one else gave the drug. You must prevent a drug overdose. Check the person's chart and the MAR.

For a PRN order, also make sure that the time between doses has passed. For example, a drug for pain relief can be given every 4 hours. If only 2 hours have passed, you cannot give the drug. Remember to record PRN drugs at once on both the MAR and the progress notes.

Right Dose

You must give the right dose. The **dose** is the amount of drug to give. The person may suffer harm if too much or too little of a drug is given. To give the right dose:

- Compare the dose on the pharmacy label against the MAR.
- Use the correct measuring device for drugs in liquid form. A medicine cup and medicine dropper are examples.
- Report nausea and vomiting.

Calculating Drug Dosages. Sometimes the nursing team must calculate a drug dosage. For example, a drug is supplied in 25 mg tablets. The doctor ordered 50 mg of the drug. A drug calculation is necessary to determine how many tablets to give.

Some states and agencies do not allow MA-Cs to do any drug calculations. Other states and agencies allow MA-Cs to do or check simple drug calculations. See Appendix A for a review of arithmetic.

See *Promoting Safety and Comfort: Calculating Drug Dosages.*

Right Person

To make sure you have the right person, compare the information on the MAR against the person's ID bracelet. Do not check only the person's name. Some people have the same names or similar names. John Smith is a very common name. A similar name is Jon Smith.

The Joint Commission requires using at least two identifiers. An identifier cannot be the person's room or bed number. Some agencies require that the person state his or her name and birth date. Others require using the person's ID number. Always follow agency policy.

When identifying the person, also check for allergies. The person wears another bracelet for drug allergies.

See *Focus on Older Persons: Right Person.*

See *Promoting Safety and Comfort: Right Person.*

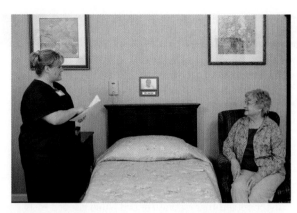

Fig. 9-8 The person's photo is at the headboard. Her name is under the photo. The nursing assistant is using the photo to identify the person.

Right Route

The drug order states the route for administration. The **route** means how and where the drug enters the body. Box 9-1, on p. 116 lists the routes of drug administration.

Not every drug can be given by every route. Never change the route of administration. And never change the dosage form. Only the doctor can make such changes by changing the drug order.

The absorption rate varies with the route used.

- Intravenous (IV)—the drug is given directly into the bloodstream. This route has the most rapid onset of action. It also presents the greatest risk for adverse affects.
- Intramuscular (IM)—after the IV route, the IM route provides the next fastest onset of action.
- Subcutaneous (subcut; subcutaneously)—after the IV and IM routes, it provides the next fastest onset of action.
- Intradermal—a small volume of drug is injected into the dermal skin layer. Absorption is slow.

As an MA-C, you can only give drugs by certain routes. You must know what your state and agency allow you to do. A nurse gives the drugs that you are not allowed to give. Remember the following:

- Always give the drug by the route stated on the order, the MAR, and the pharmacy label. Make sure the information from the three sources is the same. If not, check with the nurse.
- Never change the route.
- Never give a drug by a route not allowed by your state and agency. For example, your state and agency do not allow MA-Cs to give IV drugs. Therefore you never give a drug IV. Or your state and agency do not allow you to give injections. Therefore you never give drugs by the intramuscular, subcutaneous, and intradermal routes.

See *Promoting Safety and Comfort: Right Route,* p. 116.

BOX 9-1 Routes for Giving Drugs

ROUTE	NAME
Mouth	Oral
Skin	Topical
Under the tongue	Sublingual
Between the cheek and molar teeth	Buccal
Eye	Ophthalmic
Ear	Otic
Nose	Nasal
Respiratory tract	Inhalation
Vagina	Vaginal
Stomach	Gastric
Rectum	Rectal
Dermal skin layer	Intradermal
Between the dermis and muscle layer	Subcutaneous
Muscle	Intramuscular
Vein	Intravenous

BOX 9-2 Rules for "Right Documentation"

- Follow the rules for recording. See Chapter 4.
- Follow agency policy for recording drugs.
- Record as soon as possible after giving the drug.
- Record the following for every drug you give:
  - Date and time you gave the drug
  - The name of the drug
  - The dose
  - The route
  - The site of administration
- Record PRN drugs on the MAR or on the PRN or unscheduled medication record. Also record PRN drugs in the progress notes. See Chapter 8 for recording PRN drugs.
- Record when a drug was not given and why.
- Record the person's refusal to take a drug. Also include the reason for the refusal.
- Do not record a drug until after it is taken by the person.
- Follow agency policy for reporting drug errors.

PROMOTING SAFETY AND COMFORT
Right Route

SAFETY

The oral route is usually safe if the person is conscious and can swallow. It is not safe if the person is unconscious or has *dysphagia* (difficulty swallowing). To safely swallow oral drugs, the person must be awake, alert, able to understand, and able to swallow. Tell the nurse at once if the person shows signs of an altered level of consciousness, confusion, disorientation, or problems swallowing. The nurse will give the drug or ask the doctor to change the route ordered.

Right Documentation

You must record giving a drug as soon as possible. Otherwise it is assumed the drug was not given. A nurse or another MA-C may give another dose thinking that the drug was not given. The overdose can cause the person serious harm or even death.

With unit dose and computer charting systems, you record right after giving the drug. You record on the MAR or make a computer entry. For the "right documentation," follow the rules in Box 9-2.

THE SELF-ADMINISTRATION OF DRUGS

In some agencies and settings, patients and residents take their own drugs. This is called *self-directed medication management*. The person knows his or her drugs by name, color, or shape. The person knows what drugs to take, the correct doses, and when and how to take them. The person is able to question changes in the usual drug routine. For example, the person comments

that a pill is not broken in half. Or the person says that a pill looks different. Report comments or questions to the nurse.

Your role may involve one or more of the following:
- Reminding the person it is time to take a drug
- Reading the drug label to the person
- Opening containers for persons who cannot do so
- Checking the dosage against the drug label
- Providing water, juice, milk, crackers, applesauce, or other food and fluids as needed
- Making sure the person takes the right drug, the right amount, at the right time, and by the right route
- Charting that the person took or refused to take the drug (right documentation)
- Storing drugs

Many people find that drug organizers are helpful. Some people need medication reminders. A **medication reminder** means reminding the person to take drugs, observing them being taken as prescribed, and charting that they were taken.

See *Focus on Communication: The Self-Administration of Drugs*.

PREVENTING DRUG ERRORS

Drug errors can cause the person serious harm, even death. These are know as adverse drug events (ADEs). Box 9-3 lists examples of drug errors. You can prevent drug errors by following the:
- *Six Rights of Drug Administration*
- Rules listed in Box 9-4

FOCUS ON COMMUNICATION

The Self-Administration of Drugs

To remind a person to take his or her drugs, you can say:
- "Ms. Epstein, it's time to take your 8 o'clock pills."
- "Mr. Ladd, you'll need to take your pills in about 10 minutes."
- "Mrs. Young, are you ready to take your pills?"
To read a drug label to a person, read the following:
- The name of the person on the drug label
- The name of the drug
- How to take the drug (by mouth, with food, with a full glass of water, apply to the skin, rectally, and so on)
- The dosage
- When to take the drug (before meals, with meals, after meals, and so on)
- How often to take the drug
- Warnings and other information on the drug label

BOX 9-3 Examples of Drug Errors

PRESCRIBING ERRORS
- Prescribing the wrong drug for the person's diagnosis
- Prescribing a drug to which the person is allergic
- Prescribing the wrong dose for the person's diagnosis

TRANSCRIPTION ERRORS
- Misinterpreting or misunderstanding the drug ordered or the directions
- Interpreting hand-writing that is not legible
- Using unapproved abbreviations
- Omitting a drug order
- Using the wrong spelling
- Writing the wrong dates or times

DISPENSING
- Sending the wrong drug or dose to the nursing unit
- Using the wrong formulation
- Using the wrong dosage form

GIVING DRUGS
- Giving the wrong drug
- Giving the wrong dose
- Giving an extra dose
- Giving a drug not ordered for the person
- Missing or skipping a dose
- Giving a drug at the wrong time
- Giving the drug in the wrong way
- Not recording that a drug was given

BOX 9-4 Safety Rules for Giving Drugs

- Follow the *Six Rights of Drug Administration* p. 113.
- Store all drugs properly (p. 112).
- Make sure you have good lighting. You must be able to read the MAR and drug labels correctly.
- Stay focused. Do not allow yourself to become distracted. Ask other staff not to interrupt you unless the situation is critical.
- Keep your working area clean, neat, and orderly.
- Check the container label for the drug name, dose, and route.
- Check the person's chart, Kardex, MAR, and ID bracelet for allergies. Also ask the person before giving a drug if he or she has any allergies.
- Check the person's chart, Kardex, and MAR for rotation schedules for drugs applied to the skin (Chapter 11).
- Know why the drug was ordered. Also know its side effects and possible adverse reactions.
- Calculate drug dosages accurately (if allowed by your state and agency). Ask a nurse to check your calculation.
- Identify the person before giving any drug.
- Position the person for the route of administration. For example, for an oral drug the person should be in a sitting or Fowler's position to promote swallowing. Check the care plan and with the nurse for any position limits.
- Have correct fluids ready for the person to swallow oral drugs.
- Stay with the person to make sure that all drugs have been swallowed. If necessary, check the person's mouth—under the tongue and between teeth and the cheeks.
- Follow agency policy for self-administered drugs.
- Never leave a drug in the person's room for the person to take later (unless there is a doctor's order to do so). Always make sure the person takes the drug in your presence.
- Never leave a drug unattended.
- Refer any questions about the person's drug or treatment plan to the nurse.

Continued

BOX 9-4	Safety Rules for Giving Drugs—cont'd

- Do not prepare or give a drug if:
  - The container is not properly labeled
  - You cannot fully and clearly read the label
- Give only those drugs that your state and agency allow you to give.
- Give drugs prepared only by a pharmacist. Do not give drugs prepared by a nurse or another MA-C. Do not assume that the nurse or MA-C followed the six rights.
- Check the drug name, dose, how often to give the drug, and the route against the order.
- Do not return an unused portion or drug dose to a stock supply container.
- Do not give any oral drug to a person who is comatose.
- Do not mix a drug in liquid form with water or other fluid unless directed to do so.
- Ask the nurse if you have questions or if you are not sure about any aspect of giving a drug to any person.
- Practice hand hygiene:
  - Before preparing a person's drugs
  - After contact with the person or items in his or her care setting

- Never touch the actual drug with your hands.
- Do not let the drug container touch any part of a medicine cup or other device (Fig. 9-9).
- Check the drug carefully. Many drugs and drug forms look alike.
- Listen to the person. The person may know drugs by name, color, or shape. The person may know what drugs to take, the correct doses, and when and how to take them. The person may question changes in the usual drug routine. For example, the person comments that a tablet is not broken in half. Or the person says that a tablet looks different. Report comments or questions to the nurse.
- Observe the person for possible side effects or adverse reactions.
- Leave the medicine room or drug cart neat and orderly. Clean and straighten the area as needed. Restock medicine cups, straws, and other supplies.
- Make sure the drug cabinet or drug cart is locked.

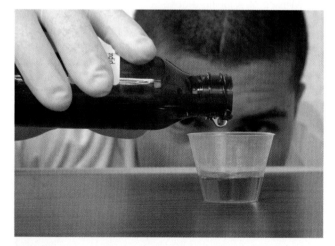

Fig. 9-9 The drug container does not touch the medicine cup. (From Perry AG, Potter PA: *Clinical nursing skills & techniques,* ed 6, St. Louis, 2006, Mosby.)

Reporting Drug Errors

If you do make a drug error, complete an incident report. Agency policy will require that you describe exactly what happened. Do not give your opinions or thoughts about why the error occurred. In the incident report, record:

- The date and time
- The time the drug was ordered

- The drug name, dosage, and route of administration
- How you found out about the error
- The person's response
- Signs and symptoms of adverse reactions
- The date and time that you reported the error to the nurse

Do not record the error in the progress notes. The nurse will contact the doctor about the error.

PREVENTING INFECTION

When giving drugs, you will have contact with many patients and residents. You will have contact with their bodies and care equipment. As you go from one person to another, you must protect them and yourself from infection. An **infection** is a disease state resulting from the invasion and growth of microbes in the body. Some microbes are harmful and can cause infections. They are called *pathogens. Non-pathogens* are microbes that do not usually cause an infection.

See *Focus on Older Persons: Infection.*

Medical Asepsis

Asepsis is being free of disease-producing microbes. Microbes are everywhere. Measures are needed to achieve asepsis. *Medical asepsis (clean technique)* is the practice used to:

- Remove or destroy pathogens. The number of pathogens is reduced.
- Prevent pathogens from spreading from one person or place to another person or place.

Surgical asepsis (sterile technique) is the practice that keeps items free of *all* microbes. *Sterile* means the absence of *all* microbes—pathogens and non-pathogens.

Sterilization is the process of destroying *all* microbes (pathogens and non-pathogens).

Contamination is the process of becoming unclean. In medical asepsis, an item or area is clean when it is free of pathogens. The item or area is contaminated if pathogens are present. A sterile item or area is contaminated when pathogens or non-pathogens are present.

Common Aseptic Practices

Aseptic practices prevent the spread of microbes. Remember to wash your hands:

- After urinating or having a bowel movement.
- After changing tampons or sanitary pads.
- After contact with your own or another person's blood, body fluids, secretions, or excretions. This includes saliva, vomitus, urine, feces, vaginal discharge, mucus, semen, wound drainage, pus, and respiratory secretions.
- After coughing, sneezing, or blowing your nose.
- Before and after handling, preparing, or eating food.
- After smoking a cigarette, cigar, or pipe.

Hand Hygiene

Hand hygiene is the easiest and most important way to prevent the spread of infection. Your hands are used for almost everything. They are easily contaminated. They can spread microbes to other persons or items. *Practice hand hygiene before and after giving drugs or other care measures.* See Box 9-5 for the rules of hand hygiene.

See *Promoting Safety and Comfort: Hand Hygiene* on p. 121.

Text continued on p. 122

BOX 9-5 Rules of Hand Hygiene

- Wash your hands (with soap and water) when they are visibly dirty or soiled with blood, body fluids, secretions, or excretions.
- Wash your hands (with soap and water) before eating and after using a restroom.
- Wash your hands (with soap and water) if exposure to the anthrax spore is suspected or proven.
- Use an alcohol-based hand rub to decontaminate your hands if they are not visibly soiled. (If an alcohol-based hand rub is not available, wash your hands with soap and water.) Follow this rule in the following clinical situations:
  - Before having direct contact with a person.
  - After contact with the person's intact skin. For example, after taking a pulse or blood pressure or after moving a person.

- After contact with body fluids or excretions, mucous membranes, non-intact skin, and wound dressings if hands are not visibly soiled.
- When moving from a contaminated body site to a clean body site during care activities.
- After contact with objects (including equipment) in the person's care setting.
- After removing gloves.
- Follow these rules for washing your hands with soap and water. See procedure: *Hand Washing*, p. 121.
  - Wash your hands under warm running water. Do not use hot water.
  - Stand away from the sink. Do not let your hands, body, or uniform touch the sink. The sink is contaminated (Fig. 9-10, p. 120).

Modified from Centers for Disease Control and Prevention: Guideline for hand hygiene in health-care settings. *Morbidity and Mortality Weekly Report*, Vol 51, No. RR-16, October 25, 2002.

Continued

BOX 9-5 **Rules of Hand Hygiene—cont'd**

- Do not touch the inside of the sink at any time.
- Keep your hands and forearms lower than your elbows. Your hands are dirtier than your elbows and forearms. If you hold your hands and forearms up, dirty water runs from your hands to your elbows. Those areas become contaminated.
- Rub your palms together to work up a good lather (Fig. 9-11). The rubbing action helps remove microbes and dirt.
- Pay attention to areas often missed during hand washing—thumbs, knuckles, sides of the hands, little fingers, and under the nails.
- Clean fingernails by rubbing the fingertips against your palms (Fig. 9-12).
- Use a nail file or orange stick to clean under fingernails (Fig. 9-13). Microbes easily grow under the fingernails.
- Wash your hands for at least 15 seconds. Wash your hands longer if they are dirty or soiled with blood, body fluids, secretions, or excretions. Use your judgment.
- Use a clean, dry paper towel to dry your hands.
- Dry your hands starting at the fingertips. Work up to your forearms. You will dry the cleanest area first.
- Use a clean, dry paper towel for each faucet to turn the water off (Fig. 9-14). Faucets are contaminated. The paper towels prevent clean hands from becoming contaminated again.
- Follow these rules when decontaminating your hands with an alcohol-based hand rub:
  - Apply the product to the palm of one hand. Follow the manufacturer's instructions for the amount to use.
  - Rub your hands together.
  - Make sure you cover all surfaces of your hands and fingers.
  - Continue rubbing your hands together until your hands are dry.
- Apply hand lotion or cream after hand hygiene. This prevents the skin from chapping and drying. Skin breaks can occur in chapped and dry skin. Skin breaks are portals of entry for microbes.

Modified from Centers for Disease Control and Prevention: Guideline for hand hygiene in health-care settings. *Morbidity and Mortality Weekly Report,* Vol 51, No. RR-16, October 25, 2002.

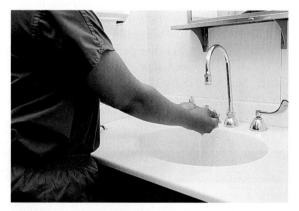

Fig. 9-10 The uniform does not touch the sink. Soap and water are within reach. Hands are lower than the elbows. Hands do not touch the inside of the sink.

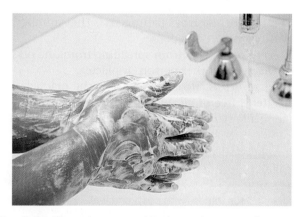

Fig. 9-11 The palms are rubbed together to work up a good lather.

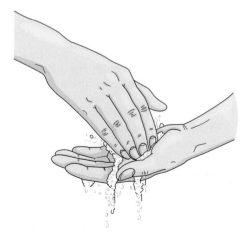

Fig. 9-12 The fingertips are rubbed against the palms to clean under the fingernails.

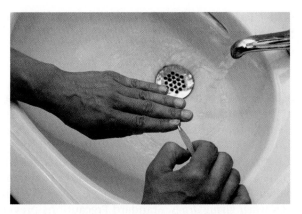

Fig. 9-13 A nail file is used to clean under the fingernails.

PROMOTING SAFETY AND COMFORT
Hand Hygiene

SAFETY
You use your hands in almost every task. They can pick up microbes from one person, place, or thing. Your hands transfer them to other people, places, and things. That is why hand hygiene is so very important.

COMFORT
You will practice hand hygiene very often during your shift. Hand lotions and hand creams help prevent chapping and dry skin. Apply hand lotion or cream as often as needed.

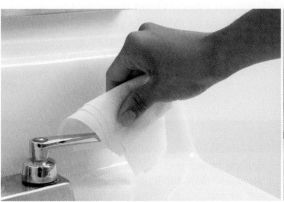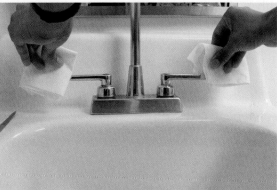

Fig. 9-14 A paper towel is used to turn off each faucet.

HAND WASHING

PROCEDURE

1 See *Promoting Safety and Comfort: Hand Hygiene.*
2 Make sure you have soap, paper towels, an orange stick or nail file, and a wastebasket. Collect missing items.
3 Push your watch up your arm 4 to 5 inches. If your uniform sleeves are long, push them up too.
4 Stand away from the sink so your clothes do not touch the sink. Stand so the soap and faucet are easy to reach (see Fig. 9-10). Do not touch the inside of the sink at any time.
5 Turn on and adjust the water until it feels warm.
6 Wet your wrists and hands. Keep your hands lower than your elbows. Be sure to wet the area 3 to 4 inches above your wrists.
7 Apply about 1 teaspoon of soap to your hands.
8 Rub your palms together and interlace your fingers to work up a good lather (see Fig. 9-11). This step should last at least 15 seconds.
9 Wash each hand and wrist thoroughly. Clean well between the fingers.

10 Clean under the fingernails. Rub your fingertips against your palms (see Fig. 9-12).
11 Clean under the fingernails with a nail file or orange stick (see Fig. 9-13). This step is done for the first hand washing of the day and when your hands are highly soiled.
12 Rinse your wrists and hands well. Water flows from the arms to the hands.
13 Repeat steps 7–12, if needed.
14 Dry your wrists and hands with a clean, dry paper towel. Pat dry starting at your fingertips.
15 Discard the paper towel into the wastebasket.
16 Turn off the faucets with clean, dry paper towels (see Fig. 9-14). Use a clean paper towel for each faucet.
17 Discard the paper towels into the wastebasket.

Isolation Precautions

Blood, body fluids, secretions, and excretions can transmit pathogens. Sometimes barriers are needed to prevent their escape. The pathogens are kept within a certain area. Usually the area is the person's room. This requires isolation procedures.

The *Guideline for Isolation Precautions: Preventing Transmission of Infectious Agents in Healthcare Settings 2007* is followed. The guideline was issued by the Centers for Disease Control and Prevention (CDC). Isolation precautions prevent the spread of *communicable diseases (contagious diseases)*. They are diseases caused by pathogens that spread easily.

Isolation precautions are based on *clean* and *dirty*. *Clean* areas or objects are free of pathogens. They are not contaminated. *Dirty* areas or objects are contaminated with pathogens. If a *clean* area or object has contact with something *dirty*, the clean area or object is now dirty. *Clean* and *dirty* also depend on how the pathogen is spread.

The CDC's isolation precautions guideline has two tiers of precautions:

- Standard Precautions
- Transmission-Based Precautions (Appendix B)

Standard Precautions. Standard Precautions are part of the CDC's *Guideline for Isolation Precautions: Preventing Transmission of Infectious Agents in Healthcare Settings 2007* (Box 9-6). They reduce the risk of spreading pathogens. They also reduce the risk of spreading known and unknown infections. *Standard Precautions are used for all persons whenever care is given. This includes when giving drugs.* Standard Precautions prevent the spread of infection from:

- Blood
- All body fluids, secretions, and excretions (except sweat) even if blood is not visible
- Non-intact skin (skin with open breaks)
- Mucous membranes

See *Promoting Safety and Comfort: Standard Precautions*, p. 124.

BOX 9-6 **Standard Precautions**

HAND HYGIENE
- Follow the rules for hand hygiene. See Box 9-5.
- Avoid unnecessary touching of surfaces close to the person. This prevents contamination of clean hands from environmental surfaces. It also prevents the transmission of pathogens from contaminated hands to other surfaces.
- Do not wear fake nails or nail extenders if you will have contact with persons at risk for infection or other adverse outcomes.

PERSONAL PROTECTIVE EQUIPMENT (PPE)
- Wear PPE when contact with blood or body fluids is likely.
- Do not contaminate your clothing or skin when removing PPE.
- Remove and discard PPE before leaving the person's room or care setting.

GLOVES
- Wear gloves when contact with the following is likely:
  - Blood
  - Potentially infectious materials (body fluids, secretions, and excretions are examples)
  - Mucous membranes
  - Non-intact skin
  - Skin that may be contaminated (for example, a person incontinent of stool or urine)

- Wear gloves that fit and are appropriate for the task:
  - Wear disposable gloves to provide direct care to the person.
  - Wear disposable gloves or utility gloves for cleaning equipment or care settings.
- Remove gloves after contact with the person or the person's care setting. The care setting includes equipment used in the person's care.
- Remove gloves after contact with care equipment.
- Do not wear the same pair of gloves to care for more than one person. Remove gloves after contact with a person and before going to another person.
- Do not wash gloves for re-use with different persons.
- Change gloves during care if your hands will move from a contaminated body site to a clean body site.

GOWNS
- Wear a gown that is appropriate to the task.
- Wear a gown to protect your skin and clothing when contact with blood, body fluids, secretions, or excretions is likely.
- Wear a gown for direct contact with a person if he or she has uncontained secretions or excretions.
- Remove the gown and perform hand hygiene before leaving the person's room or care setting.
- Do not re-use gowns even for repeated contacts with the same person.

Modified from Siegel JD, Rhinehart E, Jackson M, Chiarello L, and the Healthcare Infection Control Practices Advisory Committee: *Guideline for Isolation Precautions: Preventing Transmission of Infectious Agents in Healthcare Settings 2007*, June 2007.

Continued

BOX 9-6 Standard Precautions—cont'd

MOUTH, NOSE, AND EYE PROTECTION

- Wear PPE—masks, goggles, face shields—for procedures and tasks that are likely to cause splashes and sprays of blood, body fluids, secretions, or excretions.
- Wear PPE—mask, goggles, face shield—appropriate for the procedure or task.
- Wear gloves, a gown, and one of the following for procedures that are likely to cause sprays of respiratory secretions:
  - A face shield that fully covers the front and sides of the face
  - A mask with attached shield
  - A mask and goggles

RESPIRATORY HYGIENE/COUGH ETIQUETTE

- Instruct persons with respiratory symptoms to:
  - Cover the nose and mouth when coughing or sneezing.
  - Use tissues to contain respiratory secretions.
  - Dispose of tissues in the nearest waste container after use.
  - Perform hand hygiene after contact with respiratory secretions.
- Provide visitors with masks according to agency policy.

CARE EQUIPMENT

- Wear appropriate PPE when handling care equipment that is visibly soiled with blood, body fluids, secretions, or excretions.
- Wear appropriate PPE when handling care equipment that may have been in contact with blood, body fluids, secretions, or excretions.
- Remove organic material before disinfection and sterilization procedures. Use cleaning agents according to agency policy.

CARE OF THE ENVIRONMENT

- Follow agency policies and procedures for cleaning and maintaining surfaces. Environmental surfaces and care equipment are examples. Surfaces near the person may need more frequent cleaning and maintenance—door knobs, bed rails, overbed tables, toilet surfaces and areas, and so on.
- Clean and disinfect multi-use electronic equipment according to agency policy. This includes:
  - Items used by patients and residents
  - Items used to give care
  - Mobile devices that are moved in and out of patient or resident rooms
- Follow these rules for toys used by pediatric patients or child play toys in waiting areas:
  - Select play toys that can be easily cleaned and disinfected.
  - Do not allow use of stuffed furry toys if they will be shared.
  - Clean and disinfect large stationary toys (for example, climbing equipment) at least weekly and whenever visibly soiled.
  - Rinse toys with water after disinfection if they are likely to be mouthed by children. Or wash them in a dishwasher.
  - Clean and disinfect a toy immediately when it requires cleaning. Or store the toy in a labeled container away from toys that are clean and ready for use.

TEXTILES AND LAUNDRY

- Handle used textiles and fabrics (linens) with minimum agitation. This is done to avoid contamination of air, surfaces, and other persons.

WORKER SAFETY

- Protect yourself and others from exposure to bloodborne pathogens. This includes how to handle needles and other sharps. Follow federal and state standards and guidelines. See the Bloodborne Pathogen Standard (p. 124).
- Use a mouthpiece, resuscitation bag, or other ventilation device during resuscitation to prevent contact with the person's mouth and oral secretions.

PATIENT OR RESIDENT PLACEMENT

- A private room is preferred if the person is at risk for transmitting the infection to others.
- Follow the nurse's instructions if a private room is not available.

Modified from Siegel JD, Rhinehart E, Jackson M, Chiarello L, and the Healthcare Infection Control Practices Advisory Committee: *Guideline for Isolation Precautions: Preventing Transmission of Infectious Agents in Healthcare Settings 2007,* June 2007.

The Bloodborne Pathogen Standard

The human immunodeficiency virus (HIV) and the hepatitis B virus (HBV) are major health concerns. The health team is at risk for exposure to these viruses. The Bloodborne Pathogen Standard is intended to protect them from exposure. It is a regulation of the Occupational Safety and Health Administration (OSHA).

HIV and HBV are found in the blood. They are bloodborne pathogens. They exit the body through blood. They are spread to others by blood. Other potentially infectious materials (OPIM) also spread the viruses. See Appendix C for the Bloodborne Pathogen Standard.

⊙ GIVING DRUGS

As listed in Box 9-1, drugs can be given by different routes. No matter the route used, safe administration is always the goal. Box 9-4 lists the rules for giving drugs safely.

The procedure described here is offered as a guideline only. The order of steps depends on the drug distribution system used in your agency. For example, if drugs are prepared in a medicine room at the nurses' station, you will prepare the drug and then take it to the person's room. If using a unit dose or computer-controlled system, drugs are prepared by or in the person's room.

See *Promoting Safety and Comfort: Giving Drugs.*

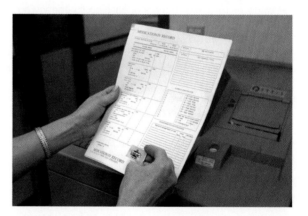

Fig. 9-15 The drug order on the MAR is compared against the pharmacy label on the drug container. (Courtesy Rick Brady, from Lilley LL and others: *Pharmacology and the nursing process,* ed 5, St Louis, 2007, Mosby.)

GIVING A DRUG

QUALITY OF LIFE

Remember to:
- Knock before entering the person's room.
- Address the person by name.
- Introduce yourself by name and title.

- Explain the procedure to the person before beginning and during the procedure.
- Protect the person's rights during the procedure.
- Handle the person gently during the procedure.

PRE-PROCEDURE

1 Check the drug order. **(First safety check.)** Focus on the:
- *Right drug*
- *Right time*
- *Right dose*
- *Right person*
- *Right route*

2 Check with the nurse if you have any questions.
3 Practice hand hygiene.
4 Collect needed items. For example, you might need a medicine or souffle cup, juice, or a straw. This will depend on the drug form and how the drug is given. See Chapters 10, 11, 12, and 13.

PROCEDURE

5 Unlock the drug cart.
6 Read the order on the MAR.
7 Select the right drug from the person's drawer (see Fig. 9-5).
8 Compare the drug order on the MAR against the pharmacy label on the drug container (Fig. 9-15). **(Second safety check.)** Check for the:
- *Right drug*
- *Right time*
- *Right dose*
- *Right person*
- *Right route*

9 Check the drug container for an expiration date.
10 Compare the drug order on the MAR against the pharmacy label on the drug container. **(Third safety check.)** Check for the:
- *Right drug*
- *Right time*
- *Right dose*
- *Right person*
- *Right route*

11 Open the container. If pouring from a bottle, pour the correct dosage. Return extra drugs to the container. (NOTE: Do not open a unit dose container until you are at the person's bedside.)

12 Close the container. Compare the drug order on the MAR against the pharmacy label on the drug container. **(Fourth safety check.)** Check for the:
- *Right drug*
- *Right time*
- *Right dose*
- *Right person*
- *Right route*

13 Return the container to the drawer.
14 Repeat steps 6–13 for each drug ordered for the person.
15 Lock the drug cart if you will leave it outside the person's room.
16 Identify the person. Check the ID bracelet against the MAR. Make sure you use at least two identifiers according to agency policy. Also call the person by name. Follow agency policy if using a bar code scanner.
17 Provide for privacy.
18 Obtain required measurements as noted on the MAR. For example: measure the person's blood pressure or pulse. Note the measurement on the MAR.
19 Position the person appropriate for the drug form. See Chapters 10, 11, 12, and 13.
20 Give the person the drugs. See Chapters 10, 11, 12, and 13.

POST-PROCEDURE

21 Discard the medicine or souffle cup or unit dose packages.
22 Provide for the person's comfort. See the inside of the front book cover.
23 Unscreen the person.
24 Complete a safety check before leaving the room. See the inside of the front book cover.
25 Practice hand hygiene.

26 Record the *right documentation* on the MAR:
- The date, time, drug name, dosage, and route of administration
- The application site
- Your name or initials

27 Report and record any specific patient or resident observations or concerns.

REVIEW QUESTIONS

Circle the **BEST** answer.

1 A drug order was received from the pharmacy. What should you do *first?*
 a Tell the nurse.
 b Compare the pharmacy label against the drug order on the MAR.
 c Give the ordered dose as soon as possible.
 d Transcribe the order on the MAR.

2 A drug is dispensed in a packet for each drug ordered. This is done with the
 a floor stock system
 b individual prescription order system
 c unit dose system
 d narcotic control system

3 The pharmacy sends a 3- to 5-day supply of an ordered drug to the nursing unit. This is done with the
 a floor stock system
 b individual prescription order system
 c unit dose system
 d computer-controlled dispensing system

4 Ordered drugs are readily available with the
 a floor stock system
 b individual prescription order system
 c unit dose system
 d narcotic control system

5 Bar codes are used with the
 a floor stock system
 b individual prescription order system
 c unit dose system
 d computer-controlled dispensing system

6 Which is used to account for each narcotic and the dose given?
 a inventory control sheet
 b MAR
 c doctor's order form
 d unscheduled medication record

7 Only a portion of a controlled substance dose is ordered. What should you do with the unused portion?
 a Return it to the pharmacy.
 b Return it to the medicine room.
 c Ask a nurse to watch you dispose of the unused portion.
 d Save the unused portion for the next dose.

8 A narcotics count is required
 a at the end of each shift
 b every week
 c every month
 d whenever a dose is removed

9 The pharmacy issued 12 doses of a controlled substance. Eight were used. How many should remain?
 a 2   c 6
 b 4   d 8

10 You need to leave a drug cart to go into a person's room. What should you do?
 a Lock the cart and take the keys with you.
 b Lock the cart and leave the keys in the lock.
 c Leave the cart open if you can see it from the bedside.
 d Ask a co-worker to guard the cart.

11 The following statements are about storing drugs. Which is *false?*
 a Drugs are stored in their original containers.
 b Refrigerated drugs are stored with food and fluids.
 c Drug containers are kept tightly closed.
 d One drug bin or drawer is open at a time.

12 Which is commonly used in assisted living residences to store drugs?
 a medicine room   c drug organizer
 b drug cart   d bedside drawer

13 Controlled substances are
 a double locked
 b kept with the nurse
 c stored in the person's drawer or bin
 d kept in the pharmacy

14 You have a drug ready to give. The person refuses to take the drug. What should you do with the drug?
 a Return it to the drug cart.
 b Send it to the pharmacy.
 c Leave it at the person's bedside.
 d Dispose of it following agency policy.

15 You dropped a drug on the floor. What should you do?
 a Dispose of the drug.
 b Decontaminate the drug.
 c Sterilize the drug.
 d Keep the drug for yourself.

16 To give the right drug, always compare the exact spelling of the drug on the label against the
 a MAR   c progress notes
 b Kardex   d doctor's order form

17 To give the right drug, you always read the drug label before the following *except*
 a removing the drug from the drug cart or from the shelf
 b preparing the prescribed dose
 c returning the drug to the shelf
 d charting that you gave the drug

18 A drug was ordered to be given one-time-only. You should
 a check to see if it was given
 b give the drug as soon as it arrives from the pharmacy
 c ask the person when he or she would like to take the drug
 d give the drug with those ordered for 0800

REVIEW QUESTIONS

19 The right dose is
   a the dosage sent by the pharmacy
   b the amount of drug to give
   c the amount of drug in the unit dose packet
   d the amount needed to maintain a blood level

20 To make sure you give the right drug to the right person, you must use
   a two identifiers
   b the person's name and room number
   c the person's name
   d the person's name and bed number

21 Before giving a drug, when should you identify the person?
   a right before giving the drug
   b when you arrive at the person's bedside
   c before you open the person's drug bin
   d after deciding how to give the drug

22 The drug route is
   a where the drug is absorbed in the body
   b how and where the drug enters the body
   c how the drug is supplied
   d the supplies used to give the drug

23 Which route provides the fastest absorption rate?
   a IV   c subcutaneous
   b IM   d oral

24 You are using a unit dose system. When should you record giving a drug?
   a when the drug is ready to give
   b after giving the drug
   c after returning to the nurses' station
   d at the end of your shift

25 Self-directed medication management means that patients and residents
   a order their own drugs
   b take their own drugs
   c buy their own drugs
   d record their own drugs

26 Your role in self-directed medication management may involve the following *except*
   a ordering drugs
   b reminding the person to take a drug
   c checking the dosage against the drug label
   d charting that the person took or refused to take a drug

27 You made a drug error. You must complete
   a an inventory control sheet
   b the MAR
   c an incident report
   d the required part of the progress notes

28 Which action is *not* safe?
   a having good lighting to read the MAR and drug labels
   b leaving drugs in a room for the person to take later
   c giving drugs prepared only by a pharmacist
   d making sure the drug cart is locked

29 When giving drugs, you must practice the following *except*
   a hand hygiene
   b Standard Precautions
   c surgical asepsis
   d the Bloodborne Pathogen Standard

30 How many safety checks are done when giving drugs?
   a 1
   b 2
   c 3
   d 4

Circle T if the statement is true. Circle F if the statement is false.

31 T F A drug is ordered for 0900 and 2100. You must give the doses exactly at 0900 and 2100.

32 T F A PRN drug is ordered to be given every 4 hours as needed. Three hours have passed since the last dose. You can give another dose.

33 T F Your state does not allow you to give IV drugs. However, you can give an IV drug in an emergency.

34 T F Giving the wrong drug is a drug error.

35 T F Skipping a dose is a drug error.

36 T F Giving the drug at the wrong time is a drug error.

37 T F Giving a drug to the wrong person is a drug error.

38 T F You did not record giving a drug. This is a drug error.

39 T F When giving drugs, you should help your co-workers give care.

40 T F Before giving any drug, you should check if the person has allergies.

41 T F You calculated a drug dosage. You should ask another MA-C to check your calculation.

42 T F Oral drugs are ordered for a person who is comatose. You can give the oral drugs.

Answers to these questions are on p. 444.

10

Oral, Sublingual, and Buccal Drugs

OBJECTIVES

- Define the key terms and key abbreviations used in this chapter.
- Identify solid and liquid oral dose forms.
- Explain how to use the equipment for giving oral dose forms.
- Know the equivalents for household, apothecary, and metric measurements.
- Explain how to give oral, sublingual, and buccal drugs.
- Perform the procedures described in this chapter.

PROCEDURES

- Giving an Oral Drug—Solid Form
- Giving an Oral Drug—Liquid Form

KEY TERMS

buccal Inside the cheek (*bucco*)

capsule A gelatin container that holds a drug in a dry powder or liquid form

elixir A clear liquid made up of a drug dissolved in alcohol and water

emulsion An oral dose form containing small droplets of water-in-oil or oil-in-water

lavage Washing out the stomach

lozenge A flat disk containing a medicinal agent with a flavored base; troche

medicine cup A plastic container with measurement scales

medicine dropper A small glass or plastic tube with a hollow rubber ball at one end

souffle cup A small paper or plastic cup used for solid drug forms

sublingual Under (*sub*) the tongue (*lingual*)

suspension A liquid containing solid drug particles

KEY TERMS—cont'd

syringe A plastic measuring device with three parts—tip, barrel, and plunger

syrup An oral dose form containing a drug dissolved in sugar

tablet A dried, powdered drug compressed into a small disk

troche See "lozenge"

KEY ABBREVIATIONS

GI Gastro-intestinal
ISMP Institute for Safe Medication Practices
PO By mouth (per os)

Oral drugs are given by mouth—the *oral route*. Drugs are given directly into the gastro-intestinal (GI) tract. The oral route is commonly used for giving drugs. The oral route has these advantages:

- Most drugs have oral dose forms.
- Oral drugs are easy to give.
- Most people can swallow oral drugs easily.
- The procedure is non-invasive. That is:
  - The skin is not pierced as for an injection.
  - A finger or administration device is not inserted into a body opening (vagina, rectum).
- The drug can be retrieved from the stomach to lessen adverse drug events. If necessary, an oro-gastric or naso-gastric tube is inserted to wash out (lavage) the stomach.

However, there are limits and some problems with oral drugs:

- They have the slowest rate of absorption and onset of action.
- Some can harm or discolor the teeth.
- Some taste or smell badly.
- Some cause nausea.
- They cannot be given if the person:
  - Is vomiting
  - Has gastric or intestinal suction
  - Is at risk for aspiration
  - Is unconscious or comatose
  - Cannot swallow

An order for an oral drug is written as one of the following:

- PO—per os (*per* means *by*; *os* means *mouth*)
- By mouth
- Orally

See p. 138 for buccal and sublingual drugs.
See *Promoting Safety and Comfort: Oral Drugs.*

| **PROMOTING SAFETY AND COMFORT** |
| **Oral Drugs** |

SAFETY

If a drug order is written as "per os," check with the nurse before giving the drug. The Institute for Safe Medication Practices (ISMP) lists "per os" as an error-prone abbreviation. This is because "os" can be mistaken for OS—*oculus sinister*—which means *left eye*. OS also is an error-prone abbreviation.

ORAL DOSE FORMS

Oral drugs come in these dose forms.

- *Capsule.* A **capsule** is a gelatin container that holds a drug in a dry powder or liquid form. This form is used for drugs that have an unpleasant odor or taste. You can identify a drug by the size, color, and shape of the capsule (Fig. 10-1, p. 130). *Timed-release capsules* contain granules (Fig. 10-2, p. 130). The granules dissolve at different rates. Over a period of time, there is a continuous release of the drug. Fewer doses are needed per day.
- *Tablets.* A **tablet** is a dried, powdered drug compressed into a small disk.
  - *Scored* tablets are grooved for use in dividing the dose (Fig. 10-3, *A*, p. 130).
  - *Layered* tablets have layers (Fig. 10-3, *B*, p. 130). More than one drug is given at the same time.
  - *Enteric-coated* tablets have a special coating (Fig. 10-3, *C*, p. 130). The coating prevents the tablet from dissolving in the stomach. The tablet dissolves in the small intestine.
- *Lozenges.* A **lozenge (troche)** is a flat disk containing a medicinal agent with a flavored base (Fig. 10-4, p. 130). The base is a hard or soft sugar candy. Lozenges are held or sucked in the mouth to slowly dissolve.
- *Elixirs.* An **elixir** is a clear liquid made up of a drug dissolved in alcohol and water (Fig. 10-5, p. 130). A flavor is added to improve the taste.
- *Emulsions.* An **emulsion** contains small droplets of water-in-oil or oil-in-water (Fig. 10-6, p. 130). This form is used to mask bitter tastes or to increase the ability to dissolve.
- *Suspensions.* A **suspension** is a liquid containing solid drug particles (Fig. 10-7, p. 131). Before giving a suspension, shake the bottle well to thoroughly mix the particles.
- *Syrups.* A **syrup** contains drugs dissolved in sugar (Fig. 10-8, p. 131). The sugar helps mask the drug's bitter taste. Syrups are often used for children.

See *Focus on Communication: Oral Dose Forms,* p. 131.

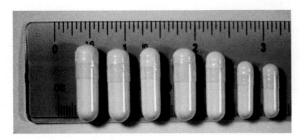

Fig. 10-1 Capsules.

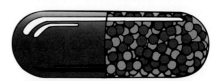

Fig. 10-2 Timed-release capsule.

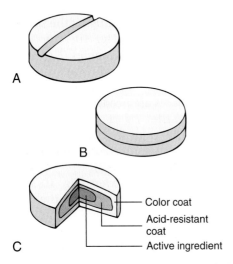

Color coat

Acid-resistant coat

Active ingredient

Fig. 10-3 A, Scored tablet. **B,** Layered tablet. **C,** Enteric-coated tablet.

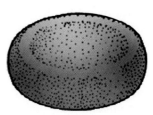

Fig. 10-4 Lozenge. (From Edmunds MW: *Introduction to clinical pharmacology,* ed 5, St Louis, 2006, Mosby.)

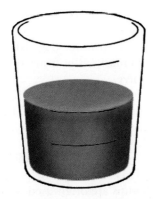

Fig. 10-5 An elixir. (From Edmunds MW: *Introduction to clinical pharmacology,* ed 5, St Louis, 2006, Mosby.)

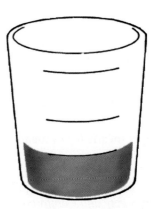

Fig. 10-6 An emulsion. (From Edmunds MW: *Introduction to clinical pharmacology,* ed 5, St Louis, 2006, Mosby.)

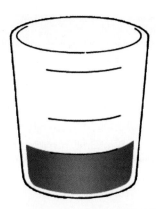

Fig. 10-7 A suspension. (From Edmunds MW: *Introduction to clinical pharmacology*, ed 5, St Louis, 2006, Mosby.)

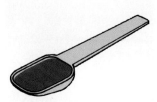

Fig. 10-8 A syrup. (From Edmunds MW: *Introduction to clinical pharmacology*, ed 5, St Louis, 2006, Mosby.)

EQUIPMENT

The equipment used to give oral drugs depends on the dose form ordered.

- *Souffle cups.* A **souffle cup** is a small paper or plastic cup used for solid drug forms (Fig. 10-9). Tablets and capsules are solid dose forms.
- *Medicine cups.* A **medicine cup** is a plastic container with measurement scales (Fig. 10-10). Check the medicine cup carefully before pouring any drug. You must use the proper scale (Table 10-1, p. 132) for the dose ordered. The medicine cup is not accurate for doses smaller than 1 teaspoonful. For small doses, use an oral syringe.

- *Medicine droppers.* A **medicine dropper** is a small glass or plastic tube with a hollow rubber ball at one end (Fig. 10-11, p. 132). Measurements are marked on the tube. Drops vary in size from dropper to dropper. *Only use the dropper supplied by the manufacturer of the drug ordered.* Once you draw the drug into the tube, do not turn the dropper upside down. When the dropper is turned upside down, some of the drug flows into the bulb. The person receives less than the amount ordered. Also, do not transfer the drug from the medicine dropper to another container. Part of the drug remains in the container. The person receives less than the amount ordered.
- *Teaspoon.* Many liquid drug doses are ordered in teaspoons. In hospitals and nursing centers, the teaspoon measure is converted into a metric measure (Table 10-1). For example, 2 teaspoons are ordered. You give 10 mL. For home use, use an oral syringe or a measuring teaspoon used for baking (Fig. 10-12, p. 132). Never use a teaspoon (kitchen spoon) that is used for eating.
- *Oral syringes.* A **syringe** is a plastic measuring device with three parts—tip, barrel, and plunger (Fig. 10-13, p. 132). Measurements are marked on the barrel. To withdraw a liquid, pull back on the plunger. To give a liquid, push the plunger forward. Oral syringes measure volumes from 0.1 mL to 15 mL. Choose the correct size syringe for the amount ordered.

See *Promoting Safety and Comfort: Equipment*, p. 132.

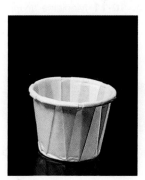

Fig. 10-9 Souffle cup.

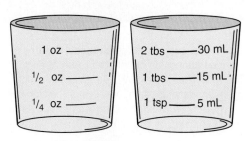

1 oz ———	2 tbs ———30 mL
1/2 oz ———	1 tbs ———15 mL
1/4 oz ———	1 tsp ———5 mL

Fig. 10-10 Medicine cup.

TABLE 10-1	Measurement Equivalents	
HOUSEHOLD MEASUREMENT	**APOTHECARY MEASUREMENT**	**METRIC MEASUREMENT**
2 tbsp (tbsp = tablespoon)	1 oz (oz = ounce)	30 mL (mL = milliliters)
1 tbsp (tbsp = tablespoon)	1/2 oz (oz = ounce)	15 mL (mL = milliliters)
2 tsp (tsp = teaspoon)	1/3 oz (oz = ounce)	10 mL (mL = milliliters)
1 tsp (tsp = teaspoon)	1/6 oz (oz = ounce)	5 mL (mL = milliliters)

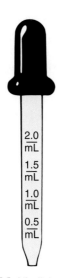

Fig. 10-11 Medicine dropper.

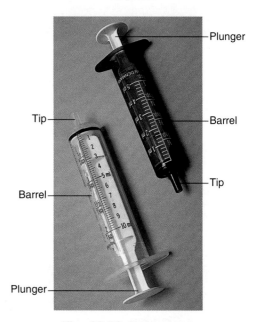

Fig. 10-13 Oral syringe.

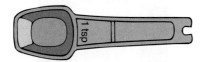

Fig. 10-12 Measuring teaspoon.

PROMOTING SAFETY AND COMFORT
Equipment

SAFETY

Always use *oral syringes* to give an oral drug by syringe. Oral syringes cannot be connected to an IV port or catheter. The ISMP has reported drug errors in which parenteral syringes were used for oral drugs. Left on the drug cart or when more than one drug was prepared, nurses gave the oral drugs by the IV route. These were serious drug errors.

GIVING ORAL DRUGS

When giving oral drugs, always practice medication safety (Chapter 9). Remember to:
* Follow the *Six Rights of Drug Administration.*
* Prevent drug errors.
* Prevent infection.
* Follow the procedure, *Giving a Drug,* described in Chapter 9.
* Follow the rules for giving oral drugs listed in Box 10-1.

See *Delegation Guidelines: Giving Oral Drugs* on p. 134.

See *Promoting Safety and Comfort: Giving Oral Drugs* on p. 134.

Text continued on p. 138

BOX 10-1 | Rules for Giving Oral Drugs

GENERAL RULES

- Give the most important drug first. Drugs affecting the heart are examples. So are antibiotics.
- Give solid drugs first. Then liquid drugs.
- Do not mix solid drugs with liquid drugs.
- Stay with the person while he or she takes the drug. Do not leave the drug at the bedside unless there is a doctor's order to do so.
- Do not let the container touch any part of a souffle cup, medicine cup, or measuring teaspoon.
- Place a container or bottle cap or lid upside down on a clean surface. Do not touch the inside of the cap or lid.

SOLID FORM

- Use the same souffle or medicine cup for all of the person's tablets and capsules with the nurse's approval.
  - Use a separate cup for a drug affecting the heart.
  - Use a separate cup for a drug affecting blood pressure.
- Check with the nurse before crushing tablets or opening capsules. To crush a tablet:
  - Wear gloves.
  - Use a mortar and pestle (Fig. 10-14, A). Place the tablet in the mortar. Use the pestle to crush the tablet. Or use a pill crusher (Fig. 10-14, B).
  - Wash (with water) and dry the mortar and pestle or pill crusher after each use. This removes powder or particles left in or on the device.
- Check with the nurse before cutting a scored tablet. To cut a scored tablet:
  - Wear gloves.
  - Use a disposable pill cutter. It should be labeled with the person's name. Do not use the person's pill cutter for another patient or resident.

- Wash (with water) and dry the pill cutter if it is not disposable. This removes powder or particles left on the device.
- Do not mix a drug with food or fluids unless ordered to do so.
- Do not give a drug with food unless ordered to do so.
- Let the person drink a small amount of water before taking a drug. This moistens the mouth to make swallowing the drug easier.
- Have the person place the drug well back on the tongue. Assist as needed. (Wear gloves if you will assist the person.)
- Give the person fluids to swallow the drug.
- Have the person keep his or head forward (like when eating) while swallowing. Tilting the head backward usually does not help the person swallow the drug.
- Encourage the person to drink a full glass of fluid. This helps the drug reach the stomach. And the fluid helps dilute the drug to decrease the risk of stomach irritation.
- Remind the person to suck on a lozenge. Lozenges are not swallowed whole.

LIQUID FORM

- Do not dilute (add water or other fluid) a liquid drug unless ordered to do so.
- Do not mix liquid drugs together. Pour each liquid into a separate medicine cup or measuring teaspoon. If using oral syringes, use a different syringe for each liquid.
- Give cough syrup last if giving more than one liquid drug. Cough syrup is given to coat and soothe the throat.
- Do not return extra liquid poured into a medicine cup or measuring teaspoon back to the bottle. Dispose of the drug according to agency policy.

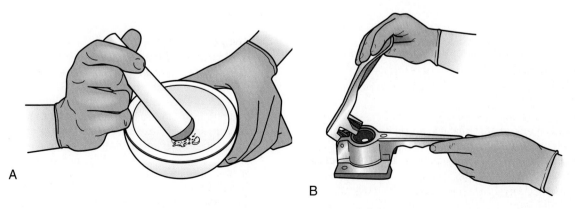

A   B

Fig. 10-14 Crushing tablets. **A,** Mortar and pestle. **B,** Pill crusher.

DELEGATION GUIDELINES
Giving Oral Drugs

When giving oral drugs is delegated to you, you need the following information from the nurse, the care plan, and the MAR:

- Which drugs to give first.
- Which tablets are crushed for a person.
- Which capsules are opened for a person.
- What to use to give crushed tablets or opened capsules—applesauce, pudding, custard, jelly, strained fruit, ice cream, and so on.
- If the sitting or Fowler's position is allowed. If not, how to position the person.
- When to report observations.
- What specific patient or resident concerns to report at once.

PROMOTING SAFETY AND COMFORT
Giving Oral Drugs

SAFETY

When crushed tablets or opened capsules are mixed with food, use a teaspoon to give the drug. Unless otherwise ordered, the teaspoon should only be one-third full. This portion is swallowed easily. Some people need smaller portions. Follow the care plan. The person must ingest all of the food used for the drug. Otherwise the person receives less than the amount of drug ordered. Therefore you may need to fill the teaspoon 2 or 3 times.

COMFORT

A crushed tablet or opened capsule does not taste good. Mix the drug with food as directed by the nurse, care plan, and MAR. (See *Delegation Guidelines: Giving Oral Drugs.*)

GIVING AN ORAL DRUG–SOLID FORM

QUALITY OF LIFE

Remember to:
- Knock before entering the person's room.
- Address the person by name.
- Introduce yourself by name and title.

- Explain the procedure to the person before beginning and during the procedure.
- Protect the person's rights during the procedure.
- Handle the person gently during the procedure.

PRE-PROCEDURE

1 Follow *Delegation Guidelines: Giving Oral Drugs.* See *Promoting Safety and Comfort: Giving Oral Drugs.*
2 Check the drug order. **(First safety check.)** Focus on the:
- *Right drug*
- *Right time*
- *Right dose*
- *Right person*
- *Right route*

3 Check with the nurse if you have any questions.
4 Practice hand hygiene.
5 Collect the following:
- MAR
- Water glass and water or other ordered liquid
- Straws
- Souffle cups

PROCEDURE

6 Unlock the drug cart.
7 Read the order on the MAR.
8 Select the right drug from the person's drawer or bin.
9 Compare the drug order on the MAR against the pharmacy label on the drug container. **(Second safety check.)** Check for the:
- *Right drug*
- *Right time*
- *Right dose*
- *Right person*
- *Right route*
10 Check the drug container for an expiration date.
11 Compare the drug order on the MAR against the pharmacy label on the drug container. **(Third safety check.)** Check for the:
- *Right drug*
- *Right time*

- *Right dose*
- *Right person*
- *Right route*
12 Prepare the drug. (NOTE: Do not open a unit dose package until you are at the person's bedside.)
  a Open the container.
  b Pour the ordered dosage into the container cap or lid. Gently tap on the container. Do not let the container touch the cap or lid. See Figure 10-15.
  c Return extra tablets or capsules back into the container. Do not let the cap or lid touch the container. For example, 1 tablet is ordered but 3 tablets are poured from the container into the cap. Return 2 tablets to the container.
  d Pour the tablet or capsule from the lid into the souffle cup.

GIVING AN ORAL DRUG—SOLID FORM—cont'd

PROCEDURE—cont'd

13 Close the container. Compare the drug order on the MAR against the pharmacy label on the drug container. **(Fourth safety check.)** Check for the:
- *Right drug*
- *Right time*
- *Right dose*
- *Right person*
- *Right route*

14 Return the container to the drawer or bin.

15 Repeat steps 7–14 for each drug ordered for the person. You can use the same souffle cup for all tablets and capsules if the nurse approves:
- Use a separate cup for a drug affecting the heart.
- Use a separate cup for a drug affecting blood pressure.

[NOTE: Do not open a unit dose package until you are at the person's bedside.]

16 Lock the drug cart if you will leave it outside the person's room.

17 Identify the person. Check the ID bracelet against the MAR. Make sure you use at least two identifiers according to agency policy. Also call the person by name. Follow agency policy if using a bar code scanner.

18 Provide for privacy.

19 Obtain required measurements as noted on the MAR. For example, measure the person's blood pressure or pulse. Note the measurement on the MAR.

20 Position the person in a sitting or Fowler's position. Or position the person as directed by the nurse, care plan, and MAR.

21 Let the person drink a small amount of water. Provide a straw if the person prefers.

22 Give the person the drugs. If using a unit dose system:
- **a** Hand the drug package to the person. Ask him or her to read the label.
- **b** Ask the person to hand the package back to you.
- **c** Open the package.
- **d** Place the contents into the person's hand.

23 Give the person a full glass of water or ordered fluid. Provide a straw if the person prefers. Encourage the person to drink all of the water or other fluid.

24 Stay with the person to make sure he or she swallows all of the drugs. If necessary, check the person's mouth—under the tongue and between the teeth and the cheeks. (Wear gloves if checking the person's mouth.)

POST-PROCEDURE

25 Discard the souffle cup or unit dose packages.

26 Provide for the person's comfort. See the inside of the front book cover.

27 Unscreen the person.

28 Complete a safety check before leaving the room. See the inside of the front book cover.

29 Practice hand hygiene.

30 Record the *right documentation* on the MAR:
- The date, time, drug name, dosage, and route of administration
- Your name or initials

31 Report and record any specific patient or resident observations or concerns.

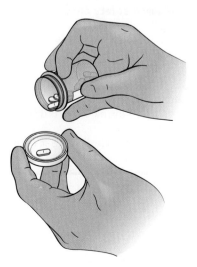

Fig. 10-15 A drug is poured from a container into the container lid. The lid does not touch the container.

GIVING AN ORAL DRUG—LIQUID FORM

QUALITY OF LIFE

Remember to:
- Knock before entering the person's room.
- Address the person by name.
- Introduce yourself by name and title.

- Explain the procedure to the person before beginning and during the procedure.
- Protect the person's rights during the procedure.
- Handle the person gently during the procedure.

PRE-PROCEDURE

1 Check the drug order. **(First safety check.)** Focus on the:
- *Right drug*
- *Right time*
- *Right dose*
- *Right person*
- *Right route*

2 Check with the nurse if you have any questions.
3 Practice hand hygiene.
4 Collect the following:
- MAR
- Medicine cup
- Oral syringe (if needed) in the correct size
- Tray (if needed)
- Paper towels

PROCEDURE

5 Unlock the drug cart.
6 Read the order on the MAR.
7 Select the right drug from the person's drawer or bin.
8 Compare the drug order on the MAR against the pharmacy label on the drug container. **(Second safety check.)** Check for the:
- *Right drug*
- *Right time*
- *Right dose*
- *Right person*
- *Right route*

9 Check the drug container for an expiration date.
10 Compare the drug order on the MAR against the pharmacy label on the drug container. **(Third safety check.)** Check for the:
- *Right drug*
- *Right time*
- *Right dose*
- *Right person*
- *Right route*

11 Prepare the drug. (NOTE: Do not open a unit dose container until you are at the person's bedside.)
   a Shake the bottle or container only if directed to do so on the label. Make sure the lid is secure before shaking a bottle.
   b Open the container.
   c Place the lid on the drug cart. The outside of the lid is down; the inside of the lid is up.
   d Hold the bottle so that the label is in the palm of your hand. This prevents the contents from running down and smearing the label during pouring.

12 *For a medicine cup:*
   a Locate the scale to be used on the medicine cup.
   b Place your fingernail at the level to be measured. For example, 15 mL are ordered. Place your fingernail at the 15 mL level.
   c Hold the medicine cup straight at eye level.
   d Pour the prescribed dose into the medicine cup. Measure the dose at the lowest level in the medicine cup (Fig. 10-16).
   e Compare the drug order on the MAR against the pharmacy label on the drug container.
   f Set the medicine cup on the drug cart.

13 *For a syringe:*
   a Follow steps 12 a–f.
   b Pull back on the plunger to withdraw the drug from the medicine cup into the barrel (Fig. 10-17).
   c Set the syringe on the tray or a paper towel.

14 Wipe off any liquid from the bottle top.
15 Replace the lid on the bottle.
16 Close the bottle. Compare the drug order on the MAR against the pharmacy label on the drug container. **(Fourth safety check.)** Check for the:
- *Right drug*
- *Right time*
- *Right dose*
- *Right person*
- *Right route*

17 Return the bottle to the drawer or bin.
18 Repeat steps 6–17 for each liquid drug ordered for the person.
19 Lock the drug cart if you will leave it outside the person's room.

GIVING AN ORAL DRUG—LIQUID FORM—cont'd

PROCEDURE—cont'd

20 Identify the person. Check the ID bracelet against the MAR. Make sure you use at least two identifiers according to agency policy. Also call the person by name. Follow agency policy if using a bar code scanner.

21 Provide for privacy.

22 Obtain required measurements as noted on the MAR. For example, measure the person's blood pressure or pulse. Note the measurement on the MAR.

23 Position the person in a sitting or Fowler's position. Or position the person as directed by the nurse, care plan, and MAR.

24 Give the person the medicine cup.

25 Have the person drink the drug.
   If using a unit dose system:
   a Hand the drug container to the person. Ask him or her to read the label.
   b Ask the person to hand the container back to you.
   c Open the container.
   d Give the container to the person.
   e Have the person drink the drug.

26 If using a medicine dropper or an oral syringe:
   a Place the dropper or syringe inside the mouth by the tongue.
   b Give the liquid in small amounts. Allow time for the person to swallow.
   c Return the dropper to the bottle.

POST-PROCEDURE

27 Discard the medicine cup, unit dose container, or oral syringe.

28 Provide for the person's comfort. See the inside of the front book cover.

29 Unscreen the person.

30 Complete a safety check before leaving the room. See the inside of the front book cover.

31 Practice hand hygiene.

32 Record the *right documentation* on the MAR:
   • The date, time, drug name, dosage, and route of administration
   • Your name or initials

33 Report and record any specific patient or resident observations or concerns.

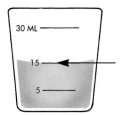

Fig. 10-16 The dose is measured at the lowest level in the medicine cup. (From Edmunds MW: *Introduction to clinical pharmacology*, ed 5, St Louis, 2006, Mosby.)

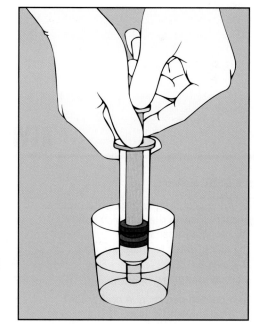

Fig. 10-17 The plunger is pulled back to withdraw a liquid drug from a medicine cup into the syringe barrel.

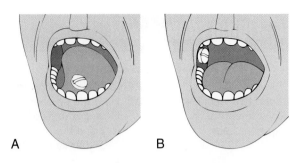

Fig. 10-18 A, A sublingual tablet is placed under the tongue. **B,** A buccal tablet is placed between the cheek and upper molar.

SUBLINGUAL AND BUCCAL DRUGS

Sublingual means under *(sub)* the tongue *(lingual).* Sublingual tablets are placed under the tongue. They are dissolved and absorbed through the many blood vessels in that area.

Buccal means inside the cheek *(bucco).* Buccal tablets are placed between the cheek and the molar teeth. A buccal tablet is absorbed by the blood vessels in the cheek.

Drugs are rapidly absorbed through the sublingual and buccal routes. Therefore the onset of action is rapid.

To give a sublingual or buccal tablet, follow the procedure, *Giving a Drug*, in Chapter 9. To give the drug, do the following:

1 Put on a glove.
2 For a sublingual drug: place the tablet under the tongue (Fig. 10-18, *A*).
3 For a buccal drug: place the tablet between the upper molar and the cheek (Fig. 10-18, *B*).
4 Do not give the person water to drink.
5 Encourage the person to:
   a Allow the drug to dissolve where placed. Remind the person not to move the drug to another part of the mouth.
   b Hold saliva in the mouth until the tablet is dissolved.
6 Remove and discard the glove.
7 Practice hand hygiene.

REVIEW QUESTIONS

Circle the BEST answer.

1 The wrong oral drug was given to a person. If necessary, how is the drug retrieved?
   a by giving an enema
   b by giving water to dilute the drug
   c by lavage
   d through surgery

2 Which person can receive oral drugs?
   a the person who is alert, oriented
   b the person who is vomiting
   c the person who is at risk for aspiration
   d the person who is comatose

3 To receive oral drugs, the person must be able to
   a state his or her name   c sit in Fowler's position
   b identify the drug   d swallow

4 Oral drug orders are written as follows. Which should you question?
   a 10 mL PO   c 10 mL orally
   b 10 mL per os   d 10 mL by mouth

5 Which dose form contains granules?
   a tablet
   b capsule
   c timed-release capsule
   d lozenge

6 Which dose form is held in the mouth to dissolve?
   a tablet
   b capsule
   c timed-release capsule
   d lozenge

REVIEW QUESTIONS

7 Another name for a lozenge is
 a elixir
 b emulsion
 c troche
 d suspension

8 Which is *not* a liquid dose form?
 a elixir
 b emulsion
 c lozenge
 d syrup

9 Which of the following prevents a tablet from dissolving in the stomach?
 a scoring
 b layering
 c granules
 d enteric coating

10 Which dose form should you shake before pouring the drug?
 a suspension
 b timed-release capsule
 c elixir
 d syrup

11 Which has a hollow rubber ball at one end?
 a souffle cup
 b medicine cup
 c medicine dropper
 d oral syringe

12 Which is *not* a part of an oral syringe?
 a tip
 b barrel
 c plunger
 d bulb

13 How many milliliters (mL) in 1 teaspoon?
 a 5
 b 10
 c 15
 d 30

14 How many milliliters (mL) in ¹/₂ ounce?
 a 5
 b 10
 c 15
 d 30

15 A person has 4 drugs ordered for 0900. Which should you give first?
 a the liquid drug
 b a drug in a unit dose package
 c a solid drug
 d the most important drug

16 Before giving a person a solid dose form, you should have the person
 a eat some food
 b drink a small amount of water
 c drink a full glass of water
 d tilt his or her head back

Circle T if the statement is true. Circle F if the statement is false.

17 T F You can mix solid dose forms with liquid dose forms.

18 T F You can mix liquid drugs together.

19 T F You can leave a drug at the bedside if there is a doctor's order to do so.

20 T F A medicine cup can touch the drug container or bottle.

21 T F A bottle cap is placed upside down on a clean surface.

22 T F A person has 4 drugs ordered for 1300. The drugs are in tablet and capsule form. You can use the same souffle cup for all the drugs if the nurse approves.

23 T F You can give all ordered drugs with food.

24 T F You are giving 2 liquid drugs. One is cough syrup. The cough syrup is given last.

25 T F You pour extra liquid into a medicine cup. You can return the extra liquid to the bottle.

Answers to these questions are on p. 444.

11

Topical Drugs

OBJECTIVES

- Define the key terms and key abbreviations used in this chapter.
- Identify the factors that affect topical drug absorption.
- List the reasons for topical drug applications.
- Describe the topical dose forms.
- Explain the rules for applying topical dose forms.
- Explain how to safely apply nitroglycerin ointment.
- Explain how to safely apply a transdermal drug delivery system.
- Perform the procedures described in this chapter.

PROCEDURES

- Applying a Cream, Lotion, Ointment, and Powder
- Applying Nitroglycerin Ointment

KEY TERMS

cream A semi-solid emulsion containing a drug

debride To remove

lotion A watery preparation containing suspended particles

ointment A semi-solid preparation containing a drug in an oily base

powder A finely ground drug in a talc base

topical Refers to a surface of a part of the body

topical medication A drug applied to the skin

transdermal Through *(trans)* the skin *(dermal)*

KEY ABBREVIATIONS

TDD Transdermal drug delivery

Topical refers to a surface of a part of the body. A **topical medication** is a drug applied to the skin. The absorption of a topical drug is affected by:

- The strength of the drug
- How long the drug is in contact with the skin
- The size of the area of application
- Skin thickness
- Amount of water in the tissues
- Amount of skin breakdown or irritation
  Drugs are applied topically to:
- Clean and debride a wound. **Debride** means to remove. Wounds are debrided to remove dirt, damaged tissue, foreign objects, and drainage. This is done to prevent infection and to promote healing.
- Hydrate (add water) the skin.
- Reduce inflammation.
- Relieve itching or a rash.
- Provide a protective barrier to the skin.
- Reduce thickening of the skin. Callous formation is an example.

TOPICAL DOSE FORMS

Creams, lotions, ointments, and powders are common topical dose forms.

- *Creams.* A **cream** is a semi-solid emulsion containing a drug. An *emulsion* contains small droplets of water-in-oil or oil-in-water. The cream base is usually non-greasy. Creams are removed with water.
- *Lotions.* A **lotion** is a watery preparation containing suspended particles. Shake all lotions before the application. Then gently but firmly pat the lotion onto the skin. Do not rub the lotion into the skin. Rubbing increases circulation and itching. Rubbing also causes friction, which can irritate the skin. Lotions are used to:
  - Soothe and protect the skin
  - Relieve rashes and itching
  - Cleanse the skin
- *Ointments.* An **ointment** is a semi-solid preparation containing a drug in an oily base. Ointments are not easily removed with water. Therefore the drug has longer contact with the skin.
- *Powders.* A **powder** is a finely ground drug in a talc base. Powders are used to absorb moisture. They also dry, cool, and protect the skin. Powder is applied to dry skin in a thin, even layer.

BOX 11-1 **Rules for Applying Creams, Lotions, Ointments, and Powders**

- Practice hand hygiene before and after the application.
- Follow Standard Precautions.
- Follow isolation precautions as ordered (Appendix B).
- Wear gloves.
- Do not let the dose form touch your skin.
- Provide for privacy.
- Position the person to expose the application site. Avoid unnecessary exposure.
- Clean and dry the skin as directed by the nurse before applying a dose form. Usually soap and water are used if the person's skin condition allows. Make sure previous applications are thoroughly removed.
- Observe the skin. Report and record your observations. See *Delegation Guidelines: Applying Creams, Lotions, Ointments, and Powders.*
- See *Promoting Safety and Comfort: Applying Creams, Lotions, Ointments, and Powders.*
- Shake lotions thoroughly. The lotion should have a uniform color throughout.
- Apply the dose form to clean, dry skin.
- Apply the correct amount. Use a sterile tongue blade or sterile cotton-tipped applicator to remove the dose from a jar. If applying the drug by hand or finger, use the tongue blade or cotton-tipped applicator to transfer the dose to your gloved hand or finger.
- Do not let the drug container touch the person's skin.
- Cover the site with gauze or other covering as directed by the nurse, care plan, and MAR. Ointments and creams may stain or soil garments and linens.
- See procedure: *Applying Nitroglycerin Ointment,* p. 145.

Applying Creams, Lotions, Ointments, and Powders

Each topical dose form is applied differently. Lotions are dabbed on the skin with gauze or a cotton ball. A tongue blade, cotton-tipped applicator, or a gloved hand or finger is used to apply ointments and creams. Powders are applied in a thin, even layer. To safely apply a topical dose form, follow the rules in Box 11-1. Also practice medication safety (Chapter 9). To apply a nitroglycerin ointment, see p. 144.

See *Focus on Older Persons: Applying Creams, Lotions, Ointments, and Powders.*

See *Delegation Guidelines: Applying Creams, Lotions, Ointments, and Powders.*

See *Promoting Safety and Comfort: Applying Creams, Lotions, Ointments, and Powders.*

FOCUS ON OLDER PERSONS

Applying Creams, Lotions, Ointments, and Powders

Dry skin occurs with aging. Soap also dries the skin. Dry skin is easily damaged. Thorough rinsing is needed when using soap. The nurse and care plan may direct you to use a different cleansing agent.

DELEGATION GUIDELINES
Applying Creams, Lotions, Ointments, and Powders

Before applying a topical dose form, you need the following information from the nurse, care plan, and MAR:
- If isolation precautions are required. If yes:
  - What type of precaution
  - What personal protective equipment is needed
- Special measures for cleaning and drying the skin.
- What cleansing agent to use.
- The exact site of application.
- What to use to apply the drug—tongue blade, cotton-tipped applicator, or gloved hand or finger.
- If you need to cover the application. If yes, how to cover the application site—gauze, see-through dressing and tape, and so on.
- What observations to report and record:
  - The color of the skin
  - The location and description of rashes
  - Dry skin
  - Bruises or open skin areas
  - Pale or reddened areas, particularly over bony parts
  - Blisters
  - Drainage or bleeding from wounds or body openings
  - Skin temperature
  - Complaints of pain or discomfort
- When to report observations.
- What specific patient or resident concerns to report at once.

PROMOTING SAFETY AND COMFORT
Applying Creams, Lotions, Ointments, and Powders

SAFETY

Use caution when applying powder. Inhaling powder can irritate the airway and lungs. Do not shake or sprinkle powder onto the person. To safely apply powder:
- Turn away from the person.
- Sprinkle a small amount of powder onto your hands or a cloth.
- Apply the powder in a thin layer.
- Make sure powder does not get on the floor. Powder is slippery and can cause falls.

COMFORT

A skin area is exposed to apply topical dose forms. Provide for privacy. Screen the person. Close doors and window coverings—drapes, shades, blinds, shutters, and so on. Avoid unnecessary exposure. Expose only the area needed.

The person may have a rash or skin lesion. A skin disorder may be contagious. The person knows the disease can be spread to others. Self-esteem may suffer. He or she may feel dirty and undesirable. Treat the person with dignity and respect.

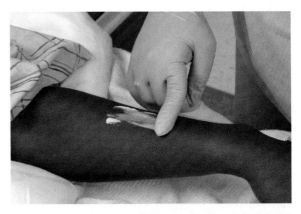

Fig. 11-1 A cream is applied with a gloved index finger. (Courtesy Rick Brady, from Lilley LL and others: *Pharmacology and the nursing process*, ed 5, St Louis, 2007, Mosby.)

APPLYING A CREAM, LOTION, OINTMENT, AND POWDER

QUALITY OF LIFE

Remember to:
- Knock before entering the person's room.
- Address the person by name.
- Introduce yourself by name and title.

- Explain the procedure to the person before beginning and during the procedure.
- Protect the person's rights during the procedure.
- Handle the person gently during the procedure.

PRE-PROCEDURE

1 Follow *Delegation Guidelines: Applying Creams, Lotions, Ointments, and Powders.* See *Promoting Safety and Comfort: Applying Creams, Lotions, Ointments, and Powders.*
2 Check the drug order. **(First safety check.)** Focus on the:
   - *Right drug*
   - *Right time*
   - *Right dose*
   - *Right person*
   - *Right route*

3 Check with the nurse if you have any questions.
4 Practice hand hygiene.
5 Collect needed items:
   - Soap or other cleansing agent
   - Washcloth and towel
   - Wash basin with warm water
   - Gauze squares or cotton balls
   - Sterile tongue blade
   - Sterile cotton-tipped applicator
   - Gloves
   - MAR

PROCEDURE

6 Unlock the drug cart.
7 Read the order on the MAR.
8 Select the right drug from the person's drawer. Lock the drug cart.
9 Compare the drug order on the MAR against the pharmacy label on the drug container. **(Second safety check.)** Check for the:
   - *Right drug*
   - *Right time*
   - *Right dose*
   - *Right person*
   - *Right route*
10 Check the drug container for an expiration date.
11 Identify the person. Check the ID bracelet against the MAR. Make sure you use at least two identifiers according to agency policy. Also call the person by name. Follow agency policy if using a bar code scanner.
12 Provide for privacy.
13 Put on gloves.
14 Position the person to expose the application site. Expose the site.
15 Clean and dry the application site.
16 Observe the application site.
17 Remove and discard the gloves. Practice hand hygiene. Put on clean gloves.
18 Compare the drug order on the MAR against the pharmacy label on the drug container. **(Third safety check.)** Check for the:
   - *Right drug*
   - *Right time*
   - *Right dose*
   - *Right person*
   - *Right route*
19 Shake the lotion thoroughly.

20 Open the container. Place the lid or cap upside down on a clean surface. For an ointment or cream:
   a *From a jar:* use a tongue blade to remove the ordered amount.
   b *From a tube:* squeeze the ordered amount onto a tongue blade or cotton-tipped applicator.
21 Close the container. Compare the drug order on the MAR against the pharmacy label on the drug container. **(Fourth safety check.)** Check for the:
   - *Right drug*
   - *Right time*
   - *Right dose*
   - *Right person*
   - *Right route*
22 Apply the topical dose form:
   a Lotion:
      (1) Hold the bottle in your non-dominant hand. The label is in the palm of your hand. This prevents the contents from running down and smearing the label during pouring.
      (2) Pour some lotion onto a cotton ball or gauze square. Do not let any part of the container touch the cotton ball.
      (3) Dab the lotion onto the skin. Do not rub.
      (4) Repeat steps 22 a (1)–(3) with a new cotton ball or gauze square until the area is covered.
   b Cream or ointment:
      (1) Transfer the cream or ointment from the tongue blade or cotton-tipped applicator to your gloved hand or index finger (if necessary).
      (2) Apply the agent to the skin with the tongue blade, cotton-tipped applicator, or your gloved hand or finger (Fig. 11-1).
      (3) Apply the agent in a thin layer in the direction of hair growth. Use firm, gentle strokes.

Continued

APPLYING A CREAM, LOTION, OINTMENT, AND POWDER—cont'd

PROCEDURE—cont'd

c Powder:
  (1) Apply in a thin, even layer with your gloved hand.
  (2) Smooth over the area for even coverage.
23 Return the container to the drawer. Lock the drug cart.

POST-PROCEDURE

24 Discard the supplies or unit dose packages.
25 Remove the gloves. Practice hand hygiene.
26 Provide for the person's comfort. See the inside of the front book cover.
27 Empty and clean the wash basin. Return it and other supplies to their proper place. (Wear gloves for this step.)
28 Unscreen the person.
29 Complete a safety check before leaving the room. See the inside of the front book cover.

30 Follow agency policy for soiled linen.
31 Practice hand hygiene.
32 Record the *right documentation* on the MAR:
  • The date, time, drug name, dosage, and route of administration
  • The application site
  • Your name or initials
33 Report and record any specific patient or resident observations or concerns.

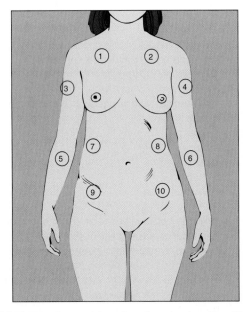

Fig. 11-2 Sites for applying nitroglycerin ointment. The sites also are used for a transdermal drug delivery system.

Applying Nitroglycerin Ointment. Nitroglycerin ointment is used to prevent angina (chest pain). It relaxes the heart's blood vessels and increases the blood and oxygen supply to the heart. See Chapter 21.

The dosage applied must be accurate. To properly apply nitroglycerin ointment, follow these rules:
• Apply the drug to clean, dry skin that has little or no hair (Fig. 11-2).
• Do not shave an area to apply the ointment. Shaving can cause skin irritation.
• Do not apply the ointment to irritated, scarred, open, broken, or calloused skin areas. Such areas can affect drug absorption.
• Wear gloves. Do not let any ointment touch any part of your skin.
• Check for an old application:
  • Check the MAR.
  • Ask the person the location of an existing application.
• Do not assume that there are no applications or that one has fallen off. Carefully check the person's skin. This is especially important if the person is confused, sedated, or non-responsive.
• Remove the old application before applying a new one. Check the person carefully to make sure there is only one old application. If you find more than one, tell the nurse at once. Remove all applications before applying a new one.

- Rotate the application site. This means that different sites are used. Rotating sites prevents skin irritation. Check the MAR or care plan for the rotation schedule.
- Do not rub or massage the ointment into the skin.
- Date, time, and sign your name and title to the tape securing the new application. Also include the drug name and dosage. Do not use a ball-point pen. A ball-point pen can puncture the application.
- Document the application site on the MAR.

See *Promoting Safety and Comfort: Applying Nitroglycerin Ointment.*

APPLYING NITROGLYCERIN OINTMENT

QUALITY OF LIFE

Remember to:
- Knock before entering the person's room.
- Address the person by name.
- Introduce yourself by name and title.

- Explain the procedure to the person before beginning and during the procedure.
- Protect the person's rights during the procedure.
- Handle the person gently during the procedure.

PRE-PROCEDURE

1 Follow *Delegation Guidelines: Applying Creams, Lotions, Ointments, and Powders,* p. 142. See *Promoting Safety and Comfort:*
   - *Applying Creams, Lotions, Ointments, and Powders,* p. 142
   - *Applying Nitroglycerin Ointment*
2 Check the drug order. **(First safety check.)** Focus on the:
   - *Right drug*
   - *Right time*
   - *Right dose*
   - *Right person*
   - *Right route*

3 Check with the nurse if you have any questions.
4 Practice hand hygiene.
5 Collect needed items:
   - Soap or other cleansing agent
   - Washcloth and towel
   - Wash basin with warm water
   - Applicator paper
   - See-through dressing
   - Non-allergic tape
   - Gloves
   - MAR

PROCEDURE

6 Unlock the drug cart.
7 Read the order on the MAR.
8 Select the nitroglycerin ointment from the person's drawer. Lock the drug cart.
9 Compare the drug order on the MAR against the pharmacy label on the drug container. **(Second safety check.)** Check for the:
   - *Right drug*
   - *Right time*
   - *Right dose*
   - *Right person*
   - *Right route*
10 Check the drug container for an expiration date.
11 Provide for privacy.

12 Identify the person. Check the ID bracelet against the MAR. Make sure you use at least two identifiers according to agency policy. Also call the person by name. Follow agency policy if using a bar code scanner.
13 Put on gloves.
14 Position the person to expose the old application site. Expose the site.
15 Remove the old application. Fold the old application in half with the sticky sides together. Discard the application according to agency policy. Make sure that no one can access the old application.
16 Clean and dry the old application site.
17 Observe the old application site.

Continued

APPLYING NITROGLYCERIN OINTMENT—cont'd

PROCEDURE—cont'd

18 Position the person to expose the new application site. Expose and observe the site.

19 Clean and dry the new application site. Follow agency policy.

20 Remove and discard the gloves. Practice hand hygiene.

21 Put on clean gloves.

22 Compare the drug order on the MAR against the pharmacy label on the drug container. **(Third safety check.)** Check for the:
- *Right drug*
- *Right time*
- *Right dose*
- *Right person*
- *Right route*

23 Use the dose-measuring paper to measure the ordered dose. The paper has a ruler along the side or in the middle (Fig. 11-3, *A*). The print side is *down.*

24 Squeeze a ribbon of ointment on the paper for the amount ordered (Fig. 11-3, *B*). For example, if the order is for 2 inches, squeeze a ribbon length of two inches.

25 Close the container. Compare the drug order on the MAR against the pharmacy label on the drug container. **(Fourth safety check.)** Check for the:
- *Right drug*
- *Right time*
- *Right dose*
- *Right person*
- *Right route*

26 Apply the paper, ointment side down, to the application site (Fig. 11-3, *C*).

27 Use the paper to spread a thin, uniform layer of ointment under the paper. *Do not rub in the ointment.*

28 Leave the paper in place.

29 Cover the paper and application site with a see-through dressing. Tape the dressing in place.

30 Date, time, and sign your name and title to the tape. Include the drug name and dosage.

31 Return the container to the drawer. Lock the drug cart.

POST-PROCEDURE

32 Discard the supplies.

33 Remove the gloves. Practice hand hygiene.

34 Provide for the person's comfort. See the inside of the front book cover.

35 Empty and clean the wash basin. Return it and other supplies to their proper place. (Wear gloves for this step.)

36 Unscreen the person.

37 Complete a safety check before leaving the room. See the inside of the front book cover.

38 Follow agency policy for soiled linen.

39 Practice hand hygiene.

40 Record the *right documentation* on the MAR:
- The removal of an old application and from what site
- The date, time, drug name, dosage, and route of administration
- The application site
- Your name or initials

41 Report and record any specific patient or resident observations or concerns.

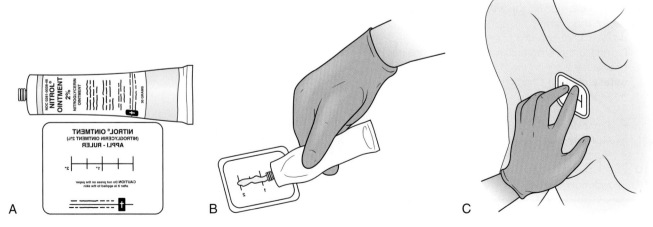

Fig. 11-3 A, Nitroglycerin ointment and application paper. **B,** The ordered amount is squeezed onto the paper. **C,** The ointment is applied to the skin. (Redrawn and modified from Edmunds MW: *Introduction to clinical pharmacology,* ed 5, St Louis, 2006, Mosby.)

TRANSDERMAL DRUG DELIVERY SYSTEM

Transdermal means through *(trans)* the skin *(dermal).* A transdermal drug delivery (TDD) system provides continuous, gradual absorption of a drug through the skin and into the bloodstream. The effect is systemic. *Systemic* relates to the whole body.

A transdermal disk or patch provides controlled release of a drug (Fig. 11-4). The drug is slowly absorbed over several hours or days. The dose released depends on the drug and the size of the skin area covered.

To apply a TDD system:
* Follow the rules in Box 11-1.
* Follow the rules listed for "Applying Nitroglycerin Ointment."
* Follow the procedure: *Applying Nitroglycerin Ointment.*
  * Do not cover the patch with a dressing unless directed by the nurse, care plan, and MAR.
  * Omit the steps for applying the ointment on the paper. The TDD system contains the drug.
* Apply the system as shown in Figure 11-5.
  See *Promoting Safety and Comfort: Transdermal Drug Delivery System.*

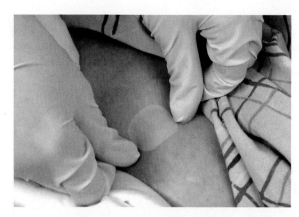

Fig. 11-4 Transdermal patch. (Courtesy Rick Brady, from Lilley LL and others: *Pharmacology and the nursing process,* ed 5, St Louis, 2007, Mosby.)

PROMOTING SAFETY AND COMFORT
Transdermal Drug Delivery System

SAFETY
Always carefully look for the old transdermal patch before applying a new one. Patches may be hard to see on the skin because:
* Many patches are clear
* The drug name printed on the patch may have rubbed off

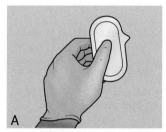 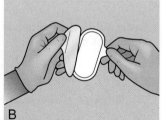 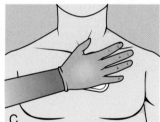 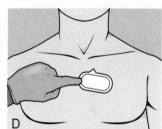

Fig. 11-5 Applying a TDD system. **A,** Pick up the system with the clear plastic backing facing you. Some systems have tabs to assist with removal. **B,** Remove the clear plastic backing. Do not touch the inside of the exposed system. **C,** Place the exposed adhesive side of the system onto the skin. Press firmly with the palm of your hand. **D,** Circle the outside edge of the system with one or two fingers. This helps secure the system to the skin.

REVIEW QUESTIONS

Circle the **BEST** answer.

1 Topical drug absorption is affected by the following *except*
   a the time of application
   b how long the drug is in contact with the skin
   c skin thickness
   d amount of water in the tissues

2 A topical drug is applied to debride a wound. Debriding is done to
   a relieve itching
   b provide a protective barrier to the skin
   c reduce inflammation
   d promote healing

3 Which of the following is a watery preparation?
   a cream
   b lotion
   c ointment
   d powder

4 Which of the following do you shake?
   a cream
   b lotion
   c ointment
   d powder

5 Lotions are used for the following reasons *except*
   a absorb moisture
   b soothe and protect the skin
   c relieve itching
   d cleanse the skin

6 Which topical dose form is dabbed on?
   a cream
   b lotion
   c ointment
   d powder

7 These statements are about applying powder. Which is *false?*
   a You shake or sprinkle powder onto the person.
   b Powder is applied in a thin layer.
   c Powder is slippery and can cause falls.
   d After applying powder, you smooth over the area for even coverage.

8 Before applying a topical dose form, *always*
   a provide for the person's privacy
   b follow isolation precautions
   c shave the application site
   d clip hair at the application site

9 An ointment is in a jar. What should you use to remove the amount ordered?
   a your hand
   b a sterile tongue blade
   c a syringe
   d a measuring spoon

10 These statements are about nitroglycerin ointment and transdermal drug delivery systems. Which is *false?*
   a An old application is removed before applying a new one.
   b You rub or massage the ointment into the skin.
   c The application site is rotated.
   d The drug is applied to a skin site with little or no hair.

11 Which is used to measure the ordered dose of nitroglycerin ointment?
   a a measuring spoon
   b a medicine cup
   c dose-measuring paper
   d a transdermal patch

Circle **T** if the statement is true. Circle **F** if the statement is false.

12 T F   You need to wear gloves to apply a topical dose form.

13 T F   A topical dose form can touch your skin.

14 T F   Topical drugs are applied to clean, dry skin.

15 T F   You can use your gloved hand to apply creams and ointments as directed by the nurse.

16 T F   Creams and ointments are applied in the direction of hair growth.

17 T F   Nitroglycerin ointment can touch your skin.

18 T F   A transdermal patch requires a dressing.

Answers to these questions are on p. 444.

12

Eye, Ear, Nose, and Inhaled Drugs

OBJECTIVES

- Define the key terms and key abbreviations used in this chapter.
- Explain the safety rules for giving eye, ear, nose, and inhaled drugs.
- Perform the procedures described in this chapter.

PROCEDURES

- Applying Medications to the Eye
- Instilling Ear Drops
- Giving Nose Medications
- Giving Inhaled Medications

KEY TERMS

cerumen Ear wax
instill To enter drop by drop
nasal Nose
ocular Pertains to the eye
ophthalmic Pertains to the eye
otic Pertains to the ear

KEY ABBREVIATIONS

ISMP Institute for Safe Medication Practices
MDI Metered-dose inhaler

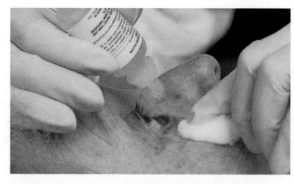

Fig. 12-1 The lower conjunctival sac is exposed. (From Elkin MK, Perry AG, Potter PA: *Nursing interventions & clinical skills*, ed 4, St Louis, 2007, Mosby.)

The eyes, ears, and nose contain mucous membranes. Drugs are well absorbed across such surfaces. So are inhaled drugs. They affect the bronchial smooth muscle. To safely give eye, ear, nose, and inhaled medications, follow the rules in Box 12-1.

EYE MEDICATIONS

Ophthalmic and **ocular** are terms that pertain to the eye (*Opthalmo* means *eye. Ocular* means *eye.*) Ocular drugs are usually in the form of drops or ointments.

See *Delegation Guidelines: Eye Medications.*
See *Promoting Safety and Comfort: Eye Medications.*

BOX 12-1 Administering Eye, Ear, Nose, and Inhaled Drugs

GENERAL RULES
- Practice hand hygiene.
- Follow Standard Precautions and the Bloodborne Pathogen Standard (Appendix C).
- Wear gloves.
- Use only the dropper supplied by the drug manufacturer.
- Do not let the dropper touch the eye, ear, nose, face, or other body part.
- Use a separate bottle or tube for each person.

EYE MEDICATIONS
- Position the person properly:
  - Supine, sitting, or Fowler's position.
  - The head is tilted back slightly. The face is directed toward the ceiling.
- Remove eye secretions with saline and gauze squares, cotton balls, or a washcloth. Clean from the inner aspect of the eye to the outer aspect.
- Give eye drops at room temperature.
- Do not allow the container tip to touch the eye, face, or other body part.
- Apply the drops or ointment to the conjunctival sac (Fig. 12-1). Do not apply the drug directly onto the eyeball.
- Have the person gently close the eye after the application.
- Use a tissue to blot medication that runs out of the eye. Do not rub or wipe the eye.

EAR MEDICATIONS
- Give ear drops at room temperature. If refrigerated, allow the container to warm to room temperature. This may take about 30 minutes.
- Position the person in a side-lying position. The affected ear is up.
- Remove excessive amounts of cerumen (ear wax). Use a wet washcloth.

NASAL MEDICATIONS
- Explain that the medication may cause a burning or stinging feeling.
- Position the person properly:
  - For nose drops: supine with the head over the edge of the mattress
  - For nasal spray: sitting or Fowler's position
- Remind the person not to blow his or her nose after receiving a nasal medication.

INHALED MEDICATIONS
- Follow the manufacturer's instructions for the inhaler used.
- Give a broncho-dilator (Chapter 24) before giving a cortico-steroid (Chapter 28).
- Check inside the inhaler after removing the cap. Look for and remove foreign matter.
- Have the person rinse his or her mouth after inhaling a cortico-steroid. This helps prevent a fungal infection in the mouth.
- Clean the inhaler and spacer after use. Follow the manufacturer's instruction.

DELEGATION GUIDELINES
Eye Medications

Before applying drugs to the eye, you need this information from the nurse, care plan, and MAR:

- If more than one eye medication is ordered
- How long to wait before applying more than one eye medication (if ordered)—usually 1 to 5 minutes between applications
- What observations to report and record:
  - The color of the sclera
  - Redness
  - Irritation
  - Drainage
  - Complaints of pain or discomfort
- When to report observations
- What specific patient or resident concerns to report at once

PROMOTING SAFETY AND COMFORT
Eye Medications

SAFETY

If a drug ordered for the eye is not labeled "ophthalmic," do not administer the drug to the eye. Check with the nurse.

The drug order should read right eye, left eye, or each eye. According to the Institute for Safe Medication Practices (ISMP), the following are error-prone abbreviations: OD (right eye), OS (left eye), and OU (each eye). If a drug order contains such abbreviations, check with the nurse before giving the drug.

APPLYING MEDICATIONS TO THE EYE

QUALITY OF LIFE

Remember to:
- Knock before entering the person's room.
- Address the person by name.
- Introduce yourself by name and title.

- Explain the procedure to the person before beginning and during the procedure.
- Protect the person's rights during the procedure.
- Handle the person gently during the procedure.

PRE-PROCEDURE

1 Follow *Delegation Guidelines: Eye Medications*. See *Promoting Safety and Comfort: Eye Medications*.
2 Check the drug order. **(First safety check.)** Focus on the:
  - *Right drug*
  - *Right time*
  - *Right dose*
  - *Right person*
  - *Right route*

3 Check with the nurse if you have any questions.
4 Practice hand hygiene.
5 Collect needed items:
  - Gauze squares, cotton balls, or a washcloth
  - Saline solution
  - Tissues
  - Gloves
  - MAR

PROCEDURE

6 Unlock the drug cart.
7 Read the order on the MAR.
8 Select the right drug from the person's drawer. Lock the drug cart.
9 Compare the drug order on the MAR against the pharmacy label on the drug container. **(Second safety check.)** Check for the:
  - *Right drug*
  - *Right time*
  - *Right dose*
  - *Right person*
  - *Right route*

10 Check the drug container for an expiration date.
11 Provide for privacy.
12 Identify the person. Check the ID bracelet against the MAR. Make sure you use at least two identifiers according to agency policy. Also call the person by name. Follow agency policy if using a bar code scanner.
13 Put on gloves.
14 Position the person supine or in a sitting position. The head is tilted back slightly.

Continued

APPLYING MEDICATIONS TO THE EYE–cont'd

PROCEDURE—cont'd

15 Remove eye drainage. Clean from the inner aspect to the outer aspect. Use a new gauze square or cotton ball with saline for each wipe. If using a washcloth, use a clean part of the washcloth for each wipe.

16 Observe the eye.

17 Compare the drug order on the MAR against the pharmacy label on the drug container. **(Third safety check.)** Check for the:
• *Right drug*
• *Right time*
• *Right dose*
• *Right person*
• *Right route*

18 Open the container. For ointment, place the lid or cap upside down on a clean surface.

19 Compare the drug order on the MAR against the pharmacy label on the drug container. **(Fourth safety check.)** This is done before applying the dose. Check for the:
• *Right drug*
• *Right time*
• *Right dose*
• *Right person*
• *Right route*

20 Ask the person to look up toward the ceiling.

21 Expose the lower conjunctival sac with your non-dominant hand. Gently pull down on the lower lid (see Fig. 12-1). Use a gauze square, cotton ball, or tissue if desired.

22 Apply eye drops:
a Hold the container in your dominant hand.
b Hold the dropper $1/2$ to $3/4$ (one-half to three-fourths) inch above the conjunctival sac.
c Drop the ordered number of drops into the conjunctival sac (Fig. 12-2, *A*).
d Release the lower lid.
e Apply gentle pressure to the inner corner of the eyelid on the bone for 1 to 2 minutes (Fig. 12-2, *B*). Use a clean cotton ball or tissue. This promotes proper absorption.

23 Apply eye ointment:
a Squeeze the ointment in a strip fashion into the conjunctival sac (Fig. 12-3). Start at the inner aspect and move toward the outer aspect.
b Release the lower lid.
c Ask the person to:
(1) Gently close his or her eyes.
(2) Move the eyes with the lids shut as if looking around the room. This spreads the medication over the eye.

24 Cap and return the container to the drawer. Lock the drug cart.

POST-PROCEDURE

25 Discard the supplies or unit dose packages.
26 Remove the gloves. Practice hand hygiene.
27 Provide for the person's comfort. See the inside of the front book cover.
28 Unscreen the person.
29 Complete a safety check before leaving the room. See the inside of the front book cover.
30 Follow agency policy for soiled linen.

31 Practice hand hygiene.
32 Record the *right documentation* on the MAR:
• The date, time, drug name, dosage, and route of administration
• The application site
• Your name or initials
33 Report and record any specific patient or resident observations or concerns.

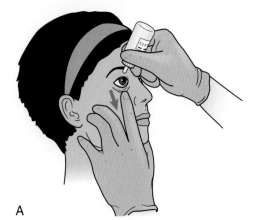
A

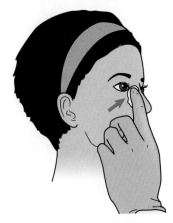
B

Fig. 12-2 Eye drops. **A,** Drops are given into the conjunctival sac. **B,** Pressure is applied to the inner corner of the eyelid on the bone.

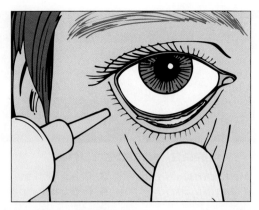

Fig. 12-3 Ointment is applied to the conjunctival sac.

EAR MEDICATIONS

Otic pertains to the ear *(oto)*. Otic (ear) drops are used to treat ear inflammations and infections. They also are used to soften ear wax **(cerumen).**

Ear drops are instilled into the ear. To **instill** means to enter drop by drop.

See *Delegation Guidelines: Ear Medications.*

See *Promoting Safety and Comfort: Ear Medications.*

DELEGATION GUIDELINES
Ear Medications

Before applying drugs to the ear, you need this information from the nurse, care plan, and MAR:
- How long to wait before instilling ear drops in the other ear (if ordered)—usually 5 to 10 minutes.
- How long the person needs to remain in the side-lying position after receiving the ear drops—usually 5 to 10 minutes.
- If you need to insert a cotton pledget or plug into the ear. If yes, how long should it remain in place—usually about 15 minutes.
- What observations to report and record:
  - Redness
  - Irritation
  - Drainage
  - Complaints of pain or discomfort
- When to report observations.
- What specific patient or resident concerns to report at once.

PROMOTING SAFETY AND COMFORT
Ear Medications

SAFETY

If a drug ordered for the ear is not labeled "otic," do not administer the drug to the ear. Check with the nurse.

The drug order should read right ear, left ear, or each ear. According to the ISMP, the following are error-prone abbreviations: AD (right ear), AS (left ear), and AU (each ear). If a drug order contains such abbreviations, check with the nurse before giving the drug.

If you can see excess ear wax, remove it with a wet washcloth. Do not insert cotton swabs or cotton-tipped applicators into the ear. If you cannot remove the wax, call for the nurse.

COMFORT

Ear drops are given at room temperature. Cold ear drops can cause nausea, pain, and dizziness.

INSTILLING EAR DROPS

PRE-PROCEDURE

1 Follow *Delegation Guidelines: Ear Medications,* p. 153. See *Promoting Safety and Comfort: Ear Medications,* p. 153.
2 Check the drug order. **(First safety check.)** Focus on the:
  - *Right drug*
  - *Right time*
  - *Right dose*
  - *Right person*
  - *Right route*

3 Check with the nurse if you have any questions.
4 Practice hand hygiene.
5 Collect needed items:
  - Wet washcloth
  - Cotton pledget or plug
  - Gloves
  - MAR

PROCEDURE

6 Unlock the drug cart.
7 Read the order on the MAR.
8 Select the right drug from the person's drawer. Lock the drug cart.
9 Compare the drug order on the MAR against the pharmacy label on the drug container. **(Second safety check.)** Check for the:
  - *Right drug*
  - *Right time*
  - *Right dose*
  - *Right person*
  - *Right route*
10 Check the drug container for an expiration date.
11 Provide for privacy.
12 Identify the person. Check the ID bracelet against the MAR. Make sure you use at least two identifiers according to agency policy. Also call the person by name. Follow agency policy if using a bar code scanner.
13 Put on gloves.
14 Position the person in a side-lying position. The affected ear is up.
15 Remove excess ear wax. Use the wet washcloth.
16 Observe the ear.
17 Compare the drug order on the MAR against the pharmacy label on the drug container. **(Third safety check.)** Check for the:
  - *Right drug*
  - *Right time*
  - *Right dose*
  - *Right person*
  - *Right route*

18 Open the container.
19 Draw medication into the dropper.
20 Compare the drug order on the MAR against the pharmacy label on the drug container. **(Fourth safety check.)** Check for the:
  - *Right drug*
  - *Right time*
  - *Right dose*
  - *Right person*
  - *Right route*
21 Apply ear drops (for persons 3 years of age and older):
  a Pull the ear upward and back (Fig. 12-4). This straightens the external auditory canal.
  b Instill the ordered number of drops along the side of the ear canal.
  c Return the dropper to the container.
22 Insert a cotton pledget or plug loosely into the ear if ordered. This prevents the medication from flowing out of the ear.
23 Have the person remain in the side-lying position for 5 to 10 minutes. Or as directed by the nurse and the care plan.
24 Remove the cotton pledget or plug.
25 Return the container to the drawer. Lock the drug cart.

INSTILLING EAR DROPS—cont'd

POST-PROCEDURE

26 Discard the supplies or unit dose packages.
27 Remove the gloves. Practice hand hygiene.
28 Provide for the person's comfort. See the inside of the front book cover.
29 Unscreen the person.
30 Complete a safety check before leaving the room. See the inside of the front book cover.
31 Follow agency policy for soiled linen.

32 Practice hand hygiene.
33 Record the *right documentation* on the MAR:
  • The date, time, drug name, dosage, and route of administration
  • The application site
  • Your name or initials
34 Report and record any specific patient or resident observations or concerns.

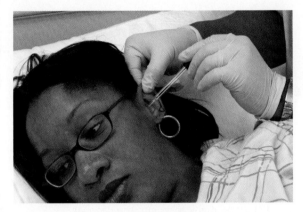

Fig. 12-4 The adult's ear is pulled upward and back. Ear drops are instilled. (Courtesy Rick Brady, from Lilley LL and others: *Pharmacology and the nursing process*, ed 5, St Louis, 2007, Mosby.)

DELEGATION GUIDELINES
Nose Medications

Before applying drugs to the nose, you need this information from the nurse, care plan, and MAR:
• If the person needs to blow his or her nose before receiving the drug.
• If the person can be positioned with his or her head over the edge of the mattress for nose drops. If not, how to position the person.
• How long the person needs to remain in the supine position after receiving nose drops—usually 5 minutes.
• How long the person must wait to blow his or her nose after receiving the drug.
• What observations to report and record:
  • Redness
  • Irritation
  • Drainage
  • Bleeding
  • Nasal congestion
  • Complaints of pain or discomfort
• When to report observations.
• What specific patient or resident concerns to report at once.

NOSE MEDICATIONS

Nasal means nose *(naso)*. Nose drops and nasal sprays are used to administer drugs to the mucous membranes of the nose.

See *Delegation Guidelines: Nose Medications.*
See *Promoting Safety and Comfort: Nose Medications.*

PROMOTING SAFETY AND COMFORT
Nose Medications

SAFETY
Certain conditions make blowing the nose unsafe. Nasal surgery and head injuries or surgeries are examples. Blowing the nose can increase pressure inside the person's head. Always check with the nurse and the care plan before asking a person to blow his or her nose.

GIVING NOSE MEDICATIONS

PRE-PROCEDURE

1 Follow *Delegation Guidelines: Nose Medications*, p. 155. See *Promoting Safety and Comfort: Nose Medications*, p. 155.

2 Check the drug order. **(First safety check.)** Focus on the:
- *Right drug*
- *Right time*
- *Right dose*
- *Right person*
- *Right route*

3 Check with the nurse if you have any questions.

4 Practice hand hygiene.

5 Collect needed items:
- Tissues
- Gloves
- MAR

PROCEDURE

6 Unlock the drug cart.

7 Read the order on the MAR.

8 Select the right drug from the person's drawer. Lock the drug cart.

9 Compare the drug order on the MAR against the pharmacy label on the drug container. **(Second safety check.)** Check for the:
- *Right drug*
- *Right time*
- *Right dose*
- *Right person*
- *Right route*

10 Check the drug container for an expiration date.

11 Provide for privacy.

12 Identify the person. Check the ID bracelet against the MAR. Make sure you use at least two identifiers according to agency policy. Also call the person by name. Follow agency policy if using a bar code scanner.

13 Put on gloves.

14 Observe the nose.

15 Compare the drug order on the MAR against the pharmacy label on the drug container. **(Third safety check.)** Check for the:
- *Right drug*
- *Right time*
- *Right dose*
- *Right person*
- *Right route*

16 Open the container. For nasal spray, place the lid or cap upside down on a clean surface.

17 Compare the drug order on the MAR against the pharmacy label on the drug container. **(Fourth safety check.)** This is done before giving the dose. Check for the:
- *Right drug*
- *Right time*
- *Right dose*
- *Right person*
- *Right route*

18 Give the drug:
 a Nose drops (for adults and older children):
   (1) Ask the person to gently blow the nose (Fig. 12-5, *A*). Provide tissues.
   (2) Position the person supine with the head over the edge of the mattress. Or position the person as directed by the nurse and the care plan.
   (3) Draw medication into the dropper (Fig. 12-5, *B*).
   (4) Hold the dropper about $1/2$ inch above the nostril.
   (5) Instill the number of drops ordered (Fig. 12-5, *C*).
   (6) Repeat steps 18 a (3)–(5) for the other nostril.
   (7) Have the person remain as positioned for 5 minutes. Or for as long as directed by the nurse and the care plan.
 b Nasal spray:
   (1) Ask the person to gently blow the nose. Provide tissues.
   (2) Position the person in a sitting or Fowler's position.
   (3) Block one nostril (Fig. 12-6, *A*).
   (4) Hold the spray bottle upright. Shake the bottle.
   (5) Insert the bottle tip into the nostril.
   (6) Ask the person to take a deep breath through the nose.
   (7) Squeeze a puff of spray into the nostril as the person is taking a deep breath (Fig. 12-6, *B*).
   (8) Wipe the bottle tip if you need to spray the other nostril. Then repeat steps 18 b (3)–(7).

19 Provide the person with tissues for blotting drainage. Remind the person not to blow his or her nose for several minutes.

20 Return the container to the drawer. Lock the drug cart.

GIVING NOSE MEDICATIONS—cont'd

POST-PROCEDURE

21 Discard the supplies or unit dose packages.

22 Remove the gloves. Practice hand hygiene.

23 Provide for the person's comfort. See the inside of the front book cover.

24 Unscreen the person.

25 Complete a safety check before leaving the room. See the inside of the front book cover.

26 Follow agency policy for soiled linen.

27 Practice hand hygiene.

28 Record the *right documentation* on the MAR:
- The date, time, drug name, dosage, and route of administration
- The application site
- Your name or initials

29 Report and record any specific patient or resident observations or concerns.

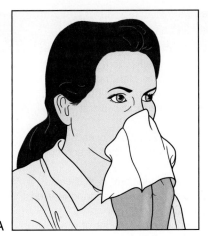
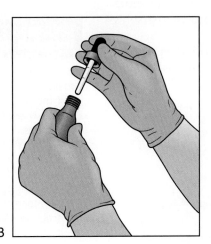
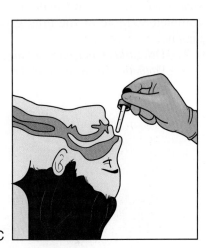

Fig. 12-5 Nose drops. **A,** The person blows her nose. **B,** Drops are drawn into the dropper. **C,** Drops are instilled into the nose.

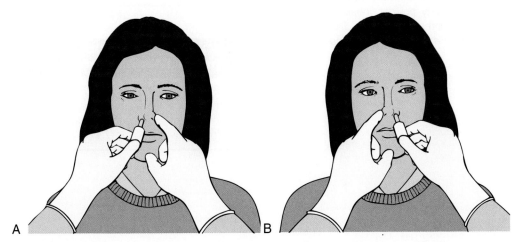

Fig. 12-6 Nasal spray. **A,** One nostril is blocked. **B,** The bottle tip is inserted into the person's nose. A puff of spray is squeezed into the nose as the person takes a deep breath.

INHALED MEDICATIONS

Some cortico-steroids (Chapter 28) and broncho-dilators (Chapter 24) are inhaled into the respiratory tract through the mouth. Inhaled drugs affect the bronchial smooth muscle. Therefore absorption and onset of action are rapid.

Metered-dose inhalers (MDIs) are commonly used (Fig. 12-7). (*Meter* means *measure*.) An MDI is a small pressurized canister that contains a spray, mist, or fine powder. A measured (metered) amount of the drug is released for inhalation each time the dispensing valve is pushed or squeezed (Fig. 12-8).

For some people, MDIs are easier to use with *spacers*. A spacer is a tube that attaches to the inhaler (Fig. 12-9). It traps or holds the dose sprayed by the MDI. Part of the dose is not sprayed into the air. And the spacer lets the person inhale more slowly and more completely. More of the drug gets into the person's airway.

See *Delegation Guidelines: Inhaled Medications*.

See *Promoting Safety and Comfort: Inhaled Medications*.

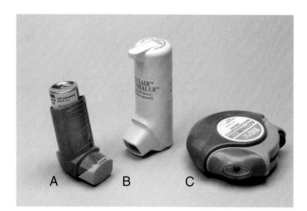

Fig. 12-7 A, Metered-dose inhaler (MDI). **B,** Automated, or breath-activated, MDI. **C,** Dry powder inhaler. It delivers powdered medication. (Courtesy Rick Brady, from Lilley LL and others: *Pharmacology and the nursing process*, ed 5, St Louis, 2007, Mosby.)

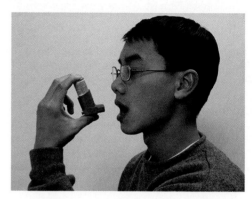

Fig. 12-8 A dose is released when the dispensing valve is pushed. (From Elkin MK, Perry AG, Potter PA: *Nursing interventions & clinical skills*, ed 4, St Louis, 2007, Mosby.)

DELEGATION GUIDELINES
Inhaled Medications

Before giving an inhaled medication, you need this information from the nurse, care plan, and MAR:

- If the person uses the MDI himself or herself.
- How many times to shake the canister—usually 4 or 5 times.
- If the person can hold his or her breath for 10 seconds. If not, how long can the person hold his or her breath.
- How long to wait if a repeat puff is ordered.
- How long to wait before giving a second inhaled drug—usually 1 to 3 minutes.
- If you need to measure the amount of medication left in the canister (Fig. 12-10).
- What observations to report and record.
- When to report observations.
- What specific patient or resident concerns to report at once.

PROMOTING SAFETY AND COMFORT
Inhaled Medications

SAFETY
Some states and agencies do not let MA-Cs give inhaled medications. Make sure you know what your state and agency allow.

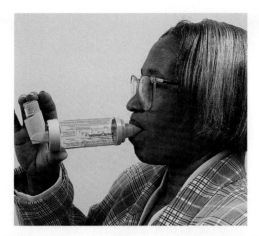

Fig. 12-9 A spacer is attached to an MDI. (From Potter PA, Perry AG: *Fundamentals of nursing,* ed 6, St Louis, 2005, Mosby.)

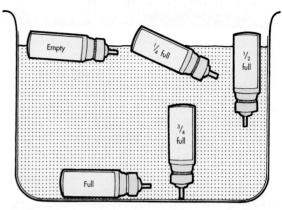

Fig. 12-10 The canister is immersed in water to measure the amount of medication remaining. (From Elkin MK, Perry AG, Potter PA: *Nursing interventions & clinical skills,* ed 4, St Louis, 2007, Mosby.)

GIVING INHALED MEDICATIONS

QUALITY OF LIFE

Remember to:
- Knock before entering the person's room.
- Address the person by name.
- Introduce yourself by name and title.

- Explain the procedure to the person before beginning and during the procedure.
- Protect the person's rights during the procedure.
- Handle the person gently during the procedure.

PRE-PROCEDURE

1 Follow *Delegation Guidelines: Inhaled Medications.* See *Promoting Safety and Comfort: Inhaled Medications.*
2 Check the drug order. **(First safety check.)** Focus on the:
   - *Right drug*
   - *Right time*
   - *Right dose*
   - *Right person*
   - *Right route*

3 Check with the nurse if you have any questions.
4 Practice hand hygiene.
5 Collect needed items:
   - Tissues
   - Gloves
   - MAR

PROCEDURE

6 Unlock the drug cart.
7 Read the order on the MAR.
8 Select the right inhaler from the person's drawer. Lock the drug cart.
9 Compare the drug order on the MAR against the pharmacy label on the inhaler. **(Second safety check.)** Check for the:
   - *Right drug*
   - *Right time*
   - *Right dose*

   - *Right person*
   - *Right route*
10 Check the inhaler for an expiration date.
11 Provide for privacy.
12 Identify the person. Check the ID bracelet against the MAR. Make sure you use at least two identifiers according to agency policy. Also call the person by name. Follow agency policy if using a bar code scanner.
13 Put on gloves.

Continued

GIVING INHALED MEDICATIONS—cont'd

PROCEDURE—cont'd

14 Compare the drug order on the MAR against the pharmacy label on the inhaler. **(Third safety check.)** Check for the:
- *Right drug*
- *Right time*
- *Right dose*
- *Right person*
- *Right route*

15 Position the person so that he or she is upright—standing, sitting, or Fowler's position.

16 Remove the cap from the inhaler. Place the lid or cap upside down on a clean surface.

17 Compare the drug order on the MAR against the pharmacy label on the inhaler. **(Fourth safety check.)** Check for the:
- *Right drug*
- *Right time*
- *Right dose*
- *Right person*
- *Right route*

18 Hold the inhaler upright (see Fig. 12-8). Use your thumb and first 1 or 2 fingers.

19 Give the drug:
  a *MDI without a spacer:*
  (1) Shake the inhaler the number of times as directed by the nurse.
  (2) Ask the person to open his or her mouth. Also ask the person to tilt his or her head back slightly.
  (3) Ask the person to exhale.
  (4) Place the inhaler 1 to 2 inches in front of the person's mouth.
  (5) Push down on or squeeze the dispensing valve. This releases the dose. Ask the person to inhale deeply and slowly for 3 to 5 seconds.
  (6) Ask the person to hold his or her breath for about 10 seconds.
  (7) Ask the person to exhale slowly through his or her mouth.
  (8) Repeat the puffs as ordered:
    (a) Shake the inhaler again.
    (b) Repeat steps 19 a (2)–(7).
  b *MDI with a spacer:*
  (1) Insert the inhaler into the spacer.
  (2) Shake the inhaler and spacer the number of times as directed by the nurse.
  (3) Ask the person to open his or her mouth. Also ask the person to tilt his or her head back slightly.
  (4) Ask the person to exhale.
  (5) Ask the person to place the spacer mouthpiece in his or her mouth. Then ask the person to close the lips around the mouthpiece.
  (6) Push down on or squeeze the dispensing valve. This releases the dose. Ask the person to inhale deeply and slowly for 3 to 5 seconds.
  (7) Ask the person to hold his or her breath for about 10 seconds.
  (8) Ask the person to exhale slowly through his or her mouth.
  (9) Repeat the puffs as ordered:
    (a) Shake the inhaler again.
    (b) Repeat steps 19 b (3)–(8).

20 Remove the spacer (if used). Replace the cap on the inhaler.

21 Have the person rinse his or her mouth with water if he or she inhaled a cortico-steroid.

22 Return the inhaler and spacer to the drawer. Lock the drug cart.

POST-PROCEDURE

23 Remove the gloves. Practice hand hygiene.

24 Provide for the person's comfort. See the inside of the front book cover.

25 Unscreen the person.

26 Clean the inhaler and spacer. Follow the manufacturer's instructions. (Wear gloves for this step.)

27 Complete a safety check before leaving the room. See the inside of the front book cover.

28 Follow agency policy for soiled linen.

29 Practice hand hygiene.

30 Record the *right documentation* on the MAR:
- The date, time, drug name, dosage, and route of administration
- Your name or initials

31 Report and record any specific patient or resident observations or concerns.

REVIEW QUESTIONS

Circle the BEST answer.

1 Otic medications are administered to the
a eye
b ear
c nose
d throat

2 To give eye, ear, or nose medications, you should wear
a gloves
b a gown
c a face mask
d a surgical cap

3 Eye drops are ordered. You should use
a a syringe
b a dropper from the supply cart
c the dropper supplied by the drug manufacturer
d a squeeze bottle

4 A person has two eye medications ordered for the same eye. You can usually give the second medication
a immediately
b after 1 to 5 minutes
c after 5 to 10 minutes
d after 10 to 15 minutes

5 Which is *not* a position for giving eye medications?
a supine
b sitting
c Fowler's
d with the head over the edge of the mattress

6 A drug order states that a medication is to be given "OS." What should you do?
a Give the drug in the left eye.
b Give the drug in the right eye.
c Give the drug in both eyes.
d Check with the nurse.

7 An eye dropper is held
a $^1/_2$ inch above the eye
b 1 inch above the eye
c $1^1/_2$ inches above the eye
d 2 inches above the eye

8 After eye ointment is applied, the person should
a wipe the eye
b rub the eye
c close the eyes gently
d stare straight ahead

9 Ear medications are given
a cold
b at room temperature
c after being heated
d directly from the refrigerator

10 To give ear drops, the person is positioned
a in a side-lying position with the affected ear up
b in a side-lying position with the affected ear down
c supine with the head over the edge of the mattress
d sitting with the head turned to one side

11 What should you use to remove excess cerumen?
a tongue blade
b cotton-tipped applicator
c gauze and saline
d wet washcloth

12 To instill a drug means to give
a a puff by squeezing a tube
b a spray by squeezing a container
c it drop by drop
d it in a strip fashion

13 Ear drops are ordered for both ears. How long should you wait before giving ear drops in the second ear?
a No waiting is required.
b Wait 1 to 5 minutes.
c Wait 5 to 10 minutes.
d Wait 10 to 15 minutes.

14 You inserted a cotton pledget after giving ear drops. How long should the pledget remain in place?
a 1 minute
b 5 minutes
c 10 minutes
d 15 minutes

15 After receiving nose drops, how long should the person remain in the supine position?
a 1 minute
b 5 minutes
c 10 minutes
d 15 minutes

16 Which is the position for giving nasal spray?
a supine
b side-lying
c Fowler's
d with the head over the edge of the mattress

17 To give a nasal spray, you give a puff of spray as the person
a blows his or her nose
b takes a deep breath
c exhales deeply
d holds his or her breath

18 Nasal spray is ordered for both nostrils. What should you do to give the drug in the second nostril?
a Get a new spray bottle.
b Wipe the bottle tip.
c Get a new dropper.
d Ask the nurse.

Continued

REVIEW QUESTIONS–cont'd

19 Before a person uses an MDI with a spacer, you should:
a squeeze the dispensing valve to remove foreign objects
b shake the MDI and spacer
c ask the person to inhale
d have the person rinse out his or her mouth with water

20 The mouthpiece of an MDI spacer is
a placed 1 to 2 inches in front of the person's mouth
b placed 3 to 4 inches in front of the person's mouth
c positioned on the person's lips
d placed in the person's mouth

21 After using an MDI, the person does the following *except*
a holds his or her breath for about 10 seconds
b exhales slowly through the mouth
c inhales more puffs immediately
d rinses the mouth with water if a cortico-steroid was inhaled

Circle T if the statement is true. Circle F if the statement is false.

22 T F Eye drops are applied to the eyeball.

23 T F Eye ointment is applied from the inner aspect of the conjunctiva to the outer aspect.

24 T F To give ear drops to an adult, the ear is pulled upward and back.

25 T F A person should blow the nose after receiving a nasal medication.

26 T F When using an MDI, you measure the dose released.

Answers to these questions are on pp. 444-445.

Vaginal and Rectal Drugs

The vagina and rectum are lined with mucous membranes. Vaginal drugs are usually given for a local effect. That is, the site of action is in the vagina. Rectal drugs are given either for local or systemic effects. They are given to treat or prevent:

- Constipation
- Anal itching
- Hemorrhoids
- Vomiting
- Fever
- Bladder spasms

Vaginal drugs are usually creams, gels, tablets, foams, or suppositories. Rectal drugs are usually in the form of suppositories. A **suppository** is a cone-shaped, solid drug that is inserted into a body opening; it melts at body temperature. As shown in Figure 13-1, vaginal suppositories are larger than rectal suppositories. Vaginal suppositories also are more oval than rectal ones.

Suppositories are stored in a cool place to prevent softening. If one becomes soft and the package is sealed, do one of the following until it hardens:

- Hold the foil-wrapped suppository under cold running water
- Place the foil-wrapped suppository in ice water

To properly administer vaginal and rectal drugs, follow the rules listed in Box 13-1.

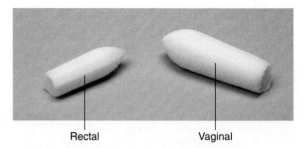

Fig. 13-1 Rectal and vaginal suppositories. (Courtesy Rick Brady, from Lilley LL and others: *Pharmacology and the nursing process*, ed 5, St Louis, 2007, Mosby.)

Rectal   Vaginal

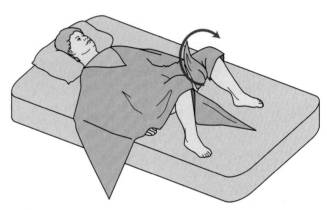

Fig. 13-2 The woman is in the lithotomy position and draped.

BOX 13-1   Administering Vaginal and Rectal Drugs

GENERAL RULES
- Practice hand hygiene before and after the application.
- Follow Standard Precautions and the Bloodborne Pathogen Standard (Appendix C).
- Follow Transmission-Based Precautions as ordered.
- Wear gloves.
- Provide for privacy.
- Insert the rounded end of the suppository first.
- Remind the person of the nurse's instructions if self-administration is allowed.

VAGINAL DRUGS
- Administer vaginal suppositories at room temperature.
- Have the woman void before the procedure. A full bladder can cause discomfort.
- Position the woman in the lithotomy position. Use a pillow to elevate her hips. Drape her as for perineal care. See Figure 13-2.

- Apply a perineal pad or panty shield after administering the drug. This protects clothing or bottom linens from soiling or staining.
- Have the woman remain supine with her hips elevated for 5 to 10 minutes. This allows a suppository to melt. It allows the drug to spread within the vagina.

RECTAL DRUGS
- Ask the person to have a bowel movement (if possible) before the procedure.
- Position the person in the Sims' position. Use the left side-lying position if the person cannot tolerate the Sims' position.
- Do not insert the suppository into feces (Fig. 13-3, *A*). The suppository must have contact with the rectal wall (Fig. 13-3, *B*).
- Have the person remain in the Sims' or a left side-lying position for 15 to 20 minutes. The suppository melts and is absorbed during this time.

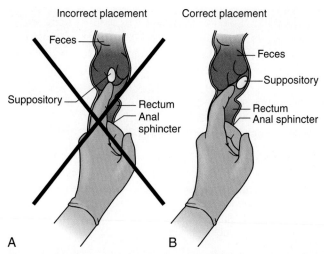

Incorrect placement   Correct placement

Feces

Suppository

Rectum
Anal sphincter

Feces

Suppository

Rectum
Anal sphincter

A   B

Fig. 13-3 A, Do not insert a rectal suppository into feces. **B,** Insert a rectal suppository along the rectal wall. (Modified from deWit SC: *Fundamental concepts and skills for nursing,* ed 2, Philadelphia, 2005, Saunders.)

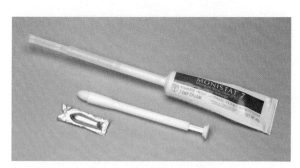

Fig. 13-4 Vaginal cream and suppository with applicators provided by the manufacturers. (Courtesy Rick Brady, from Lilley LL and others: *Pharmacology and the nursing process,* ed 5, St Louis, 2007, Mosby.)

VAGINAL DRUGS

Vaginal drugs are ordered for some gynecologic disorders. **Gynecologic** pertains to diseases of the female reproductive organs and breasts. (*Gyneco* means *woman*.)

Vaginal creams, gels, tablets, foams, and some suppositories are inserted with applicators provided by the manufacturers (Fig. 13-4). Often a gloved index finger is used to insert a suppository.

See *Delegation Guidelines: Vaginal Drugs.*

See *Promoting Safety and Comfort: Vaginal Drugs.*

DELEGATION GUIDELINES
Vaginal Drugs

Before giving a vaginal drug, you need the following information from the nurse, care plan, and MAR:
- If the woman can self-administer the drug
- If you should apply a perineal pad or panty shield after administration
- How to position the woman after administering the drug and for how long—usually the supine position with the hips elevated for 5 to 10 minutes
- If the applicator is to be discarded or washed with soap and water
- How and where to store a re-usable applicator
- What observations to report and record:
  - Redness, swelling, discharge, bleeding, or irritation
  - Color and amount of discharge or bleeding
  - Odor
  - Complaints of pain, burning, or other discomfort
  - Amount and length of symptom relief
- When to report observations
- What specific patient or resident concerns to report at once

---

PROMOTING SAFETY AND COMFORT
Vaginal Drugs

COMFORT
Often vaginal drugs are ordered to be given at bedtime. Doing so allows the drug to remain in place longer. The woman does not lose part of the dose by leakage when she sits or stands. And vaginal leakage can cause discomfort and embarrassment.

Some women prefer to self-administer vaginal drugs. Doing so is less embarrassing. The nurse, care plan, and MAR can provide information about self-administration.

GIVING VAGINAL DRUGS

PRE-PROCEDURE

1 Follow *Delegation Guidelines: Vaginal Drugs*, p. 165. See *Promoting Safety and Comfort: Vaginal Drugs*, p. 165.
2 Check the drug order. **(First safety check.)** Focus on the:
- *Right drug*
- *Right time*
- *Right dose*
- *Right person*
- *Right route*

3 Check with the nurse if you have any questions.
4 Practice hand hygiene.
5 Collect needed items:
- Vaginal applicator
- Water-soluble lubricant
- Pillow
- Perineal pad or panty shield
- Gloves
- Paper towels
- MAR

PROCEDURE

6 Unlock the drug cart or storage area.
7 Read the order on the MAR.
8 Select the right drug from the person's drawer or the storage area. Lock the drug cart or storage area.
9 Compare the drug order on the MAR against the pharmacy label on the drug container. **(Second safety check.)** Check for the:
- *Right drug*
- *Right time*
- *Right dose*
- *Right person*
- *Right route*

10 Check the drug container for an expiration date.
11 Provide for privacy.
12 Identify the person. Check the ID bracelet against the MAR. Make sure you use at least two identifiers according to agency policy. Also call the person by name. Follow agency policy if using a bar code scanner.
13 Put on gloves.
14 Position and drape the woman in the lithotomy position. Elevate her hips on a pillow.
15 Remove and discard the gloves. Practice hand hygiene. Put on clean gloves.
16 Compare the drug order on the MAR against the pharmacy label on the drug container. **(Third safety check.)** Check for the:
- *Right drug*
- *Right time*
- *Right dose*
- *Right person*
- *Right route*

17 Prepare the drug:
a *Cream, foam, or gel with an applicator:*
  (1) Open the container. Place the lid or cap upside down on a clean surface.
  (2) Attach the applicator to the container.
  (3) Squeeze the container to fill the applicator.
  (4) Lubricate the applicator tip. Use the water-soluble lubricant.
  (5) Set the applicator on a paper towel.
b *Suppository:*
  (1) Open and remove the wrapper containing the suppository.
  (2) Insert the suppository into an applicator (if using one).
  (3) Lubricate the suppository. Use the water-soluble lubricant.
  (4) Set the suppository on a paper towel.

18 Close the container. Compare the drug order on the MAR against the pharmacy label on the drug container. **(Fourth safety check.)** Check for the:
- *Right drug*
- *Right time*
- *Right dose*
- *Right person*
- *Right route*

19 Expose the perineum.
20 Observe the perineum and vaginal opening.
21 Administer the dose form:
a *Cream, foam, or gel with an applicator:*
  (1) Spread the labia to expose the vagina. Use your non-dominant hand.
  (2) Insert the applicator as far as possible into the vagina.
  (3) Push the plunger to deposit the drug (Fig. 13-5).
  (4) Remove the applicator.
  (5) Wrap the applicator in the paper towel.

GIVING VAGINAL DRUGS—cont'd

PROCEDURE—cont'd

b *Suppository:*
  (1) Lubricate your gloved index finger (if not using an applicator). Use the water-soluble lubricant.
  (2) Spread the labia to expose the vagina. Use your non-dominant hand.
  (3) Insert the suppository as far as possible into the vagina (Fig. 13-6). Use your gloved finger or an applicator.
  (4) Remove the applicator (if used).
  (5) Wrap the applicator (if used) in the paper towel.

22 Apply a perineal pad or panty shield.
23 Assist the woman to the supine position with her hips elevated. Ask her to remain in this position for 5 to 10 minutes. Or position her as directed by the nurse, care plan, or MAR.
24 Remove and discard the gloves.
25 Practice hand hygiene.
26 Return the container to the drawer or storage area. Lock the drug cart or storage area.

POST-PROCEDURE

27 Discard supplies or unit dose packages.
28 Provide for the person's comfort. See the inside of the front book cover.
29 Unscreen the person.
30 Empty and clean the applicator. Store it according to agency policy. Discard the paper towel. (Wear gloves for this step.)
31 Complete a safety check before leaving the room. See the inside of the front book cover.

32 Follow agency policy for soiled linen.
33 Practice hand hygiene.
34 Record the *right documentation* on the MAR:
  • The date, time, drug name, dosage, and route of administration
  • Your name or initials
35 Report and record any specific patient or resident observations or concerns.

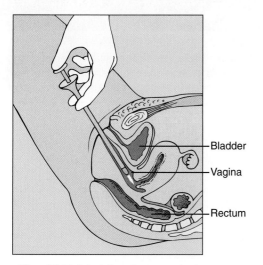

Fig. 13-5 Administering a vaginal cream.

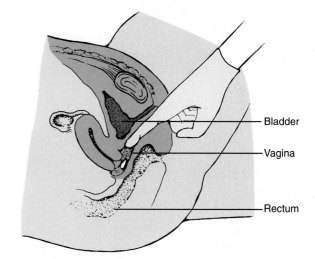

Fig. 13-6 Administering a vaginal suppository. (Modified from Lilley LL and others: *Pharmacology and the nursing process,* ed 5, St Louis, 2007, Mosby.)

RECTAL DRUGS

Suppositories are the most common rectal drugs. They generally are not used:

- After recent prostate surgery
- After recent rectal surgery
- After recent rectal trauma
- If the person has rectal bleeding
- If the person has diarrhea
  See *Delegation Guidelines: Rectal Drugs.*
  See *Promoting Safety and Comfort: Rectal Drugs.*

Before giving a rectal drug, you need the following information from the nurse, care plan, and MAR:

- If the person can self-administer the drug
- How to position the person after administering the drug and for how long—usually the Sims' or left side-lying position for 15 to 20 minutes
- What observations to report and record (for the drug ordered):
  - Redness, swelling, discharge, bleeding, or irritation
  - Color and amount of discharge or bleeding
  - Odor
  - Complaints of pain, burning, or other discomfort
  - Nausea
  - Vomiting
  - Respiratory rate
  - Temperature
  - Color, amount, consistency, shape, and odor of stools
  - Amount and length of relief from pain, nausea, or vomiting
- When to report observations
- What specific patient or resident concerns to report at once

PROMOTING SAFETY AND COMFORT
Rectal Drugs

COMFORT
Some people prefer to self-administer rectal drugs. Doing so is less embarrassing. The nurse, care plan, and MAR can provide information about self-administration.

GIVING A RECTAL SUPPOSITORY

QUALITY OF LIFE

Remember to:
- Knock before entering the person's room.
- Address the person by name.
- Introduce yourself by name and title.

- Explain the procedure to the person before beginning and during the procedure.
- Protect the person's rights during the procedure.
- Handle the person gently during the procedure.

PRE-PROCEDURE

1 Follow *Delegation Guidelines: Rectal Drugs.* See *Promoting Safety and Comfort: Rectal Drugs.*
2 Check the drug order. **(First safety check.)** Focus on the:
- *Right drug*
- *Right time*
- *Right dose*
- *Right person*
- *Right route*

3 Check with the nurse if you have any questions.
4 Practice hand hygiene.
5 Collect needed items:
- Water-soluble lubricant
- Gloves
- Paper towels
- Toilet tissue
- MAR

PROCEDURE

6 Unlock the drug cart or the storage area.
7 Read the order on the MAR.
8 Select the right drug from the storage area. Lock the storage area.
9 Compare the drug order on the MAR against the pharmacy label on the drug container. **(Second safety check.)** Check for the:
- *Right drug*
- *Right time*
- *Right dose*
- *Right person*
- *Right route*
10 Check the drug container for an expiration date.
11 Provide for privacy.
12 Identify the person. Check the ID bracelet against the MAR. Make sure you use at least two identifiers according to agency policy. Also call the person by name. Follow agency policy if using a bar code scanner.
13 Put on gloves.
14 Position and drape the person in Sims' position or a left side-lying position. Bend the uppermost leg toward the waist.
15 Compare the drug order on the MAR against the pharmacy label on the drug container. **(Third safety check.)** Check for the:
- *Right drug*
- *Right time*
- *Right dose*
- *Right person*
- *Right route*
16 Open and remove the wrapper containing the suppository (Fig. 13-7, *A,* p. 170).

17 Lubricate the suppository (Fig. 13-7, *B,* p. 170).
18 Set the suppository on a paper towel.
19 Compare the drug order on the MAR against the pharmacy label on the drug container. **(Fourth safety check.)** Check for the:
- *Right drug*
- *Right time*
- *Right dose*
- *Right person*
- *Right route*
20 Expose the rectal area.
21 Observe the rectal area.
22 Insert the suppository:
a Raise the upper buttock to expose the anus (Fig. 13-8, p. 170).
b Ask the person to take a deep breath.
c Place the rounded tip of the suppository into the anus and rectum. Insert it about 1 inch into the rectum along the rectal wall (see Fig. 13-3, *B*).
23 Wipe the anus to remove excess lubricant. Use the toilet tissue.
24 Ask the person to remain in a left side-lying position for 15 to 20 minutes. Or position him or her as directed by the nurse, care plan, or MAR.

Continued

GIVING A RECTAL SUPPOSITORY—cont'd

POST-PROCEDURE

25 Discard supplies or unit dose packages. Dispose of toilet tissue.

26 Remove and discard the gloves. Practice hand hygiene.

27 Provide for the person's comfort. See the inside of the front book cover.

28 Unscreen the person.

29 Complete a safety check before leaving the room. See the inside of the front book cover.

30 Follow agency policy for soiled linen.

31 Practice hand hygiene.

32 Record the *right documentation* on the MAR:
  • The date, time, drug name, dosage, and route of administration
  • Your name or initials

33 Report and record any specific patient or resident observations or concerns.

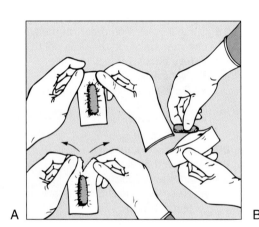
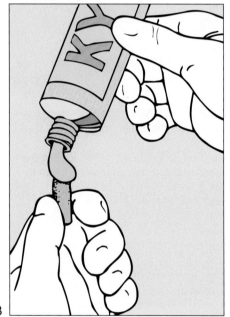

Fig. 13-7 A, The rectal suppository is unwrapped. **B,** The suppository is lubricated with water-soluble lubricant.

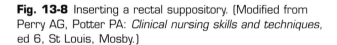
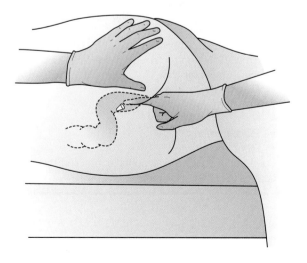

Fig. 13-8 Inserting a rectal suppository. (Modified from Perry AG, Potter PA: *Clinical nursing skills and techniques,* ed 6, St Louis, Mosby.)

REVIEW QUESTIONS

Circle the BEST answer.

1 A cone-shaped, solid drug inserted into a body opening is called a
a tablet
b foam
c gel
d suppository

2 Vaginal drugs are given for
a constipation
b bladder spasms
c vomiting
d gynecologic disorders

3 When giving vaginal or rectal drugs, you should always
a wear gloves
b wear a gown
c wear a mask
d wear gloves, a gown, and a mask

4 For a vaginal drug, the woman is positioned in
a the lithotomy position
b Sims' position
c a left side-lying position
d the supine position

5 After receiving a vaginal drug, the woman is positioned in
a the lithotomy position
b Sims' position
c a left side-lying position
d the supine position

6 Which is used to give a vaginal cream, gel, or foam?
a a gloved finger
b an applicator provided by the manufacturer
c a cotton-tipped swab
d a suppository

7 To protect garments and bed linens after giving a vaginal drug, you can
a apply a perineal pad or panty shield
b place a waterproof pad under the buttocks
c elevate the woman's hips on pillows
d ask the woman to use the bedpan or toilet

8 To give a rectal drug, the person is positioned in
a the lithotomy position
b Sims' position
c a right side-lying position
d the supine position

9 A rectal suppository usually melts in
a 5 to 10 minutes
b 15 to 20 minutes
c 20 to 25 minutes
d 25 to 30 minutes

10 A rectal suppository can be given
a for fever
b after rectal surgery
c after prostate surgery
d if the person has diarrhea

11 Which is used to give a rectal suppository?
a a gloved finger
b an applicator provided by the manufacturer
c a cotton-tipped applicator
d an enema tube

Circle T if the statement is true. Circle F if the statement is false.

12 T F Suppositories are stored in a cool place.

13 T F The rounded end of a suppository is inserted first.

14 T F Vaginal suppositories are given at room temperature.

15 T F A rectal suppository can be inserted into feces.

Answers to these questions are on p. 445.

Drugs Affecting the Nervous System

OBJECTIVES

- Define the key terms and key abbreviations used in this chapter.
- Review the structures and functions of the nervous system.
- Describe adrenergic agents and their uses.
- Explain how to assist with the nursing process when adrenergic agents are used.
- Describe alpha- and beta-adrenergic blocking agents and their uses.
- Explain how to assist with the nursing process when beta-adrenergic blocking agents are used.
- Describe cholinergic agents and their uses.
- Explain how to assist with the nursing process when cholinergic agents are used.
- Describe anti-cholinergic agents and their uses.
- Explain how to assist with the nursing process when anti-cholinergic agents are used.
- Describe sedative-hypnotic drugs and their uses.
- Describe barbiturates and their uses.
- Explain how to assist with the nursing process when barbiturates are used.
- Describe the benzodiazepines.
- Explain how to assist with the nursing process when benzodiazepines are used.
- Describe non-barbiturate, non-benzodiazepine sedative-hypnotic agents.

- Explain how to assist with the nursing process when non-barbiturate, non-benzodiazepine sedative-hypnotic agents are used.
- Describe the drugs used for Parkinson's disease.
- Explain how to assist with the nursing process when drugs for Parkinson's disease are used.
- Describe the drugs used to treat Alzheimer's disease.
- Explain how to assist with the nursing process when drugs to treat Alzheimer's disease are used.

KEY TERMS

adrenergic fibers Nerve endings that release norepinephrine (a neurotransmitter)

adrenergic blocking agent A drug that inhibits adrenergic effects

agonist A drug that acts on a certain type of cell to produce a predictable response

anti-cholinergic agent A drug that blocks or inhibits cholinergic activity

barbiturate A drug that depresses the central nervous system, respirations, blood pressure, and temperature

cholinergic fibers Nerve endings that release acetylcholine (a neurotransmitter)

homeostasis A constant internal environment

hypnotic A drug that produces sleep

inhibitor A drug that prevents or restricts a certain action

insomnia A chronic condition in which the person cannot sleep or stay asleep all night

neuron The basic nerve cell of the nervous system

neurotransmitter A chemical substance that transmits nerve impulses

sedative A drug that quiets the person; it gives a feeling of relaxation and rest

synapse The junction between one neuron and the next

KEY ABBREVIATIONS

AD Alzheimer's disease
CNS Central nervous system
COMT Catechol O-methyltransferase
g Gram
GI Gastro-intestinal
IM Intramuscular
IV Intravenous
mcg Microgram
mg Milligram
MI Myocardial infarction
mL Milliliter
mm Hg Millimeters of mercury
ODT Orally disintegrating tablet

The nervous system regulates the body's on-going activities. See Box 14-1 for a review of the structures and functions of the nervous system.

See *Delegation Guidelines: Drugs Affecting the Nervous System.*

DELEGATION GUIDELINES
Drugs Affecting the Nervous System

Some drugs affecting the nervous system are given parenterally—by subcutaneous, intramuscular, or intravenous injection. Because you do not give parenteral dose forms, they are not included in this chapter. Should a nurse delegate the administration of such to you, you must:

- Remember that parenteral dosages are often very different from dosages for other routes.
- Refuse the delegation. Make sure you explain why. Do not just ignore the request. Make sure the nurse knows that you cannot give the drug and why.

BOX 14-1 | The Nervous System: Body Structure and Function

The nervous system controls, directs, and coordinates body functions. Its two main divisions are:

- The *central nervous system* (CNS). It consists of the brain and spinal cord (Fig. 14-1, p. 174)
- The *peripheral nervous system*. It involves the *nerves* throughout the body (Fig. 14-2, p. 174).

Nerves carry messages or impulses to and from the brain. Nerves connect to the spinal cord. They are easily damaged and take a long time to heal. Some nerve fibers have a protective covering called a *myelin sheath*. The myelin sheath also insulates the nerve fiber. Nerve fibers covered with myelin conduct impulses faster than those fibers without it.

THE CENTRAL NERVOUS SYSTEM

The *brain* and *spinal cord* make up the central nervous system. The brain is covered by the skull. The three main parts of the brain are the *cerebrum*, the *cerebellum*, and the *brainstem* (Fig. 14-3, p. 175).

The cerebrum is the largest part of the brain. It is the center of thought and intelligence. The cerebrum is divided into two halves called the *right* and *left hemispheres*. The right hemisphere controls movement and activities on the body's left side. The left hemisphere controls the right side.

The outside of the cerebrum is called the *cerebral cortex*. It controls the highest functions of the brain. These include reasoning, memory, consciousness, speech, voluntary muscle movement, vision, hearing, sensation, and other activities.

The cerebellum regulates and coordinates body movements. It controls balance and the smooth movements of voluntary muscles. Injury to the cerebellum results in jerky movements, loss of coordination, and muscle weakness.

The brainstem connects the cerebrum to the spinal cord. The brainstem contains the *midbrain, pons,* and *medulla*. The midbrain and pons relay messages between the medulla and the cerebrum. The medulla is below the pons. The medulla controls heart rate, breathing, blood vessel size, swallowing, coughing, and vomiting. The brain connects to the spinal cord at the lower end of the medulla.

The spinal cord lies within the spinal column. The cord is 17 to 18 inches long. It contains pathways that conduct messages to and from the brain.

The brain and spinal cord are covered and protected by three layers of connective tissue called meninges:

- The outer layer lies next to the skull. It is a tough covering called the *dura mater*.
- The middle layer is the *arachnoid*.
- The inner layer is the *pia mater*.

Continued

BOX 14-1 **The Nervous System: Body Structure and Function—cont'd**

The space between the middle layer (arachnoid) and inner layer (pia mater) is the *arachnoid space*. The space is filled with *cerebrospinal fluid*. It circulates around the brain and spinal cord. Cerebrospinal fluid protects the central nervous system. It cushions shocks that could easily injure brain and spinal cord structures.

THE PERIPHERAL NERVOUS SYSTEM

The peripheral nervous system has 12 pairs of *cranial nerves* and 31 pairs of *spinal nerves*. Cranial nerves conduct impulses between the brain and the head, neck, chest, and abdomen. They conduct impulses for smell, vision, hearing, pain, touch, temperature, and pressure. They also conduct impulses for voluntary and involuntary muscles. Spinal nerves carry impulses from the skin, extremities, and the internal structures not supplied by cranial nerves.

Some peripheral nerves form the *autonomic nervous system*. This system controls involuntary muscles and certain body functions. The functions include the heartbeat, blood pressure, intestinal contractions, and glandular secretions. These functions occur automatically.

The autonomic nervous system is divided into the *sympathetic nervous system* and the *parasympathetic nervous system*. They balance each other. The sympathetic nervous system speeds up functions. The parasympathetic nervous system slows functions. When you are angry, scared, excited, or exercising, the sympathetic nervous system is stimulated. The parasympathetic system is activated when you relax or when the sympathetic system is stimulated for too long.

THE SENSE ORGANS

The five senses are *sight*, *hearing*, *taste*, *smell*, and *touch*. Receptors for taste are in the tongue. They are called *taste buds*. Receptors for smell are in the nose. Touch receptors are in the dermis, especially in the toes and fingertips.

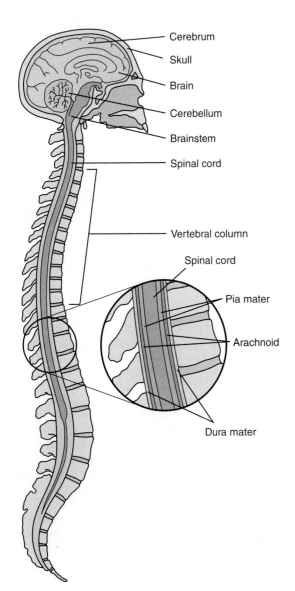

Fig. 14-1 Central nervous system.

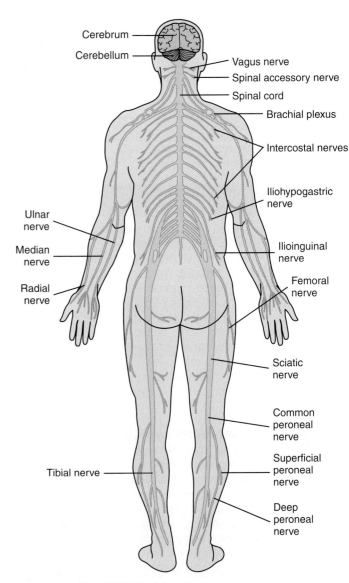

Fig. 14-2 Peripheral nervous system.

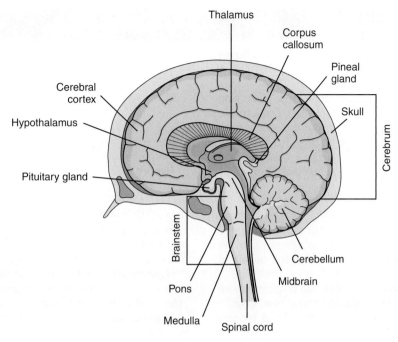

Fig. 14-3 The brain.

DRUGS AFFECTING THE AUTONOMIC NERVOUS SYSTEM

A **neuron** is the basic nerve cell of the nervous system. Each nerve is composed of a series of segments called neurons. The junction between one neuron and the next is called a **synapse.** Chemical substances called **neurotransmitters** (transmitters of nerve impulses) cause nerve signals or impulses:

- A neurotransmitter is released into the synapse at the end of a neuron.
- Receptors on the next neuron in the chain or at the end of the nerve chain are activated.
- The target organ is stimulated. For example, the heart is activated.

Neurotransmitters are excitatory (excite) or inhibitory (inhibit). *Excite* means to stimulate. If excitatory, the neuron is stimulated. *Inhibit* means to slow down, interfere with, or reduce chemical activity. If the neurotransmitter is inhibitory, the neuron's action is slowed. A single neuron releases only one type of neurotransmitter. Therefore different types of neurons secrete separate neurotransmitters. Neurotransmitter regulation with drugs is a way to control diseases caused by an excess or deficiency of neurotransmitters.

Except for skeletal muscle, the autonomic nervous system controls most tissue functions. Blood pressure, gastro-intestinal (GI) secretion and motility, urinary bladder function, sweating, and body temperature are examples. The autonomic nervous system maintains a constant internal environment (**homeostasis**) and responds to emergencies. Its two major neurotransmitters are:

- *Norepinephrine* (nohr ep' in ef' rin). Nerve endings that release norepinephrine are called **adrenergic** (ad' rin er' gek) **fibers.** Drugs that cause effects like those produced by the adrenergic neurotransmitters are called *adrenergic, sympathomimetic,* or *catecholamine drugs.* They mimic the action produced by stimulation of the sympathetic nervous system. Those that inhibit adrenergic effects are called **adrenergic blocking agents.**
- *Acetylcholine* (ah se' til koh' leen). Nerve endings that release acetylcholine are called **cholinergic** (koh' lin er' gek) **fibers.** Drugs that cause effects like those produced by acetylcholine are called *cholinergic* or *parasympathomimetic drugs.* They cause the same action produced by stimulation of the parasympathetic nervous system. Drugs that block or inhibit cholinergic activity are called **anti-cholinergic agents.**

Most organs have both adrenergic and cholinergic fibers. The fibers produce opposite responses. For example, adrenergic agents increase the heart rate. Cholinergic agents slow the heart rate. In the eyes, adrenergic agents cause the pupils to dilate. Cholinergic agents cause the pupils to constrict.

See Box 14-2 on p. 176 for the clinical uses of drugs affecting the autonomic nervous system.

BOX 14-2   Clinical Uses of Drugs Affecting the Autonomic Nervous System

Angina. Angina *(pain)* is chest pain. It is from reduced blood flow to part of the heart muscle *(myocardium)*. It occurs when the heart needs more oxygen. Chest pain is described as a tightness, pressure, squeezing, or burning in the chest. Pain can occur in the shoulders, arms, neck, jaw, or back. Pain in the jaw, neck, and down one or both arms is common. The person may be pale, feel faint, and perspire. Dyspnea is common. Nausea, fatigue, and weakness may occur. Some persons complain of "gas" or indigestion.

Arrhythmia. This is an abnormal heart rhythm.

Asthma. The airway becomes inflamed and narrow. Extra mucus is produced. Dyspnea results. Wheezing and coughing are common. So are pain and tightening in the chest. Symptoms are mild to severe. Asthma usually is triggered by allergies.

Biliary colic. This is smooth muscle pain associated with the passing of stones through the bile ducts. See "Colic."

Broncho-spasm. The smooth muscles of the bronchi and bronchioles contract. The contraction is excessive and prolonged. This results in acute airway narrowing and obstruction. A cough and wheezing occur. See "Asthma."

Colic. This is sharp pain caused by obstruction or smooth muscle spasm of a tube. See "Biliary colic" and "Urethral colic."

Emphysema. Emphysema is a lung disease. The alveoli enlarge and become less elastic. They do not expand and shrink normally with breathing in and out. As a result, some air is trapped in the alveoli when exhaling. Trapped air is not exhaled. Over time, more alveoli are involved. Oxygen and carbon dioxide exchange cannot occur in affected alveoli. The person has shortness of breath and a cough. At first, shortness of breath occurs with exertion. Over time, it occurs at rest. Sputum may contain pus. Fatigue is common. The person works hard to breathe in and out. And the body does not get enough oxygen. Breathing is easier when the person sits upright and slightly forward.

Enuresis. Enuresis is urinary incontinence in bed at night.

Heart failure. Heart failure or congestive heart failure occurs when the heart is weakened and cannot pump normally. Blood backs up. Tissue congestion occurs.

- When the left side of the heart cannot pump blood normally, blood backs up into the lungs. Respiratory congestion occurs. The person has dyspnea, increased sputum, cough, and gurgling sounds in the lungs. Also, the rest of the body does not get enough blood. Signs and symptoms occur from the effects on other organs. Poor blood flow to the brain causes confusion, dizziness, and fainting. The kidneys produce less urine. The skin is pale. Blood pressure falls. A very severe form of left-sided heart failure is *pulmonary edema* (fluid in the lungs). It is an emergency. The person can die.

- When the right side of the heart cannot pump blood normally, blood backs up into the venous system. Feet and ankles swell. Neck veins bulge. Liver congestion affects liver function. The abdomen becomes congested with fluid. The right side of the heart pumps less blood to the lungs. Normal blood flow does not occur from the lungs to the left side of the heart. The left side has less blood to pump to the body. As with left-sided heart failure, organs receive less blood. The signs and symptoms described for left-sided failure occur.

Hypertension. With hypertension *(high blood pressure)*, the resting blood pressure is too high. The systolic pressure is 140 mm Hg (millimeters of mercury) or higher *(hyper)*. Or the diastolic pressure is 90 mm Hg or higher. Such measurements must occur several times. Narrowed blood vessels are a common cause. The heart pumps with more force to move blood through narrowed vessels.

Hypertrophic subaortic stenosis. The left ventricle is enlarged *(hyper)*. There is constriction or narrowing *(stenosis)* in the aortic valve.

Hypotension. This is when the systolic blood pressure is below *(hypo)* 90 mm Hg and the diastolic pressure is below 60 mm Hg.

Indigestion. This is a vague feeling of discomfort above the stomach after eating. Fullness, heartburn, bloating, and nausea are common symptoms.

Irritable bowel syndrome. This disorder comes and goes. Nerves that control muscles in the GI tract are too active. The GI tract becomes sensitive to food, feces, gas, and stress. The person has abdominal pain, bloating, and constipation or diarrhea.

Migraine. A migraine is a recurring vascular headache. The person has an intense pulsing or throbbing pain in one area of the head. During a migraine, the person may be sensitive to light and sound. He or she may have nausea and vomiting.

Myasthenia gravis. *Myasthenia gravis* means *grave muscle weakness*. It is a neuromuscular disease. The person has weakness of the skeletal muscles. Muscle weakness increases during activity and improves with rest. Muscles that control the eye and eyelid movement, facial expression, chewing, talking, and swallowing are commonly involved. Muscles that control breathing and neck, arm, and leg movement may be affected.

Myocardial infarction (MI). *Myocardial* refers to the heart muscle. *Infarction* means tissue death. With MI, part of the heart muscle dies. Sudden cardiac death *(sudden cardiac arrest)* can occur. In MI, blood flow to the heart muscle is suddenly blocked. A thrombus (blood clot) blocks blood flow in an artery with atherosclerosis. The area of damage may be small or large. The person usually has severe chest pain, usually on the left side. The pain is often described as crushing, stabbing, or squeezing. Some describe it as someone sitting on the chest. Pain or numbness in one or both arms, the back, neck, jaw, or stomach may occur. Indigestion, dyspnea, nausea, dizziness, perspiration, and cold, clammy skin are other signs and symptoms.

Mydriasis. Mydriasis is dilation of the pupil of the eye.

BOX 14-2 **Clinical Uses of Drugs Affecting the Autonomic Nervous System—cont'd**

Parkinson's disease. The area of the brain that controls muscle movement is affected. See "Drugs Used for Parkinson's Disease" on p. 186.

Peptic ulcer. A peptic ulcer is a sore in the lining of the esophagus, stomach, or duodenum of the small intestine.

Pylorospasm. This is a spasm of the pyloric sphincter in the stomach.

Tremors. Tremors are quivering movements that result from the involuntary contraction and relaxation of skeletal muscles.

Urethral colic. This is sharp pain caused by obstruction or smooth muscle spasm of the urethra. See "Colic."

Ventricular dysrhythmia. This is an abnormal heart rhythm that occurs in the heart's ventricles.

DRUG CLASS: **Adrenergic Agents**

Two broad classes of adrenergic agents are *catecholamines* (kat eh col' ah meens) and *non-catecholamines*. Naturally occurring catecholamines are:

- Norepinephrine—secreted from the nerve terminals
- Epinephrine—secreted from the medulla
- Dopamine—secreted at selected sites within the brain, kidneys, and GI tract

These three agents are given to produce the same effects as those secreted naturally. Non-catecholamines have actions similar to the catecholamines. Non-catecholamines are more selective for certain types of receptors, do not act as fast, and have a longer duration.

The autonomic nervous system has *alpha, beta,* and *dopaminergic* (doh' pah min er' gek) receptors. When stimulated by chemicals of certain shapes, the receptors produce a certain action.

- Alpha-1 receptors—stimulation causes the blood vessels to constrict.
- Alpha-2 receptors—prevent further release of norepinephrine.
- Beta-1 receptors—increase the heart rate.
- Beta-2 receptors—relax the smooth muscle in the bronchi (broncho-dilation), uterus, and peripheral arterial blood vessels (vaso-dilation).
- Dopaminergic receptors:
  - In the brain—improve the symptoms of Parkinson's disease (p. 186).
  - In the kidneys—increase urine output because of better renal blood flow.

Many drugs act on more than one type of adrenergic receptor. However, each agent can be used for a certain purpose without many adverse effects. If recommended doses are exceeded, certain receptors may be stimulated excessively. That causes serious adverse effects. For example, terbutaline is primarily a beta stimulant. With normal doses, it is an effective broncho-dilator. Besides broncho-dilation, higher doses of terbutaline cause CNS stimulation. Insomnia and wakefulness result. See Table 14-1 on p. 178 for clinical uses of adrenergic agents.

Assisting With the Nursing Process

When giving adrenergic drugs, you assist the nurse with the nursing process.

ASSESSMENT

- Measure heart rate and blood pressure.
- See "Assisting with the Nursing Process" for respiratory tract diseases, broncho-dilators, and decongestants (Chapter 24).

PLANNING

See Table 14-1 (p. 178) for "Dose Forms."

IMPLEMENTATION

See Table 14-1 (p. 178) for "Action" and "Clinical Use."

EVALUATION

Side effects are usually dose related. They resolve when the dosage is reduced or the drug is discontinued. Persons with liver disease, thyroid disease, hypertension, and heart disease are at risk for side effects. Persons with diabetes may have more frequent episodes of hyperglycemia. Also report and record the following:

- *Palpitations, tachycardia, skin flushing, dizziness, and tremors.* These are usually mild and tend to resolve with continued therapy.
- *Orthostatic hypotension.* This is generally mild when it occurs. Dizziness and weakness may occur when the drug is started. Blood pressure is measured daily in the supine and standing positions. Provide for safety. Remind the person to rise slowly from a supine or sitting position. Have the person sit or lie down if he or she feels faint.
- *Dysrhythmias, chest pain, severe hypotension, hypertension, angina, nausea, vomiting.* Report such side effects at once. The nurse needs to tell the doctor.

DRUG CLASS: **Alpha- and Beta-Adrenergic Blocking Agents**

Alpha- and beta-adrenergic blocking agents plug alpha or beta receptors. This prevents other agents (usually naturally occurring catecholamines) from stimulating specific receptors.

There are non-selective and selective beta blockers.

- *Non-selective blocking agents.* Inhibit beta-1 and beta-2 receptors.
- *Selective beta-1 blocking agents.* Act against the heart's beta-1 receptors (cardio-selective).

TABLE 14-1	Adrenergic Agents					
GENERIC NAME	**BRAND NAME**	**DOSE FORMS**	**ADRENERGIC RECEPTOR**	**ACTION**	**CLINICAL USE**	
albuterol	Proventil, Ventolin	Aerosol: 90 mcg per puff Tablets: 2, 4 mg Syrup: 2 mg/5 mL Tablets: extended-release 4, 8 mg	Beta-2	Broncho-dilator	Asthma, emphysema	
ephedrine		Capsules: 25 mg	Alpha, beta	Broncho-dilator, vaso-constrictor	Nasal decongestant, hypotension	
metaproterenol	Alupent	Aerosol: 0.65 mg/ puff Nebulization: 0.4, 0.6, 5% solution	Beta-2	Broncho-dilator	Broncho-spasm	
phenylephrine	Neo-Synephrine	Ophthalmic drops: 0.12, 2.5, 10% Nasal solutions: 0.125, 0.25, 0.5, 1% Tablets: 10 mg	Alpha-1	Vaso-constrictor	Shock, hypotension, nasal decongestant, ophthalmic vaso-constrictor, mydriatic	
terbutaline	Brethine, Bricanyl	Tablets: 2.5, 5 mg	Beta-2	Broncho-dilator, uterine relaxant	Emphysema, asthma, premature labor	

The primary action of alpha-receptor stimulants is vaso-constriction (blood vessels constrict.) Therefore alpha blocking agents (alpha blockers) are used in persons with diseases associated with vaso-constriction. Alpha blockers cause vaso-dilation (blood vessels dilate). Some alpha blockers are used to treat hypertension.

Beta blocking agents (beta blockers) are commonly used after myocardial infarction (MI) and to treat angina, dysrhythmias, and hyperthyroidism. Beta blockers must be used with extreme caution in persons with respiratory disorders. Bronchitis, emphysema, asthma, and allergies are examples. Beta blockers can produce severe broncho-constriction. They may increase wheezing, especially during the pollen season.

Assisting With the Nursing Process
When giving beta blockers, you assist the nurse with the nursing process.

ASSESSMENT
- Measure heart rate and rhythm.
- Measure blood pressure.
- See "Assisting with the Nursing Process" for persons with:
  - Hypertension (Chapter 19)
  - Anti-dysrhythmic therapy (Chapter 20)

PLANNING
See Table 14-2 for "Oral Dose Forms."
IMPLEMENTATION
- See Table 14-2 for "Adult Dosage Range."
- The onset of action is fairly rapid. However, it may take several days or weeks for the desired level of improvement and to stabilize on the lowest dose needed to control the disorder. Angina and MI are risks if the drug is suddenly discontinued. To discontinue the drug, the doctor reduces the dosage over 1 to 2 weeks.

EVALUATION
Most adverse effects from beta blockers are dose related. They resolve when the dosage is adjusted. Also report and record the following:
- Cardiovascular—bradycardia, peripheral vaso-constriction (purple, mottled skin)
- Respiratory—broncho-spasm, wheezing
- Persons with diabetes—signs and symptoms of hypoglycemia: headache, weakness, decreased coordination, general apprehension, sweating, hunger, or blurred or double vision
- Persons with heart failure—increase in edema, dyspnea, bradycardia, and orthopnea

TABLE 14-2 Beta-Adrenergic Blocking Agents

GENERIC NAME	BRAND NAME	ORAL DOSE FORMS	CLINICAL USE	ADULT DOSAGE RANGE
acebutolol	Sectral	Capsules: 200, 400 mg	Hypertension, ventricular dysrhythmias	Initial, 400 mg daily; maintenance, 800-1200 mg daily
atenolol	Tenormin	Tablets: 25, 50, 100 mg	Hypertension, angina, after myocardial infarction	Initial, 50 mg daily; maintenance, up to 200 mg daily
betaxolol	Kerlone	Tablets: 10, 20 mg	Hypertension	Initial, 10 mg daily; maintenance, 20 mg daily
bisoprolol	Zebeta	Tablets: 5, 10 mg	Hypertension	Initial, 5 mg daily; maintenance, 10-20 mg daily
carteolol	Cartrol	Tablets: 2.5, 5 mg	Hypertension	Initial, 2.5, 5 mg daily; maintenance, 2.5-10 mg daily
carvedilol	Coreg	Tablets: 3.125, 6.25, 12.5, 25 mg	Hypertension, heart failure, myocardial infarction	Initial, 6.25 mg twice daily; maintenance, up to 50 mg daily
labetalol	Normodyne, Trandate	Tablets: 100, 200, 300 mg	Hypertension	Initial, 100 mg two times daily; maintenance, up to 2400 mg daily
metoprolol	Lopressor, Toprol XL	Tablets: 50, 100 mg Tablets, extended release: 25, 50, 100, 200 mg	Hypertension, myocardial infarction, angina, heart failure	Initial, 100 mg daily; maintenance, 100-450 mg daily
nadolol	Corgard	Tablets: 20, 40, 80, 120, 160 mg	Angina pectoris, hypertension	Initial, 40 mg once daily; maintenance, 80-320 mg daily; maximum, 640 mg/day
penbutolol	Levatol	Tablets: 20 mg	Hypertension	Initial, 20 mg daily; maintenance, 20 mg daily
pindolol	Visken	Tablets: 5, 10 mg	Hypertension	Initial, 5 mg twice daily; maximum, 60 mg/day
propranolol	Inderal Inderal LA	Tablets: 10, 20, 40, 60, 80 mg Sustained-release capsules: 60, 80, 120, 160 mg	Dysrhythmias, hypertension, angina pectoris, myocardial infarction, migraine, tremors, hypertrophic subaortic stenosis	Initial, 40 mg two times daily; maintenance, 120-640 mg daily
sotalol	Betapace	Tablets: 80, 120, 160, 240 mg	Dysrhythmias	Initial, 80 mg two times daily; maintenance, up to 320 mg daily
timolol	Blocadren	Tablets: 5, 10, 20 mg	Hypertension, myocardial infarction, migraine, angina pectoris	Initial, 10 mg twice daily; maintenance, up to 30 mg twice daily

DRUG CLASS: Cholinergic Agents

Cholinergic (parasympathomimetic) agents produce effects similar to acetylcholine. Some cholinergic agents directly stimulate the parasympathetic nervous system. Others inhibit acetylcholinesterase—the enzyme that metabolizes acetylcholine when released by a nerve ending. Such agents are *indirect-acting cholinergic agents*.

Some cholinergic actions are:
- Slow heart beat
- Increased GI motility and secretions
- Increased urinary bladder contractions with relaxation of muscle sphincter
- Increased secretions and contractility of bronchial smooth muscle
- Sweating
- Miosis of the eye, which reduces intra-ocular pressure (*Miosis* comes from the Greek word that means *becoming less.* With miosis, a muscle of the iris contracts. This causes the pupil to become smaller.)
- Increased force of skeletal muscle contractions
- Sometimes decreased blood pressure

TABLE 14-3	Cholinergic Agents		
GENERIC NAME	**BRAND NAME**	**ORAL DOSE FORMS**	**CLINICAL USE**
ambenonium	Mytelase	Tablets: 10 mg	Treatment of myasthenia gravis
bethanechol	Urecholine	Tablets: 5, 10, 25, 50 mg	Restore bladder tone and urination
guanidine	Guanidine	Tablets: 125 mg	Treatment of myasthenia gravis
neostigmine	Prostigmin	Tablets: 15 mg	Treatment of myasthenia gravis
pilocarpine	Isopto Carpine, Pilocar, Adsorbocarpine		See Chapter 31
pyridostigmine	Mestinon	Tablets: 60 mg Syrup: 60 mg/5 mL Sustained-release tablets: 180 mg	Treatment of myasthenia gravis

Cholinergic agents are used to diagnose and treat myasthenia gravis.

Assisting With the Nursing Process

When giving cholinergic agents, you assist the nurse with the nursing process.

ASSESSMENT
- Measure heart rate and blood pressure.
- See "Assisting With the Nursing Process" for persons with:
  - Respiratory tract disease (Chapter 24)
  - Urinary disorders (Chapter 30)
  - Eye disorders (Chapter 31)

PLANNING
See Table 14-3 for "Oral Dose Forms."

IMPLEMENTATION
See Table 14-3 for "Clinical Use."

EVALUATION
Cholinergic fibers are throughout the body. Therefore most body systems are affected. Because all receptors do not respond to the same dosage, adverse effects are not always seen. The risk for adverse effects increases with higher dosages. Also report and record the following:
- *Nausea, vomiting, diarrhea, abdominal cramping.* These symptoms are dose related.
- *Dizziness, hypotension.* The person's pulse and blood pressure are monitored. The person should rise slowly from a supine or sitting position. He or she should perform exercises to prevent blood pooling while standing or sitting in one position for prolonged periods. The person needs to sit or lie down if feeling faint.
- *Broncho-spasm, wheezing, bradycardia.* The nurse may tell you to with-hold the next dose until the doctor can evaluate the person.

DRUG CLASS: **Anti-Cholinergic Agents**

Anti-cholinergic agents are also called *cholinergic blocking agents* or *parasympatholytic agents*. They block the action of acetylcholine in the parasympathetic nervous system. These drugs occupy receptor sites at parasympathetic nerve endings. By doing so, they prevent the action of acetylcholine. The parasympathetic response is reduced.

Some anti-cholinergic effects are:
- Dilation of the pupil with increased intra-ocular pressure in persons with glaucoma
- Dry, thick secretions of the mouth, nose, throat, and bronchi
- Decreased secretions and motility of the GI tract
- Increased heart rate
- Decreased sweating

Anti-cholinergic agents are used to treat GI and eye disorders, bradycardia, Parkinson's disease, and genito-urinary disorders. They are used pre-operatively to:
- Decrease respiratory secretions to prevent aspiration
- Prevent vagal stimulation from skeletal muscle relaxants or placement of an endo-tracheal tube

Assisting With the Nursing Process

When giving anti-cholinergic agents, you assist the nurse with the nursing process.

ASSESSMENT
- Measure heart rate and blood pressure
- See "Assisting With the Nursing Process" for:
  - Drugs used for Parkinson's disease (p. 186)
  - Persons taking antihistamines (Chapter 24)
  - Persons with eye disorders (Chapter 31)

PLANNING
See Table 14-4 for "Oral Dose Forms."

IMPLEMENTATION
See Table 14-4 for "Clinical Use."

TABLE 14-4 Anti-Cholinergic Agents

GENERIC NAME	BRAND NAME	ORAL DOSE FORMS	CLINICAL USE
atropine	Atropine sulfate	Tablets: 0.4 mg	Treatment of pyloro-spasm and spastic conditions of the GI tract Treatment of urethral and biliary colic
belladonna	Belladonna tincture	Tincture: 30 mg/100 mL	Indigestion, peptic ulcer Enuresis Parkinson's disease
dicyclomine	Bentyl, Antispas, Dibent	Tablets: 20 mg Capsules: 10 mg Syrup: 10 mg/5 mL	Irritable bowel syndrome
glycopyrrolate	Robinul	Tablets: 1, 2 mg	Peptic ulcer disease
mepenzolate	Cantil	Tablets: 25 mg	Peptic ulcer disease
propantheline	Pro-Banthine	Tablets: 7.5, 15 mg	Peptic ulcer disease

EVALUATION

Cholinergic fibers are throughout the body. Therefore most body systems are affected. Because all receptors do not respond to the same dosage, adverse effects are not always seen. The risk for adverse effects increases with higher dosages. Also report and record the following:

- *Blurred vision; constipation; urinary retention; dryness of the mouth, nose, and throat.* Provide for safety if the person has blurred vision. Follow the care plan for constipation and urinary retention. For mouth, nose, and throat dryness, the nurse may allow the person to suck on hard candy or ice chips or chew gum.
- *Confusion, depression, nightmares, hallucinations.* Provide for safety.
- *Orthostatic hypotension.* This is generally mild when it occurs. Dizziness and weakness may occur when the drug is started. Blood pressure is measured daily in the supine and standing positions. Provide for safety. Remind the person to rise slowly from a supine or sitting position. Have the person sit or lie down if he or she feels faint.
- *Palpitations, dysrhythmias.* Tell the nurse at once.

SEDATIVE-HYPNOTIC DRUGS

Insomnia is a chronic condition in which the person cannot sleep or stay asleep all night. Common causes are changes in life-style or environment. Pain, illness, excess caffeine or alcohol, eating a large meal before bedtime, and stress are common causes.

Sedative-hypnotics are drugs used for altered sleep patterns. A **hypnotic** is a drug that produces sleep. A **sedative** is a drug that quiets the person. It gives a feeling of relaxation and rest. Most sedative-hypnotics increase total sleeping time.

Sedatives and hypnotics are not always different drugs. Their effects depend on the dose and the person's condition. A small dose may act as a sedative. A larger dose of the same drug may act as a hypnotic and produce sleep.

Sedative-hypnotics are used to:

- Treat insomnia and improve sleep
- Decrease anxiety level, increase relaxation, and promote sleep before diagnostic or surgical procedures

See *Promoting Safety and Comfort: Sedative-Hypnotic Drugs.*

PROMOTING SAFETY AND COMFORT
Sedative-Hypnotic Drugs

SAFETY

Sedative-hypnotic drugs depress the central nervous system. Assist the nurse with assessment of the person's level of alertness, orientation, and ability to perform motor functions. Practice safety measures and follow the care plan to provide for the person's safety.

Working around machines, driving a car, pouring and giving drugs and performing other duties require mental alertness. A person should not take these drugs while performing any of these functions.

Many of these drugs can cause severe allergic reactions. They also can cause sleep-related behaviors including sleep-driving. Sleep-driving is driving while not fully awake after taking a sedative-hypnotic. The person has no memory of the event. Follow the care plan to provide for safety.

DRUG CLASS: **Barbiturates**

A **barbiturate** is a drug that depresses the central nervous system, respirations, blood pressure, and temperature. It acts as a sedative or hypnotic. Some barbiturates are used in anesthesia and to treat seizures (Chapter 16).

CNS depression can range from mild sedation to deep coma and death. It depends on the dose, route of administration, tolerance from previous use, CNS excitability, and the person's condition. The risk of addiction is high.

Barbiturates are rarely used for sleep or sedation. Short-acting barbiturates (pentobarbital, secobarbital) are used for sedation before diagnostic procedures. The long-acting barbiturate, phenobarbital, is also used as an anti-convulsant (Chapter 16).

Assisting With the Nursing Process

When giving barbiturates, you assist the nurse with the nursing process.

ASSESSMENT
- Measure pulse, respirations, and blood pressure.
- Observe the person's level of alertness.
- Ask the person about pain or discomfort.

PLANNING

See Table 14-5 for "Oral Dose Forms."

IMPLEMENTATION
- See Table 14-5 for "Adult Oral Dose."
- Rapidly discontinuing the drug after long-term use of high dosages may cause symptoms similar to alcohol withdrawal. These vary from weakness and anxiety to delirium and grand mal seizures. Withdrawal of the drug should be gradual over 2 to 4 weeks.

TABLE 14-5 Barbiturates

GENERIC NAME	BRAND NAME	ORAL DOSE FORMS	ADULT ORAL DOSE	COMMENTS
butabarbital	Butisol	Tablets: 15, 30, 50, 100 mg Elixir: 30 mg/5 mL	Sedation: 15-30 mg three or four times daily Hypnosis: 50-100 mg at bedtime	Intermediate acting; Schedule III Elixir contains 7.5% alcohol Used primarily as a daytime sedative and bedtime hypnotic
mephobarbital	Mebaral	Tablets: 32, 50, 100 mg	Sedation: 32-100 mg three or four times daily Anti-convulsant: 400-600 mg daily	Long acting; Schedule IV Used primarily as an anti-convulsant; may also be used as a daytime sedative
pentobarbital	Nembutal	Capsules: 100 mg Elixir: 20 mg/5 mL	Sedation: 30 mg three or four times daily Hypnosis: 100 mg at bedtime	Short acting; Schedule II Used primarily as a daytime sedative and bedtime hypnotic; may also be used as a pre-anesthetic sedative Elixir contains 18% alcohol
phenobarbital	Luminal, Solfoton	Tablets: 8, 15, 30, 60, 100 mg Capsules: 16 mg Elixir: 15, 20 mg/5 mL	Sedation: 8-30 mg two or three times daily Hypnosis: 100-320 mg Anti-convulsant: 60-100 mg two or three times daily	Long acting; Schedule IV Used most commonly now as an anti-convulsant; may also be used as a daytime sedative, pre-anesthetic, or hypnotic agent Elixir contains 13.5% alcohol
secobarbital	Seconal	Capsules: 100 mg	Hypnosis: 100-200 mg at bedtime	Short acting; Schedule II Used primarily as a daytime sedative or bedtime hypnotic Therapy is not recommended for longer than 14 days

EVALUATION

Barbiturates can cause drowsiness, lethargy, headache, muscle or joint pain, and mental depression. Also report and record the following:

- *Hangover, sedation, lethargy.* Patients may complain of "morning hangover," blurred vision, or dizziness on arising. *Lethargy* is a state of feeling dull, sleepy, sluggish, or very drowsy. The person may have problems with coordination. Have the person rise to a sitting position, gain balance, and then stand. Assist with walking as needed.
- *Excitement, restlessness, confusion.* Older persons and those in severe pain may respond in ways opposite to sedation or sleep. Provide for safety, and help calm and orient the person to person, time, and place.
- *Allergic reactions.* Report hives, itching (pruritus), rash, fever, or inflammation of mucous membranes at once. Do not give the drug again until the nurse gives approval.

DRUG CLASS: **Benzodiazepines**

Benzodiazepines have actions similar to CNS depressants. However they act more selectively at specific sites. This allows for a variety of uses—sedative-hypnotic, muscle relaxant, anti-anxiety, and anti-convulsant.

Benzodiazepines are the most commonly used sedative-hypnotics. When therapy is started, the person feels a sense of deep or refreshing sleep. Over time the quality of sleep decreases. When therapy is discontinued, the person may have strange dreams and insomnia. These agents should be used for no more than 4 weeks.

Drugs in this class are used:

- To produce mild sedation
- For short-term use to produce sleep
- For pre-operative sedation (IM and IV dose forms)

Assisting With the Nursing Process

When giving benzodiazepines, you assist the nurse with the nursing process.

ASSESSMENT

- Measure vital signs.
- Measure blood pressure in the sitting and supine positions.
- Ask the person to rate his or her pain using the agency's pain rating scale.

PLANNING

See Table 14-6 for "Oral Dose Forms."

IMPLEMENTATION

- See Table 14-6 for "Adult Oral Dose."
- The habitual use of these drugs results in physical and psychologic dependence. Rapidly discontinuing the drug after long-term use may cause symptoms similar to alcohol withdrawal. They include weakness, anxiety, delirium, and seizures. The symptoms may not appear for several days. Treatment consists of gradual withdrawal of the drug over 2 to 4 weeks.

EVALUATION

Drugs in this class can cause drowsiness, hangover, sedation, and lethargy. Also report and record the following:

- *Confusion, agitation, hallucinations, amnesia.* All drugs in this class can cause these symptoms. Older persons who have taken high doses for a prolonged time are at risk.
- *Liver toxicity.* Symptoms include anorexia, nausea, vomiting, jaundice, and abnormal liver function tests.

TABLE 14-6	Benzodiazepines Used for Sedation-Hypnosis			
GENERIC NAME	BRAND NAME	ORAL DOSE FORMS	ADULT ORAL DOSE	COMMENTS
estazolam	ProSom	Tablets: 1, 2 mg	Hypnosis: 1-2 mg at bedtime	Intermediate acting; Schedule IV Used to treat insomnia Tapering therapy recommended to reduce rebound insomnia Minimal morning hangover
flurazepam	Dalmane	Capsules: 15, 30 mg	Hypnosis: 15-30 mg at bedtime	Long acting; Schedule IV Used for short-term treatment of insomnia, up to 4 weeks Morning hangover may be significant Rebound insomnia and REM (rapid eye movement) sleep occur less frequently

Continued

TABLE 14-6	Benzodiazepines Used for Sedation-Hypnosis—cont'd			
GENERIC NAME	**BRAND NAME**	**ORAL DOSE FORMS**	**ADULT ORAL DOSE**	**COMMENTS**
lorazepam	Ativan	Tablets: 0.5, 1, 2 mg Oral solution: 2 mg/mL Syrup: 2 mg/mL	Hypnosis: 2-4 mg at bedtime	Used primarily to treat insomnia but may also be used for anxiety
quazepam	Doral	Tablets: 7.5, 15 mg	Hypnosis: 7.5-15 mg at bedtime	Long acting; Schedule IV Used to treat insomnia Tapering therapy recommended to reduce rebound insomnia Morning hangover may be significant Dangerous to use in older persons
temazepam	Restoril	Capsules: 7.5, 15, 22.5, 30 mg	Hypnosis: 15-30 mg at bedtime	Intermediate acting; Schedule IV Used to treat insomnia Minimal if any morning hangover Rebound insomnia may occur
triazolam	Halcion	Tablets: 0.125, 0.25 mg	Hypnosis: 0.125-0.5 mg at bedtime	Short acting; Schedule IV Used to treat insomnia but tends to lose effectiveness within 2 weeks Tapering therapy is recommended to reduce rebound insomnia Rapid onset of action No morning hangover

DRUG CLASS: **Non-Barbiturate, Non-Benzodiazepine Sedative-Hypnotic Agents**

These drugs depress the central nervous system. They are used to produce sleep. Daytime drowsiness is generally not a problem with these agents.

Drugs in this class are used:

- To produce mild sedation
- For short-term use to produce sleep

Assisting With the Nursing Process

When giving drugs in this class, you assist the nurse with the nursing process.

ASSESSMENT

- Measure vital signs.
- Measure blood pressure in the sitting and supine positions.
- Ask the person to rate his or her pain using the agency's pain rating scale.

PLANNING

See Table 14-7 for "Dose Forms."

IMPLEMENTATION

- See Table 14-7 for "Adult Oral Dose."
- Zaleplon, zolpidem, and eszopiclone have a very rapid onset of action. The dose should be taken right before going to bed. Or the dose is taken after the person has gone to bed and has problems falling asleep.

EVALUATION

General side effects include drowsiness, lethargy, headache, muscle or joint pain, and mental depression. Some persons have short-term restlessness and anxiety before falling asleep. Dullness, moodiness, and coordination problems may occur. Also report and record the following:

- *Hangover, sedation, lethargy.* Patients may complain of "morning hangover," blurred vision, or dizziness on arising. *Lethargy* is a state of feeling dull, sleepy, sluggish, or very drowsy. The person may have problems with coordination. Have the person rise to a sitting position, gain balance, and then stand. Assist with walking as needed.
- *Restlessness, anxiety.* These are usually mild.
- *Excitement, restlessness, confusion.* Older persons and those in severe pain may respond in ways opposite to sedation or sleep. Provide for safety, and help calm and orient the person to person, time, and place.

TABLE 14-7 Non-Barbiturate, Non-Benzodiazepine Sedative-Hypnotic Agents

GENERIC NAME	BRAND NAME	DOSE FORMS	ADULT ORAL DOSE	COMMENTS
chloral hydrate	Aquachloral	Capsules: 500 mg Syrup: 250, 500 mg/5 mL Suppositories: 324, 648 mg	Sedation: 250 mg three times daily after meals Hypnosis: 500 mg to 1 g 15-30 minutes before bedtime	Schedule IV Used primarily as a bedtime hypnotic, but also is used as a pre-operative sedative because it does not depress respirations or cough reflex May cause nausea; administer with full glass of water; do not chew capsules
diphenhydramine	Benadryl	Tablets: 12.5, 25, 50 mg Capsules: 25, 50 mg Liquid: 12.5 mg/5 mL	Sedation: 25-50 mg at bedtime	Over-the-counter availability Used for mild insomnia for up to 1 week. Tolerance develops, increased dosage causes more side effects with no more efficacy
doxylamine	Unisom	Tablets: 25 mg	Sedation: 25 mg at bedtime	Over-the-counter availability Morning hangover may be significant See "diphenhydramine"
eszopiclone	Lunesta	Tablets: 1, 2, 3 mg	Hypnosis: 2-3 mg	Onset within 45 minutes; duration 5-8 hours Older adult patients should start with 1 mg
paraldehyde	Paral	Liquid: 30 mL (for oral or rectal use)	Sedation: 4-8 mL	Schedule IV Bitter tasting, unpleasant odor; administer in milk or iced fruit juice to mask taste and odor Dispense only in a glass container; do not use a plastic spoon or container Used predominantly as a sedative in treating delirium tremens This agent imparts a strong, foul odor to the breath for up to 24 hours after administration; the patient is often unaware of the foul smell
ramelteon	Rozerem	Tablets: 8 mg	Hypnosis: 8 mg within 30 minutes of bedtime	Do not take with or immediately after a high-fat meal
zaleplon	Sonata	Capsules: 5, 10 mg	Hypnosis: 10 mg at bedtime	Schedule IV Short acting; onset within 30 minutes; duration 2-4 hours Older adult or low-weight patients should start with 5 mg
zolpidem	Ambien	Tablets: 5, 10 mg	Hypnosis: 10 mg at bedtime	Schedule IV Short acting; onset within 30 minutes; duration 3-5 hours
	Ambien CR	Controlled-release tablets: 6.25, 12.5 mg	Hypnosis: 12.5 mg at bedtime	Older adult patients should start with 5 mg immediate-release tablets or 6.25 mg controlled-release tablets

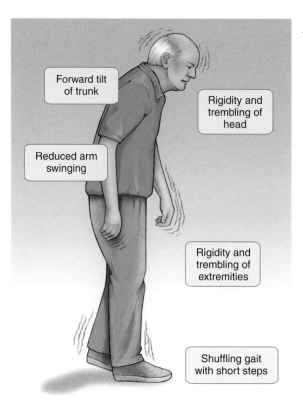

Fig. 14-4 Signs of Parkinson's disease. (From Thibodeau GA, Patton KT: *The human body in health and disease,* ed 4, St Louis, 2005, Mosby.)

DRUGS USED FOR PARKINSON'S DISEASE

Parkinson's disease is a slow, progressive disorder with no cure. The area of the brain that controls muscle movement is affected. Persons over the age of 50 are at risk. Signs and symptoms become worse over time (Fig. 14-4). They include:

- *Tremors*—often start in one finger and spread to the whole arm. Pill-rolling movements—rubbing the thumb and index finger—may occur. The person may have trembling in the hands, arms, legs, jaw, and face.
- *Rigid, stiff muscles*—in the arms, legs, neck, and trunk.
- *Slow movements*—the person has a slow, shuffling gait.
- *Stooped posture and impaired balance*—it is hard to walk. Falls are a risk.
- *Mask-like expression*—the person cannot blink and smile. A fixed stare is common.

Other signs and symptoms develop over time. They include swallowing and chewing problems, constipation, and bladder problems. Sleep problems, depression, and emotional changes (fear, insecurity) can occur. So can memory loss and slow thinking. The person may have slurred, monotone, and soft speech. Some people talk too fast or repeat what they say.

Symptoms are caused by a deficiency of dopamine. Dopamine is an inhibitory neurotransmitter. With a deficiency of dopamine, there is an increase in acetylcholine activity.

Parkinson's disease has no cure. All drugs prescribed for Parkinson's disease affect the central nervous system. The goals of treatment are to:

- Relieve signs and symptoms to the extent possible
- Restore dopamine activity to as close to normal as possible

The lowest dosages possible are used. As the disease progresses, dosages are increased. Other drugs are added as needed.

See *Promoting Safety and Comfort: Drugs Used for Parkinson's Disease.*

PROMOTING SAFETY AND COMFORT
Drugs Used for Parkinson's Disease

SAFETY

Orthostatic hypotension is common with most drugs used to treat Parkinson's disease. Safety measures are needed. Remind the person to rise slowly from a supine or sitting position. Have the person sit or lie down if he or she feels faint.

DRUG CLASS: **Dopamine Agonists**

An **agonist** is a drug that acts on a certain type of cell. It produces a predictable response. These dopamine agonists are used in the treatment of Parkinson's disease:

- amantadine hydrochloride (ah man' ta deen); Symmetrel (sim' eh trel)
- bromocriptine mesylate (bro mo krip' teen); Parlodel (par' lo del)
- carbidopa (kar bi doe' pa), levodopa (lee voe doe' pa); Sinemet (sin' eh met) and Parcopa (par' koe pa)
- pergolide mesylate (per' go lide); Permax (per' maks)
- pramipexole (pra mi pex' ole); Mirapex (mihr' ah pex)
- ropinirole (roh pin' ihr ol); Requip (re' kwip)

amantadine hydrochloride (Symmetrel)

Amantadine hydrochloride (Symmetrel) seems to slow the destruction of dopamine. This makes the small amount of dopamine present more effective. It may also help release dopamine from its storage sites. The drug is used to relieve the symptoms of Parkinson's disease.

Assisting With the Nursing Process

When giving amantadine hydrochloride (Symmetrel), you assist the nurse with the nursing process.
ASSESSMENT
Measure blood pressure in the supine and standing positions.
PLANNING
The oral dose forms are:
- 100 mg capsules
- 50 mg/5 mL syrup

IMPLEMENTATION
- At first for an adult, 100 mg are given two times a day.
- The maximum daily adult dose is 400 mg.
- Insomnia is a side effect. Therefore the last dose is usually ordered for late in the afternoon rather than at bedtime.

EVALUATION
Most adverse effects are dose related. They can be reversed. Report and record the following:
- *Confusion, disorientation, hallucinations, mental depression.* Provide for safety.
- *Dizziness, light-headedness, anorexia, nausea, abdominal discomfort.* These are usually mild and tend to resolve with continued therapy. Provide for safety when the person is light-headed or dizzy.
- *Skin mottling.* Mottling means mixed colors. The person has rose-colored mottling of the skin usually in the extremities. Often there is ankle edema. Mottling is worse when the person is standing or exposed to cold.

- *Liver disease.* Signs and symptoms include anorexia, nausea, vomiting, jaundice, and abnormal liver function tests.
- *Seizure disorders, psychosis.* Provide for safety.
- *Dyspnea and edema.* The person with heart failure is weighed regularly.

bromocriptine mesylate (Parlodel)

This drug stimulates dopamine receptors in the brain. It is used to relieve rigidity, tremors, and loss of movement.

Assisting With the Nursing Process

When giving bromocriptine mesylate (Parlodel), you assist the nurse with nursing process.
ASSESSMENT
Measure blood pressure in the supine and standing positions.
PLANNING
The oral dose forms are 2.5 and 5 mg tablets.
IMPLEMENTATION
- When the drug is started, 1.25 mg are given two times a day with meals (adult dosage).
- The dosage is increased 2.5 mg per day every 2 to 4 weeks (adult dosage).
- The dosage is adjusted according to the person's response and tolerance.

EVALUATION
Starting with small doses can minimize side effects. The dosage is increased gradually. Report and record the following:
- *GI effects.* Give the drug with food. Stool softeners or stimulant laxatives are ordered for constipation (Chapter 26).
- *Mouth dryness, double vision, nasal congestion, and a metallic taste.*
- *Nervous system side effects.* These often occur with higher doses. Observe the person's level of alertness and orientation to person, time, and place. Provide for safety.
- *Orthostatic hypotension.* See *Promoting Safety and Comfort: Drugs Used for Parkinson's Disease.*
- *Hypertension.* This may start the first or second week of therapy. Measure blood pressure. Report headaches.
- *Sudden sleep events.* These are described as sleep attacks or sleep episodes, including daytime sleep. Sudden sleep events can cause accidents.

carbidopa, levodopa (Sinemet and Parcopa)

Sinemet and Parcopa are a combination of carbidopa and levodopa. Carbidopa reduces the metabolism of levodopa. This lets more levodopa reach the desired receptor sites. Carbidopa has no effect when used alone. It must be used with levodopa. The intent of these drugs is to deliver more dopamine to brain cells.

Assisting With the Nursing Process

When giving carbidopa, levodopa (Sinemet or Parcopa), you assist the nurse with the nursing process.

ASSESSMENT

Ask the nurse about the person's signs and symptoms and response to therapy.

PLANNING

Sinemet and Parcopa contain carbidopa and levodopa. For example, Sinemet 10/100 mg tablets have 10 mg of carbidopa and 100 mg of levodopa.

- Sinemet oral dose forms:
  - 10/100 mg tablets
  - 25/100 mg tablets
  - 25/250 mg tablets
- Sinemet CR oral dose forms:
  - 25/100 mg tablets
  - 50/200 mg tablets
- Parcopa oral dose forms:
  - 10/100 mg orally disintegrating tablets (ODTs)
  - 25/100 mg ODTs
  - 25/250 mg ODTs

IMPLEMENTATION

Sinemet CR tablets are sustained-released. They must be swallowed whole. Do not crush the tablet or have the person chew the tablet.

Parcopa ODTs are placed on the tongue. They are allowed to dissolve, then swallowed. The tablets are not given with water or other liquids.

EVALUATION

Carbidopa has no effect when used alone. It must be used with levodopa. The carbidopa allows more levodopa to reach the brain.

The many side effects are dose related. Side effects also depend on the stage of the disease. Report and record the following:

- *Nausea, vomiting, anorexia.* Give the drug with food or with antacids (Chapter 25) if they are ordered.
- *Orthostatic hypotension.* This may occur when therapy is started. It may resolve after a few weeks of therapy. See *Promoting Safety and Comfort: Drugs Used for Parkinson's Disease*, p. 186.
- *Chewing motions, bobbing, facial grimacing, rocking movements.* These are involuntary movements.
- *Nightmares, depression, confusion, hallucinations.* Orient the person to person, time, and place. Provide for safety.
- *Tachycardia, palpitations.* Take the person's pulse. Note its rhythm and force.

pramipexole (Mirapex)

The drug stimulates dopamine receptors in the brain. The intent of the drug is to increase motor function and the person's ability to perform activities of daily living.

Assisting With the Nursing Process

When giving pramipexole (Mirapex), you assist the nurse with the nursing process.

ASSESSMENT

- Measure vital signs.
- Report hallucinations, nightmares, or anxiety.

PLANNING

The oral dose forms of pramipexole (Mirapex) are:

- 0.125 mg tablets
- 0.25 mg tablets
- 0.5 mg tablets
- 1 mg tablets
- 1.5 mg tablets

IMPLEMENTATION

- The dosage is adjusted according to the person's response and tolerance.
- Therapy is started with small doses. The dosage is gradually increased.
- The drug is usually given 3 times a day.
- Give the drug with food or milk to reduce stomach irritation.

EVALUATION

The many side effects are dose related. Side effects depend on the stage of the disease and other drugs the person takes. Report and record the following:

- *Nausea, vomiting, anorexia.* Give the drug with food or milk.
- *Orthostatic hypotension.* See *Promoting Safety and Comfort: Drugs Used for Parkinson's Disease*, p. 186.
- *Chewing motions, bobbing, facial grimacing, rocking movements.* These are involuntary movements.
- *Nightmares, depression, confusion, hallucinations.* Orient the person to person, time, and place. Provide for safety.
- *Tachycardia, palpitations.* Take the person's pulse. Note its rhythm and force.
- *Sudden sleep events.* These are described as sleep attacks or sleep episodes, including daytime sleep. Sudden sleep events can cause accidents.

ropinirole (Requip)

This drug stimulates dopamine receptors. It is used alone to manage the early signs and symptoms of Parkinson's disease. It is also used with levodopa to manage signs and symptoms when the disease is advanced. The intent of the drug is to increase motor function and the person's ability to perform activities of daily living.

Assisting With the Nursing Process

When giving ropinirole (Requip), you assist the nurse with the nursing process.

ASSESSMENT

- Measure vital signs.
- Report hallucinations, nightmares, or anxiety.

PLANNING

The oral dose forms of ropinirole (Requip) are:

- 0.25 mg tablets
- 0.5 mg tablets
- 1 mg tablets
- 2 mg tablets
- 5 mg tablets

IMPLEMENTATION

- The dosage is adjusted according to the person's response and tolerance.
- Therapy is started with small doses. The dosage is gradually increased.
- The drug is usually given 3 times a day.
- Give the drug with food or milk to reduce stomach irritation.

EVALUATION

The many side effects are dose related. Side effects depend on the stage of the disease and other drugs the person takes. Report and record the following:

- *Nausea, vomiting, anorexia.* Give the drug with food or milk.
- *Orthostatic hypotension.* See *Promoting Safety and Comfort: Drugs Used for Parkinson's Disease,* p. 186.
- *Chewing motions, bobbing, facial grimacing, rocking movements.* These are involuntary movements.
- *Nightmares, depression, confusion, hallucinations.* Orient the person to person, time, and place. Provide for safety.
- *Tachycardia, palpitations.* Take the person's pulse. Note its rhythm and force.
- *Sudden sleep events.* These are described as sleep attacks or sleep episodes, including daytime sleep. Sudden sleep events can cause accidents.

DRUG CLASS: **COMT Inhibitor**

COMT stands for catechol O-methyltransferase. It is the enzyme that breaks down levodopa. An **inhibitor** is a drug that prevents or restricts a certain action. By preventing or restricting the breakdown of levodopa, the duration of levodopa is longer. Remember, levodopa replaces the dopamine deficiency in the brain. Therefore a COMT inhibitor allows more dopamine to reach the brain.

These COMT inhibitors are used to treat Parkinson's disease:

- entacapone (en ta' ka pone); Comtan (com' tan) and Stalevo (stah lee' voh)

entacapone (Comtan and Stalevo)

These drugs reduce the destruction of dopamine in peripheral tissues. More dopamine can reach the brain. Comtan is given with carbidopa-levodopa. It does not affect Parkinson's disease when given alone. Stalevo contains carbidopa, entacapone, and levodopa.

Assisting With the Nursing Process

When giving entacapone (Comtan and Stalevo), you assist the nurse with the nursing process.

ASSESSMENT

- Measure blood pressure in the supine and sitting positions.
- Observe the person's level of alertness and orientation to person, time, and place.
- Report bowel or GI symptoms.

PLANNING

Oral dose forms are:

- Comtan: 200 mg tablets
- Stalevo:
    - 25/200/100 mg tablets
    - 37.5/200/150 mg tablets
    - 50/200/200 mg tablets
    - 12.5/200/50 mg tablets

IMPLEMENTATION

The dosage is adjusted according to the person's response and tolerance.

EVALUATION

Side effects can be reduced by controlling the dosage of levodopa. Report and record the following:

- *Diarrhea.* May develop 1 to 2 weeks after therapy is started.
- *Drowsiness and lethargy.* Observe the person's level of alertness, orientation, and ability to perform motor functions. Provide for safety. People working around machines, driving a car, pouring and giving drugs, or performing other duties that require mental alertness should not take these drugs while working.
- *Brownish-orange urine.* This is harmless.
- *Confusion and hallucinations.* Provide for safety.
- *Chorea. Chorea* means *to dance.* The person has rapid, involuntary movements that have no purpose. Flexing and extending the fingers, raising and lowering the shoulders, and grimacing may occur. Provide for safety.
- *Orthostatic hypotension.* See *Promoting Safety and Comfort: Drugs Used for Parkinson's Disease,* p. 186.

DRUG CLASS: **Anti-Cholinergic Agents**

With Parkinson's disease there is a dopamine deficiency. This leaves an excess of acetylcholine—a cholinergic neurotransmitter. Anti-cholinergic agents are used to reduce the over stimulation caused by excess amounts of acetylcholine.

Anti-cholinergic agents are used to reduce drooling and tremors. They are more useful for persons with minor symptoms and no cognitive impairment. These agents have little effect on stiff and rigid muscles, slow movements, and stooped posture.

Assisting With the Nursing Process

When giving anti-cholinergic drugs, you assist the nurse with the nursing process.

ASSESSMENT

- Report the person's urinary and bowel elimination patterns.
- Measure blood pressure in the supine and sitting positions.
- Measure the pulse. Note the rhythm and if it is regular or irregular.
- Observe the person's level of alertness and orientation to person, time, and place.

PLANNING

See Table 14-8 for "Oral Dose Forms."

IMPLEMENTATION

- See Table 14-8 for "Initial Adult Dose" and "Maximum Daily Dose."
- Give the drug with food or milk to prevent stomach irritation.

EVALUATION

Report and record the following:

- *Constipation.* Give stool softeners if ordered (Chapter 26). Encourage fluid intake and exercise.
- *Urinary retention.* Record intake and output.
- *Blurred vision.* Provide for safety if the person has blurred vision.
- *Dryness of the mouth, throat, and nose.* The nurse may allow the person to suck on hard candy or ice chips or chew gum.
- *Confusion, depression, nightmares, hallucinations.* Provide for safety.

- *Orthostatic hypotension.* See *Promoting Safety and Comfort: Drugs Used for Parkinson's Disease*, p. 186.
- *Palpitations, dysrhythmias.* Tell the nurse at once. The nurse needs to tell the doctor.

OTHER AGENTS

The following also are used to treat Parkinson's disease:

- selegiline (she ledge' ah leen); Eldepryl (el' deh pril) and Zelapar (zel' a par)

Selegiline (Eldepryl and Zelapar) reduce the destruction of dopamine in the brain. Therefore it allows greater dopamine activity.

As Parkinson's disease progresses, it is often necessary to add other drugs. Selegiline (Eldepryl and Zelapar), along with carbidopa-levodopa, improves memory and allows the person to move faster.

Selegiline (Eldepryl and Zelapar) helps slow the development of symptoms and disease progress. Levodopa therapy can be delayed.

Assisting With the Nursing Process

When giving selegiline (Eldepryl and Zelapar), you assist the nurse with the nursing process.

ASSESSMENT

- Report GI symptoms.
- Measure blood pressure in the supine and sitting positions.
- Observe the person's level of alertness and orientation to person, time, and place.

TABLE 14-8 Anti-Cholinergic Agents Used to Treat Parkinson's Disease				
GENERIC NAME	BRAND NAME	ORAL DOSE FORMS	INITIAL ADULT DOSE	MAXIMUM DAILY DOSE (mg)
benztropine mesylate	Cogentin	Tablets: 0.5, 1, 2 mg	0.5-1 mg at bedtime	6
biperiden hydrochloride	Akineton	Tablets: 2 mg	2 mg three or four times daily	16
diphenhydramine hydrochloride	Benadryl	Tablets: 12.5, 25, 50 mg Capsules: 25, 50 mg Elixir: 12.5 mg/5 mL Syrup: 12.5 mg/5 mL	25-50 mg three or four times daily	400
orphenadrine citrate	Banflex, Norflex	Tablets: 100 mg Sustained-release tablets: 100 mg	50 mg three times daily	150-250
procyclidine hydrochloride	Kemadrin	Tablets: 5 mg	2.5 mg three times daily	15-20
trihexyphenidyl hydrochloride	Artane	Tablets: 2, 5 mg Elixir: 2 mg/5 mL Sustained-release capsules: 5 mg	1-2 mg daily	12-15

PLANNING

The oral dose forms are:

- Eldepryl: 5 mg capsules
- Zelapar: 1.25 mg ODT

IMPLEMENTATION

The dosage is adjusted according to the person's response and tolerance.

Do not push the Zelapar ODT through the foil packing. Instead, pull back the packing with dry, gloved hands. Place the tablet or tablets on the tongue. The drug will disintegrate in a few seconds. The person should not swallow the tablet. The person should not ingest food or fluids for 5 minutes before or after taking an ODT.

EVALUATION

Report and record the following:

- *Chorea, confusion, and hallucinations.* Provide for safety.
- *Orthostatic hypotension.* See *Promoting Safety and Comfort: Drugs Used for Parkinson's Disease*, p. 186.

DRUGS USED FOR ALZHEIMER'S DISEASE

Alzheimer's disease (AD) is a brain disease. Nerve cells that control intellectual and social function are damaged. Memory, thinking, reasoning, judgment, language, behavior, mood, and personality are affected. The person has problems with work and everyday functions. Problems with family and social relationships occur. There is a steady decline in memory and mental function.

The disease is gradual in onset. It gets worse and worse over time. AD usually occurs after the age of 60. The risk increases with age. It is often diagnosed around the age of 80. Nearly half of the persons age 85 and older have AD.

The classic sign of AD is *gradual loss of short-term memory.* At first, the only symptom may be forgetfulness. Signs and symptoms become more severe as the disease progresses. The disease ends in death. The Alzheimer's Association describes seven stages:

- *No impairment.* The person does not show signs of memory problems.
- *Very mild cognitive decline.* The person thinks that he or she has memory lapses. Familiar words or names are forgotten. The person does not know where to find keys, eyeglasses, or other objects. These problems are not apparent to family, friends, or the health team.
- *Mild cognitive decline.* Family, friends, and others notice problems. The person has problems with memory or concentration and with words or names. The person loses or misplaces something valuable. Functioning in social or work settings declines.

- *Moderate cognitive decline.* Memory of recent or current events declines. There are problems with shopping, paying bills, and managing money. The person may withdraw or be quiet in social situations.
- *Moderately severe decline.* The person has major memory problems. There may be confusion about the date or day of the week. He or she may need help choosing the correct clothing to wear. The person knows his or her own name, a partner's name, and children's names. Usually help is not needed with eating or elimination.
- *Severe cognitive decline.* Memory problems are worse. Personality and behavior changes develop—delusions, hallucinations, repetitive behavior. The person needs much help with daily activities, including dressing and elimination. Names may be forgotten, but faces may be recognized. Sleep problems, incontinence (urinary and fecal), and wandering are common.
- *Very severe decline.* The person cannot respond to his or her environment, speak, or control movement. The person cannot walk without help. Over time, he or she cannot sit up without support or hold the head up. Muscles become rigid. Swallowing is impaired.

The following drugs are used in the treatment of AD:

- donepezil (don ep' ih zil); Aricept (air' ih sept)
- memantine (mem' an teen); Namenda (nam en' dah)
- galantamine (gah lan' tah meen); Razadyne (raz' a dine)
- rivastigmine (ri va stig' meen); Exelon (ex' a lon)

donepezil (Aricept)

With AD there is a loss of cholinergic neurons. This results in memory loss and dementia. Donepezil (Aricept) inhibits acetylcholinesterase—the enzyme that metabolizes acetylcholine when released by a nerve ending. The drug enhances cholinergic function. However, its effects lessen as more neurons are lost.

The drug is used in mild to moderate dementia. The goals of therapy are to improve cognitive skills—word recall, naming objects, language, word finding, and ability to do tasks.

Assisting With the Nursing Process

When giving donepezil (Aricept), you assist the nurse with the nursing process.

ASSESSMENT

- Measure vital signs.
- Observe cognitive function.
- Observe for GI symptoms.

PLANNING

The oral dose forms are:

- 5 and 10 mg tablets
- 5 and 10 mg orally disintegrating tablets

IMPLEMENTATION
- The initial dose is 5 mg daily at bedtime. After 4 to 6 weeks, the dosage may be increased to 10 mg daily.
- The drug is given with or without food.

EVALUATION
Report and record:
- *Nausea, vomiting, indigestion, diarrhea*. Symptoms are less with lower doses. They tend to subside after 2 to 3 weeks of therapy.
- *Bradycardia*. Tell the nurse at once if the person's pulse is less than 60 beats per minute.

memantine (Namenda)

Memantine (Namenda) blocks a receptor in the CNS that is activated in AD. The drug is used alone or with other drugs to treat moderate to severe AD. Cognitive function and behaviors are improved. The decline in activities of daily living is slower. However, the drug does not prevent or slow the progress of AD.

Assisting With the Nursing Process

When giving memantine (Namenda), you assist the nurse with the nursing process.

ASSESSMENT
- Measure vital signs.
- Observe cognitive function.

PLANNING
The oral dose forms are 5 and 10 mg tablets.

IMPLEMENTATION
- The oral dose is 5 mg once a day.
- The dosage is increased by 5 mg every 7 days to 10 mg daily, 15 mg daily, and 20 mg daily.
- The drug is given with or without food.

EVALUATION
Report and record:
- *Headache, dizziness, insomnia, restlessness, increased motor activity, excitement, agitation*. These tend to decline with continued therapy. The dosage may need adjustment.

galantamine (Razadyne)

Galantamine (Razadyne) prevents the breakdown of acetylcholine. More acetylcholine is released in the brain. The drug is used to treat mild to moderate symptoms of AD.

Assisting With the Nursing Process

When giving galantamine (Razadyne), you assist the nurse with the nursing process.

ASSESSMENT
- Measure vital signs.
- Measure weight.
- Observe cognitive function.

PLANNING
The oral dose forms are:
- 4, 8, and 12 mg tablets
- 16 and 24 mg extended-release capsules

IMPLEMENTATION
- The initial dose is 4 mg two times a day (8 mg once a day).
- After 4 weeks, the dose is increased to 8 mg two times a day (16 mg once a day).
- After another 4 weeks, the dose is increased to 12 mg two times a day (24 mg once a day).
- The drug is given with food.

EVALUATION
Report and record:
- *Nausea, vomiting, diarrhea, weight loss*. The doctor may discontinue the drug for several doses.

rivastigmine (Exelon)

Rivastigmine (Exelon) prevents the breakdown of acetylcholine. More acetylcholine is released in the brain. The drug is used to treat mild to moderate symptoms of AD.

Assisting With the Nursing Process

When giving rivastigmine (Exelon), you assist the nurse with the nursing process.

ASSESSMENT
- Measure vital signs.
- Measure weight.
- Observe cognitive function.
- Observe for muscle weakness.

PLANNING
The dose forms are:
- Oral
  - 1.5, 3, 4.5, and 6 mg capsules
  - 2 mg/mL solution
- Transdermal patch
  - 4.6 mg/24 hours
  - 9.5 mg/24 hours

IMPLEMENTATION
- The initial dose for 4 weeks is:
  - Oral: 1.5 mg two times a day with food
  - Transdermal patch: 4.6 mg once a day
- After 4 weeks:
  - The oral dose is increased by 1.5 mg two times a day every 2 weeks. The usual maintenance dose is 3 to 6 mg two times a day.
  - Transdermal patch: 9.5 mg once a day.

EVALUATION
Report and record:
- *Nausea, vomiting, weight loss, GI upset, muscle weakness*. The doctor may discontinue the drug for several doses.

REVIEW QUESTIONS

Circle the BEST answer.

1 Nerve signals or impulses are caused by
a neurons
c agonists
b synapses
d neurotransmitters

2 Which is *not* an adrenergic agent?
a levodopa
c epinephrine
b dopamine
d norepinephrine

3 Most adrenergic agents cause
a vaso-constriction
c broncho-spasm
b vaso-dilation
d hypotension

4 Beta blocking agents are commonly used to treat
a hypotension
c vaso-constriction
b hypertension
d respiratory disorders

5 When giving a beta blocker, you assist with assessment by
a measuring heart rate and blood pressure
b observing the color of urine
c asking the person to use a pain rating scale
d observing the person's level of alertness

6 Cholinergic agents are used in the treatment of
a myocardial infarction
c myasthenia gravis
b Parkinson's disease
d heart failure

7 Anti-cholinergic actions include the following *except*
a increasing the heart rate
b drying respiratory secretions
c increasing GI motility
d dilating the pupil

8 Which of the following drugs is an anti-cholinergic?
a carvedilol (Coreg)
b terbutaline (Brethine)
c bethanechol (Urecholine)
d atropine (Atropine Sulfate)

9 When giving an anti-cholinergic agent, you assist with assessment by
a measuring heart rate and blood pressure
b observing the color of urine
c asking the person to use a pain rating scale
d observing the person's level of alertness

10 Sedative-hypnotic drugs are used to
a produce sleep
b dry respiratory secretions before surgery
c decrease drooling and tremors
d stimulate the central nervous system

11 All of the following are barbiturates *except*
a phenobarbital (Luminal)
b pentobarbital (Nembutal)
c secobarbital (Seconal)
d flurazepam (Dalmane)

12 The benzodiazepines are used for the following reasons *except*
a to dry respiratory secretions
b to produce mild sedation
c to produce sleep
d for pre-operative sedation

13 The following are benzodiazepines *except*
a zolpidem (Ambien)
c estazolam (ProSom)
b lorazepam (Ativan)
d triazolam (Halcion)

14 Which drug is *not* used to promote sleep?
a chloral hydrate (Aquachloral)
b diphenhydramine (Benadryl)
c zaleplon (Sonata)
d carbidopa, levodopa (Sinemet)

15 Which is a common side effect of drugs used to treat Parkinson's disease?
a drooling
c orthostatic hypotension
b rigid, stiff muscles
d tremors

16 Signs and symptoms of Parkinson's disease are caused by a deficiency of
a levodopa
c carbidopa
b dopamine
d norepinephrine

17 The following drugs are used to treat Parkinson's disease *except*
a pramipexole (Mirapex)
c secobarbital (Seconal)
b ropinirole (Requip)
d selegiline (Eldepryl)

18 Drugs used to treat Parkinson's disease
a depress the central nervous system
b increase the amount of dopamine available to brain cells
c cure the disease
d inhibit the use of dopamine

Circle **T** if the statement is true. Circle **F** if the statement is false.

19 T F Side effects of adrenergic agents resolve when the dosage is reduced.

20 T F Most body systems are affected by cholinergic drugs.

21 T F Anti-cholinergic agents are used pre-operatively.

22 T F Sedative-hypnotics are used pre-operatively.

23 T F Barbiturates stimulate the central nervous system.

24 T F Barbiturate use can lead to addiction.

25 T F Donepezil (Aricept) can stop the progress of Alzheimer's disease.

26 T F Memantine (Namenda) is given to improve cognitive function in persons with dementia.

Answers to these questions are on p. 445.

Drugs Used for Mental Health Disorders

OBJECTIVES

- Define the key terms and key abbreviations used in this chapter.
- Describe the common mental health disorders.
- Describe the drugs used to treat anxiety.
- Explain how to assist with the nursing process when giving drugs to treat anxiety.
- Describe the drugs used to treat mood disorders.
- Explain how to assist with the nursing process when giving drugs to treat mood disorders.
- Describe the drugs used in alcohol rehabilitation.
- Explain how to assist with the nursing process when giving drugs used in alcohol rehabilitation.

KEY TERMS

antagonist A drug that exerts an opposite action to that of another; or it competes for the same receptor sites

anti-anxiety drugs Drugs used to treat anxiety

anti-depressants Several classes of drugs used to treat mood disorders

anxiety A vague, uneasy feeling in response to stress

psychosis A state of severe mental impairment; the person does not view the real or unreal correctly

tranquilizers Anti-anxiety drugs

KEY ABBREVIATIONS

CNS Central nervous system
GI Gastro-intestinal
MAOI Monoamine oxidase inhibitor
mg Milligram
mL Milliliter
OCD Obsessive-compulsive disorder
PO Per os (orally)
PTSD Post-traumatic stress disorder
SSRI Selective serotonin re-uptake inhibitor
TCA Tri-cyclic anti-depressant

Physical illnesses range from mild to severe. The common cold is at one extreme. A life-threatening illness is at the other extreme. Mental health problems have the same extremes.

Mental relates to the mind. It is something that exists in the mind or is done by the mind. Therefore mental health involves the mind. The mentally healthy person copes with and adjusts to everyday stresses in ways accepted by society. The person with a *mental health disorder* has problems with coping or adjusting to stress.

Causes of mental health disorders include:
• Not being able to cope or adjust to stress
• Chemical imbalances
• Genetics
• Drug or substance abuse
• Social and cultural factors

Common mental health disorders are described in Box 15-1. Psycho-therapy, drugs, and other treatments and therapies are used to treat mental health disorders. Many of the drugs used affect the central nervous system (CNS). See Chapter 14 for a review of the nervous system.

See *Delegation Guidelines: Drugs Used for Mental Health Disorders* on p. 197.

BOX 15-1 **Common Mental Health Disorders**

ANXIETY DISORDERS

Obsessive-Compulsive Disorder. An *obsession* is a recurrent, unwanted thought, idea, or image. *Compulsion* is repeating an act over and over again (a ritual). The act may not make sense. However, the person has much anxiety if the act is not done. Common rituals are hand washing, constant checking to make sure the stove is off, cleaning, and counting things to a certain number. Such activities can take over an hour every day. They are very distressing and affect daily life. Some persons with obsessive-compulsive disorder (OCD) also have depression, eating disorders, substance abuse, and other anxiety disorders.

Panic Disorder. Panic is the highest level of anxiety. *Panic* is an intense and sudden feeling of fear, anxiety, terror, or dread. Onset is sudden with no obvious reason. The person cannot function. Signs and symptoms of anxiety (p.197) are severe. The person may also have:
• Chest pain
• Shortness of breath
• Rapid heart rate ("heart pounding")
• Numbness and tingling in the hands
• Dizziness
• A smothering sensation
• Feeling of impending doom or loss of control

The person may feel that he or she is having a heart attack, losing his or her mind, or on the verge of death. Attacks can occur at any time, even during sleep.

Panic attacks can last for 10 minutes or longer. They can occur often. Panic disorder can last for a few months or for many years.

Many people avoid places where panic attacks occurred. For example, a person had a panic attack in a shopping mall. Malls are avoided.

Phobias. *Phobia* means an intense fear. The person has an intense fear of an object, situation, or activity that has little or no actual danger. The person avoids what is feared. When faced with the fear, the person has high anxiety and cannot function. Common phobias are fear of:
• Being in an open, crowded, or public place (agoraphobia—*agora* means marketplace)
• Being in pain or seeing others in pain (algophobia—*algo* means pain)
• Water (aquaphobia—*aqua* means water)
• Being in or being trapped in an enclosed or narrow space (claustrophobia—*claustro* means closing)
• The slightest uncleanliness (mysophobia—*myso* means anything that is disgusting)
• Night or darkness (nyctophobia—*nycto* means night or darkness)
• Fire (pyrophobia—*pyro* means fire)
• Strangers (xenophobia—*xeno* means strange)

Continued

BOX 15-1 **Common Mental Health Disorders—cont'd**

Post-Traumatic Stress Disorder. Post-traumatic stress disorder (PTSD) occurs after a terrifying ordeal. The ordeal involved physical harm or the threat of physical harm. Signs and symptoms of PTSD are listed in Box 15-2. PTSD can develop:

- After being harmed
- After a loved one was harmed
- After seeing a harmful event happen to loved ones or strangers

PTSD can result from many traumatic events. They include:

- War
- A terrorist attack
- Mugging
- Rape
- Torture
- Kidnapping
- Being held captive
- Child abuse
- A crash—vehicle, train, plane
- Bombing
- A natural disaster—flood, tornado, hurricane

Most people with PTSD have flashbacks. A *flashback* is reliving the trauma in thoughts during the day and in nightmares during sleep. A flashback may involve images, sounds, smells, or feelings. They are often triggered by everyday things. A door slamming is an example. During a flashback, the person may lose touch with reality. He or she may believe that the trauma is happening all over again.

Signs and symptoms usually develop about 3 months after the harmful event. However, they may not emerge until years later. Some people recover within 6 months. PTSD lasts longer in other people. The condition may become chronic.

PTSD can develop at any age including during childhood. The person may also suffer from depression, substance abuse, and other anxiety disorders.

MOOD DISORDERS

Bipolar Disorder. *Bipolar* means two *(bi)* poles or ends *(polar)*. The person with bipolar disorder has severe extremes in mood, energy, and ability to function. There are emotional lows *(depression)* and emotional highs *(mania)*. The disorder also is called manic-depressive illness. The person may:

- Be more depressed than manic
- Be more manic than depressed
- Alternate between depression and mania

The disorder tends to run in families. It usually develops in the late teens or in early adulthood. The disorder requires life-long management.

See Box 15-3 for the signs and symptoms of mania and depression. They can range from mild to severe. Mood changes are called "episodes." Bipolar disorder can damage relationships and affect school or work performance. Some people are suicidal.

Major Depression. Depression involves the body, mood, and thoughts. Symptoms (see Box 15-3) affect work, study, sleep, eating, and other activities. The person is very sad. He or she loses interest in daily activities.

Depression may occur because of a stressful event such as death of a partner, parent, or child. Divorce and loss of job are other stressful events. Some physical disorders can cause depression. Stroke, myocardial infarction (heart attack), cancer, and Parkinson's disease are examples. Hormonal factors may cause depression in women—menstrual cycle changes, pregnancy, miscarriage, after birth (post-partum depression), and before and during menopause.

Schizophrenia. *Schizophrenia* means split *(schizo)* mind *(phrenia)*. It is a severe, chronic, disabling brain disorder. The person with schizophrenia has severe mental impairment *(psychosis)*. Thinking and behavior are disturbed. The person has false beliefs *(delusions)*. He or she also has *hallucinations*. That is, the person sees, hears, smells, or feels things that are not real. The person has problems relating to others. He or she may be *paranoid*. That is, the person is suspicious about a person or situation. The person may have difficulty organizing thoughts. Responses are inappropriate. Communication is disturbed. The person may ramble or repeat what another says. Sometimes speech cannot be understood. He or she may make up words. The person may withdraw. That is, the person lacks interest in others. He or she is not involved with people or society.

Disorders of movement occur. These include:

- Being clumsy and uncoordinated
- Involuntary movements
- Grimacing
- Unusual mannerisms
- Sitting for hours without moving, speaking, or responding

Some persons regress. To *regress* means to retreat or move back to an earlier time or condition. For example, a 5-year-old wets the bed when there is a new baby. This is normal. Healthy adults do not act like infants or children.

In men, the symptoms usually begin in the late teens or early 20s. In women, symptoms usually begin in the mid-20s and early 30s. People with schizophrenia do not tend to be violent. However, if a person with paranoid schizophrenia becomes violent, it is often directed at family members. The violence usually occurs at home. Some persons with schizophrenia attempt suicide.

DELEGATION GUIDELINES
Drugs Used for Mental Health Disorders

Some drugs used to treat mental health disorders are given parenterally (by injection). Because you do not give parenteral dose forms, they are not included in this chapter. Should a nurse delegate the administration of such to you, you must:

- Remember that parenteral dosages are often very different from dosages for other routes.
- Refuse the delegation. Make sure you explain why. Do not just ignore the request. Make sure the nurse knows that you cannot give the drug and why.

BOX 15-2 Signs and Symptoms of Post-Traumatic Stress Disorder

- Startles easily
- Emotionally numb—especially to those with whom the person used to be close
- Difficulty trusting people
- Difficulty feeling close to people
- Loss of interest in things he or she used to enjoy
- Problems being affectionate
- Feelings of intense guilt
- Irritability
- Avoiding situations that are reminders of the harmful event
- Difficulty around the anniversary of the harmful event
- Gets mad easily
- Outbursts of anger
- Problems sleeping
- Increasingly aggressive
- Becoming more violent
- Physical symptoms:
  - Headache
  - Gastro-intestinal (GI) distress
  - Immune system problems
  - Dizziness
  - Chest pain
  - Discomfort in other body parts

BOX 15-3 Signs and Symptoms of Bipolar Disorder

MANIA (MANIC EPISODE)
Increased energy, activity, and restlessness
Excessively "high," overly good mood
Extreme irritability
Racing thoughts and talking very fast
Jumping from one idea to another
Easily distracted; problems concentrating
Little sleep needed
Unrealistic beliefs in one's abilities and powers
Poor judgment
Spending sprees
A lasting period of behavior that is different from usual
Increased sexual drive
Drug abuse (particularly cocaine, alcohol, and sleeping pills)
Aggressive behavior
Denial that anything is wrong

DEPRESSION (DEPRESSIVE EPISODE)
Lasting sad, anxious, or empty mood
Feelings of hopelessness
Feelings of guilt, worthlessness, or helplessness
Loss of interest or pleasure in activities once enjoyed
Loss of interest in sex
Decreased energy; a feeling of fatigue or being "slowed down"
Problems concentrating, remembering, or making decisions
Restlessness or irritability
Sleeping too much, or unable to sleep
Change in appetite
Unintended weight loss or gain
Chronic pain or other symptoms not caused by physical illness or injury
Thoughts of death or suicide
Suicide attempts

DRUGS USED FOR ANXIETY DISORDERS

Anxiety is a vague, uneasy feeling in response to stress. The person may not know why or the cause. The person senses danger or harm—real or imagined. The person acts to relieve the unpleasant feeling. Often anxiety occurs when needs are not met.

Some anxiety is normal. Persons with mental health disorders have higher levels of anxiety. Signs and symptoms depend on the degree of anxiety

(Box 15-4, p. 198). A person has an anxiety disorder when his or her responses to stressful situations are:
- Abnormal or irrational
- Impair normal daily function

Anxiety disorders last at least 6 months. They can get worse if not treated. Anxiety disorders commonly occur with other physical illnesses involving the cardiovascular, pulmonary, digestive, and endocrine systems. It also is a major symptom of many mental health disorders. Schizophrenia, mania, depression, dementia, and substance abuse are examples. The anxious person is evaluated to determine if the anxiety is due to a physical or mental health problem.

Anti-anxiety drugs are used to treat anxiety. They also are known as **tranquilizers.**

BOX 15-4 Signs and Symptoms of Anxiety

- A "lump" in the throat
- "Butterflies" in the stomach
- Pulse: rapid
- Respirations: rapid
- Blood pressure: increased
- Speech: rapid
- Voice changes
- Mouth: dry
- Sweating
- Nausea
- Diarrhea
- Urinary frequency and urgency
- Attention span: poor
- Directions: difficulty following
- Sleep: difficulty
- Appetite: loss of

DRUG CLASS: Benzodiazepines

Benzodiazepines are commonly used to treat anxiety disorders (Table 15-1). They are:

- Consistently effective
- Less likely to interact with other drugs
- Less likely to cause overdose
- Have a lower risk for abuse than barbiturates and other anti-anxiety drugs

These drugs stimulate the action of an inhibitory neurotransmitter. (A *neurotransmitter* is a chemical substance that transmits nerve impulses. Something that *inhibits* prevents or restricts a certain action. See Chapter 14). They can lower anxiety within a short time. The intent is to decrease anxiety so that:

- Coping is improved
- Physical signs are reduced (see Box 15-4)

These drugs are usually ordered for a short time. If taken for weeks or months, drug tolerance and dependence may occur. Abuse and withdrawal symptoms are possible.

See *Promoting Safety and Comfort: Benzodiazepines*.

TABLE 15-1 Benzodiazepines Used to Treat Anxiety

GENERIC NAME	BRAND NAME	ORAL DOSE FORMS	INITIAL ADULT DOSE	MAXIMUM DAILY DOSE (mg)
alprazolam	Xanax Niravam	Tablets: 0.25, 0.5, 1, 2 mg Tablets, orally disintegrating: 0.25, 0.5, 1, 2 mg	0.25-0.5 mg three times daily	10
	Xanax XR	Tablets, extended-release: 0.5, 1, 2, 3 mg Solution: 1 mg/mL	0.5-1 mg daily	6
chlordiazepoxide	Librium	Capsules: 5, 10, 25 mg	5-10 mg three or four times daily	300
clorazepate	Tranxene	Tablets: 3.75, 7.5, 11.25, 15, 22.5 mg	7.5-15 mg two to four times daily	60
	Tranxene XR	Extended-release tablets: 11.25 and 22.5 mg		
diazepam	Valium	Tablets: 2, 5, 10 mg Liquid: 5 mg/5 mL	2-10 mg two to four times daily	40
lorazepam	Ativan	Liquid: 2 mg/mL Tablets: 0.5, 1, 2 mg	2-3 mg two or three times daily	10
oxazepam	Serax	Tablets: 15 mg Capsules: 10, 15, 30 mg	10-15 mg three or four times daily	120

Assisting With the Nursing Process

When giving benzodiazepines, you assist the nurse with the nursing process.

ASSESSMENT
- Measure blood pressure in the sitting and supine positions.
- Observe for signs and symptoms of anxiety.

PLANNING
See Table 15-1 for "Oral Dose Forms."

IMPLEMENTATION
- See Table 15-1 for "Initial Adult Dose" and "Maximum Daily Dose."
- Long-term use may cause physical and psychological dependence. Mild withdrawal signs and symptoms can occur after taking the drug for 4 to 6 weeks. Restlessness, worsening of anxiety, insomnia, tremors, muscle tension, rapid pulse, and hearing sensitivity are common. Delirium and seizures can occur. Signs and symptoms may not appear for several days after the drug is discontinued.

EVALUATION
Report and record:
- *Drowsiness, hangover, sedation, lethargy.* Provide for safety.
- *Orthostatic hypotension.* Provide for safety. Remind the person to rise slowly from a supine or sitting position. Have the person sit or lie down if he or she feels faint.
- *Excessive use or abuse.* This may cause physical and psychological dependence.
- *Anorexia, nausea, vomiting, and jaundice.* These may signal liver toxicity.

OTHER ANTI-ANXIETY AGENTS

Other drugs used to treat anxiety disorders include:
- buspirone (byoo spy' rone); BuSpar (byoo sphar')
- fluvoxamine (fluv ox' ah meen); Luvox (loo' vox)
- hydroxyzine (hi drox' ee zeen); Vistaril (vis tar' il) and Atarax (at' a raks')

buspirone (BuSpar)

This drug causes less sedation than other anti-anxiety agents. And it does not alter psycho-motor function. Improvement is seen after 7 to 10 days of treatment. The person may need 3 to 4 weeks of therapy. The risk for abuse is low.

Assisting With the Nursing Process

When giving buspirone (BuSpar), you assist the nurse with the nursing process.
ASSESSMENT
Observe for signs and symptoms of anxiety.
PLANNING
The oral dose forms are:
- 5, 10, 15, and 30 mg tablets
- 15 and 30 mg tablets are scored to divide into 2 or 3 doses

IMPLEMENTATION
- The adult initial dose is 5 to 7.5 mg orally 2 times a day.
- The dosage may be increased by 5 mg every 2 to 3 days.
- The maximum daily dose is 60 mg.

EVALUATION
Report and record:
- *Insomnia, nervousness, drowsiness, and light-headedness.* Provide for safety.
- *Slurred speech, dizziness.* These are signs of excess dosing.

fluvoxamine (Luvox)

This drug is used to treat OCD. Symptoms are reduced, but obsessions and compulsions are not prevented. The person may have more control over them. The intent is to:
- Decrease anxiety
- Improve coping with obsessions
- Reduce the frequency of compulsive activity

Assisting With the Nursing Process

See p. 203 for "Selective Serotonin Re-Uptake Inhibitors."

hydroxyzine (Vistaril and Atarax)

These drugs produce sedation and reduce anxiety. Other uses include preventing vomiting and controlling allergic reactions.

Mild tranquilizers, Vistaril and Atarax are used to:
- Decrease anxiety
- Produce sedation and relaxation before surgery
- Reduce the amount of pain-relief drugs needed after surgery
- Prevent vomiting
- Control itching from allergic reactions

Assisting With the Nursing Process

When giving hydroxyzine (Vistaril or Atarax), you assist the nurse with the nursing process.

ASSESSMENT

Observe for signs and symptoms of anxiety.

PLANNING

The oral dose forms are:

- Vistaril
  - 25 and 50 mg capsules
  - 25 mg/5 mL suspension
- Atarax
  - 10, 25, 50, and 100 mg tablets
  - 10 mg/5 mL syrup

IMPLEMENTATION

For an adult, 25 to 100 mg are given orally 3 to 4 times a day.

EVALUATION

Report and record:

- *Blurred vision; constipation; dryness of the mouth, nose, and throat.* Provide for safety if the person has blurred vision. Give stool softeners as ordered. The nurse may allow the person to suck on hard candy or ice chips or chew gum.
- *Sedation.* See *Promoting Safety and Comfort: Benzodiazepines,* p. 199.
- *Dizziness, slurred speech.* These signal excess dosing.

DRUGS USED FOR MOOD DISORDERS

Mood or *affect* relates to feelings and emotions. Mood (or affective) disorders involve feelings, emotions, and moods.

Before regaining full function, most persons pass through three therapy phases:

- *Acute phase.* The time from diagnosis to the first treatment response. Symptoms are reduced. This phase may take 6 to 8 weeks. It can take longer if the person does not take prescribed drugs and follow other therapies. Some people simply stop treatment.
- *Continuation phase.* This phase involves preventing a relapse and reaching a full recovery. The person should be symptom-free for 6 months.
- *Maintenance phase.* The goal of this phase is to prevent the mood disorder from recurring.

Mood disorders are treated with several classes of drugs called **anti-depressants.** They prolong the action of neurotransmitters—norepinephrine, dopamine, and serotonin. The drug classes are:

- Monoamine oxidase inhibitors (MAOIs)
- Tri-cyclic anti-depressants (TCAs)
- Selective serotonin re-uptake inhibitors (SSRIs)
- Other agents

See *Focus on Older Persons: Drugs Used for Mood Disorders.*

See *Promoting Safety and Comfort: Drugs Used for Mood Disorders.*

FOCUS ON OLDER PERSONS

Drugs Used for Mood Disorders

Depression is common in older persons. They have many losses—death of family and friends, loss of health, loss of body functions, loss of independence. Loneliness and the side effects of some drugs also are causes. See Box 15-5 for the signs and symptoms of depression in older persons.

Depression in older persons is often over-looked or a wrong diagnosis is made. Often the person is thought to have dementia. Therefore depression is often not treated.

PROMOTING SAFETY AND COMFORT
Drugs Used for Mood Disorders

SAFETY

Anti-depressants may increase the risk of suicidal thinking and behavior. When started on anti-depressants, observe the person carefully. Observe for agitation, changes in behavior, objects that could cause harm, making a will, giving away belongings, and statements or comments about death. Report your observations and concerns to the nurse. Follow suicide precautions according to the care plan.

BOX 15-5 Signs and Symptoms of Depression in Older Persons

- Fatigue and lack of interest
- Inability to experience pleasure
- Feelings of uselessness, hopelessness, and helplessness
- Decreased sexual interest
- Increased dependency
- Anxiety
- Slow or unreliable memory
- Paranoia
- Agitation
- Focus on the past
- Thoughts of death and suicide
- Difficulty completing activities of daily living
- Changes in sleep patterns
- Poor grooming
- Withdrawal from people and interests
- Muscle aches, abdominal pain, and headaches
- Nausea and vomiting
- Dry mouth

From Meiner SB, Lueckenotte AG: *Gerontologic nursing,* ed 3, St Louis, 2006, Mosby.

DRUG CLASS:
Monoamine Oxidase Inhibitors

Monoamine oxidase inhibitors (MAOIs) are listed in Table 15-2. They prevent the breakdown of neurotransmitters—epinephrine, norepinephrine, dopamine, and serotonin. These neurotransmitters are involved in areas of the brain that control mood and emotion. Drug effects are seen within 2 to 4 weeks.

MAOIs have serious side effects when taken with certain drugs, food, and fluids. Doctors usually order other anti-depressants first. MAOIs may be used when other drugs fail.

See *Promoting Safety and Comfort: Drug Class—Monoamine Oxidase Inhibitors*, p. 202.

TABLE 15-2	Anti-Depressants					
GENERIC NAME	BRAND NAME	DOSE FORMS	INITIAL ADULT DOSE	DAILY MAINTENANCE DOSE (mg)	MAXIMUM DAILY DOSE (mg)
MONOAMINE OXIDASE INHIBITORS (MAOIs)					
phenelzine	Nardil	Tablets: 15 mg	15 mg three times daily	15-60	90
tranylcypromine	Parnate	Tablets: 10 mg	10 mg twice daily	30	60
isocarboxazid	Marplan	Tablets: 10 mg	10 mg twice daily	40	60
selegiline	Emsam	Transdermal patch: 6, 9, 12 mg	6 mg patch daily	6	12
TRI-CYCLIC ANTI-DEPRESSANTS					
amitriptyline	Elavil	Tablets: 10, 25, 50, 75, 100, 150 mg	25 mg three times daily	150-250	300
amoxapine		Tablets: 25, 50, 100, 150 mg	50 mg three times daily	200-300	400 (out-patients) 600 (in-patients)
clomipramine	Anafranil	Capsules: 25, 50, 75 mg	25 mg three times daily	100-150	250
desipramine	Norpramin	Tablets: 10, 25, 50, 75, 100, 150 mg	25 mg three times daily	75-200	300
doxepin	Sinequan	Capsules: 10, 25, 50, 75, 100, 150 mg Oral concentrate 10 mg/mL	25 mg three times daily	at least 150	300
imipramine	Tofranil	Tablets: 10, 25, 50 mg	30-75 mg daily at bedtime	150-250	300
nortriptyline	Aventyl, Pamelor	Capsules: 10, 25, 50, 75 mg Solution: 10 mg/5 mL	25 mg three or four times daily	50-75	100
protriptyline	Vivactil	Tablets: 5, 10 mg	5-10 mg three or four times daily	20-40	60
trimipramine	Surmontil	Capsules: 25, 50, 100 mg	25 mg three times daily	50-150	200 (out-patients) 300 (in-patients)
SELECTIVE SEROTONIN RE-UPTAKE INHIBITORS (SSRIs)					
citalopram	Celexa	Tablets: 10, 20, 40 mg Liquid: 10 mg/5 mL	20 mg daily	20-40	60
duloxetine	Cymbalta	Sustained-release capsules: 20, 30, 60 mg	40 mg daily	60	60

Continued

TABLE 15-2 Anti-Depressants—cont'd

GENERIC NAME	BRAND NAME	DOSE FORMS	INITIAL ADULT DOSE	DAILY MAINTENANCE DOSE (mg)	MAXIMUM DAILY DOSE (mg)
SELECTIVE SEROTONIN RE-UPTAKE INHIBITORS (SSRIs)—cont'd					
escitalopram	Lexapro	Tablets: 5, 10, 20 mg Liquid: 5 mg/5 mL	10 mg daily	10-20	20
fluoxetine	Prozac	Capsules: 10, 20, 40 mg Tablets: 10, 20 mg Solution: 20 mg/5 mL Weekly capsule: 90 mg	20 mg daily	20-60	80
fluvoxamine	Luvox	Tablets: 25, 50, 100 mg	90 mg at bedtime	100-300	300
paroxetine	Paxil Paxil CR	Tablets: 10, 20, 30, 40 mg Suspension: 10 mg/5 mL Sustained-release tablets: 12.5, 25, 37.5 mg	20 mg daily	20-50	50
sertraline	Zoloft	Tablets: 25, 50, 100 mg Oral concentrate: 20 mg/mL	50 mg daily	50-200	200

PROMOTING SAFETY AND COMFORT
Drug Class—Monoamine Oxidase Inhibitors

SAFETY

MAOIs can cause serious hypertension if taken with foods or fluids that contain tyramine. *Tyramine* stimulates the release of epinephrine and norepinephrine. The person taking an MAOI should avoid the following:
- Aged cheese—Camembert, Edam, Roquefort, Parmesan, cheddar, Swiss, blue
- Smoked or pickled meats, poultry, and fish—corned beef, herring, salami, pepperoni, sausage
- Aged or fermented meats—chicken or beef pâté, game fish, poultry
- Meat extracts—bouillon, consommé
- Products containing yeast
- Red wines
- Beer
- Avocados
- Chicken livers
- Sauerkraut
- Fava beans

Signs and symptoms of a hypertensive crisis include severe headache, stiff neck, sweating, nausea, vomiting, and very high blood pressure.

Assisting With the Nursing Process

When giving MAOIs, you assist the nurse with the nursing process.

ASSESSMENT
- Measure pulse rate.
- Measure blood pressure in the supine and standing positions.
- Measure blood glucose.
- Ask about foods and fluids consumed during the past few days.

PLANNING
See Table 15-2 for "Oral Dose Forms."

IMPLEMENTATION
- See Table 15-2 for "Initial Adult Dose," "Daily Maintenance Dose," and "Maximum Daily Dose."
- MAOIs are given 2 or 3 times a day. The last dose is given no later than 1800 (6:00 PM) to prevent insomnia.

EVALUATION
Report and record:
- *Orthostatic hypotension.* This is the most common side effect of MAOIs. Dizziness and weakness may occur when the drug is started. Blood pressure is measured daily in the supine and standing positions. Provide for safety. Remind the person to rise slowly from a supine or sitting position. Have the person sit or lie down if he or she feels faint.

- *Drowsiness, sedation.* These tend to disappear with dosage adjustment and continued therapy. Provide for safety. Remind the person to use caution when performing tasks that require alertness.
- *Restlessness, agitation, insomnia.* These resolve when the dosage is adjusted. The last dose should be given before 1800 (6:00 PM).
- *Blurred vision; constipation; urinary retention; dryness of the mouth, nose, and throat.* Provide for safety if the person has blurred vision. Follow the care plan for constipation and urinary retention. For mouth, nose, and throat dryness, the nurse may allow the person to suck on hard candy or ice chips or chew gum.
- *Hypertension.* Many drugs, foods, and fluids can cause serious hypertension. See *Promoting Safety and Comfort: Drug Class—Monoamine Oxidase Inhibitors.*

DRUG CLASS: Selective Serotonin Re-Uptake Inhibitors

Selective serotonin re-uptake inhibitors (SSRIs) affect serotonin. *Re-uptake* means re-absorption. SSRIs block certain nerve cells from re-absorbing serotonin. Therefore the brain has more serotonin available. Mood is improved because the sending of nerve impulses is improved.

SSRIs are used to improve the person's mood and reduce depression. They are the most widely used anti-depressants (see Table 15-2). They are safer than the other classes of anti-depressants. Drug effects are seen within 2 to 4 weeks.

Assisting With the Nursing Process

When giving SSRIs, you assist the nurse with the nursing process.

ASSESSMENT
- Measure blood pressure in the supine and standing positions.
- Weigh the person weekly.
- Observe for insomnia, nervousness, and other CNS signs and symptoms.
- Ask the person about GI symptoms.

PLANNING
See Table 15-2 for oral "Dose Forms."

IMPLEMENTATION
See Table 15-2 for "Initial Adult Dose," "Daily Maintenance Dose," and "Maximum Daily Dose."

EVALUATION
Report and record:
- *Restlessness, agitation, anxiety, insomnia.* These usually occur early in therapy. The drug should be given before 1800 (6:00 PM). The doctor may order a sedative-hypnotic agent.
- *Sedative effects.* Remind the person to use caution when performing tasks that require alertness.
- *GI effects.* Give the drug with food. The doctor may adjust the dose.
- *Suicidal actions.* See *Promoting Safety and Comfort: Drugs Used for Mood Disorders,* p. 200.

DRUG CLASS: Tri-Cyclic Anti-Depressants

Tri-cyclic anti-depressants (TCAs) prolong the action of norepinephrine, dopamine, and serotonin. They do so by blocking the re-uptake (re-absorption) of these neurotransmitters in the synapses between the neurons.

This class of drugs produces anti-depressant and tranquilizing effects. After 2 to 4 weeks of therapy, they elevate mood, improve appetite, and increase alertness.

Some TCAs also are used to treat other disorders. They include:
- Phantom limb pain
- Chronic pain
- Cancer pain
- Peripheral neuropathy with pain
- Arthritic pain
- Eating disorders
- Pre-menstrual symptoms

Assisting With the Nursing Process

When giving TCAs, you assist the nurse with the nursing process.

ASSESSMENT
- Ask about bowel movements. Constipation is common when taking these drugs.
- Measure blood pressure in the supine and sitting positions.
- Measure pulse rate and rhythm. Report tachycardia or an irregular pulse.

PLANNING
See Table 15-2 for "Oral Dose Forms."

IMPLEMENTATION
- See Table 15-2 for "Initial Adult Dose," "Daily Maintenance Dose," and "Maximum Daily Dose."
- Dose increases are usually started in the evening. This is because of sedation.

EVALUATION

Report and record:

- *Blurred vision; constipation; urinary retention; dryness of the mouth, nose, and throat.* Provide for safety if the person has blurred vision. Follow the care plan for constipation and urinary retention. For mouth, nose, and throat dryness, the nurse may allow the person to suck on hard candy or ice chips or chew gum.
- *Orthostatic hypotension.* All drugs in this class may cause some degree of orthostatic hypotension. Dizziness and weakness may occur when the drug is started. Blood pressure is measured daily in the supine and standing positions. Provide for safety. Remind the person to rise slowly from a supine or sitting position. Have the person sit or lie down if he or she feels faint.
- *Sedative effects.* Provide for safety.
- *Tremors, numbness, tingling, Parkinson-like symptoms.* Provide for safety.
- *Tachycardia, dysrhythmias, signs and symptoms of heart failure.* See Chapters 20 and 21.
- *Seizures.* Provide for safety. See Chapter 16.
- *Suicidal actions.* See *Promoting Safety and Comfort: Drugs Used for Mood Disorders,* p. 200.

OTHER ANTI-DEPRESSANTS

Other anti-depressant agents include:

- bupropion hydrochloride (byoo pro' pee on); Wellbutrin (wel byoo' trihn)
- maprotiline hydrochloride (ma proe' ti leen)
- mirtazapine (mer taz' ah peen); Remeron (rem' er on)
- nefazodone (nehf as' oh doan)
- trazodone hydrochloride (tray' zoh doan); Desyrel (dez' er el)
- venlafaxine (vehn lah fax' een); Effexor (eef ex' ohr)

With these drugs, symptoms of depression may improve within a few days. Appetite, sleep, and psychomotor activity may increase. However, depression still exists. It usually takes several weeks before improvement is noted.

bupropion hydrochloride (Wellbutrin)

Wellbutrin is a weak inhibitor of the re-uptake (reabsorption) of serotonin, norepinephrine, and dopamine.

The drug is used for persons who:

- Do not respond to TCAs
- Cannot tolerate the adverse effects of TCAs

Assisting With the Nursing Process

When giving bupropion (Wellbutrin), you assist the nurse with the nursing process.

ASSESSMENT

Weigh the person.

PLANNING

Oral dose forms are:

- 75 and 100 mg tablets
- 100, 150, and 200 mg sustained-release tablets
- 150 and 300 mg extended-release tablets

IMPLEMENTATION

- The initial adult dose is usually 100 mg twice daily. This may be increased to 100 mg three times a day (at least every 6 hours) after several days of therapy.
- The maximum dose in one day is 450 mg. Avoid a dose shortly before bedtime.

EVALUATION

Report and record:

- *GI effects.* Give with food. Give stool softeners as ordered for constipation.
- *Restlessness, agitation, anxiety, and insomnia.* Bedtime doses are avoided if the person has insomnia. The doctor may order a sedative-hypnotic.
- *Seizures.* Provide for safety. See Chapter 16.
- *Suicidal actions.* See *Promoting Safety and Comfort: Drugs Used for Mood Disorders,* p. 200.

maprotiline

Maprotiline enhances norepinephrine and serotonin at the nerve endings. The drug elevates mood and reduces symptoms of depression. It is used:

- To treat depression
- To treat the depressive phase of bipolar disorder
- For relief of anxiety associated with depression

Assisting With the Nursing Process

When giving maprotiline, you assist the nurse with the nursing process.

ASSESSMENT

- Measure blood pressure in the supine, sitting, and standing positions.
- Weigh the person weekly.

PLANNING

Oral dose forms are 25, 50, and 75 mg tablets.

IMPLEMENTATION

- The adult starting dose is 75 mg daily in 2 or 3 divided doses.
- The usual maintenance dose is 150 mg daily.
- The maximum dose in one day is 225 mg.
- Dosage increases are usually made in the evening because of increased sedation.

EVALUATION

See "Tri-Cyclic Anti-Depressants" on p. 203.

mirtazapine (Remeron)

Remeron is a serotonin antagonist. An antagonist is a drug that exerts an opposite action to that of another. Or it competes for the same receptor sites. Mirtazapine's response is like that of the TCAs. The drug elevates mood and reduces symptoms of depression.

Assisting With the Nursing Process

When giving mirtazapine (Remeron), you assist the nurse with the nursing process.

ASSESSMENT

- Measure blood pressure in the supine, sitting, and standing positions.
- Weigh the person weekly.

PLANNING

Oral dose forms are:

- 15, 30, and 45 mg tablets
- 15 mg Soltabs (Dissolves on the tongue. It is swallowed with saliva. No water is needed.)

IMPLEMENTATION

- The adult starting dose is 15 mg daily.
- Every 1 to 2 weeks, the dosage may be increased up to a maximum of 45 mg daily.
- Dosage increases are usually made in the evening because of increased sedation.

EVALUATION

See "Tri-Cyclic Anti-Depressants" on p. 203.

nefazodone

Nefazodone inhibits serotonin and norepinephrine reuptake. It also blocks some serotonin receptors. The drug elevates mood and reduces symptoms of depression. It carries the risk of life-threatening liver failure.

Assisting With the Nursing Process

When giving nefazodone, you assist the nurse with the nursing process.

ASSESSMENT

- Measure blood pressure in the supine, sitting, and standing positions.
- Measure heart rate.
- Ask about GI symptoms.
- Observe for CNS symptoms.

PLANNING

Oral dose forms are 50, 100, 150, 200, and 250 mg tablets.

IMPLEMENTATION

- The adult starting dose is 100 mg two times a day.
- The dosage may be increased by 100 to 200 mg twice a day.
- The normal dose range is 300 to 600 mg daily.

EVALUATION

Report and record:

- *Drowsiness, sedation.* These symptoms tend to disappear with continued therapy or dosage adjustment. The person needs to exercise caution when working around machines, driving a car, pouring and giving drugs, or performing other duties that require mental alertness.
- *Blurred vision; constipation; urinary retention; dryness of the mouth, nose, and throat.* Provide for safety if the person has blurred vision. Follow the care plan for constipation and urinary retention. The nurse may allow the person to suck on hard candy or ice chips or chew gum.
- *Orthostatic hypotension.* Provide for safety. Remind the person to rise slowly from a supine or sitting position. Have the person sit or lie down if he or she feels faint.
- *Sedative effects.* Remind the person to use caution when performing tasks that require alertness.

trazodone hydrochloride (Desyrel)

This drug elevates mood and reduces symptoms of depression. It is useful in treating:

- Depression
- Depression associated with schizophrenia
- Depression, tremors, and anxiety associated with alcohol dependence
- Insomnia in persons with substance abuse

Assisting With the Nursing Process

When giving trazodone hydrochloride (Desyrel), you assist the nurse with the nursing process.

ASSESSMENT

Measure blood pressure in the supine, sitting, and standing positions.

PLANNING

Oral dose forms are 50, 100, 150, and 300 mg tablets.

IMPLEMENTATION

- The starting dose is 150 mg in 3 divided doses.
- The drug is increased by 50 mg daily every 3 to 4 days.
- The maximum daily dose is 400 mg for outpatients; 600 mg daily for hospital patients.
- Dosage increases are usually made in the evening because of sedation.
- Give the drug after a meal or with a light snack to reduce adverse effects.

EVALUATION

Report and record:

- *Confusion, dizziness, and light-headedness.* Provide for safety.
- *Drowsiness.* The person needs to exercise caution when working around machines, driving a car, pouring and giving drugs, or performing other duties that require mental alertness.
- *Orthostatic hypotension.* Provide for safety. Remind the person to rise slowly from a supine or sitting position. Have the person sit or lie down if he or she feels faint.
- *Dysrhythmias, tachycardia.* Report tachycardia or an irregular pulse.

venlafaxine (Effexor)

This drug is a strong inhibitor of the re-uptake of serotonin and norepinephrine. The drug is used to treat depression and anxiety. The drug elevates mood. It also reduces symptoms of depression and anxiety.

Assisting With the Nursing Process

When giving venlafaxine (Effexor), you assist the nurse with the nursing process.

ASSESSMENT

- Measure blood pressure.
- Measure weight.
- Ask about GI symptoms.
- Observe for CNS symptoms such as insomnia or nervousness.

PLANNING

Oral dose forms are:

- 25, 37.5, 50, 75, and 100 mg tablets
- 37.5, 75, and 150 mg sustained-release capsules

IMPLEMENTATION

- The daily adult dose is 75 mg in 2 or 3 doses.
- Dosages may be increased by 75 mg daily after every 4 days.
- The maximum dose is 375 mg in one day—usually in 3 divided doses.
- The drug is given with food.

EVALUATION

Report and record:

- *Dizziness, drowsiness.* The person needs to exercise caution when working around machines, driving a car, pouring and giving drugs, or performing other duties that require mental alertness.
- *Nausea, anorexia.* Give the drug with food. The doctor may reduce the dosage.
- *Restlessness, agitation, anxiety, insomnia.* These usually occur early in therapy. Bedtime doses are avoided. The doctor may order a sedative-hypnotic agent.
- *Suicidal actions.* See *Promoting Safety and Comfort: Drugs Used for Mood Disorders*, p. 200.

ANTI-MANIC AGENTS

Eskalith (esk' ah lith) and Lithane (lith' ane) are brand names for lithium carbonate (lith' ee um). Lithium is used to treat acute mania. It also is used to prevent manic and depressive episodes in bipolar disorder. In persons with bipolar disorder, lithium is more effective in preventing signs and symptoms of mania than those of depression. The goal of therapy is to maintain the person at an optimal level of functioning with few mood swings.

Acute anti-manic effect usually occurs within 5 to 7 days. Full therapeutic effect often takes 10 to 21 days.

Lithium may cause a loss of sodium. The person must:

- Maintain a normal dietary intake of sodium.
- Drink 10 to 12 eight-ounce glasses of water daily

Assisting With the Nursing Process

When giving lithium, you assist the nurse with the nursing process.

ASSESSMENT

- Measure blood pressure in the supine, sitting, and standing positions.
- Measure weight.
- Record intake and output.
- Measure blood glucose.

PLANNING

Oral dose forms are:

- 150, 300, and 600 mg capsules and tablets
- 300 and 450 mg slow-release tablets
- 300 mg/5 mL syrup

IMPLEMENTATION

- The daily adult dose is 300 to 600 mg three or four times a day.
- Give the drug with food or milk.

EVALUATION

Report and record:

- *Nausea, vomiting, anorexia, abdominal cramps.* These are usually mild. They tend to resolve with continued therapy. Give the drug with food or milk to prevent stomach irritation.
- *Excess thirst and urination, fine hand tremor.* These are usually mild. They tend to resolve with continued therapy.
- *Vomiting, diarrhea, increased reflex reactions, lethargy, weakness.* These signal toxicity. Tell the nurse at once. Give the next dose only with the nurse's permission.
- *Progressive fatigue, weight gain.* These are early signs of a thyroid problem.
- *Itching, ankle edema, metallic taste, hyperglycemia.* These are rare.
- *Increased or decreased urinary output.* These may signal renal toxicity.

DRUGS USED FOR PSYCHOSES

Psychosis is a state of severe mental impairment. The person does not view the real or unreal correctly. The following symptoms are common with psychosis.

- *Delusion*—a false belief. For example, the person believes that a radio station is broadcasting the person's thoughts.
- *Hallucination*—seeing, hearing, smelling, or feeling something that is not real. A person may see animals, insects, or people that are not real. "Voices" are the most common type of hallucination in schizophrenia. "Voices" may comment on behavior, order the person to do things, warn of danger, or talk to other voices.
- *Paranoia*—a disorder *(para)* of the mind *(noia)*. The person has false beliefs (delusions). He or she is suspicious about a person or situation. For example, a person may believe that others are cheating, harassing, poisoning, spying upon, or plotting against him or her.
- *Delusion of grandeur*—an exaggerated belief about one's importance, wealth, power, or talents. For example, a man believes he is Superman. Or a woman believes she is the Queen of England.

- *Delusion of persecution*—the false belief that one is being mistreated, abused, or harassed. For example, a person believes that someone is "out to get" him or her.

Schizophrenia is the most common psychotic disorder. Psychotic symptoms also can occur from medical problems:

- *Dementia and delirium.* The underlying cause may be an infection or a metabolic or endocrine disorder.
- *Mood disorders.* Major depression and bipolar disorder are examples.
- *Drugs and substance abuse.* Opiates (Chapter 17), amphetamines, cocaine, hallucinogens, and alcohol are examples.

Drug and non-drug therapies are used to treat psychoses. The goal is to restore behaviors, cognitive function, and psycho-social processes and skills to as close to normal as possible. Unless the psychosis is caused by a medical problem, symptoms will re-occur most of the person's life.

Anti-psychotic drugs (Table 15-3) are classified as:

- *Typical or first-generation anti-psychotic agents.* These drugs antagonize dopamine in the central nervous system.
- *Atypical or second-generation anti-psychotic agents.* These drugs inhibit dopamine receptors. To a certain degree, they also inhibit serotonin receptors.

TABLE 15-3 Anti-Psychotic Agents			
GENERIC NAME	**BRAND NAME**	**DOSE FORMS**	**ADULT DOSAGE RANGE (mg)**
TYPICAL (FIRST-GENERATION) ANTI-PSYCHOTIC AGENTS			
Phenothiazines			
chlorpromazine	Thorazine	Tablets: 10, 25, 50, 100, 200 mg Syrup: 100 mg/mL Suppository: 100 mg	30-1000
fluphenazine	Prolixin	Tablets: 1, 2.5, 5, 10 mg Elixir: 2.5 mg/5 mL	0.5-20
perphenazine		Tablets: 2, 4, 8, 16 mg Concentrate: 16 mg/5 mL	12-64
prochlorperazine	Compazine	Tablets: 5, 10, 25 mg Sustained-release capsules: 30 mg Syrup: 5 mg/mL Suppository: 2.5, 5, 25 mg	15-150
thioridazine		Tablets: 10, 15, 25, 50, 100, 150, 200 mg	150-800
trifluoperazine		Tablets: 1, 2, 5, 10 mg	2-40

Continued

TABLE 15-3	Anti-Psychotic Agents—cont'd		
GENERIC NAME	**BRAND NAME**	**DOSE FORMS**	**ADULT DOSAGE RANGE (mg)**
Thioxanthenes			
thiothixene	Navane	Capsules: 1, 2, 5, 10, 20 mg	6-60
Non-Phenothiazines			
haloperidol	Haldol	Tablets: 0.5, 1, 2, 5, 10, 20 mg Concentrate: 2 mg/mL	1-15
loxapine	Loxitane	Capsules: 5, 10, 25, 50 mg	20-250
molindone	Moban	Tablets: 5, 10, 25, 50 mg	15-225
ATYPICAL (SECOND-GENERATION) ANTI-PSYCHOTIC AGENTS			
aripiprazole	Abilify	Tablets: 5, 10, 15, 20, 30 mg	10-15
clozapine	Clozaril	Tablets: 12.5, 25, 100 mg Tablets, orally disintegrating: 25, 100 mg	300-900
olanzapine	Zyprexa	Tablets: 2.5, 5, 7.5, 10, 15, 20 mg Tablets, orally disintegrating: 5, 10, 15, 20 mg	10-15
quetiapine	Seroquel	Tablets: 25, 100, 200, 300 mg	50-800
risperidone	Risperdal	Tablets: 0.25, 0.5, 1, 2, 3, 4 mg Tablets, orally disintegrating: 0.5, 1, 2 mg Solution: 1 mg/mL	4-16
ziprasidone	Geodon	Capsules: 20, 40, 60 mg	100-160

The drugs also affect other neurotransmitter receptors. This accounts for the many adverse effects of therapy.

The initial goals of therapy are to:
- Calm the agitated person. That person may be a threat to himself or herself or to others.
- Begin treatment of the psychosis and thought disorder.

Often therapy involves benzodiazepines (often lorazepam; Ativan) and anti-psychotic agents. This allows lower doses of the anti-psychotic agent. This reduces the risk of serious adverse effects common with higher-dose therapy. Some therapeutic effects occur within 1 week of therapy. Reduced agitation and insomnia are examples. Other symptoms often require 6 to 8 weeks for full therapeutic effects. They include hallucinations, delusions, and thought disorders. Increasing the dose of anti-psychotic drugs does not reduce the response time.

The need for maintenance therapy depends on the psychotic disorder and the person's tolerance of drug side effects. Most psychotic disorders are treated with low maintenance doses. This lowers the risk of the disorder re-occurring.

Anti-psychotic drugs can cause many adverse effects (Box 15-6). Other classes of drugs may be needed to control involuntary body movements and other side effects.

DRUG CLASS: ANTI-PSYCHOTIC AGENTS

Anti-psychotic agents are listed in Table 15-3. All act by blocking the action of dopamine in the brain. The atypical (not typical) anti-psychotic agents also block serotonin receptors.

All the anti-psychotic agents work at different sites within the brain. Therefore side effects are observed in different body systems. Atypical anti-psychotic agents tend to be more effective. They have fewer side effects than the typical anti-psychotic agents.

The intent of therapy is to:
- Maintain the person at an optimal level of function
- Reduce the re-occurrence of psychotic symptoms
- Have few adverse effects from drug therapy

Assisting With the Nursing Process
When giving anti-psychotic drugs, you assist the nurse with the nursing process.

ASSESSMENT
- Measure blood pressure in the supine, sitting, and standing positions.
- Measure weight and height.
- Measure blood glucose.

PLANNING
See Table 15-3 for oral and rectal "Dose Forms."

BOX 15-6   Adverse Effects From Anti-Psychotic Drugs

INVOLUNTARY BODY MOVEMENTS
- Tongue protrusion
- Rolling back of the eyes
- Jaw spasm
- Head turned to one side
- Parkinson-like symptoms
  - Tremors
  - Muscle rigidity
  - Mask-like expression
  - Shuffling gait
  - Loss or weakness of motor function
- Pacing
- Rocking
- Not being able to sit or stand in one place
- Tongue movements
  - Forward, backward, lateral
  - Thrusting
  - Rolling
  - Fly-catching
- Chewing
- Jaw movements that produce smacking noises
- Problems chewing, speaking, or swallowing
- Blinking
- Brow arching
- Grimacing
- Upward movement of the eyes

OTHER ADVERSE EFFECTS
- Allergic reactions
- Appetite: increased
- Dysrhythmias
- Blood cells: changes in
- Blurred vision
- Constipation
- Drowsiness
- Dry mouth
- Endocrine disorders
- Hyperglycemia
- Hypotension
- Liver toxicity
- Sedation
- Seizures
- Sexual dysfunction
- Urinary retention
- Weight gain

IMPLEMENTATION
- See Table 15-3 for "Adult Dosage Range."
- The dosage is adjusted according to the degree of mental and emotional disturbance. It often takes several weeks for the person to show desired improvement.

EVALUATION
Report and record:
- *Fatigue, drowsiness.* The dose is usually ordered for bedtime. The person needs to exercise caution when working around machines, driving a car, pouring and giving drugs, or performing other duties that require mental alertness.
- *Orthostatic hypotension.* Provide for safety. Remind the person to rise slowly from a supine or sitting position. Have the person sit or lie down if he or she feels faint.
- *Blurred vision; constipation; dryness of the mouth, nose, and throat.* Provide for safety if the person has blurred vision. Give stool softeners as ordered. The nurse may allow the person to suck on hard candy or ice chips or chew gum.
- *Seizures.* Provide for safety. See Chapter 16.
- *Parkinson-like symptoms.* Provide for safety.
- *Involuntary body movements* (see Box 15-6). Provide for safety.

- *Anorexia, nausea, jaundice.* These signal liver toxicity.
- *Hives, itching, rash.* These signal an allergic reaction. Tell the nurse at once. Do not give the next dose unless approved by the nurse.

DRUGS USED FOR ALCOHOL REHABILITATION

Alcohol slows down brain activity. It affects alertness, judgment, coordination, and reaction time. Over time, heavy drinking damages the brain, CNS, liver, heart, kidneys, and stomach. It causes changes in the heart and blood vessels. It also can cause forgetfulness and confusion.

Alcoholism is a chronic disease. It lasts throughout life. Life-style and genetics are risk factors. Some people turn to alcohol for relief from life stresses—retirement, lowered income, loss of job, failing health, loneliness, or the deaths of loved ones or friends. The craving for alcohol can be as strong as the need for food or water. An alcoholic will continue to drink despite serious family, health, or legal problems.

There is no cure. However, alcoholism can be treated. Counseling and drugs are used to help the person stop drinking. The person must avoid all alcohol to avoid a relapse.

The following drugs are used in alcohol rehabilitation:

- acamprosate (a kamp' roh sait) Campral (kam' prahl)
- disulfiram (di sul' fi ram); Antabuse (ant' ah buse)

The goal of therapy is that the person will not drink alcohol.

acamprosate (Campral)

Acamprosate (Campral) is used for chronic alcohol patients who want to maintain a sober state. It enhances the person's ability to not drink. The drug reduces drinking rates in persons who are alcohol-dependent and are not drinking at the start of treatment. The drug does not treat withdrawal symptoms.

Assisting With the Nursing Process

When giving acamprosate (Campral), you assist the nurse with the nursing process.

ASSESSMENT

- Observe the person's level of alertness and orientation to person, time, and place.
- Measure vital signs.
- Ask about GI symptoms.

PLANNING

The oral dose form is 333 mg delayed-release tablets.

IMPLEMENTATION

- The adult dose is two 333 mg tablets (666 mg) three times a day.
- Tablets may be taken without regard to meals.

EVALUATION

Report and record:

- *Diarrhea.* This is usually mild and tends to resolve with continued therapy.
- *Suicidal actions.* Observe for negative thoughts, feelings, behaviors, depression, or suicidal thinking. Report your observations and concerns to the nurse. Follow suicide precautions according to the care plan.

disulfiram (Antabuse)

Disulfiram (Antabuse) produces a very unpleasant reaction when taken before alcohol. Nausea, severe vomiting, sweating, throbbing headache, dizziness, blurred vision, and confusion occur.

The level of reaction depends on the person and the amount of alcohol consumed. How long the reaction lasts depends on the presence of alcohol in the blood. Mild reactions may last from 30 to 60 minutes. Severe reactions may last for several hours.

Taking the drug over a prolonged period of time does not produce tolerance. Rather, the person becomes more sensitive to alcohol the longer he or she remains on therapy.

The drug is used for chronic alcohol patients who want to maintain a sober state. As little as 10 to 15 mL of alcohol may produce a reaction. The person must not drink or apply alcohol in any form. This includes over-the-counter products such as sleep aids, cough and cold products, after-shave lotions, mouthwashes, and rubbing alcohol. The person must not eat sauces, vinegars, and other foods containing alcohol.

Assisting With the Nursing Process

When giving disulfiram (Antabuse), you assist the nurse with the nursing process.

ASSESSMENT

- Observe the person's level of alertness and orientation to person, time, and place.
- Measure vital signs.
- Ask about GI symptoms.

PLANNING

The oral dose form is 250 mg tablets.

IMPLEMENTATION

- The adult initial dose is 500 mg once a day for 1 to 2 weeks.
- The maintenance dose ranges from 125 to 500 mg daily. The maximum daily dose is 500 mg.
- The drug is never given to persons who are intoxicated.
- The drug is given after the person has not had alcohol for at least 12 hours.

EVALUATION

Report and record:

- *Drowsiness, fatigue, headache, impotence, metallic taste.* These are usually mild and tend to resolve with continued therapy.
- *Anorexia, nausea, vomiting, jaundice.* These may signal liver toxicity.
- *Hives, rash, itching.* These signal an allergic reaction. Tell the nurse at once. Do not give the next dose unless approved by the nurse.

REVIEW QUESTIONS

Circle the **BEST** answer.

1 A state of severe mental impairment is called
- a anxiety
- b depression
- c a mood disorder
- d psychosis

2 Many of the drugs used to treat mental health disorders affect the
- a central nervous system
- b endocrine system
- c respiratory system
- d cardiovascular system

3 Which of the following are used to treat anxiety?
- a benzodiazepines
- b monoamine oxidase inhibitors
- c selective serotonin re-uptake inhibitors
- d anti-manic agents

4 The following drugs are used to treat anxiety *except*
- a alprazolam (Xanax)
- b diazepam (Valium)
- c clorazepate (Tranxene)
- d fluoxetine (Prozac)

5 The following drugs are used to treat anxiety *except*
- a hydroxyzine (Vistaril)
- b paroxetine (Paxil)
- c hydroxyzine (Atarax)
- d fluvoxamine (Luvox)

6 Which of the following is used to produce sedation before surgery?
- a hydroxyzine (Vistaril)
- b chlordiazepoxide (Librium)
- c lorazepam (Ativan)
- d clorazepate (Tranxene)

7 Mood disorders are treated with
- a anti-anxiety drugs
- b anti-depressant drugs
- c anti-psychotic drugs
- d sedative-hypnotics

8 Which of the following have severe side effects when taken with aged cheese and other foods?
- a monoamine oxidase inhibitors
- b tri-cyclics
- c selective serotonin re-uptake inhibitors
- d benzodiazepines

9 The last dose of an MAOI is usually given no later than
- a 1400
- b 1600
- c 1800
- d 2000

10 What is the most common side effect of an MAOI?
- a orthostatic hypotension
- b sedation
- c insomnia
- d mouth dryness

11 Which of the following is an MAOI?
- a doxepin (Sinequan)
- b fluoxetine (Prozac)
- c sertraline (Zoloft)
- d phenelzine (Nardil)

12 Selective serotonin re-uptake inhibitors are used to treat
- a anxiety
- b depression
- c bipolar disorder
- d schizophrenia

13 How long does it usually take to see the effects of SSRIs?
- a 1 week
- b 1 to 2 weeks
- c 2 to 4 weeks
- d 4 to 6 weeks

14 Which is an SSRI?
- a sertraline (Zoloft)
- b amitriptyline hydrochloride (Elavil)
- c phenelzine (Nardil)
- d doxepin (Sinequan)

15 Which is *not* an anti-depressant?
- a bupropion hydrochloride (Wellbutrin)
- b mirtazapine (Remeron)
- c buspirone (BuSpar)
- d trazodone hydrochloride (Desyrel)

16 Which is an anti-manic agent?
- a lithium carbonate (Lithium)
- b paroxetine (Paxil)
- c fluoxetine (Prozac)
- d sertraline (Zoloft)

17 Anti-manic agents are used to treat
- a psychosis
- b bipolar disorder
- c anxiety
- d depression

18 The full effect of anti-manic agents are usually seen in
- a 5 to 7 days
- b 7 to 14 days
- c 10 to 21 days
- d 6 months

19 Lithium can cause a loss of
- a sodium
- b calories
- c protein
- d potassium

20 The most common psychotic disorder is
- a hallucinations
- b delusions
- c schizophrenia
- d post-traumatic stress disorder

21 Anti-psychotic drugs often cause
- a involuntary body movements
- b severe hypertension
- c suicide actions
- d sedation

22 The following are anti-psychotic agents *except*
- a diazepam (Valium)
- b chlorpromazine (Thorazine)
- c prochlorperazine (Compazine)
- d haloperidol (Haldol)

Circle **T** if the statement is **true**. Circle **F** if the statement is **false**.

23 T F Drugs used to treat anxiety can lead to dependence.

24 T F Drowsiness is a common side effect of anti-anxiety agents.

25 T F Monoamine oxidase inhibitors can cause severe hypotension.

26 T F Tri-cyclic anti-depressants have tranquilizing effects.

27 T F Acamprosate (Campral) can cause a reaction with as little as 10 mL of alcohol.

28 T F The person taking disulfiram (Antabuse) can use over-the-counter products that contain alcohol.

Answers to these questions are given on p. 445.

16

Drugs Used for Seizure Disorders

OBJECTIVES

- Define the key terms and key abbreviations used in this chapter.
- Describe the causes and types of seizure disorders.
- Describe the major types of seizures.
- Identify the factors that affect the anti-convulsant therapy ordered for a person.
- Describe the drugs used to control seizures.
- Explain how to assist with the nursing process when giving drugs to control seizures.

KEY TERMS

anti-convulsants Drugs used to prevent or reduce seizures

epilepsy A brain disorder in which clusters of nerve cells sometimes signal abnormally

seizure Violent and sudden contractions or tremors of muscle groups; convulsion

KEY ABBREVIATIONS

g Gram
kg Kilogram
mg Milligram
mL Milliliter

A *seizure* (convulsion) involves violent and sudden contractions or tremors of muscle groups. Movements are uncontrolled. The person may lose consciousness. They are caused by abnormal electrical activity in brain neurons. Causes include head injury during birth or from trauma, high fever, brain tumors, poisoning, drug overdose or withdrawal, and nervous system disorders. Lack of blood flow to the brain, seizure disorders, and epilepsy are other causes.

Epilepsy is a brain disorder in which clusters of nerve cells sometimes signal abnormally. There are brief changes in the brain's electrical function. The person can have strange sensations, emotions, and behaviors. Sometimes there are seizures, muscle spasms, and loss of consciousness. A single seizure does not mean epilepsy. In epilepsy, seizures recur. The person has a permanent brain injury or defect.

Children and young adults are commonly affected. However, epilepsy can develop at any time in a person's life. It can occur with any problem affecting the brain. Such causes include:

* Brain injury before, during, or after birth
* Problems with brain development before birth
* The mother having an injury or infection during pregnancy
* Head injury (accidents, gun shot wounds, sports injuries, falls, blows to the head)
* Poor nutrition
* Brain tumor
* Childhood fevers
* Poison—such as lead and alcohol
* Infection—such as meningitis and encephalitis
* Stroke

There is no cure for seizure disorders at this time. Doctors order drugs to prevent seizures. The drugs control seizures in many people. For others, drug therapy does not work.

When controlled, epilepsy usually does not affect learning and activities of daily living. Activity and job limits occur in severe cases. For example, a person has seizures at any time. The person may not be allowed to drive. This may limit job choices. Also the person is at risk for accidents and injuries. Safety measures are needed. They are needed for the home, workplace, transportation, and recreation.

The major types of seizures are:

* *Partial seizure.* Only one part of the brain is involved. A body part may jerk. Or the person has a hearing or vision problem or stomach discomfort. The person does not lose consciousness.
* *Generalized tonic-clonic seizure (grand mal seizure).* This type has two phases. In the *tonic phase,* the person loses consciousness. If standing or sitting, the person falls to the floor. The body is rigid because all muscles contract at once. The *clonic phase* follows. Muscle groups contract and relax. This causes jerking and twitching movements. Urinary and fecal incontinence may occur. A deep sleep is common after the seizure. Confusion and headache may occur on awakening.
* *Generalized absence (petit mal) seizure.* This type usually lasts a few seconds. There is loss of consciousness, twitching of the eyelids, and staring. No first aid is necessary. However, you should guide the person away from dangers—stairs, streets, a hot stove, fireplaces, and so on.

ANTI-CONVULSANT THERAPY

Seizure treatment must include the cause. If caused by an infection, the infection is treated. If seizures continue after treating the cause, anti-convulsant therapy is the main treatment.

Anti-convulsants are drugs used to prevent or reduce seizures. The goals of therapy are to:

* Reduce the frequency of seizures
* Reduce injury from seizure activity
* Have few adverse effects from therapy
  The drug ordered for a person depends on:
* The type of seizure
* The person's age and gender (male, female)
* Other health problems
* Potential adverse effects from the drugs

The ordered drug is discontinued if it does not control seizures. Another drug is ordered. The process continues until a drug or a combination of drugs controls seizure activity.

Anti-convulsant drugs control seizures by:

* Inhibiting the processes that excite the neurons
* Enhancing the processes that inhibit the neurons
* Preventing the seizure from spreading to other neurons

See *Delegation Guidelines: Anti-Convulsant Therapy.*

> ### DELEGATION GUIDELINES
> #### Anti-Convulsant Therapy
>
> Some anti-convulsant drugs are given parenterally. Because you do not give parenteral dose forms, they are not included in this chapter. Should a nurse delegate the administration of such to you, you must:
> * Remember that parenteral dosages are often very different from dosages for other routes.
> * Refuse the delegation. Make sure you explain why. Do not just ignore the request. Make sure the nurse knows that you cannot give the drug and why.

TABLE 16-1	Anti-Convulsants		
GENERIC NAME	**BRAND NAME**	**DOSE FORMS**	**ADULT DOSAGE RANGE**
BENZODIAZEPINES			
clonazepam	Klonopin	Tablets: 0.5, 1, 2 mg Tablets, orally disintegrating: 0.125, 0.25, 0.5, 1, 2 mg	Up to 20 mg/day
clorazepate	Tranxene	Tablets: 3.75, 7.5, 11.25, 15, 22.5 mg	Up to 90 mg/day
diazepam	Valium	Tablets: 2, 5, 10 mg Liquid: 1, 5 mg/mL Gel, rectal: 2.5, 5, 10, 15, 20 mg	Initially 5-10 mg, up to 30 mg
HYDANTOINS			
ethotoin	Peganone	Tablets: 250 mg	2-3 g/day
phenytoin	Dilantin	Tablets: 50 mg Capsules: 30, 100 mg Suspension: 125 mg/5 mL	300-600 mg/day
SUCCINIMIDES			
ethosuximide	Zarontin	Capsules: 250 mg Syrup: 250 mg/5 mL	1000-1250 mg/day
methsuximide	Celontin	Capsules: 150, 300 mg	900-1200 mg/day

DRUG CLASS: Benzodiazepines

The benzodiazepines used for anti-convulsant therapy are listed in Table 16-1. How they control seizures is not fully understood. They might inhibit neurotransmission.

Assisting With the Nursing Process

When giving benzodiazepines for anti-convulsant therapy, you assist the nurse with the nursing process.

ASSESSMENT

Observe the person's:
- Speech pattern
- Degree of alertness
- Orientation to person, time, and place

PLANNING

See Table 16-1 for oral and rectal "Dose Forms."

IMPLEMENTATION

- See Table 16-1 for "Adult Dosage Range."
- Rapidly discontinuing these drugs after long-term use may cause symptoms similar to alcohol withdrawal. These may vary from weakness and anxiety to delirium and seizures. Signs and symptoms may not appear for several days after the drug is discontinued. Benzodiazepines are withdrawn over 2 to 4 weeks.

EVALUATION

Report and record:
- *Sedation, drowsiness, dizziness, blurred vision, fatigue, lethargy.* These resolve with dosage adjustment or when the drug is discontinued. Provide for safety. The person must use caution when working around machines, driving a car, pouring and giving drugs, or performing other duties that require mental alertness.
- *Behavior disturbances.* The person may be aggressive and agitated. Provide for safety.
- *Sore throat, fever, jaundice, weakness.* These may signal changes in red blood cells and white blood cells.
- *Anorexia, nausea, vomiting, jaundice.* These may signal liver toxicity.

DRUG CLASS: Hydantoins

The action of hydantoins is not known.

Assisting With the Nursing Process

When giving hydantoins, you assist the nurse with the nursing process.

ASSESSMENT

- Measure blood glucose.
- Observe the person's:
  - Speech pattern
  - Degree of alertness
  - Orientation to person, time, and place

PLANNING

See Table 16-1 for oral "Dose Forms."

IMPLEMENTATION

- See Table 16-1 for "Adult Dosage Range."
- Give the drug with food or milk to reduce stomach irritation.
- If an oral suspension is ordered, shake the container well. Use an oral syringe to measure the dose.

EVALUATION

Report and record:

- *Nausea, vomiting, indigestion.* Give the drug with food or milk.
- *Sedation, drowsiness, dizziness, blurred vision, fatigue, lethargy.* These resolve with dosage adjustment or when the drug is discontinued. Provide for safety. The person must use caution when working around machines, driving a car, pouring and giving drugs, or performing other duties that require mental alertness.
- *Confusion.* Provide for safety.
- *Gum over-growth.* Provide good oral hygiene.
- *Hyperglycemia.* Measure blood glucose.
- *Sore throat, fever, jaundice, weakness.* These may signal changes in red blood cells and white blood cells.
- *Anorexia, nausea, vomiting, jaundice.* These may signal liver toxicity.
- *Rash, itching.* These may signal an allergic reaction. Tell the nurse at once. Do not give the next dose unless approved by the nurse.

DRUG CLASS: **Succinimides**

The action of succinimides is not known. They are used to control generalized absence (petit mal) seizures.

Assisting With the Nursing Process

When giving succinimides, you assist the nurse with the nursing process.

ASSESSMENT

Observe the person's:

- Speech pattern
- Degree of alertness
- Orientation to person, time, and place

PLANNING

See Table 16-1 for oral "Dose Forms."

IMPLEMENTATION

See Table 16-1 for "Adult Dosage Range."

EVALUATION

Report and record:

- *Nausea, vomiting, indigestion.* Give the drug with food or milk.

- *Sedation, drowsiness, dizziness, fatigue, lethargy.* Provide for safety. The person must use caution when working around machines, driving a car, pouring and giving drugs, or performing other duties that require mental alertness.

OTHER ANTI-CONVULSANTS

The following are other anti-convulsant agents:

- carbamazepine (kar bah maz' e peen); Tegretol (teg' reh tol)
- gabapentin (gah bah pen' tin); Neurontin (nuhr on' tin)
- lamotrigine (lah mot' rah geen); Lamictal (lah mik' tahl)
- levetiracetam (lehv et tihr see' tahm); Keppra (kep' rah)
- oxcarbazepine (ox karb az' e peen); Trileptal (tri lehp' tahl)
- phenobarbital (fee' no barb' it al); Luminal (loom' in al)
- primidone (prih' mih doan); Mysoline (my' so leen)
- tiagabine (tee ag' ah bean); Gabitril (gab' ah tril)
- topiramate (toh peer' ah mate); Topamax (toh' pah max)
- valproic acid (val proe' ik ah' sid); Depakene (dep' ah keen)
- zonisamide (zoh nis' am eyd); Zonegran (zoh' negh grahn)

carbamazepine (Tegretol)

This drug blocks the re-uptake of norepinephrine and the release of norepinephrine. It also affects dopamine. The drug is often used with other anti-convulsants.

Assisting With the Nursing Process

When giving carbamazepine (Tegretol), you assist the nurse with the nursing process.

ASSESSMENT

- Measure blood pressure in the supine and standing positions.
- Measure weight daily.
- Measure intake and output.
- Observe the person's:
  - Speech pattern
  - Degree of alertness
  - Orientation to person, time, and place

PLANNING

Oral dose forms are:

- Tablets: 100 and 200 mg
- Extended-release tablets: 100, 200, and 400 mg
- Extended-release capsules: 100, 200, and 300 mg
- Suspension: 100 mg/5 mL

IMPLEMENTATION
- The initial adult dose is 200 mg two times a day during the first day.
- The drug is gradually increased by 200 mg/day in divided doses every 6 to 8 hours.
- Total daily dosage should not exceed 1600 mg.

EVALUATION
Report and record:
- *Nausea, vomiting, drowsiness, dizziness.* Provide for safety. The person must use caution when working around machines, driving a car, pouring and giving drugs, or performing other duties that require mental alertness.
- *Hypertension, orthostatic hypotension.* Provide for safety. Remind the person to rise slowly from a supine or sitting position. Have the person sit or lie down if he or she feels faint.
- *Dyspnea, edema.* Measure intake and output.
- *Kidney toxicity.* Check urine color.
- *Sore throat, fever, jaundice, weakness.* These may signal changes in red blood cells and white blood cells.
- *Anorexia, nausea, vomiting, jaundice.* These may signal liver toxicity.
- *Rash, itching.* These may signal an allergic reaction. Tell the nurse at once. Do not give the next dose unless approved by the nurse.

gabapentin (Neurontin)

This drug is usually used with other anti-convulsants to reduce the frequency of partial seizures.

Assisting With the Nursing Process
When giving gabapentin (Neurontin), you assist the nurse with the nursing process.

ASSESSMENT
Observe the person's:
- Speech pattern
- Degree of alertness
- Orientation to person, time, and place

PLANNING
Oral dose forms are:
- 100, 300, and 400 mg capsules
- 100, 300, 400, 600, and 800 mg tablets
- 250 mg/5 mL suspension

IMPLEMENTATION
- The adult dosage is 900 to 1800 mg daily.
- The dosage is usually adjusted as follows:
  - Day 1 at bedtime: 300 mg.
  - Day 2: 300 mg two times a day.
  - Day 3: 300 mg three times a day.
  - The dosage is increased to no more than 1800 mg daily in 3 divided doses.

- If antacids (Chapter 25) are ordered for the person, give the gabapentin (Neurontin) at least two hours after the last dose of antacid. Antacids reduce the absorption of the drug.

EVALUATION
Report and record:
- *Sedation, drowsiness, dizziness, blurred vision.* These resolve with dosage adjustment or when the drug is discontinued. Provide for safety. The person must use caution when working around machines, driving a car, pouring and giving drugs, or performing other duties that require mental alertness.
- *Speech, alertness, and orientation to person, time, and place.* Observe for changes.

lamotrigine (Lamictal)

The drug stabilizes neuron membranes. It inhibits the release of some excitatory neurotransmitters. The drug is used in combination with other anti-convulsants to treat partial and generalized seizures.

Assisting With the Nursing Process
When giving lamotrigine (Lamictal), you assist the nurse with the nursing process.

ASSESSMENT
Observe the person's:
- Speech pattern
- Degree of alertness
- Orientation to person, time, and place

PLANNING
Dose forms are:
- 25, 100, 150, 200 mg tablets
- 2, 5, and 25 mg chewable tablets

IMPLEMENTATION
- The adult dosage is started at 50 mg once a day for 2 weeks. It is followed by 50 mg twice a day for 2 weeks.
- The usual maintenance dose is 300 to 500 mg per day in 2 divided doses.

EVALUATION
Report and record:
- *Nausea, vomiting, indigestion.* Give the drug with food or milk.
- *Sedation, drowsiness, dizziness, blurred vision.* These resolve with dosage adjustment or when the drug is discontinued. Provide for safety. The person must use caution when working around machines, driving a car, pouring and giving drugs, or performing other duties that require mental alertness.
- *Rash, itching.* Slower increases in dosage adjustment may resolve the problem. Rash and itching may signal an allergic reaction. Tell the nurse at once. Do not give the next dose unless approved by the nurse.

levetiracetam (Keppra)

This drug is used in combination with other anti-convulsants to treat partial seizures.

Assisting With the Nursing Process

When giving levetiracetam (Keppra), you assist the nurse with the nursing process.

ASSESSMENT

Observe the person's:

- Speech pattern
- Degree of alertness
- Orientation to person, time, and place

PLANNING

Dose forms are:

- 250, 500, 750, and 1000 mg tablets
- 100 mg/mL oral solution

IMPLEMENTATION

- The initial adult dose is 500 mg two times a day.
- Dosage may be increased every 2 weeks by 500 mg two times a day.
- The maximum daily dose is 3000 mg in divided doses.

EVALUATION

Report and record:

- *Weakness, drowsiness, dizziness.* These are usually mild and resolve with continued therapy. Provide for safety. The person must use caution when working around machines, driving a car, pouring and giving drugs, or performing other duties that require mental alertness.
- *Speech, alertness, and orientation to person, time, and place.* Observe for changes.

oxcarbazepine (Trileptal)

This drug stabilizes neurons. It prevents repeated firing of electrical impulses thought to produce seizures. The drug is used alone or in combination with other anti-convulsants to treat partial seizures.

Assisting With the Nursing Process

When giving oxcarbazepine (Trileptal), you assist the nurse with the nursing process.

ASSESSMENT

Observe the person's:

- Speech pattern
- Degree of alertness
- Orientation to person, time, and place

PLANNING

Dose forms are:

- 150, 300, and 600 mg tablets
- 300 mg/5 mL suspension

IMPLEMENTATION

- The adult initial dosage is 300 mg two times a day for the first 3 days.
- The dosage may be increased by 300 mg/day every 3 days to a dosage of 1200 mg a day.
- Dosages of 2400 mg/day are effective in some persons.

EVALUATION

Report and record:

- *Confusion, poor coordination, drowsiness, dizziness.* These are usually mild and resolve with continued therapy. Provide for safety. The person must use caution when working around machines, driving a car, pouring and giving drugs, or performing other duties that require mental alertness.
- *Speech, alertness, and orientation to person, time, and place.* Observe for changes.
- *Nausea, headache, lethargy, confusion, reduced level of consciousness, weakness.* These are signs of low sodium.

phenobarbital (Luminal)

This drug is a long-acting barbiturate (Chapter 15). It prevents the spread of seizure activity. The drug is used in combination with other anti-convulsants to treat partial and generalized seizures.

The drug has sedative effects. Therefore it is used when non-sedating anti-convulsants do not control seizures.

Assisting With the Nursing Process

See Chapter 15.

primidone (Mysoline)

This drug is related to the barbiturates. The drug is used in combination with other anti-convulsants to treat partial and generalized seizures.

Assisting With the Nursing Process

When giving primidone (Mysoline), you assist the nurse with the nursing process.

ASSESSMENT

Observe the person's:

- Speech pattern
- Degree of alertness
- Orientation to person, time, and place

PLANNING

The oral dose forms are 50 and 250 mg tablets.

IMPLEMENTATION

- For an adult, the drug is ordered as follows:
  - Days 1, 2, and 3 at bedtime: 100 to 125 mg daily.
  - Days 4, 5, and 6: the dosage is increased to 100 to 125 mg two times a day.

- Days 7, 8, and 9: the dosage is increased to 100 to 125 mg three times a day.
  - Every 3 or 4 days: the dosage is increased by 100 to 125 mg until the person responds or tolerance develops.
- The typical dosage is 750 to 1500 mg in one day. The dosage should not exceed 2000 mg in one day.

EVALUATION

Report and record:

- *Sedation, drowsiness, dizziness, blurred vision.* These resolve with continued therapy or with dosage adjustment. Provide for safety. The person must use caution when working around machines, driving a car, pouring and giving drugs, or performing other duties that require mental alertness.
- *Sore throat, fever, jaundice, weakness.* These may signal changes in red blood cells and white blood cells.

tiagabine (Gabitril)

The drug is used in combination with other anti-convulsants to treat partial seizures.

Assisting With the Nursing Process

When giving tiagabine (Gabitril), you assist the nurse with the nursing process.

ASSESSMENT

Observe the person's:

- Speech pattern
- Degree of alertness
- Orientation to person, time, and place

PLANNING

The oral dose forms are 2, 4, 12, and 16 mg tablets.

IMPLEMENTATION

Initially for an adult, 4 mg are given daily. The daily dosage is increased by 4 to 8 mg every week until:

- The person responds.
- A total daily dose of 56 mg is given. A total daily dosage of 32 to 56 mg may be given in 2 to 4 divided doses.

EVALUATION

Report and record:

- *Sedation, drowsiness, dizziness.* These resolve with continued therapy or with dosage adjustment. Provide for safety. The person must use caution when working around machines, driving a car, pouring and giving drugs, or performing other duties that require mental alertness.
- *Speech, alertness, memory loss, and orientation to person, time, and place.* Observe for changes.

topiramate (Topamax)

The drug is used in combination with other anti-convulsants to treat:

- Partial and generalized seizures
- Migraine headaches

Assisting With the Nursing Process

When giving topiramate (Topamax), you assist the nurse with the nursing process.

ASSESSMENT

- Observe the person's:
  - Speech pattern
  - Degree of alertness
  - Orientation to person, time, and place
- Measure weight.
- Measure intake and output.
- Ask about headaches.

PLANNING

Oral dose forms are:

- 25, 50, 100, and 200 mg tablets
- 15 and 25 mg sprinkle capsules

IMPLEMENTATION

- As an anti-convulsant:
  - The adult initial dose is 25 mg twice a day.
  - The daily dosage is increased by 50 mg at weekly intervals until the person responds.
  - The usually daily dosage is 400 mg two times a day.
- To prevent migraine headaches in an adult:
  - Week 1: 25 mg daily in the evening
  - Week 2: 25 mg morning and evening
  - Week 3: 25 mg in the morning; 50 mg in the evening
  - Week 4 and after: 50 mg in the morning; 50 mg in the evening
- Note the following when giving this drug:
  - Tablets should not be broken. They taste bitter.
  - Sprinkle capsules can be swallowed whole. If sprinkle capsules are not swallowed whole, open the capsule carefully. Sprinkle the entire contents on a teaspoon of soft food. Ask the person to swallow the drug/food mixture at once. Tell the person not to chew the drug/food mixture.

EVALUATION

Report and record:

- *Sedation, drowsiness, dizziness.* These resolve with continued therapy or with dosage adjustment. Provide for safety. The person must use caution when working around machines, driving a car, pouring and giving drugs, or performing other duties that require mental alertness.

- *Speech, alertness, and orientation to person, time, and place.* Observe for changes.
- *Decreased sweating, over-heating.* These may occur with vigorous activity or exposure to warm or hot temperatures.

valproic acid (Depakene)

The action of this drug is not known. It may inhibit neurotransmitter activity. The drug is used to treat:
- Partial and generalized seizures
- Migraine headaches

Assisting With the Nursing Process

When giving valproic acid (Depakene), you assist the nurse with the nursing process.

ASSESSMENT

Observe the person's:
- Speech pattern
- Degree of alertness
- Orientation to person, time, and place

PLANNING

The oral dose forms are:
- 250 mg capsules
- 125 mg capsules containing coated particles
- 125, 250, and 500 mg sustained-release tablets
- 250 mg/5 mL syrup

IMPLEMENTATION
- The adult dosage is based on the person's body weight—5 mg/kg every 8 hours.
- The dosage is increased by 5 to 10 mg/kg at weekly intervals.
- Give the drug with food or milk to reduce gastric irritation.

EVALUATION

Report and record:
- *Sedation, drowsiness, dizziness.* These resolve with continued therapy or with dosage adjustment. Provide for safety. The person must use caution when working around machines, driving a car, pouring and giving drugs, or performing other duties that require mental alertness.
- *Nausea, vomiting, and indigestion.* Give the drug with food or milk.
- *Sore throat, fever, jaundice, weakness.* These may signal changes in red blood cells and white blood cells.
- *Anorexia, nausea, vomiting, jaundice.* These may signal liver toxicity.
- *Abdominal pain, nausea, vomiting, anorexia.* These are symptoms of pancreatitis.

zonisamide (Zonegran)

This drug is used in combination with other anticonvulsants to treat partial seizures.

Assisting With the Nursing Process

When giving zonisamide (Zonegran), you assist the nurse with the nursing process.

ASSESSMENT
- Observe the person's:
  - Speech pattern
  - Degree of alertness
  - Orientation to person, time, and place
- Measure vital signs

PLANNING

The oral dose forms are 25, 50, and 100 mg capsules.

IMPLEMENTATION
- The initial adult dose is 100 mg daily.
- After 2 weeks, the dosage may be increased to 200 mg/day for at least 2 weeks. The 200 mg may be taken at the same time.
- The dosage can be increased up to 600 mg per day. Two weeks should pass between dosage changes.
- Note the following when giving this drug:
  - It is taken with or without food.
  - Due to sedative effects, it may be taken at bedtime.
  - The person should drink 6 to 8 glasses of water each day.

EVALUATION

Report and record:
- *Sedation, drowsiness, dizziness.* These resolve with continued therapy or with dosage adjustment. Provide for safety. The person must use caution when working around machines, driving a car, pouring and giving drugs, or performing other duties that require mental alertness.
- *Speech, alertness, and orientation to person, time, and place.* Observe for changes.
- *Back pain, abdominal pain, pain on urination.* These may signal kidney problems.
- *Sore throat, fever, jaundice, weakness.* These may signal changes in red blood cells and white blood cells.
- *Rash, itching.* Slower increases in dosage adjustment may resolve the problem. Rash and itching may signal an allergic reaction. Tell the nurse at once. Do not give the next dose unless approved by the nurse.

REVIEW QUESTIONS

Circle the **BEST** answer.

1 A body part may jerk. The person does not lose consciousness. This is
 a epilepsy
 b a partial seizure
 c a generalized seizure
 d a petit mal seizure

2 Seizure treatment must always include
 a anti-convulsant therapy
 b benzodiazepines
 c the cause of the seizures
 d treatment of epilepsy

3 Anti-convulsant drugs control seizures by affecting
 a neurons in the brain
 b nerves in the central nervous system
 c voluntary muscles
 d involuntary muscles

4 Which is a benzodiazepine?
 a diazepam (Valium)
 b ethotoin (Peganone)
 c phenytoin (Dilantin)
 d ethosuximide (Zarontin)

5 When giving a benzodiazepine you must
 a give the drug with food or milk
 b provide for safety
 c give good oral hygiene
 d measure blood pressure

6 Which is a hydantoin?
 a phenobarbital (Luminal)
 b diazepam (Valium)
 c phenytoin (Dilantin)
 d methsuximide (Celontin)

7 Succinimides are given
 a with food or milk
 b at bedtime
 c before meals
 d after meals

8 Before giving carbamazepine (Tegretol), you
 a measure blood glucose
 b give good oral hygiene
 c measure weight
 d give the person food

9 When giving most anti-convulsants, you observe the following *except*
 a the person's speech pattern
 b the person's urine color
 c the person's degree of alertness
 d the person's orientation to person, time, and place

10 The first dose of gabapentin (Neurontin) is given
 a with food or milk
 b at bedtime
 c before meals
 d after meals

11 Which is a barbiturate?
 a phenobarbital (Luminal)
 b lorazepam (Ativan)
 c phenytoin (Dilantin)
 d ethosuximide (Zarontin)

12 Before giving topiramate (Topamax), you
 a observe urine color
 b give good oral hygiene
 c measure weight
 d measure blood pressure

13 Which drug's dosage is based on the person's body weight?
 a valproic acid (Depakene)
 b tiagabine (Gabitril)
 c topiramate (Topamax)
 d zonisamide (Zonegran)

14 Before giving zonisamide (Zonegran), you
 a provide food or milk
 b give good oral hygiene
 c measure weight
 d measure vital signs

Circle **T** if the statement is **true**. Circle **F** if the statement is **false**.

15 T F Many anti-convulsant drugs cause sedation.

16 T F Phenytoin (Dilantin) is given with food or milk.

17 T F The person with a seizure disorder can take only one anti-convulsant.

18 T F Lamotrigine (Lamictal) is given before meals.

19 T F The first doses of primidone (Mysoline) are given in the morning.

20 T F A dose form of topiramate (Topamax) is sprinkle capsules. The person can chew the capsule contents.

Answers to these questions are given on p. 445.

Drugs Used to Manage Pain

OBJECTIVES

- Define the key terms and key abbreviations used in this chapter.
- Explain how to assist the nurse in assessing a person's pain.
- Describe the different types of pain.
- Describe the factors that affect a person's reaction to pain.
- Describe the drugs used for pain management.
- Explain how to assist with the nursing process when giving drugs for pain management.

KEY TERMS

analgesic A drug that relieves pain; *an* means *without* and *algesic* means *pain*

euphoria An exaggerated feeling or state of physical or mental well-being

opiate A drug that contains opium, is derived from opium, or has opium-like activity

opium The milky substance from unripe poppy seed pods; *opion* means *poppy juice*

pain To ache, hurt, or be sore; discomfort

semi-synthetic A natural substance that has been partially altered by chemicals

synthetic A substance that is made rather than naturally occurring

KEY ABBREVIATIONS

CNS Central nervous system
g Gram
GI Gastro-intestinal
h Hour
MAR Medication administration record
mcg Microgram
mg Milligram
MI Myocardial infarction
mL Milliliter
NSAID Non-steroidal anti-inflammatory drug
PG Prostaglandin
PO Per os (orally)
PRN When necessary, as needed
q Every
STAT At once, immediately

Pain *(discomfort)* means to ache, hurt, or be sore. It is unpleasant. Pain is subjective (Chapter 4). That is, you cannot see, hear, touch, or smell pain. You must rely on what the person says. Report complaints to the nurse. The information is used for the nursing process.

Pain is personal. It differs for each person. What *hurts* to one person may *ache* to another. What one person calls *sore,* another may call *aching.* If a person complains of pain, the person *has* pain. You must believe the person. You cannot see, hear, feel, or smell the pain.

Pain is a warning from the body. It means there is tissue damage. Pain often causes the person to seek health care.

There are different types of pain. The doctor uses the type of pain when diagnosing and ordering drugs for pain relief. The nurse uses it for the nursing process.

- *Acute pain* is felt suddenly from injury, disease, trauma, or surgery. There is tissue damage. Acute pain lasts a short time, usually less than 6 months. It lessens with healing.
- *Chronic pain* lasts longer than 6 months. Pain is constant or occurs off and on. There is no longer tissue damage. Chronic pain remains long after healing. Arthritis and cancer are common causes.
- *Radiating pain* is felt at the site of tissue damage and in nearby areas. Pain from a heart attack is often felt in the left chest, left jaw, left shoulder, and left arm. Gallbladder disease can cause pain in the right upper abdomen, the back, and the right shoulder.
- *Phantom pain* is felt in a body part that is no longer there. A person with an amputated leg may still sense leg pain.

A person may handle pain well one time and poorly the next time. Many factors affect reactions to pain.

- *Past experience.* We learn from past experiences. They help us know what to do or what to expect. A person may have had pain before. The severity of pain, its cause, how long it lasted, and if relief occurred all affect the person's current response to pain. Knowing what to expect can help or hinder how the person handles pain. Some people have not had pain. When it occurs, pain can cause fear and anxiety. They can make pain worse.
- *Anxiety.* Anxiety relates to feelings of fear, dread, worry, and concern. The person is uneasy and tense. The person may feel troubled or threatened. Pain and anxiety are related. Pain can cause anxiety. Anxiety increases how much pain the person feels. Reducing anxiety helps lessen pain. For example, the nurse explains to Mr. Smith that he will have pain after surgery. The nurse also explains that he will receive drugs for pain relief. Mr. Smith knows the cause of the pain. And he knows what to expect. This helps reduce his anxiety and therefore the amount of pain felt.
- *Rest and sleep.* Rest and sleep restore energy. They reduce body demands, and the body repairs itself. Lack of needed rest and sleep affects thinking and coping with daily life. Sleep and rest needs increase with illness and injury. Pain seems worse when tired or restless. Also, the person tends to focus on pain when tired and unable to rest or sleep.
- *Attention.* The more a person thinks about the pain, the worse it seems. Sometimes severe pain is all the person thinks about. However, even mild pain can seem worse if the person thinks about it all the time. Pain often seems worse at night. Activity is less, and it is quiet. There are no visitors. The radio or TV is off. Others are asleep. When unable to sleep, the person has time to think about the pain.
- *Personal and family duties.* Often pain is ignored when there are children to care for. Some people go to work with pain. Others deny pain if a serious illness is feared. The illness can interfere with a job, going to school, or caring for children, a partner, or ill parents.
- *The value or meaning of pain.* To some people, pain is a sign of weakness. It may mean a serious illness and the need for painful tests and treatments. Therefore pain is ignored or denied. Sometimes pain gives pleasure. The pain of childbirth is one example. For some persons, pain means not having to work or assume daily routines. Pain is used to avoid certain people or things. The pain is useful. Some people like doting and pampering by others. The person values and wants such attention.
- *Support from others.* Dealing with pain is often easier when family and friends offer comfort and support. The use of touch by a valued person is very comforting. Just being nearby also helps. Some people do not have caring family or friends. They deal with pain alone. Being alone can increase anxiety. The person has more time to think about the pain.

- *Culture.* Culture affects pain responses. In some cultures, the person in pain is *stoic*. To be stoic means to show no reaction to joy, sorrow, pleasure, or pain. Strong verbal and nonverbal reactions to pain are seen in other cultures. Non-English speaking persons may have problems describing pain. The agency must know who these persons are. Someone must be available to interpret the person's needs. All persons have the right to be comfortable and as pain-free as possible.
- *Illness.* Some diseases cause decreased pain sensations. Central nervous system (CNS) disorders are examples. The person may not feel pain. Or it may not feel severe. The person is at risk for undetected disease or injury. Pain occurs with tissue damage. The pain is an alert to illness or injury. If pain is not felt, the person does not know to seek health care.
- *Age.* Children may not understand pain. They know it feels bad. They have fewer pain experiences. They do not know what to expect. Children do not know how to relieve their own pain. They rely on adults for help. Adults must be alert to behaviors and situations that signal a child's pain. Infants cry, fuss, and are restless. Toddlers and preschoolers may not have the words to express pain. See *Focus on Older Persons: Factors Affecting Pain.*

FOCUS ON OLDER PERSONS

Factors Affecting Pain

Older persons may have decreased pain sensations. They may not feel pain. Or it may not feel severe. The person is at risk for undetected disease or injury. Pain occurs with tissue damage. The pain signals illness or injury. If pain is not felt, the person does not know to seek health care.

Some older persons have many painful health problems. Chronic pain may mask new pain. Older persons may ignore or deny new pain. They may think it relates to a known health problem. Older persons often deny or ignore pain because of what it may mean.

Thinking and reasoning are affected in some older persons. Some cannot verbally communicate pain. Changes in usual behavior may signal pain. A person who normally moans and groans may become quiet and withdrawn. A person who is friendly and outgoing may become agitated and aggressive. One who is nonverbal and quiet may become restless and cry easily. Loss of appetite also signals pain.

Report any changes in a person's usual behavior to the nurse. All persons have the right to correct pain management. The nurse needs to do a pain assessment when the person's behavior changes.

You cannot see, hear, feel, or smell the person's pain. You must rely on what the person tells you. Promptly report any information you collect about pain. Write down what the person says. Use the person's exact words when reporting and recording. The nurse needs this information to assess the person's pain:

- *Location.* Where is the pain? Ask the person to point to the area of pain. Pain can radiate. Ask the person if the pain is anywhere else and to point to those areas.
- *Onset and duration.* When did the pain start? How long has it lasted?
- *Intensity.* Does the person complain of mild, moderate, or severe pain? Ask the person to rate the pain on a scale of 1 to 10, with 10 as the most severe (Fig. 17-1). Or use the Wong-Baker Faces Pain Rating Scale (Fig. 17-2, p. 224). Designed for children, the scale is useful for persons of all ages. To use the scale, tell the person that each face shows how a person is feeling. Read the description for each face. Then ask the person to choose the face that best describes how he or she feels.
- *Description.* Ask the person to describe the pain. If the person cannot describe the pain, offer some of the words listed in Box 17-1, p. 224.
- *Factors causing pain.* These are called *precipitating* factors. *To precipitate* means *to cause.* Such factors include moving or turning in bed, coughing or deep breathing, and exercise. Ask what the person was doing before the pain started and when it started.
- *Factors affecting pain.* Ask the person what makes the pain better. Also ask what makes it worse.
- *Vital signs.* Measure the person's pulse, respirations, and blood pressure. Increases in these vital signs often occur with acute pain. Vital signs may be normal with chronic pain.
- *Other signs and symptoms.* Does the person have other symptoms—dizziness, nausea, vomiting, weakness, numbness or tingling, or others? Box 17-2, p. 224, lists the signs and symptoms that often occur with pain.

PAIN: Ask person to rate pain on scale of 0-10										
No pain									Worst pain imaginable	
0	1	2	3	4	5	6	7	8	9	10

Fig. 17-1 Pain rating scale. (Modified from deWit SC: *Fundamental concepts and skills for nursing*, ed 2, Philadelphia, 2005, Saunders.)

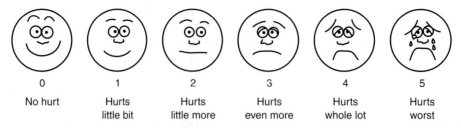

0	1	2	3	4	5
No hurt	Hurts little bit	Hurts little more	Hurts even more	Hurts whole lot	Hurts worst

Fig. 17-2 Wong-Baker Faces Pain Rating Scale. (From Hockenberry MJ, Wilson D: *Wong's nursing care of infants and children,* ed 8, St Louis, 2007, Mosby.)

BOX 17-1 Words Used to Describe Pain

- Aching
- Burning
- Cramping
- Crushing
- Dull
- Gnawing
- Knife-like
- Piercing
- Pressure
- Sharp
- Sore
- Squeezing
- Stabbing
- Throbbing
- Vise-like

BOX 17-2 Signs and Symptoms of Pain

BODY RESPONSES
- Appetite: changes in
- Dizziness
- Nausea
- Numbness
- Pulse, respirations, and blood pressure: increased
- Skin: pale (pallor)
- Sleep: difficulty with
- Sweating (diaphoresis)
- Tingling
- Vomiting
- Weakness

BEHAVIORS
- Crying
- Gasping
- Grimacing
- Groaning
- Grunting
- Holding the affected body part (splinting; guarding)
- Irritability
- Moaning
- Mood: changes in
- Positioning: maintaining one position; refusing to move
- Quietness
- Restlessness
- Rubbing
- Screaming
- Speech: slow or rapid; loud or quiet

PAIN MANAGEMENT

An **analgesic** is a drug that relieves pain. (*An* means *without. Algesic* means *pain.*) The goals of pain management are to:

- Relieve the intensity of pain and how long the person complains of pain
- Prevent the pain from becoming chronic
- Prevent suffering and disability associated with pain
- Prevent psychologic and socio-economic consequences from inadequate pain management
- Control the side effects from pain management
- Improve the person's ability to perform activities of daily living to an optimal level

Pain is transmitted from the site of injury to the brain. First, pain receptors are stimulated at the site of damage. Neurotransmitters send nerve impulses from the site of damage to the spinal cord. The impulses travel up the spinal cord to various areas of the brain.

Opiate receptors within the CNS control pain. When opiates stimulate these receptors, pain sensation is blocked. An **opiate** is a drug that contains opium, is derived from opium, or has opium-like activity. Opiate comes from the Greek word *opion,* which means *poppy juice.* **Opium** is the milky substance from unripe poppy seed pods.

When cells are damaged, other chemicals are released that stimulate pain receptors. Other drugs block such chemicals and stop pain.

Most drugs for pain management are given PRN (when necessary, as needed). *The nurse decides when a PRN drug is needed.*

See *Delegation Guidelines: Pain Management.*

DRUG CLASS: **Opiate Agents**

The term *opiate* once referred to drugs derived from opium. Morphine and heroine (a morphine-like drug) are examples. (*Morphine* comes from the Greek name *Morpheus.* It means *god of sleep.*) Other analgesics not related to morphine act at the same sites in the brain.

Opiate agonists are a group of semi-synthetic or synthetic drugs that can relieve severe pain without

DELEGATION GUIDELINES
Pain Management

Some drugs used for pain management are given parenterally—by subcutaneous, intramuscular, or intravenous injection. Because you do not give parenteral dose forms, they are not included in this chapter. Should a nurse delegate the administration of such to you, you must:

- Remember that parenteral dosages are often very different from doses for other routes.
- Refuse the delegation. Make sure you explain why. Do not just ignore the request. Make sure the nurse knows that you cannot give the drug and why.

loss of consciousness. (*Synthetic* means *to put together*.) A **synthetic** is a substance that is made rather than naturally occurring. A **semi-synthetic** is a natural substance that has been partially altered by chemicals.

Remember, an *agonist* is a drug that acts on a certain type of cell to produce a predictable response

(Chapter 14). Opiate agonists are listed in Table 17-1. They stimulate opiate receptors in the CNS and cause the following effects:

- Analgesia
- Respiratory depression
- Cough reflex suppression
- Drowsiness
- Sedation
- Mental clouding
- Euphoria (**Euphoria** is an exaggerated feeling or state of physical or mental well-being.)
- Nausea and vomiting

Most opiate agonists can produce addiction. They are considered controlled substances under the Federal Controlled Substances Act of 1970. If used for recreational purposes, addiction may develop after 3 to 6 weeks of continuous use. Addiction from the use of opiates for acute pain management is not a frequent problem. The addicted person has the signs and symptoms listed in Box 17-3, p. 226, when the drug is withdrawn. The symptoms become increasingly severe and peak in 36 to 72 hours. They disappear over the next 5 to 14 days.

TABLE 17-1 Opiate Agonists

GENERIC NAME	BRAND NAME	DOSE FORMS	INITIAL ADULT DOSE
MORPHINE AND MORPHINE-LIKE DERIVATIVES			
codeine	Codeine Sulfate Codeine Phosphate	Tablets: 15, 30, 60 mg Oral solution: 15 mg/5 mL	Analgesic: 15-60 mg q4-6h Antitussive: 10-20 mg q4-6h
hydromorphone	Dilaudid, Dilaudid-HP	Tablets: 2, 4, 8 mg Capsules, extended-release: 12, 16, 24, 32 mg Liquid: 1 mg/mL Suppositories: 3 mg	PO: 2 mg q4-6h Rectal: 3 mg q6-8h
levorphanol	Levo-Dromoran	Tablets: 2 mg	2 mg
morphine	Roxanol, Morphine Sulfate, MSIR, Duramorph, MS Contin, Kadian	Tablets: 15, 30 mg Capsules: 15, 30 mg Sustained-release tablets: 15, 30, 60, 100, 200 mg Solution: 10, 20, 100 mg/5 mL; 20 mg/mL Suppositories: 5, 10, 20, 30 mg	PO: 10-30 mg q4h Rectal: 10-20 mg q4h
oxycodone	Roxicodone Oxycontin	Tablets: 5 mg Tablets, controlled-release: 10, 20, 40, 80, 160 mg Oral solution: 5 mg/5 mL; 20 mg/mL	5 mg q6h
	Percodan (with aspirin)	Tablets: 5 mg	5 mg q6h
oxymorphone	Numorphan	Suppositories: 5 mg	Rectal: 5 mg q4-6h

Continued

TABLE 17-1	Opiate Agonists—cont'd		
GENERIC NAME	**BRAND NAME**	**DOSE FORMS**	**INITIAL ADULT DOSE**
MEPERIDINE-LIKE DERIVATIVES			
fentanyl	Actiq	Lozenges: 200, 400, 600, 800, 1200, 1600 mcg Buccal: 100, 200, 300, 400, 600, 800 mcg	Buccal: 200 mcg
	Duragesic	Transdermal patch: 12, 25, 50, 75, 100 mcg/hour	Upper torso: 25 mcg/hour every 72 hours
meperidine	Demerol	Tablets: 50, 100 mg Syrup: 50 mg/5 mL	50-150 mg q3-4h
METHADONE-LIKE DERIVATIVES			
methadone	Methadone, Dolophine	Tablets: 5, 10, 40 mg Solution: 5, 10 mg/5 mL Oral concentrate: 10 mg/mL	Analgesia: 2.5-10 mg q3-4h Maintenance: 20-40 mg; up to 120 mg daily
OTHER OPIATE AGONISTS			
tramadol	Ultram	Tablets: 50 mg	50-100 mg

BOX 17-3	Signs and Symptoms of Opiate Withdrawal

- Restlessness
- Perspiration
- Goose-flesh
- Tears
- Nose: runny
- Pupils: dilated
- Muscle spasms
- Pain: severe back, abdominal, and leg
- Cramps: muscle and abdominal
- Flashes: hot and cold
- Insomnia
- Nausea
- Vomiting
- Diarrhea
- Sneezing: severe
- Vital signs: increased temperature, heart rate, respiratory rate, and blood pressure

Uses

Opiate agonists are used:

- To relieve acute or chronic moderate to severe pain. Pain from acute injury, surgery, renal or biliary colic, myocardial infarction (MI), and cancer are examples.
- For pre-operative sedation.
- To supplement anesthesia.
- To reduce anxiety in persons with acute pulmonary edema.

Assisting With the Nursing Process

Many states and agencies do not let MA-Cs give controlled substances by any route. Others let MA-Cs give oral, rectal, and transdermal dose forms.

Opiate agonists are given PRN for pain relief. For other uses, they may be ordered as a STAT (at once, immediately) order (MI, pulmonary edema) or a one-time order (pre-operative sedation). Oral dose forms are usually PRN.

When a person receives an opiate agonist, you assist the nurse with the nursing process.

ASSESSMENT

- Observe the person's speech pattern, degree of alertness, and orientation to person, time, and place.
- Measure vital signs. Tell the nurse at once if the person's respirations are below 12 per minute.
- Ask the person to rate his or her pain. Use a pain rating scale.
- Check the medication administration record (MAR) for when the person last received an analgesic.

PLANNING

- See Table 17-1 for "Dose Forms."
- Many opiate agonists are available for subcutaneous, intramuscular, or intravenous injection. You do not give drugs by those routes.

TABLE 17-2 — Salicylates

GENERIC NAME	BRAND NAME	DOSE FORMS	USES AND ADULT DOSAGES	MAXIMUM DAILY DOSE (mg)
SALICYLATES				
aspirin	Zorprin, ASA, Empirin	Tablets: 81, 165, 325, 500, 650 mg Suppositories: 120, 200, 300, 600 mg	Minor aches and pains: 325-600 mg q4h Arthritis: 2.6-5.2 g/day in divided doses Acute rheumatic fever: 7.8 g/day Myocardial infarction prophylaxis: 81-325 mg daily	—
choline salicylate	Arthropan	Liquid: 870 mg/5 mL	Mild pain: 870 mg q3-4h (fewer GI side effects)	7000
diflunisal	Dolobid	Tablets: 250, 500 mg	Mild to moderate pain: Initially, 1000 mg, then 500 mg q8h Osteoarthritis and rheumatoid arthritis: 250-500 mg twice daily	1500
magnesium salicylate	Magan, Mobidin	Tablets: 467, 500, 545, 580, 600 mg	Mild aches and pains: 500-600 mg three or four times daily	9600
salsalate	Salsitab Artha-G	Tablets: 500, 750 mg	Mild pain: 500-750 mg four to six times daily	3000
sodium salicylate	Sodium Salicylate	Enteric-coated tablets: 325, 650 mg	Mild analgesia: 325-650 mg q4-8h (less effective than equal doses of aspirin)	3900

IMPLEMENTATION

See Table 17-1 for "Initial Adult Dose."

EVALUATION

Report and record:

- *Light-headedness, dizziness, sedation, nausea, vomiting, sweating.* These tend to occur with the first dose. The supine position helps reduce these symptoms. Provide for safety.
- *Confusion, disorientation.* Observe the person's alertness and orientation to person, time, and place. Provide for safety.
- *Orthostatic hypotension.* The person may have dizziness and weakness with the first dose. Provide for safety. Measure blood pressure. Do not allow the person to sit up.
- *Constipation.* This may occur from continued use. Follow the care plan for fluid intake and diet. Give stool softeners or laxatives as ordered (Chapter 26).
- *Respiratory depression.* Tell the nurse at once if the person's respiratory rate is 12 per minute or less. Also observe the depth of respirations. Tell the nurse at once if the person has shallow breathing.

- *Urinary retention.* Opiate agonists can cause ureter and bladder spasms. Urine is retained. The person may have problems starting a urine stream. Measure intake and output. Ask about problems urinating. Follow the care plan to promote urination.
- *Excess use or abuse.* The person often complains of pain or requests a drug for pain relief. The report of pain may be well before the next dose can be given. Always report complaints of pain or drug requests to the nurse at once. See Box 17-3 for signs and symptoms of withdrawal.

DRUG CLASS: Salicylates

Salicylates (sahl ih sil' ates) are the most commonly used analgesics for slight to moderate pain. See Table 17-2.

Drugs in this class inhibit the production of prostaglandins. Prostaglandins (PGs) are fatty acids that cause various responses.

- *Analgesic effect.* Salicylates inhibit the formation of PGs affecting pain receptors.
- *Anti-inflammatory effect.* Salicylates inhibit PGs that produce signs and symptoms of inflammation. Redness, swelling, and warmth are examples.
- *Anti-pyretic effect. Anti* means against. *Pyretic* comes from the Greek word that means *fever.* Salicylates inhibit the formation and release of PGs in the brain that cause body temperature to rise. An anti-pyretic is a drug given to reduce fever.

Drugs in this class do not dull alertness. They do not cause mental sluggishness or affect memory. They do not cause hallucinations, euphoria, or sedation.

aspirin

Aspirin inhibits platelet activity (Chapter 23). Platelets are needed for blood clotting. By inhibiting platelet activity, aspirin reduces blood clotting. Therefore aspirin is used to:

- Reduce the risk of transient ischemic attacks or stroke in men
- Reduce the risk of MI in persons with previous MI or unstable angina

Assisting With the Nursing Process

When a person receives salicylates, you assist the nurse with the nursing process.

ASSESSMENT
- Observe the person's speech pattern, degree of alertness, and orientation to person, time, and place.
- Measure vital signs.
- Ask the person to rate his or her pain. Use a pain rating scale.
- Check the MAR for when the person last received the ordered drug.

PLANNING
See Table 17-2 for "Dose Forms."

IMPLEMENTATION
- See Table 17-2 for "Uses and Adult Dosages" and for "Maximum Daily Dose."
- To prevent blood clotting, the oral dose is 81 to 1300 mg daily. Larger doses are usually divided into 325 mg in 2, 3, or 4 doses daily.

EVALUATION
Report and record:
- *Stomach irritation.* Give the drug with food or milk or with large amounts of water. If antacids (Chapter 25) are ordered, they are given 1 hour later. Enteric forms are often ordered to reduce stomach irritation.

- *GI bleeding.* Vomitus that looks like coffee grounds ("coffee ground emesis"), red vomitus, and black or dark tarry stools are signs of GI bleeding. Test stools for occult blood as directed by the nurse and care plan.
- *Tinnitus (ringing in the ears), impaired hearing, dimmed vision, sweating, fever, lethargy, dizziness, confusion, nausea, vomiting.* These signal salicylate toxicity. This can occur from the continuous use of high doses. The condition resolves when the dose is reduced.

DRUG CLASS: Non-Steroidal Anti-Inflammatory Drugs

Non-steroidal anti-inflammatory drugs (NSAIDs) are known as "aspirin-like" drugs. They are prostaglandin inhibitors. They have varying degrees of analgesic, anti-inflammatory, and anti-pyretic effects.

NSAIDs are used to reduce pain, inflammation, and fever. Over-the-counter NSAIDs are used to:
- Reduce fever
- Relive minor aches and pains from the common cold
- Relieve headaches, toothaches, muscle aches, backaches, joint pain from arthritis, and menstrual cramps

Side effects tend to be less than those from the salicylates. However, there is a risk of MI, stroke, and life-threatening GI bleeding from NSAIDs.

NSAIDs are not given to persons allergic to aspirin.

Assisting With the Nursing Process

When a person receives NSAIDs, you assist the nurse with the nursing process.

ASSESSMENT
- Observe the person's speech pattern, degree of alertness, and orientation to person, time, and place.
- Measure vital signs.
- Ask the person to rate his or her pain. Use a pain rating scale.

PLANNING
See Table 17-3 for "Dose Forms."

IMPLEMENTATION
See Table 17-3 for "Uses and Adult Dosages" and for "Maximum Daily Dose."

TABLE 17-3 Non-Steroidal Anti-Inflammatory Agents

GENERIC NAME	BRAND NAME	DOSE FORMS	USES AND ADULT DOSAGES	MAXIMUM DAILY DOSE (mg)
celecoxib	Celebrex	Capsules: 100, 200, 400 mg	Rheumatoid and osteoarthritis: 100-200 mg twice daily Ankylosing spondylitis: 200-400 mg daily Acute pain and primary dysmenorrhea: 400 mg initially, followed by 200 mg on the first day, then 200 mg twice daily	400
diclofenac	Cataflam, Voltaren	Tablets: 50 mg Tablets, delayed-release: 25, 50, 75, 100 mg	Rheumatoid and osteoarthritis, ankylosing spondylitis: 25-75 mg two or three times daily Primary dysmenorrhea: 50 mg three times daily	200
etodolac	Lodine, Lodine XL	Capsules: 200, 300 mg Tablets: 400, 500 mg Tablets, extended-release: 400, 500, 600 mg	Osteoarthritis, pain: 300-400 mg three or four times daily	1200
fenoprofen	Nalfon	Capsules: 200, 300 mg Tablets: 600 mg	Rheumatoid and osteoarthritis: 300-600 mg three or four times daily Mild to moderate pain: 200 mg q4-6h	3200
flurbiprofen	Ansaid	Tablets: 50, 100 mg	Rheumatoid and osteoarthritis: 50-100 mg two or three times daily	300
ibuprofen	Motrin, Advil	Tablets: 50, 100, 200, 400, 600, 800 mg Capsules: 200 mg Suspension: 100 mg/2.5 mL, 100 mg/5 mL	Rheumatoid and osteoarthritis: 300-600 mg three or four times daily Mild to moderate pain: 400 mg q4-6h Primary dysmenorrhea: 400 mg q4h	2400
indomethacin	Indocin	Capsules: 25, 50 mg Sustained-release capsules: 75 mg Oral suspension: 25 mg/5 mL Suppository: 50 mg	Rheumatoid and osteoarthritis, ankylosing spondylitis: 25-50 mg three or four times daily Acute painful shoulder: 25-50 mg two or three times daily Acute gouty arthritis: 50 mg three times daily	200

Continued

TABLE 17-3 Non-Steroidal Anti-Inflammatory Agents—cont'd

GENERIC NAME	BRAND NAME	DOSE FORMS	USES AND ADULT DOSAGES	MAXIMUM DAILY DOSE (mg)
ketoprofen	Orudis	Tablets: 12.5 mg Capsules: 50, 75 mg Extended-release capsules: 100, 150, 200 mg	Rheumatoid and osteoarthritis: Initially 75 mg three times daily or 50 mg four times daily; reduce initial dose by $1/2$ to $1/3$ in elderly patients or those with impaired renal function Mild pain, primary dysmenorrhea: 25-50 mg three or four times daily	300
ketorolac	Toradol, Acular	Tablets: 10 mg	40 mg or less/24 hours; do not exceed 5 days of therapy	40
meclofenamate		Capsules: 50, 100 mg	Rheumatoid and osteoarthritis: 200-400 mg daily in 3 or 4 equal doses Mild to moderate pain: 50-100 mg three or four times daily Primary dysmenorrhea: 100 mg three times daily	400
mefenamic acid	Ponstel	Capsules: 250 mg	Moderate pain or primary dysmenorrhea: Initially 500 mg, then 250 mg q6h; do not exceed 7 days of therapy	1000
meloxicam	Mobic	Tablets: 7.5, 15 mg Liquid: 7.5 mg/5 mL	Osteoarthritis: 7.5-15 mg daily	15
nabumetone	Relafen	Tablets: 500, 750 mg	Rheumatoid and osteoarthritis: 1000-1500 mg daily in 1 or 2 doses	2000
naproxen	Naprosyn	Tablets: 200, 250, 375, 500 mg Extended-release tablets: 375, 500 mg Oral suspension: 125 mg/5 mL	Rheumatoid and osteoarthritis, ankylosing spondylitis: 250-375 mg twice daily	1000
naproxen sodium	Anaprox, Anaprox DS	Tablets: 275 mg Tablets, extended-release: 550 mg	Acute gout: 750-825 mg initially, followed by 250-275 mg q8h Moderate pain, primary dysmenorrhea, acute tendonitis, bursitis: 500-550 mg followed by 250-275 mg	1100
oxaprozin	Daypro	Caplets: 600 mg	Rheumatoid arthritis, osteoarthritis: 1200 mg once daily	1800
piroxicam	Feldene	Capsules: 10, 20 mg	Rheumatoid and osteoarthritis: 20 mg once daily	200
sulindac	Clinoril	Tablets: 150, 200 mg	Rheumatoid and osteoarthritis, ankylosing spondylitis: 150 mg twice daily Acute painful shoulder: 200 mg twice daily	400
tolmetin	Tolectin	Tablets: 200, 600 mg Capsules: 400 mg	Rheumatoid and osteoarthritis: 400-600 mg three times daily	2000

EVALUATION

Report and record:

- *Stomach irritation.* Give the drug with food or milk.
- *Constipation.* This may occur from continued use. Follow the care plan for fluid intake and diet. Give stool softeners or laxatives as ordered.
- *Dizziness, drowsiness.* Provide for safety. The person must use caution when working around machines, driving a car, pouring and giving drugs, or performing other duties that require mental alertness.
- *GI bleeding.* Vomitus that looks like coffee grounds ("coffee ground emesis"), red vomitus, and black or dark tarry stools are signs of GI bleeding. Test stools for occult blood as directed by the nurse and care plan.
- *Confusion.* Observe the person's alertness and orientation to person, time, and place. Provide for safety.
- *Rash, hives, itching.* These may signal an allergic reaction. Tell the nurse at once. Do not give the next dose unless approved by the nurse.
- *Decreased urine output, red or smoky-colored urine.* These signal kidney problems.
- *Anorexia, nausea, vomiting, jaundice.* These may signal liver toxicity.
- *Sore throat, fever, jaundice, weakness.* These may signal changes in red blood cells and white blood cells.

DRUG CLASS: **Other Analgesic Agents**

Other drugs are used to relieve pain. Some are combination products (Table 17-4). Others are single preparations:

- acetaminophen (a seat a min' o fen); Tylenol (ty' le nol), Datril (day' tril), and Tempra (tem' pra)
- propoxyphene (proe pox' eh feen); Darvon (dar' von)
- pentazocine (pen ta' zoh seen); Talwin (tall' win)

acetaminophen (Tylenol, Datril, and Tempra)

Acetaminophen is a synthetic non-opiate analgesic. Like aspirin, it is an effective analgesic and antipyretic. The drug has no anti-inflammatory activity. Its analgesic-antipyretic effects are useful for fever and discomfort from bacterial and viral infections. It also is useful for headaches and musculoskeletal pain.

Assisting With the Nursing Process

When a person receives acetaminophen, you assist the nurse with the nursing process.

ASSESSMENT

- Measure vital signs.
- Ask the person to rate his or her pain. Use a pain rating scale.
- Check the MAR for when the person last received the ordered drug.

TABLE 17-4 Selected Analgesic Combination Products

| PRODUCT | NON-CONTROLLED SUBSTANCE | | | CONTROLLED SUBSTANCE | |
	ASPIRIN (mg)	ACETAMINOPHEN (mg)	OTHER (mg)	CODEINE (mg)	OTHER (mg)
Anacin Tablets	400		caffeine 32		
Anacin Maximum Strength	500		caffeine 32		
BC Powder	650		caffeine 33 salicylamide 195		
Darvocet-N 50		325			propoxyphene napsylate 50
Darvocet-N 100		650			propoxyphene napsylate 100
Darvon Compound-65	389		caffeine 32		propoxyphene HCl 65
Empirin Codeine #3 Codeine #4	325 325			30 60	
Excedrin Extra-strength	250	250	caffeine 65		

Continued

TABLE 17-4 Selected Analgesic Combination Products—cont'd					
	NON-CONTROLLED SUBSTANCE			CONTROLLED SUBSTANCE	
PRODUCT	ASPIRIN (mg)	ACETAMINOPHEN (mg)	OTHER (mg)	CODEINE (mg)	OTHER (mg)
Fioricet		325	caffeine 40		butalbital 50
Fiorinal	325		caffeine 40		butalbital 50
Fiorinal w/Codeine	325		caffeine 40	30	butalbital 50
Lortab 10/500		500			hydrocodone 10
Percocet 7.5		500			oxycodone 7.5
Percodan	325				oxycodone 4.5
Percogesic		325	phenyltoloxamine 30		
Talwin Compound Caplets	325				pentazocine 12.5
Tylenol					
Codeine #2		300		15	
Codeine #3		300		30	
Codeine #4		300		60	
Vicodin		500			hydrocodone 5

PLANNING

- Oral dose forms:
  - 160, 325, 500, 650 mg tablets
  - 80 and 160 mg chewable tablets
  - 325 and 500 mg capsules
  - 80 and 160 mg sprinkle capsules
  - 80 mg/0.8 mL drops
  - 80 mg/2.5 mL elixir
  - 80 mg/5 mL, 120 mg/5 mL, 160 mg/5 mL elixir
  - 500 mg/15 mL liquid
  - 80 mg/1.66 mL, 100 mg/mL solution
- Rectal dose forms:
  - 80, 120, 125, 300, 325, and 650 mg suppositories

IMPLEMENTATION

- The usual adult oral dose is 325 to 650 mg every 4 to 6 hours.
- Doses up to 1000 mg may be given 4 times a day for short-term therapy.

EVALUATION

Report and record:

- *Stomach irritation.* Give the drug with food, milk, or large amounts of water.
- *Anorexia, nausea, vomiting, low blood pressure, drowsiness, confusion, abdominal pain, jaundice.* These signal liver toxicity.

propoxyphene (Darvon)

Propoxyphene (Darvon) is a synthetic opiate agonist. It is used to relieve mild to moderate pain from muscle cramps, pre-menstrual cramps, minor surgery and trauma, and headache.

Assisting With the Nursing Process

When a person receives propoxyphene (Darvon), you assist the nurse with the nursing process.

ASSESSMENT

- Observe the person's speech pattern, degree of alertness, and orientation to person, time, and place.
- Measure vital signs.
- Measure intake and output.
- Ask the person to rate his or her pain. Use a pain rating scale.

PLANNING

- Oral dose forms are:
  - 65 mg capsules
  - 100 mg tablets
- Propoxyphene (Darvon) is available in combination with other drugs:
  - propoxyphene and acetaminophen (Darvocet)
  - propoxyphene, aspirin, caffeine (Darvon Compound)

IMPLEMENTATION

The usual adult dose is 65 mg (capsules) or 100 mg (tablets) every 4 hours as needed.

EVALUATION

Report and record:

- *Stomach irritation.* Give the drug with food or milk.
- *Sedation, dizziness.* Sedation is usually mild. It tends to resolve with continued therapy. Provide for safety. The person must use caution when working around machines, driving a car, pouring and giving drugs, or performing other duties that require mental alertness.
- *Excess use or abuse.* The person often complains of pain or requests a drug for pain relief. The report of pain may be well before the next dose can be given. Always report complaints of pain or drug requests to the nurse at once.
- *Rash.* This may signal an allergic reaction. Tell the nurse at once. Do not give the next dose unless approved by the nurse.

pentazocine (Talwin)

Pentazocine (Talwin) is an opiate partial agonist. If the person has not received opiate agonists, pentazocine (Talwin) is an effective analgesic. When used within the first few weeks of therapy, the effect is similar to morphine. Tolerance may develop after prolonged use. Increasing the dosage does not increase analgesia. However, side effects increase.

Pentazocine (Talwin) is used for short-term relief (up to 3 weeks) of moderate to severe pain. Such pain may be associated with cancer, burns, and renal colic.

(NOTE: Other opiate partial agonists are given by subcutaneous, intramuscular, or intravenous injection. Like other opiate partial agonists, pentazocine [Talwin] is a controlled substance. Many states and agencies do not let MA-Cs give controlled substances by any route. Others let MA-Cs give oral, rectal, and transdermal dose forms.)

Assisting With the Nursing Process

When a person receives pentazocine (Talwin), you assist the nurse with the nursing process.

ASSESSMENT

- Observe the person's speech pattern, degree of alertness, and orientation to person, time, and place.
- Measure vital signs.
- Ask the person to rate his or her pain. Use a pain rating scale.

PLANNING

The oral dose form is 50 mg tablets.

IMPLEMENTATION

The adult oral dose is 50 to 100 mg every 3 to 4 hours.

EVALUATION

Report and record:

- *Clamminess, dizziness, sedation, nausea, vomiting, dry mouth, sweating.* These tend to occur with the first dose. The supine position helps reduce these symptoms. Provide for safety.
- *Constipation.* This may occur from continued use. Follow the care plan for fluid intake and diet. Give stool softeners or laxatives as ordered.
- *Confusion, disorientation, hallucinations.* Observe the person's alertness and orientation to person, time, and place. Provide for safety.
- *Respiratory depression.* Tell the nurse at once if the person's respiratory rate is 12 per minute or less. Also observe the depth of respirations. Tell the nurse at once if the person has shallow breathing.
- *Excess use or abuse.* The person often complains of pain or requests a drug for pain relief. The report of pain may be well before the next dose can be given. Always report complaints of pain or drug requests to the nurse at once. See Box 17-3 for signs and symptoms of withdrawal.

REVIEW QUESTIONS

Circle the **BEST** answer.

1 A person complains of pain. What should you do?
a Ask to see the pain.
b Tell the nurse.
c Give an analgesic.
d Decide if the pain is acute or chronic.

2 A pain rating scale is used
a to describe pain
b for the location of pain
c for the intensity of pain
d to describe the duration of pain

3 Who decides when you should give an analgesic?
a the patient or resident
b the nurse
c the doctor
d you

4 An opiate acts as an analgesic by
a transmitting pain to the brain
b releasing chemicals that stimulate pain receptors
c blocking the pain sensation
d producing sleep

5 Opiate agonists can cause euphoria. Euphoria is
a an exaggerated feeling of well-being
b drowsiness and sedation
c mental clouding
d addiction

6 Opiate agonists are given for
a chronic pain
b moderate to severe pain
c moderate to mild pain
d any type of pain

7 Which are given to reduce fever?
a opiate agonists
b salicylates
c methadone-like derivatives
d opiate partial agonists

8 Which of the following signals respiratory depression?
a a respiratory rate of 12 per minute or less
b a respiratory rate of 14 per minute
c a respiratory rate of 16 per minute
d a respiratory rate of 18 per minute

9 The following are opiate agonists *except*
a Codeine and Morphine Sulfate
b Oxycontin and Percodan
c Talwin and Darvon
d Dilaudid and Demerol

10 Salicylates are given for
a severe pain
b moderate to severe pain
c moderate to mild pain
d slight to moderate pain

11 Salicylates have the following effects *except*
a analgesia
b anti-inflammatory
c anti-pyretic
d dulling alertness

12 Which of the following is used to reduce blood clotting?
a aspirin
b Tylenol
c Darvon
d Motrin

13 To prevent stomach irritation from salicylates or NSAIDs, you should give the drug
a with food or milk
b before meals
c after meals
d at bedtime

14 NSAIDS are given for the following reasons *except* to reduce
a pain
b inflammation
c fever
d euphoria

15 Which has the strongest analgesic effect?
a Talwin
b aspirin
c Darvon
d Tylenol

Circle **T** if the statement is true. Circle **F** if the statement is false.

16 T F Anxiety can increase a person's pain.

17 T F Vital signs often decrease when the person has pain.

18 T F Older persons feel pain at the same intensity as younger persons do.

19 T F Opiate agonists are controlled substances.

20 T F Addiction from the use of opiates for pain management is a common problem.

21 T F A person was given an opiate agonist. You must provide for safety.

22 T F Acetaminophen has an anti-inflammatory effect.

Answers to these questions are given on p. 445.

Drugs Used to Lower Lipids

OBJECTIVES

- Define the key terms and key abbreviations used in this chapter.
- Identify the main lipids in the blood.
- Explain how lipids can cause coronary artery disease.
- Explain the difference between low-density and high-density lipo-proteins.
- Describe the drugs used to lower blood lipid levels.
- Explain how to assist with the nursing process when giving drugs to reduce blood lipid levels.

KEY TERMS

cholesterol A waxy, fat-like substance found in all body cells

dyslipidemia An abnormality of one or more of the blood fats (lipids)

hyperlipidemia Excess *(hyper)* lipids *(fats)* in the blood *(emia)*

lipids Fats

triglycerides Fatty compounds that come from animal and vegetable fats

KEY ABBREVIATIONS

CAD Coronary artery disease
g Gram
HDL High-density lipo-protein
LDL Low-density lipo-protein
mg Milligram
MI Myocardial infarction
TLC Therapeutic Lifestyle Changes

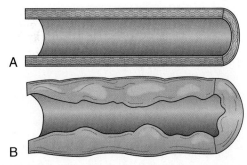

Fig. 18-1 A, Normal artery. **B,** Plaque on the artery wall in atherosclerosis.

Lipids are fats. (*Lipos* is the Greek work meaning *fat*.) **Hyperlipidemia** (hi per lip' id e' me ah) means excess *(hyper)* lipids *(fats)* in the blood *(emia)*. The main lipids in the blood are:

- **Cholesterol** is a waxy, fat-like substance found in all body cells. The body produces the cholesterol it needs to make hormones, vitamin D, and substances used for food digestion. Cholesterol also is found in foods from animal sources—egg yolks, meat, and cheese. The body converts excess dietary fat into cholesterol.
- **Triglycerides** are fatty compounds that come from animal and vegetable fats. A source of energy, they are stored in the body's fatty tissues.

When there are too many lipids in the blood, fat can build up on the walls of arteries and arterioles throughout the body. This is called *atherosclerosis*. (*Athero* means an *abnormal mass of fat or lipids*. *Sclerosis* means *hardening*.) Often called "hardening of the arteries," atherosclerosis blocks blood flow (Fig. 18-1). When it occurs in the heart's coronary arteries, it causes coronary artery disease (CAD). CAD can lead to angina or myocardial infarction (MI). CAD is a leading cause of death in the United States in men and women.

Blood is a liquid. Lipids are fatty. Liquids and fat do not mix. To travel in the bloodstream, fats are carried in the blood by lipo-proteins. *Lipo-proteins* are made up of fat *(lipo)* and proteins.

- *Low-density lipo-protein (LDL) cholesterol.* This is often called "bad cholesterol." It leads to the build-up of plaque in the arteries. The higher the LDL level, the greater the risk of CAD.
- *High-density lipo-protein (HDL) cholesterol.* This is often called "good cholesterol." HDL carries cholesterol from other body parts to the liver. The liver removes it from the body. The higher the HDL level, the lower the risk of CAD.

Dyslipidemia (dis lip' id e' me ah) is an abnormality of one or more of the blood fats (lipids). Causes include:

- *Heredity.* High blood cholesterol can run in families.
- *A diet high in fat, cholesterol, carbohydrates, calories, and alcohol.*

- *Weight gain and being over-weight.* Losing weight can lower LDL ("bad cholesterol"). It can raise HDL ("good cholesterol").
- *Lack of regular exercise.* Regular exercise can lower LDL ("bad cholesterol") and raise HDL ("good cholesterol").
- *Age and gender.* According to the National Heart, Lung, and Blood Institute, men have lower levels of HDL ("good cholesterol") than women. As men and women age, LDL levels ("bad cholesterol") rise. Younger women have lower LDL levels than men. After age 55, women have higher LDL levels than men.

Hyperlipidemia is treated by Therapeutic Lifestyle Changes (TLC). This involves losing weight, regular exercise, and a diet low in cholesterol and fat. For some persons, TLC and drug therapy are needed. *Anti-lipemic drugs* are used to reduce *(anti)* fats *(lip)* in the blood *(emic)*. The intent is to decrease cholesterol levels and reduce the risk of atherosclerosis leading to CAD. They are used only if diet, exercise, and weight loss do not lower LDL ("bad cholesterol").

DRUG CLASS: Bile Acid-Binding Resins

Bile is a yellow-green liver secretion. It is stored in the gallbladder. Bile is released into the duodenum to prepare fats for digestion. *Bile acid* is produced when cholesterol is metabolized. *Resins* are solid or semi-solid substances.

Bile acid-binding resins interrupt the normal circulation of bile acids between the liver and intestines. More bile acids are excreted into the feces. The liver produces bile acids from cholesterol. Because there are fewer bile acids, the liver takes more LDL cholesterol from the blood to replace them. Therefore LDL cholesterol levels in the blood decrease.

Bile acid-binding resins may be used along with statins to lower LDL. The bile acid-binding resins are:

- cholestyramine (koe less teer' a meen); Questran
- colestipol (koe les' ti pole); Colestid
- colesevelam (koh leh sevv' eh lam); Welchol

Assisting With the Nursing Process

When giving bile acid-binding resins, you assist the nurse with the nursing process.

ASSESSMENT

Ask the person about abdominal pain, nausea, and flatus.

PLANNING

Oral dose forms are:

- cholestyramine (Questran):
  - 4 g powder packets
  - 210 and 378 g cans
- colestipol (Colestid) forms include:
  - 1 g tablets
  - 5 g granule packets
  - 300 and 500 g containers
- colesevelam (Welchol):
  - 625 mg tablets

IMPLEMENTATION

The adult dosages are:

- cholestyramine (Questran):
  - 4 g one to six times daily.
  - The initial dose is 4 g daily.
  - Maintenance dose is 16 g daily.
  - The maximum daily dose is 24 g.
- colestipol (Colestid):
  - Granules: 5 to 30 g of granules per day in divided doses. The initial dose is 5 g one or two times a day.
  - Tablets: 2 to 16 g per day. The initial dose is 2 g one or two times a day.
- colesevelam (Welchol):
  - 6 tablets once a day or in 2 divided doses.
  - The drug is given with liquid at meals.
- Preparing and giving these drugs:
  - Do not give the person dry powder to swallow.
  - Mix granules or powder with 2 to 6 ounces of water, juice, soup, applesauce, or crushed pineapple as the person prefers. Stir well until mixed. The powder will not dissolve. Allow it to stand for a few minutes. After the person drinks the mixture, fill the glass with water. Have the person drink all the water. This ensures that the person receives the full dose.
  - Have the person swallow tablets whole. Do not crush or cut them. The person must not chew the tablet.
  - Doses are usually given with meals. Other drugs are given 1 hour before or at least 4 hours after giving bile acid-binding resins.

EVALUATION

Report and record:

- *Constipation, abdominal pain, bloating, fullness, nausea, flatulence.* These side effects can be reduced by:
  - Starting with a low dose
  - Mixing the drug with non-carbonated drinks, pulpy juices, or sauces
- Having the person swallow without gulping air
- Drinking several glasses of water or other liquids throughout the day
- Having a diet adequate in fiber

DRUG CLASS: **Niacin**

Niacin (nicotinic acid) is vitamin B_3. Niacin limits the liver's ability to produce LDL cholesterol. Niacin can be used with bile acid–producing resins or statins to lower cholesterol and triglyceride levels. Niacin also causes vaso-dilation and increases blood flow.

Assisting With the Nursing Process

When giving niacin, you assist the nurse with the nursing process.

ASSESSMENT

- Measure blood pressure and heart rate.
- Ask the person about abdominal pain, nausea, and flatus.

PLANNING

Oral dose forms are:

- 50, 100, 250, and 500 mg tablets
- 125, 250, 400, and 500 mg timed-release capsules
- 250, 500, 750, 1000 mg timed-release tablets

IMPLEMENTATION

- The initial adult dose is 100 mg three times a day.
- The dose is increased by 300 mg weekly until the therapeutic level is attained.
- The usual daily dose ranges from 1 to 6 g daily. Some persons need 9 g daily.
- The drug is given with food.

EVALUATION

Report and record:

- *Flushing, itching, rash, tingling, headache.* These are common when therapy is started.
- *Nausea, gas, abdominal discomfort or pain.* Give all doses with food.
- *Dizziness, faintness, hypotension.* Provide for safety. The person must use caution when working around machines, driving a car, pouring and giving drugs, or performing other duties that require mental alertness.
- *Fatigue, anorexia, nausea, malaise, jaundice.* These may signal liver toxicity.
- *Muscle aches, soreness, weakness.* These may signal changes in muscle tissue.

TABLE 18-1	Statins				
GENERIC NAME	**BRAND NAME**	**ORAL DOSE FORMS**	**DAILY ADULT DOSE**	**MAXIMUM DAILY DOSE**	
HMG-CoA REDUCTASE INHIBITORS (STATINS)					
atorvastatin	Lipitor	Tablets: 10, 20, 40, 80 mg	10-40 mg daily at any time	Up to 80 mg daily	
fluvastatin	Lescol	Capsules: 20, 40 mg	20 mg at bedtime	Up to 80 mg at bedtime	
	Lescol XL	Tablets, extended-release: 80 mg	80 mg at bedtime		
lovastatin	Mevacor	Tablets: 10, 20, 40 mg	20-40 mg with evening meal	80 mg daily	
	Altoprev	Tablets, extended-release: 10, 20, 40, 60 mg	10-60 mg daily at bedtime	60 mg daily at bedtime	
pravastatin	Pravachol	Tablets: 10, 20, 40, 80 mg	40 mg daily at anytime	Up to 80 mg daily	
rosuvastatin	Crestor	Tablets: 5, 10, 20, 40 mg	5-40 mg daily at any time	Up to 40 mg daily	
simvastatin	Zocor	Tablets: 5, 10, 20, 40, 80 mg	5-20 mg daily at bedtime	Up to 80 mg at bedtime	
HMG-CoA REDUCTASE INHIBITOR COMBINATION PRODUCTS					
atorvastatin-amlodipine	Caduet	atorvastatin/amlodipine (10/5 to 80/10 mg)		atorvastatin 80 mg amlodipine 10 mg	
lovastatin-niacin (extended-release)	Advicor	lovastatin/niacin (20/500, 20/750, 20/1000 mg)		lovastatin 40 mg niacin 2000 mg	
pravastatin-aspirin	Pravigard PAC	pravastatin/aspirin (20/81 to 80/325 mg)		pravastatin 80 mg aspirin 325 mg	
simvastatin-ezetimibe	Vytorin	simvastatin/ezetimibe (10/10 to 80/10 mg)		simvastatin 80 mg ezetimibe 10 mg	

DRUG CLASS: **Statins**

Statins are the strongest anti-lipemic drugs available. They block the enzyme the liver needs to produce cholesterol. This reduces the amount of cholesterol in the liver. Therefore the liver has to remove cholesterol from the blood. The goal of therapy is to reduce LDL and lower total cholesterol levels.

Statins also reduce inflammation and blood clotting. Thus they reduce risk factors for MI and stroke.

Assisting With the Nursing Process

When giving statins, you assist the nurse with the nursing process.

ASSESSMENT

Ask the person about abdominal pain, nausea, and flatus.

PLANNING

See Table 18-1 for "Oral Dose Forms."

IMPLEMENTATION

- See Table 18-1 for "Daily Adult Dose" and "Maximum Daily Dose."
- Do not give the drug with grapefruit juice. Grapefruit juice inhibits the metabolism of some statins.

EVALUATION

Report and record:

- *Fatigue, anorexia, nausea, malaise, jaundice.* These may signal liver problems.
- *Muscle aches, soreness, weakness.* These may signal changes in muscle tissue.

DRUG CLASS: **Fibric Acids**

Fibric acids lower triglyceride and LDL levels. They raise HDL levels. They are used for persons who have not responded to weight loss, diet therapy, or other anti-lipemic drugs.

Fibric acid drugs are:

- gemfibrozil (gem fi' broe zil); Lopid
- fenofibrate (fen oh fye' brate); Tricor

Assisting With the Nursing Process

When giving fibric acids, you assist the nurse with the nursing process.

ASSESSMENT

Ask the person about abdominal pain, nausea, and flatus.

PLANNING

Oral dose forms are:
- gemfibrozil (Lopid): 600 mg tablets
- fenofibrate (Tricor): 48 and 145 mg tablets

IMPLEMENTATION

The adult dosages are:
- gemfibrozil (Lopid):
  - 1200 mg per day in 2 divided doses.
  - The drug is given 30 minutes before the morning and evening meals.
- fenofibrate (Tricor):
  - The initial dose is 48 to 145 mg per day.
  - The dosage is increased every 4 to 8 weeks up to 145 mg daily.
  - The drug is given with meals.

EVALUATION

Report and record:
- *Nausea, diarrhea, flatulence, bloating, abdominal distress*. These are common. A lower dose taken between meals may reduce these effects.
- *Fatigue, anorexia, nausea, malaise, jaundice*. These signal gallbladder disease and liver toxicity.
- *Muscle aches, soreness, weakness*. These may signal changes in muscle tissue.

DRUG CLASS: Other Anti-Lipemic Drugs

Other anti-lipemic drugs are:
- ezetimibe (ehz et' tih meeb'); Zetia (zeh te' ah)
- Omacor (oh' mah cor)

ezetimibe (Zetia)

The small intestine absorbs dietary cholesterol and releases it into the blood. Cholesterol absorption inhibitors block the absorption of cholesterol from the small intestine. Thus they lower cholesterol levels. The drug may be used along with statins.

Assisting With the Nursing Process

When giving ezetimibe (Zetia), you assist the nurse with the nursing process.

ASSESSMENT

Ask the person about abdominal pain, nausea, and flatus.

PLANNING

The oral dose form is 10 mg tablets.

IMPLEMENTATION

The usual adult dose is 10 mg once a day. It may be taken with or without meals.

EVALUATION

Report and record:
- *Abdominal pain, diarrhea*. These are generally mild and do not affect therapy.

Omacor

Omacor contains fatty acids that are sometimes called "fish oils." The drug reduces the synthesis of triglycerides in the liver. It lowers triglyceride levels with small increases in HDL.

Assisting With the Nursing Process

When giving Omacor, you assist the nurse with the nursing process.

ASSESSMENT

Ask the person about abdominal pain, nausea, and flatus.

PLANNING

The oral dose form is 1 g capsules.

IMPLEMENTATION

The adult dose is 4 g once a day or 2 g two times a day.

EVALUATION

Report and record the side effects listed in Box 18-1.

BOX 18-1   Side Effects from Omacor

Report the following at once:
- Arm, back, or jaw pain
- Chest pain or discomfort
- Chest tightness or heaviness
- Breathing: difficult or labored, shortness of breath
- Heartbeat: fast or irregular
- Nausea
- Sweating
- Wheezing

Other side effects:
- Appetite: loss of
- Belching
- Bloating
- Chills
- Cough
- Diarrhea
- Fever
- Discomfort
- Headache
- Hoarseness
- Joint pain
- Pain: lower back, side
- Muscles: aches and pains
- Urination: difficulty or painful
- Rash
- Runny nose
- Shivering
- Sore throat
- Sweating
- Sleep problems
- Taste: unusual or unpleasant, change in
- Tiredness
- Weakness
- Vomiting

REVIEW QUESTIONS

Circle the BEST answer.

1 These statements are about cholesterol. Which is *false?*
   a Cholesterol is found in all body cells.
   b The body produces cholesterol.
   c Cholesterol is needed by the body.
   d Cholesterol is a source of energy.

2 Triglycerides are stored in the body's
   a muscle tissue
   b fatty tissue
   c bones
   d nerve cells

3 Foods high in cholesterol include the following *except*
   a vegetables
   b egg yolks
   c meat
   d cheese

4 Which is called "bad cholesterol?"
   a atherosclerosis
   b bile
   c low-density lipo-protein (LDL)
   d high-density lipo-protein (HDL)

5 Which are the strongest anti-lipemic drugs?
   a bile acid-binding resins
   b fibric acids
   c statins
   d Zetia and Omacor

6 You are giving a bile-acid resin in powdered form. What should you do?
   a Give the person the dry powder to swallow.
   b Mix the powder with 2 to 6 ounces of water or juice.
   c Give the drug before meals.
   d Give the drug after meals.

7 You are giving a bile-acid resin in tablet form. Which is *true?*
   a The tablet must be swallowed whole.
   b You can cut the tablet.
   c You can crush the tablet.
   d The person can chew the tablet.

8 Niacin acts as an anti-lipemic because it
   a excretes bile acids into the feces
   b limits the liver's ability to produce LDL
   c blocks the enzyme needed to produce cholesterol
   d lowers triglyceride levels

9 Niacin can cause hypotension because of
   a vaso-constriction
   b vaso-dilation
   c atherosclerosis
   d coronary artery disease

10 Statins lower LDL and total cholesterol levels because they
   a excrete bile acids into the feces
   b limit the liver's ability to produce LDL
   c block the enzyme needed to produce cholesterol
   d block the absorption of cholesterol from the small intestine

11 The following are statins *except*
   a fenofibrate (Tricor)
   b atorvastatin (Lipitor)
   c simvastatin (Zocor)
   d fluvastatin (Lescol)

12 Common side effects from anti-lipemic drugs are
   a chest pain
   b nausea
   c hypotension
   d dizziness

Circle T if the statement is true. Circle F if the statement is false.

13 T F   Niacin is given with food.

14 T F   Statins reduce inflammation and blood clotting.

15 T F   Statins are given with grapefruit juice.

Answers to these questions are on p. 445.

Drugs Used to Treat Hypertension

OBJECTIVES

- Define the key terms and key abbreviations used in this chapter.
- Explain the factors that affect blood pressure.
- Explain the factors that cause high blood pressure.
- Describe the drugs used to treat hypertension.
- Explain how to assist with the nursing process when giving drugs to treat hypertension.

KEY TERMS

aldosterone A substance that causes the kidneys to retain sodium

angiotensin A substance that causes vaso-constriction, increased blood pressure, and the release of aldosterone

anti-hypertensive agents Drugs that reduce blood pressure

blood pressure The amount of force exerted against the walls of an artery by the blood

cardiac output The amount of blood pumped with each heartbeat

diuretic A drug that promotes the formation and excretion of urine; *dia* means *through*; *ur* means *urine*

hypertension The systolic pressure is 140 mm Hg or higher *(hyper)*, or the diastolic pressure is 90 mm Hg or higher; high blood pressure

pre-hypertension When the systolic pressure is between 120 and 139 mm Hg or the diastolic pressure is between 80 and 89 mm Hg

renin An enzyme that affects blood pressure

KEY ABBREVIATIONS

ACE Angiotensin-converting enzyme
ARB Angiotensin II receptor blocker
g Gram
mg Milligram
MI Myocardial infarction
mm Hg Millimeters of mercury
PO Per os (orally)

Blood pressure is the amount of force exerted against the walls of an artery by the blood (Chapter 4). Blood pressure is controlled by:

- The force of heart contractions
- The amount of blood pumped with each heartbeat (**cardiac output**)
- How easily blood flows through the blood vessels
  Blood pressure can change from minute to minute. Factors affecting blood pressure are listed in Box 19-1. Because it can vary so easily, blood pressure has normal ranges:

- *Systolic pressure*—less than 120 mm Hg (millimeters of mercury)
- *Diastolic pressure*—less than 80 mm Hg

  With **hypertension** *(high blood pressure)*, the blood pressure is too high. The systolic pressure is 140 mm Hg or higher *(hyper)*. Or the diastolic pressure is 90 mm Hg or higher. Such measurements must occur several times. **Pre-hypertension** is when the systolic pressure is between 120 and 139 mm Hg or the diastolic pressure is between 80 and 89 mm Hg. The person with pre-hypertension will likely develop hypertension in the future. Most people have high blood pressure sometime during their lives. See Box 19-2 for risk factors.

Narrowed blood vessels are a common cause. The heart pumps with more force to move blood through narrowed vessels. Kidney disorders, head injuries, some pregnancy problems, and adrenal gland tumors are causes.

A person can have high blood pressure for many years without knowing it. That is why hypertension is called "the silent killer." Usually hypertension is found when blood pressure is measured. Signs and symptoms develop over time. Headache, blurred vision, dizziness, and nose bleeds occur. Hypertension can lead to stroke, hardening of the arteries, myocardial infarction (MI), heart failure, kidney failure, and blindness.

Life-style changes can lower blood pressure. A diet low in fat and salt, a healthy weight, and regular exercise are needed. No smoking is allowed. Alcohol and caffeine are limited. Managing stress and sleeping well also lower blood pressure.

Drug therapy is not necessary if life-style changes control blood pressure. Even if life-style changes do

---

BOX 19-1 Factors Affecting Blood Pressure

- *Age.* Blood pressure increases with age. It is lowest in infancy and childhood. It is highest in adulthood.
- *Gender (male or female).* Women usually have lower blood pressures than men do. Blood pressures rise in women after menopause.
- *Blood volume.* This is the amount of blood in the system. Severe bleeding lowers the blood volume. Therefore blood pressure lowers. Giving intravenous fluids rapidly increases the blood volume. The blood pressure rises.
- *Stress.* Stress includes anxiety, fear, and emotions. Blood pressure increases as the body responds to stress.
- *Pain.* Pain generally increases blood pressure. However, severe pain can cause *shock*. Blood pressure is seriously low in the state of shock.
- *Exercise.* Blood pressure increases. Do not measure blood pressure right after exercise.
- *Weight.* Blood pressure is higher in over-weight persons. It lowers with weight loss.
- *Race.* Black persons generally have higher blood pressures than white persons do.
- *Diet.* A high-sodium diet increases the amount of water in the body. The extra fluid volume increases blood pressure.
- *Drugs.* Drugs can be given to raise or lower blood pressure. Other drugs have the side effects of high or low blood pressure.
- *Position.* Blood pressure is lower when lying down. It is higher in the standing position. Sudden changes in position can cause a sudden drop in blood pressure (orthostatic hypotension). When standing suddenly, the person may have a sudden drop in blood pressure. Dizziness and fainting can occur.
- *Smoking.* Blood pressure increases. Nicotine in cigarettes causes blood vessels to narrow. The heart must work harder to pump blood through narrowed vessels.
- *Alcohol.* Excessive alcohol intake can raise blood pressure.

---

not adequately control hypertension, they may reduce the number and doses of drugs needed. Once drug therapy is started, it may take months to control hypertension. The dosage may be increased. Or another drug may be tried or a second one added. Many people require two or more anti-hypertensive agents. Some are able to take a combination product—contains two drugs (p. 252). This makes drug therapy easier for the person.

Anti-hypertensive agents are drugs that reduce blood pressure. Drug therapy depends on the person's:

- Age
- Gender
- Race

FACTORS YOU *CANNOT* CHANGE
- Age—45 years or older for men; 55 years or older for women
- Gender—younger men are at greater risk than younger women; the risk increases for women after menopause
- Race—African-Americans are at greater risk than whites
- Family history—tends to run in families

FACTORS YOU *CAN* CHANGE
- Being over-weight—related to diet, lack of exercise, and atherosclerosis
- Stress—increased sympathetic nervous system activity
- Tobacco use—nicotine narrows blood vessels
- High-salt diet—sodium causes fluid retention; increased fluid raises blood volume
- Excessive alcohol—increases chemical substances in the body that increase blood pressure
- Lack of exercise—increases the risk of being over-weight
- Atherosclerosis—arteries narrow because of fatty build-up in the vessels
- Pre-hypertension—blood pressure can be controlled with life-style changes and drugs

DELEGATION GUIDELINES
Drugs Used to Treat Hypertension

Some drugs used to treat hypertension are given parenterally. Because you do not give parenteral dose forms, they are not included in this chapter. Should a nurse delegate the administration of such to you, you must:
- Remember that parenteral dosages are often very different from dosages for other routes.
- Refuse the delegation. Make sure you explain why. Do not just ignore the request. Make sure the nurse knows that you cannot give the drug and why.

- Other health problems
- Risk factors
- Previous therapy—what has or has not worked
- Drug therapy for other health problems
- Cost

See *Delegation Guidelines: Drugs Used to Treat Hypertension.*

DRUG CLASS: **Diuretics**

A **diuretic** is a drug that promotes the formation and excretion of urine. (*Dia* means *through*. *Ur* means *urine.*) Diuretics:
- Reduce the amount of extra-cellular fluid
- Promote sodium excretion
- Cause vaso-dilation (widening) of peripheral arterioles

Diuretics are commonly prescribed alone or with other anti-hypertensive drugs to treat hypertension. The risk of adverse effects is low. They are less expensive than other anti-hypertensive drugs.

Diuretics are discussed in Chapter 22.

DRUG CLASS:
Beta-Adrenergic Blocking Agents

Beta-adrenergic blocking agents (beta blockers) inhibit the heart's response to sympathetic nerve stimulation (Chapter 14). They do so by blocking beta receptors. Beta receptors increase the heart rate. By blocking the beta receptors, the heart rate and cardiac output are reduced. In turn, blood pressure is reduced.

Beta blockers also block renin release from the kidneys. **Renin** is an enzyme that affects blood pressure. Renin release results in processes that increase blood pressure:
- Vaso-constriction, which narrows blood vessels
- Sodium retention, which causes the body to retain water

Assisting With the Nursing Process
When giving beta blockers, you assist the nurse with the nursing process.
ASSESSMENT
- Measure heart rate and rhythm. Use the apical pulse.
- Measure blood pressure.
- See "Assisting with the Nursing Process" for dys-rhythmic therapy (Chapter 20)
PLANNING
See Table 14-2 in Chapter 14 for "Oral Dose Forms."
IMPLEMENTATION
- See Table 14-2 in Chapter 14 for "Adult Dosage Range."
- The onset of action is fairly rapid. However, it may take several days or weeks for the desired level of improvement and to stabilize on the lowest dose needed.
- Angina and MI are risks if the drug is suddenly discontinued. To discontinue the drug, the doctor reduces the dosage over 1 to 2 weeks.
EVALUATION
Most adverse effects from beta blockers are dose related. They resolve when the dosage is adjusted. Report and record:
- *Bradycardia, peripheral vaso-constriction (purple, mottled skin).* The nurse may tell you to with-hold the next dose until the doctor can evaluate the person.
- *Broncho-spasm, wheezing.* The nurse may tell you to with-hold the next dose until the doctor can evaluate the person.

- *Headache, weakness, decreased coordination, general apprehension, sweating, hunger, or blurred or double vision.* These signal hypoglycemia.
- *Edema, dyspnea, bradycardia, and orthopnea.* Observe persons with heart failure.

DRUG CLASS: Angiotensin-Converting Enzyme Inhibitors

Angiotensin-converting enzyme (ACE) inhibitors reduce blood pressure by affecting the renin-angiotensin-aldosterone system.

- *Renin* is secreted by the kidneys when blood pressure, sodium levels, or kidney blood flow is reduced. Renin causes vaso-constriction and sodium retention.
- **Angiotensin** is a substance that causes vaso-constriction, increased blood pressure, and the release of aldosterone.
- **Aldosterone** is a substance that causes the kidneys to retain sodium.

The renin-angiotensin-aldosterone system regulates blood pressure as follows:

- Renin is secreted by the kidneys when blood pressure, sodium levels, or kidney blood flow is reduced. Renin causes vaso-constriction and sodium retention. Both increase blood pressure.
- *Angiotensinogen* is secreted by the liver. Renin converts (changes) angiotensinogen to *angiotensin I*.
- The angiotensin-converting enzyme then converts (changes) angiotensin I to *angiotensin II*.
- Angiotensin II:
  - Acts on receptors in the blood vessels to produce strong vaso-constriction. Narrowing of the blood vessels increases blood pressure.
  - Promotes aldosterone secretion. This causes sodium retention. Increased sodium causes the body to retain water. This increases blood pressure.

ACE inhibitors affect the angiotensin-converting enzyme. Therefore the conversion (change) of angiotensin I to angiotensin II is inhibited. When ACE inhibitors are used:

- Blood levels of angiotensin II are reduced. There is less vaso-constriction. This lowers blood pressure.
- Aldosterone levels are lower. Less sodium and therefore less water are retained. This lowers blood pressure.

ACE inhibitors may be used alone to control blood pressure. They are more effective when combined with diuretic therapy.

Assisting With the Nursing Process

When giving ACE inhibitors, you assist the nurse with the nursing process.

ASSESSMENT

- Measure heart rate and rhythm. Use the apical pulse.
- Measure blood pressure in the supine and standing positions.
- Measure intake and output.
- Measure weight daily.
- Ask about bowel elimination.
- Ask if the person has a cough.

PLANNING

See Table 19-1 for "Oral Dose Forms."

IMPLEMENTATION

See Table 19-1 for "Adult Dosage Range."

EVALUATION

Report and record:

- *Hypotension with dizziness, tachycardia, and fainting.* These may occur within the first 3 hours after the first several doses. They are more common in persons who also receive diuretics. Check the person often until blood pressure is stable. Measure blood pressure in the supine and standing positions. Provide for safety. Remind the person to rise slowly from a supine or sitting position. Have the person sit or lie down if symptoms develop.
- *Nausea, fatigue, headache, diarrhea.* These are usually mild and tend to resolve with continued therapy.
- *Swelling of the face, eyes, lips, tongue; difficulty breathing.* These may signal a drug allergy. Tell the nurse at once. Do not give the next dose unless approved by the nurse.
- *Sore throat, fever, jaundice, weakness.* These may signal changes in white blood cells.
- *Intake and output.* These are used to monitor kidney function.
- *Changes in alertness, disorientation, confusion.* Provide for safety. These may signal changes in potassium levels.
- *Changes in muscle strength, muscle cramps, tremors, nausea, drowsiness, anxiety, lethargy.* These may signal changes in potassium levels.
- *Chronic, dry, non-productive, persistent cough.* This may appear 1 week to 6 months after the start of therapy.

DRUG CLASS: Angiotensin II Receptor Blockers

Angiotensin II receptor blockers (ARBs) bind to angiotensin II receptor sites. Therefore they block angiotensin II from binding to the receptors sites. Such sites are in the blood vessels, brain, heart, kidneys, and adrenal glands. By blocking angiotensin II receptor sites, ARBs lower blood pressure because:

- Vaso-constriction does not occur. Blood vessels do not narrow.
- Aldosterone secretion is blocked. This prevents sodium retention. The body does not retain excess water.

TABLE 19-1	Angiotensin-Converting Enzyme (ACE) Inhibitors			
GENERIC NAME	**BRAND NAME**	**ORAL DOSE FORMS**	**APPROVED USES**	**ADULT DOSAGE RANGE**
benazepril	Lotensin	Tablets: 5, 10, 20, 40 mg	Hypertension	Initial—10 mg once daily Maintenance—20-40 mg daily
captopril	Capoten	Tablets: 12.5, 25, 50, 100 mg	Hypertension; heart failure; diabetic nephropathy	Initial—25 mg two or three times daily 1 hour before meals Maintenance—75-450 mg daily 1 hour before meals
enalapril	Vasotec	Tablets: 2.5, 5, 10, 20 mg	Hypertension; heart failure	Initial—2.5-5 mg once daily Maintenance—10-40 mg daily
fosinopril	Monopril	Tablets: 10, 20, 40 mg	Hypertension; heart failure	Initial—10 mg once daily Maintenance—20-80 mg daily
lisinopril	Prinivil, Zestril	Tablets: 2.5, 5, 10, 20, 40 mg	Hypertension; heart failure; post-myocardial infarction	Initial—5-10 mg once daily Maintenance—20-40 mg daily
moexipril	Univasc	Tablets: 7.5, 15 mg	Hypertension	Initial—with diuretic, 3.75 mg; without diuretic, 7.5 mg Maintenance—7.5-30 mg in one or two divided doses 1 hour before meals
perindopril	Aceon	Tablets: 2, 4, 8 mg	Hypertension	Initial—4 mg daily Maintenance—4-16 mg daily
quinapril	Accupril	Tablets: 5, 10, 20, 40 mg	Hypertension, heart failure	Initial—10-20 mg daily Maintenance—20-80 mg daily
ramipril	Altace	Capsules: 1.25, 2.5, 5, 10 mg	Hypertension; heart failure	Initial—1.25-2.5 mg daily Maintenance—2.5-20 mg daily
trandolapril	Mavik	Tablets: 1, 2, 4, mg	Hypertension; heart failure	Initial—1 mg daily Maintenance—4-8 mg daily

ARBs may be used alone to control blood pressure. The blood pressure-lowering effect is seen within 1 week. It may take 3 to 6 weeks for the full therapeutic effect. Sometimes a low-dose diuretic is needed.

Assisting With the Nursing Process

When giving ARBs, you assist the nurse with the nursing process.

ASSESSMENT
- Measure heart rate and rhythm. Use the apical pulse.
- Measure blood pressure in the supine and standing positions.
- Measure intake and output.
- Measure weight daily.
- Ask about bowel elimination patterns.
- Ask about gastro-intestinal symptoms.

PLANNING
See Table 19-2 on p. 246 for "Oral Dose Forms."

IMPLEMENTATION
See Table 19-2 on p. 246 for "Adult Dosage Range."

EVALUATION
Report and record:
- *Headache, heartburn, indigestion, cramps, diarrhea.* These are mild and tend to resolve with continued therapy.
- *Hypotension, dizziness, weakness, and fainting.* These may occur within the first 3 hours after the first several doses. They are more common in persons who also receive diuretics. Check the person often until blood pressure is stable. Measure blood pressure in the supine and standing positions. Provide for safety. Remind the person to rise slowly from a supine or sitting position. Have the person sit or lie down if symptoms develop.
- *Changes in alertness, disorientation, confusion.* Provide for safety. These may signal changes in potassium levels.
- *Changes in muscle strength, muscle cramps, tremors, nausea, drowsiness, anxiety, lethargy.* These may signal changes in potassium levels.

TABLE 19-2	Angiotensin II Receptor Blockers (ARBs)		
GENERIC NAME	**BRAND NAME**	**ORAL DOSE FORMS**	**ADULT DOSAGE RANGE**
candesartan	Atacand	Tablets: 4, 8, 16, 32 mg	Initial—16 mg once daily; adjust over 4-6 weeks with total daily dose from 8-32 mg Dose may be administered once or twice daily for optimal control
eprosartan	Teveten	Tablets: 400, 600 mg	Initial—600 mg once daily; adjust over 2-3 weeks with total daily dose of 400-800 mg daily Dose may be administered once or twice daily for optimal control
irbesartan	Avapro	Tablets: 75, 150, 300 mg	Initial—150 mg once daily; adjust over 3-4 weeks with a total daily dose of 300 mg daily
losartan	Cozaar	Tablets: 25, 50, 100 mg	50 mg once daily; adjust over 4-6 weeks with a total daily dose from 25-100 mg administered once or twice daily for optimal control
olmesartan	Benicar	Tablets: 5, 20, 40 mg	Initial—20 mg once daily; adjust over 2 weeks with total daily dose of 20-40 mg daily Twice daily dosing offers no benefit
telmisartan	Micardis	Tablets: 20, 40, 80 mg	Initial—40 mg once daily; adjust over 4-6 weeks with total daily dose from 20-80 mg
valsartan	Diovan	Capsules: 40, 80, 160, 320 mg	Initial—80 mg once daily; adjust over 4-6 weeks with total daily dose from 80-320 mg

DRUG CLASS: Aldosterone Receptor Blocking Agent

The renin-angiotensin-aldosterone system regulates blood pressure as follows:

- Renin is secreted by the kidneys when blood pressure, sodium levels, or kidney blood flow is reduced. Renin causes vaso-constriction and sodium retention. Both increase blood pressure.
- *Angiotensinogen* is secreted by the liver. Renin converts (changes) angiotensinogen to *angiotensin I.*
- The angiotensin-converting enzyme then converts (changes) angiotensin I to *angiotensin II.*
- Angiotensin II:
  - Acts on receptors in the blood vessels to produce strong vaso-constriction. Narrowing of the blood vessels increases blood pressure.
  - Promotes aldosterone secretion. This causes sodium retention. Increased sodium causes the body to retain water. This increases blood pressure.

The aldosterone receptor blocking agent blocks aldosterone receptors. This prevents sodium from being re-absorbed. The following is an aldosterone receptor blocking agent used alone. Or it is used with other anti-hypertensive drugs.

- eplerenone (ep lehr' en own); Inspra (in' sprah)

Assisting With the Nursing Process

When giving eplerenone (Inspra), you assist the nurse with the nursing process.

ASSESSMENT

- Measure blood pressure in the supine and standing positions.
- Measure intake and output.
- Measure weight daily.
- Ask about bowel elimination patterns.

PLANNING

Oral dose forms are 25 and 50 mg tablets.

IMPLEMENTATION

- The initial dose is 50 mg daily with or without food.
- The full therapeutic effect should be seen within 4 weeks.
- If necessary, the dosage may be increased to 50 mg two times a day.

EVALUATION

Report and record:

- *Nausea, fatigue, headache, diarrhea.* These tend to be mild and resolve with continued therapy.

- *Hypotension, dizziness, weakness, and fainting.* These are more common in persons who also receive diuretics. Check the person often until blood pressure is stable. Measure blood pressure in the supine and standing positions. Provide for safety. Remind the person to rise slowly from a supine or sitting position. Have the person sit or lie down if symptoms develop.
- *Changes in alertness, disorientation, confusion.* Provide for safety. These may signal changes in potassium levels.
- *Changes in muscle strength, muscle cramps, tremors, nausea, drowsiness, anxiety, lethargy.* These may signal changes in potassium levels.
- *Intake and output.* These are used to monitor kidney function.
- *Anorexia, nausea, vomiting, jaundice.* These may signal liver toxicity.

DRUG CLASS: **Calcium Ion Antagonists**

To understand how calcium ion antagonists lower blood pressure, you need to know these terms:
- *Ion*—an atom with an electrical charge.
- *Atom*—the smallest part of an element.
- *Element*—a simple substance that cannot be broken down into another substance.
- *Calcium*—an element. The body needs calcium ions for the transmission of nerve impulses, muscle contractions, blood clotting, and heart functions.
- *Calcium channel*—the way calcium ions pass through the cell membrane.
- *Antagonist*—a drug that exerts an opposite action to that of another. Or it competes for the same receptor sites.

Calcium ion antagonists inhibit the movement of calcium ions across a cell membrane. They also are called *calcium antagonists* and *calcium channel blockers.* These drugs relax the smooth muscle of blood vessels. That results in vaso-dilation (widening of blood vessels) and reduced blood pressure. These drugs also are used to treat dysrhythmias (Chapter 20) and angina (Chapter 21).

Assisting With the Nursing Process

When giving calcium ion antagonists, you assist the nurse with the nursing process.

ASSESSMENT
- Measure heart rate and rhythm. Use the apical pulse.
- Measure blood pressure in the supine and standing positions.
- Measure intake and output.
- Measure weight daily.

PLANNING
See Table 19-3 for "Oral Dose Forms."

IMPLEMENTATION
See Table 19-3 for "Adult Dosage Range."

EVALUATION
Report and record:
- *Hypotension and fainting.* These may occur during the first week. They decline once the dosage is stabilized. Provide for safety. Remind the person to rise slowly from a supine or sitting position. Have the person sit or lie down if he or she feels faint.
- *Edema.* Measure weight daily. Measure intake and output.

TABLE 19-3 Calcium Ion Antagonists (Calcium Channel Blockers) Used to Treat Hypertension			
GENERIC NAME	**BRAND NAME**	**ORAL DOSE FORMS**	**ADULT DOSAGE RANGE**
amlodipine	Norvasc	Tablets: 2.5, 5, 10 mg	Initial—5 mg daily; adjust over 7-14 days to a maximum of 10 mg/day
diltiazem	Cardizem	Tablets: 30, 60, 90, 120 mg Tablets, extended-release: 120, 180, 240, 300, 360, 420 mg Capsules, sustained-release: 60, 90, 120, 180, 240, 300, 360, 420 mg	Initial—60-120 mg sustained-release capsule twice daily; adjust as needed after 14 days Maintenance—240-360 mg daily Maximum—540 mg once daily
felodipine	Plendil	Tablets: 5, 10 mg Tablets, extended-release: 2.5 mg	Initial—5 mg daily; adjust after 14 days Maintenance—5-10 mg daily Maximum—10 mg daily

Continued

TABLE 19-3	**Calcium Ion Antagonists (Calcium Channel Blockers) Used to Treat Hypertension—cont'd**			
GENERIC NAME	**BRAND NAME**	**ORAL DOSE FORMS**		**ADULT DOSAGE RANGE**
isradipine	DynaCirc	Capsules: 2.5, 5 mg Tablets, extended-release: 5, 10 mg		Initial—2.5 mg twice daily Maximal response may require 2-4 weeks Maintenance—10 mg daily Maximum—20 mg daily
nicardipine	Cardene	Capsules: 20, 30 mg Capsules, extended-release: 30, 45, 60 mg		Initial—20 mg three times daily Maximal response may require 2 weeks of therapy Adjust dose by measuring blood pressure about 8 hours after last dose Peak effect is determined by measuring blood pressure 1-2 hours after dosage administration Maintenance—20-40 mg three times daily
nifedipine	Procardia	Capsules: 10, 20 mg Tablets, sustained-release: 30, 60, 90 mg		Initial—10 mg three times daily Adjust over 7-14 days to balance anti-anginal and hypotensive activity Maintenance—10-20 mg three to four times daily Sustained-release tablets are administered once daily Maximum—capsules: 180 mg daily; sustained-release tablets: 120 mg daily
nisoldipine	Sular	Tablets: Sustained-release: 10, 20, 30, 40 mg		Initial—20 mg once daily; adjust over 7-14 days by 10 mg/week Maintenance—20-60 mg once daily
verapamil	Calan, Isoptin	Tablets: 40, 80, 120 mg Tablets, sustained-release: 120, 180, 240, 360 mg Capsules, sustained-release: 100, 120, 180, 200, 240, 300, 360 mg		Initial—80 mg three or four times daily Sustained-release tablets and capsules: 120-240 mg once daily in the morning Maintenance—240-480 mg daily Administer with food

DRUG CLASS: **Alpha-1 Adrenergic Blocking Agents**

Alpha-1 receptors in the nervous system cause blood vessels to constrict (Chapter 14). Alpha-1 adrenergic blocking agents (alpha-1 blockers) block alpha-1 receptors. By blocking receptors that cause blood vessels to constrict (narrow), the blood vessels dilate (widen). Such vaso-dilation reduces blood pressure.

Alpha-1 blockers may be used alone or with other anti-hypertensive drugs.

Alpha-1 blockers also are used to treat benign prostatic hyperplasia (Chapter 29). They relax the smooth muscles of the bladder and prostate.

Assisting With the Nursing Process

When giving alpha-1 blockers, you assist the nurse with the nursing process.

ASSESSMENT
- Measure heart rate and rhythm. Use the apical pulse.
- Measure blood pressure in the supine and standing positions.

PLANNING
See Table 19-4 for "Oral Dose Forms."

IMPLEMENTATION
See Table 19-4 for "Adult Dosage Range."

EVALUATION
Report and record:
- *Hypotension with dizziness, tachycardia, and fainting.* These may occur within 15 to 90 minutes after the first several doses. They are more common in persons who also receive diuretics. Check the person often until blood pressure is stable. Measure blood pressure in the supine and standing positions. Provide for safety. Remind the person to rise slowly from a supine or sitting position. Have the person sit or lie down if symptoms develop.
- *Drowsiness, headache, dizziness, weakness, lethargy.* These may resolve with continued therapy.

TABLE 19-4 Alpha-1 Adrenergic Blocking Agents			
GENERIC NAME	**BRAND NAME**	**ORAL DOSE FORMS**	**ADULT DOSAGE RANGE**

doxazosin	Cardura	Tablets: 1, 2, 4, 8 mg	Hypertension:
			    Initial—1 mg daily AM or PM; hypotensive effects are most
			        likely within 2-6 hours; monitor standing blood pressure
			    Maintenance—increase to 2 mg, then, if needed, 4, 8, and
			        16 mg to achieve desired reduction in blood pressure
			Benign prostatic hyperplasia:
			    Initial—as for hypertension; increase dosage at weekly
			        intervals to 2 mg, then 4 and 8 mg once daily
			    Maintenance—8 mg daily; monitor blood pressure

prazosin	Minipress	Capsules: 1, 2, 5 mg	Hypertension:
			    Initial—1 mg two or three times daily with first dose at
			        bedtime to reduce syncopal episodes
			    Maintenance—6-15 mg/day in 2 or 3 divided doses
			    Maximum dose—20-40 mg/day

terazosin	Hytrin	Capsules: 1, 2, 5, 10 mg
		Tablets: 1, 2, 5, 10 mg
			Hypertension:
			    Initial—1 mg at bedtime; measure blood pressure
			        2-3 hours after dosing and evaluate for symptoms of
			        dizziness or tachycardia; if response is substantially
			        diminished at 24 hours, increase dosage
			    Maintenance—1-5 mg daily
			    Maximum dose—20 mg/day
			Benign prostatic hyperplasia:
			    Initial—as for hypertension; gradually increase dosage in
			        stepwise fashion to 2, 5, or 10 mg daily for acceptable
			        urinary output
			    Maintenance—10 mg daily for 4-6 weeks to assess urinary
			        response
			    Maximum dose—20 mg/day

DRUG CLASS: Central-Acting Alpha-2 Agonists

Alpha-2 receptors prevent the further release of norepinephrine (Chapter 14). Norepinephrine stimulates the sympathetic nervous system. The sympathetic nervous system speeds up body functions.

An *agonist* is a drug that acts on a certain type of cell. It produces a predictable response. Central-acting alpha-2 agonists stimulate the alpha-adrenergic receptors in the brainstem. This reduces sympathetic nervous system activity. Heart rate and peripheral vascular resistance are reduced. This results in lower systolic and diastolic blood pressures.

Alpha-2 agonists are used in combination with other anti-hypertensive agents.

Assisting With the Nursing Process

When giving alpha-2 agonists, you assist the nurse with the nursing process.

ASSESSMENT
- Measure heart rate and rhythm. Use the apical pulse.
- Measure blood pressure in the supine and standing positions.
- Observe for signs and symptoms of depression (Chapter 15).
- Observe the person's sleep patterns (Chapter 14).

PLANNING
See Table 19-5, p. 250, for "Dose Forms."

IMPLEMENTATION
- See Table 19-5, p. 250, for "Adult Dosage Range."
- If a transdermal patch becomes loose, apply the adhesive overlay directly over the patch.

TABLE 19-5	Central-Acting Alpha-2 Agonists		
GENERIC NAME	**BRAND NAME**	**DOSE FORMS**	**ADULT DOSAGE RANGE**

clonidine	Catapres
	Catapres-TTS
		Tablets: 0.1, 0.2, 0.3 mg
		Transdermal patch:
		  TTS-1: 0.1 mg/24 hours
		  TTS-2: 0.2 mg/24 hours
		  TTS-3: 0.3 mg/24 hours
			PO: Initial—0.1 mg twice daily
			Maintenance—0.2-0.8 mg daily in divided doses
			Maximum—2.4 mg daily
			Transdermal—apply to a hairless area of intact skin on upper arm or torso once every 7 days; use a different site each week
			Initial—TTS-1: Adjust dosage every 1-2 weeks
			NOTE: Anti-hypertensive effect starts 2-3 days after initiation of therapy

guanabenz	Wytensin	Tablets: 4, 8 mg	Initial—4 mg twice daily; increase 4-8 mg daily every 1-2 weeks Maximum—32 mg twice daily
guanfacine	Tenex	Tablets: 1, 2 mg	Initial—1 mg daily at bedtime Maintenance—1-2 mg Maximum—3 mg daily
methyldopa	Aldomet	Tablets: 250, 500 mg	Initial—250 mg 2 or 3 times daily Maintenance—500 mg to 2 g daily in 2-4 doses

EVALUATION

Report and record:

- *Drowsiness, dizziness, dry mouth.* These tend to resolve with continued therapy. Provide for safety. Provide oral hygiene and offer fluids as directed by the nurse and the care plan.
- *Dark urine.* This is harmless.
- *Depression.* See Chapter 15 for the signs and symptoms of depression.
- *Rash.* This may occur at the site of a transdermal patch.

DRUG CLASS: Peripheral-Acting Adrenergic Antagonists

Peripheral-acting adrenergic antagonists lower norepinephrine levels. Such drugs are:

- guanadrel (gwan' a drel); Hylorel (hi lor' el)
- guanethidine sulfate (gwan eth' i deen); Ismelin (is' meh lin)
- reserpine (res' er peen); Serpasil (ser' pah sil)

guanadrel (Hylorel)

Guanadrel (Hylorel) causes the release of norepinephrine from nerve endings. Nerve endings have less norepinephrine. This causes smooth muscles of the blood vessels to relax. Peripheral vascular resistance is decreased. Blood pressure lowers. Venous blood return to the heart decreases. This can lead to fluid retention and edema.

Guanadrel (Hylorel) is used with diuretics.

Assisting With the Nursing Process

When giving guanadrel (Hylorel), you assist the nurse with the nursing process.

ASSESSMENT

- Measure blood pressure in the supine and standing positions.
- Measure daily weight.
- Measure intake and output.

PLANNING

The oral dose forms are 10 and 25 mg tablets.

IMPLEMENTATION

- The initial adult dose is 10 mg daily in 2 divided doses.
- The dosage is adjusted weekly to monthly as needed.
- The usual dosage range is 20 to 75 mg daily in 2 to 3 divided doses.

EVALUATION

Report and record:

- *Orthostatic hypotension.* Blood pressure is measured in the supine and standing positions. Provide for safety. Remind the person to rise slowly from a supine or sitting position. Have the person sit or lie down if he or she feels faint.

- *Sedation and lethargy.* These may occur when therapy is started or the dosage is increased. They tend to subside with time.
- *Edema.* Measure weight daily. Measure intake and output. Check the legs for swelling. Observe for dyspnea, wheezing, and frothy or blood-tinged sputum. See Chapter 21 for the signs and symptoms of heart failure.

guanethidine sulfate (Ismelin)

Guanethidine sulfate (Ismelin) depletes norepinephrine from the nerves. It also inhibits the release of norepinephrine in response to sympathetic nerve stimulation. Blood pressure decreases because:

- Cardiac output is less.
- Vaso-constriction is blocked. Peripheral vascular resistance is decreased.

Guanethidine sulfate (Ismelin) is used with diuretics.

Assisting With the Nursing Process

When giving guanethidine sulfate (Ismelin), you assist the nurse with the nursing process.

ASSESSMENT
- Measure blood pressure in the supine and standing positions.
- Measure daily weight.
- Measure intake and output.

PLANNING
The oral dose forms are 10 and 25 mg tablets.

IMPLEMENTATION
- The initial adult dose is 10 mg daily.
- The dose is increased 10 mg every 5 to 7 days as needed.
- The usual dosage range is between 25 and 50 mg. Sometimes much higher doses are needed.

EVALUATION
Report and record:
- *Orthostatic hypotension.* Blood pressure is measured in the supine and standing positions. Provide for safety. Remind the person to rise slowly from a supine or sitting position. Have the person sit or lie down if he or she feels faint.
- *Light-headedness, weakness.* Because blood vessels dilate, blood can collect in the lower legs. This causes reduced blood flow to the brain. These symptoms often disappear during the day. Remind the person to rise slowly from a supine position and to sit for a few minutes. Have the person perform leg, foot, and toe exercises before standing.
- *Edema.* Measure weight daily. Measure intake and output. Check the legs for swelling. Observe for dyspnea, wheezing, and frothy or blood-tinged sputum. See Chapter 21 for the signs and symptoms of heart failure.

reserpine (Serpasil)

Reserpine (Serpasil) reduces norepinephrine levels in peripheral nerve endings, the brain, and other organs. The heart rate slows and peripheral vascular resistance decreases. Blood pressure decreases.

Reserpine (Serpasil) has a long duration of action. It may take 2 to 6 weeks before the desired therapeutic effect is seen.

Assisting With the Nursing Process

When giving reserpine (Serpasil), you assist the nurse with the nursing process.

ASSESSMENT
- Measure blood pressure in the supine and standing positions.
- Measure daily weight.
- Measure intake and output.
- Observe for signs and symptoms of depression (Chapter 15).
- Observe the person's sleep patterns (Chapter 14).

PLANNING
The oral dose forms are 0.1 and 0.25 mg tablets.

IMPLEMENTATION
- The initial adult dose is 0.5 mg daily for 1 to 2 weeks.
- The usual dosage range is 0.1 to 0.25 mg daily.

EVALUATION
Report and record:
- *Nasal congestion.* This tends to resolve with continued therapy.
- *Diarrhea, stomach cramps.* These tend to resolve with continued therapy.
- *Depression.* See Chapter 15 for the signs and symptoms of depression.
- *Nightmares, insomnia.* Drug therapy may need to be changed.
- *Stomach burning or pain, nausea, vomiting.* Ulcers are a risk.

DRUG CLASS: **Direct Vaso-Dilators**

Direct vaso-dilators act directly on the smooth muscles of arterioles. The arterioles relax. This reduces peripheral vascular resistance. Blood pressure lowers. Direct vaso-dilators are:

- hydralazine (hy dral' ah zeen); Apresoline (ah pres' o leen)
- minoxidil (min ox' i dil); Loniten (lon' i ten)

hydralazine (Apresoline)

Hydralazine (Apresoline) causes the smooth muscles of arterioles to relax. This reduces peripheral vascular resistance causing lower blood pressure. However, the following increase:

- Cardiac output
- Renin release (p. 244)
- Sodium and water retention

Hydralazine (Apresoline) is used in combination with diuretics and other drugs.

Assisting With the Nursing Process

When giving hydralazine (Apresoline), you assist the nurse with the nursing process.

ASSESSMENT

- Measure heart rate and rhythm. Use the apical pulse.
- Measure blood pressure in the supine and standing positions.
- Measure daily weight.
- Measure intake and output.

PLANNING

The oral dose forms are 10, 25, 50, and 100 mg tablets.

IMPLEMENTATION

- The initial adult dose is 10 mg four times a day for the first 2 to 4 days. Then 25 mg are given four times a day.
- The second week, the dosage is increased to 50 mg four times a day as blood pressure is brought under control.

EVALUATION

Report and record:

- *Nausea, dizziness, tachycardia, numbness and tingling in the legs, nasal congestion.* The dosage may need adjustment.
- *Orthostatic hypotension.* Blood pressure is measured in the supine and standing positions. Provide for safety. Remind the person to rise slowly from a supine or sitting position. Have the person sit or lie down if he or she feels faint.
- *Fever, chills, joint and muscle pain, skin problems.* These may signal changes in white blood cells.

minoxidil (Loniten)

Minoxidil (Loniten) causes the smooth muscles of arterioles to relax. This reduces peripheral vascular resistance causing lower blood pressure. However, the following increase:

- Cardiac output
- Renin release (p. 244)
- Sodium and water retention

Minoxidil (Loniten) is used in combination with diuretics and other drugs.

Assisting With the Nursing Process

When giving minoxidil (Loniten), you assist the nurse with the nursing process.

ASSESSMENT

- Measure heart rate and rhythm. Use the apical pulse.
- Measure blood pressure in the supine and standing positions.
- Measure daily weight.
- Measure intake and output.

PLANNING

The oral dose forms are 2.5 and 10 mg tablets.

IMPLEMENTATION

- The initial adult dose is 5 mg daily.
- The dosage may be gradually increased after at least 3-day intervals to 10 mg, 20 mg, and then 40 mg daily in 1 or 2 doses.
- The dosage range is 10 to 40 mg daily.
- The dose should not exceed 100 mg daily.

EVALUATION

Report and record:

- *Hair growth.* This is seen in both men and women. Fine body hair becomes long, thick, and dark. It occurs on the face first within 3 to 6 weeks of therapy. Later it is seen on the back, arms, legs, and scalp.
- *Sodium and water retention.* Measure weight daily. Measure intake and output. Observe for swelling of the face, hands, and ankles.
- *Increased resting pulse rate.*
- *Light-headedness, fainting, dizziness.* Provide for safety.
- *Orthostatic hypotension.* Blood pressure is measured in the supine and standing positions. Provide for safety. Remind the person to rise slowly from a supine position.
- *Signs and symptoms of heart failure.* See Chapter 21.
- *Swelling of the breasts in men.*

COMBINATION DRUGS

Some persons take more than one anti-hypertensive drug. Often the second drug is a diuretic. For simple and easy use, a combination drug may be ordered. See Table 19-6.

TABLE 19-6 Combination Drugs Used to Treat Hypertension	
COMBINATION TYPE	**TRADE NAME**
Angiotensin-converting enzyme inhibitors and calcium channel blockers	Lotrel Lexxel Tarka
Angiotensin-converting enzyme inhibitors and diuretics	Lotensin HCT Capozide Vaseretic Prinzide Uniretic Accuretic
Angiotensin-receptor blockers and diuretics	Atacand HCT Teveten HCT Avalide Hyzaar Micardis HCT Diovan HCT
Beta blockers and diuretics	Tenoretic Ziac Inderide Lopressor HCT Corzide Timolide
Central-acting drug and diuretics	Aldoril Diupres Hydropres
Diuretic and diuretic	Moduretic Aldactazide Dyazide Maxzide

Modified from The Seventh Report of the Joint National Commission on Prevention, Detection, Evaluation, and Treatment of High Blood Pressure, National Institutes of Health, Publication No. 03-5233, May 2003 as in Clayton BD, Stock YN, Harroun RD: *Basic pharmacology for nurses,* ed 14, St Louis, 2007, Mosby.

REVIEW QUESTIONS

Circle the BEST answer.

1   Which lowers blood pressure?
   a   vaso-constriction
   b   vaso-dilation
   c   cardiac output
   d   heart rhythm

2   Life-style changes to lower blood pressure include the following *except*
   a   drug therapy
   b   a low-fat, low-salt diet
   c   a healthy weight
   d   regular exercise

3   When a person requires two or more anti-hypertensive drugs, one drug is usually
   a   a beta blocker
   b   a calcium channel blocker
   c   an ACE inhibitor
   d   a diuretic

4   Which promote the formation and excretion of urine?
   a   beta blockers
   b   calcium channel blockers
   c   ACE inhibitors
   d   diuretics

5   Beta blockers lower blood pressure because
   a   heart rate and cardiac output are reduced
   b   aldosterone levels increase
   c   vaso-constriction occurs
   d   the body retains sodium and water

6   Which is a beta blocker?
   a   carvedilol (Coreg)
   b   enalapril (Vasotec)
   c   quinapril (Accupril)
   d   benazepril (Lotensin)

Continued

REVIEW QUESTIONS—cont'd

7 Before giving any anti-hypertensive drug, you should
   a give the person food
   b measure the person's blood pressure
   c ask the person to void
   d ask about bowel elimination patterns

8 Which produces strong vaso-constriction?
   a renin   c angiotensin II
   b angiotensin I   d aldosterone

9 ACE inhibitors affect the conversion of
   a angiotensin I to angiotensin II
   b renin to angiotensin I
   c renin to aldosterone
   d aldosterone to angiotensin II

10 Which ACE inhibitor is given before meals?
   a benazepril (Lotensin)   c enalapril (Vasotec)
   b captopril (Capoten)   d quinapril (Accupril)

11 Hypotension as a side effect from ACE inhibitors
   a may occur within the first 3 hours when therapy is started
   b is seen after several weeks of therapy
   c can be prevented with diuretics
   d is not a concern

12 Besides preventing vaso-constriction, angiotensin II receptor blockers prevent
   a sodium retention
   b the release of renin
   c decreased cardiac output
   d abnormal heart rhythms

13 Hypotension as a side effect from angiotensin II receptor blockers
   a may occur within the first 3 hours when therapy is started
   b is seen after several weeks of therapy
   c can be prevented with diuretics
   d is not a concern

14 Which is an aldosterone receptor blocking agent?
   a hydralazine (Apresoline)
   b guanethidine sulfate (Ismelin)
   c reserpine (Serpasil)
   d eplerenone (Inspra)

15 Calcium channel blockers lower blood pressure because they
   a lower the heart rate
   b increase cardiac output
   c increase aldosterone levels
   d relax the smooth muscle of blood vessels

16 Hypotension and fainting from calcium channel blockers may occur
   a within the first 15 to 90 minutes when therapy is started
   b within the first 3 hours when therapy is started
   c during the first week
   d after several weeks

17 Which is a calcium channel blocker?
   a irbesartan (Avapro)   c amlodipine (Norvasc)
   b olmesartan (Benicar)   d prazosin (Minipress)

18 Alpha-1 adrenergic blocking agents lower blood pressure by
   a slowing the heart rate
   b increasing cardiac output
   c causing vaso-dilation
   d relaxing the smooth muscle of blood vessels

19 Central-acting alpha-2 agonists prevent the release of
   a norepinephrine   c angiotensin II
   b renin   d aldosterone

20 Central-acting alpha-2 agonists stimulate receptors in the
   a brainstem   c liver
   b kidneys   d heart

21 Which central-acting alpha-2 agonist comes in a transdermal patch?
   a clonidine (Catapres)   c guanfacine (Tenex)
   b guanabenz (Wytensin)   d methyldopa (Aldomet)

22 Peripheral-acting adrenergic antagonists lower levels of
   a norepinephrine   c angiotensin II
   b renin   d aldosterone

23 Which is *not* a peripheral-acting adrenergic antagonist?
   a guanadrel (Hylorel)
   b guanethidine sulfate (Ismelin)
   c reserpine (Serpasil)
   d hydralazine (Apresoline)

24 Direct vasodilators lower blood pressure because they
   a prevent the release of norepinephrine
   b cause arterioles to relax
   c prevent the release of renin
   d increase cardiac output

Circle T if the statement is true. Circle F if the statement is false.

25 T F   Renin causes vaso-dilation.

26 T F   Renin causes sodium retention.

27 T F   Aldosterone causes the kidneys to excrete water and sodium.

28 T F   Calcium channel blockers are used to treat angina.

Answers to these questions are on pp. 445-446.

Drugs Used to Treat Dysrhythmias

KEY TERMS

anti-dysrhythmic agents Drugs used to prevent or correct abnormal heart rhythms

arrhythmia Without *(a)* a rhythm *(rhythmia)*; dysrhythmia

dysrhythmia An abnormal *(dys)* rhythm *(rhythmia)*; arrhythmia

KEY ABBREVIATIONS

AV bundle Atrio-ventricular bundle
AV node Atrio-ventricular node
ECG Electrocardiogram
g Gram
GI Gastro-intestinal
mg Milligram
PAC Premature atrial contraction
PAT Paroxysmal atrial tachycardia
PVC Premature ventricular contraction
SA node Sino-atrial node
VF Ventricular fibrillation
V fib Ventricular fibrillation
VT Ventricular tachycardia

The heart pumps blood to itself through the coronary arteries and to the rest of the body's tissues. There are two phases of heart action. During *diastole,* the resting phase, heart chambers fill with blood. The heart relaxes during this phase. During *systole,* the working phase, the heart contracts. Blood is pumped through the blood vessels when the heart contracts. Systole and diastole make up the cardiac cycle.

The conduction system (electrical system) controls the cardiac cycle. The heart muscle must relax (fill with blood) and contract (pump blood) in a coordinated fashion. Otherwise cells do not get enough blood and oxygen.

To coordinate the cardiac cycle, the heart's muscle fibers are linked together. An electrical impulse starts in the wall of the right atrium. It passes through (is conducted or transmitted to) muscle fibers in the right and left atria, causing the atria to contract. Then the impulse moves to the ventricles, causing the ventricles to contract. For every heartbeat, an electrical impulse is conducted through the heart.

Four structures in the heart wall make up the conduction system (Fig. 20-1). They are the sino-atrial node, atrio-ventricular node, atrio-ventricular bundle, and the Purkinje fibers.

- *Sino-atrial node (SA node)* starts the impulse in the right atrium. The SA node is also called the *pacemaker.* It sets the pace (beat) of the heart.
- The electrical impulse travels from the SA node to the right and left atria.
- The right and left atria contract as the impulse travels through them. Blood is pumped to the ventricles.
- The electrical impulse reaches the *atrio-ventricular node (AV node).* It is at the bottom of the right atrium *(atrio)* near the right ventricle *(ventricular).*
- The impulse travels through the AV node to the *atrio-ventricular bundle (AV bundle)* in the wall separating the right and left ventricles. (The AV bundle is also called the *bundle of His.*)
- The AV bundle has right and left branches. The branches extend to all parts of the ventricular wall. The *right bundle branch* conducts the impulse to the right ventricle. The *left bundle branch* conducts the impulse to the left ventricle.
- *Purkinje fibers* branch into the myocardium (heart muscle) from the right and left bundle branches. When the impulse reaches the ventricular muscle, the ventricles contract.
- After contracting, the ventricles relax.

An **arrhythmia** means without *(a)* a rhythm *(rhythmia).* Another term for arrhythmia is **dysrhythmia**—an abnormal *(dys)* rhythm *(rhythmia).* There is a disturbance in the normal electrical conduction causing:

- An abnormal heart muscle contraction
- An abnormal heart rate

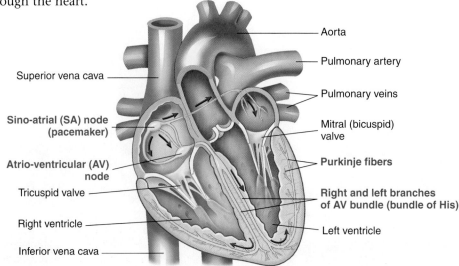

Superior vena cava

Sino-atrial (SA) node
(pacemaker)

Atrio-ventricular (AV)
node

Tricuspid valve

Right ventricle

Inferior vena cava

Aorta

Pulmonary artery

Pulmonary veins

Mitral (bicuspid)
valve

Purkinje fibers

**Right and left branches
of AV bundle (bundle of His)**

Left ventricle

Fig. 20-1 Conduction system of the heart. (Modified from Thibodeau GA, Patton KT: *Structure and function of the body,* ed 13, St Louis, 2008, Mosby.)

Areas outside the SA node can act as a pacemaker. That is, they can start an impulse. This causes an irregular heart beat. Some rhythms are life-threatening. Blocks can occur in the conduction system. A block prevents the impulse from traveling through the conduction system in a normal manner. Blocks also can be life-threatening.

Electrocardiograms (ECGs) record the electrical activity of the conduction system. The electrical activity is recorded in waves. The waves give the cardiac cycle a distinct appearance (Fig. 20-2). Each wave represents electrical activity in a certain part of the heart. The *P wave, QRS complex,* and *T wave* are the major parts of the cardiac cycle.

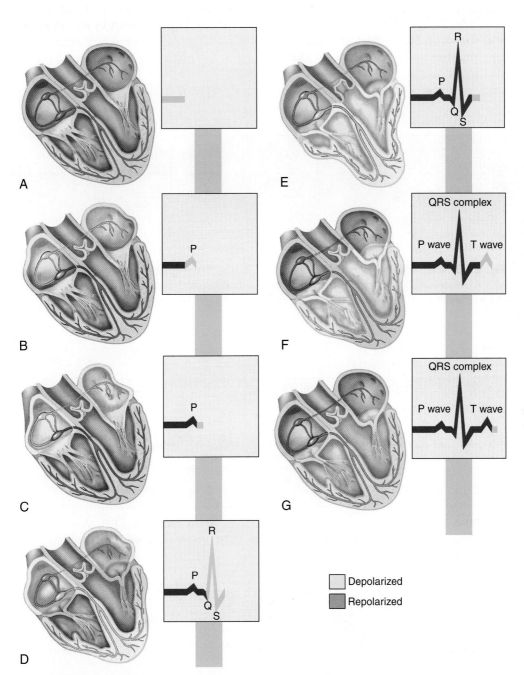

Fig. 20-2 Electrical activity in the heart. **A,** The impulse starts in the SA node. **B,** The impulse spreads to the right and left atrium. **C,** The atria contract. The *P wave* is formed. **D,** The impulse reaches the AV node and the AV bundle. The atria relax. **E,** The ventricles contract. The *QRS complex* forms. **F,** The ventricles start to relax. **G,** The ventricles relax. The *T wave* forms. (From Thibodeau GA, Patton KT: *Structure and function of the body,* ed 13, St Louis, 2008, Mosby.)

If a problem occurs in a part of the conduction system, the wave for that part appears abnormal. Problems can occur in any part of the conduction system. ECG changes also occur if the heart muscle is damaged. By studying the ECG, the doctor determines the site of the problem in the conduction system or the area of heart muscle damage.

TYPES OF DYSRHYTHMIAS

A normal rhythm is shown in Figure 20-3. It is called *normal sinus rhythm*. Impulses start in the SA node. The heart rate is between 60 and 100 beats per minute. Various heart diseases cause changes in the conduction system. Dysrhythmias are classified by origin within the heart tissues.

- *Supraventricular dysrhythmias.* Those that develop above *(supra)* the bundle of His.
  - *Sinus tachycardia*—the heart rate is rapid (Fig. 20-4). Impulses start in the SA node.
  - *Sinus bradycardia*—the heart rate is slow (Fig. 20-5). Impulses start in the SA node.

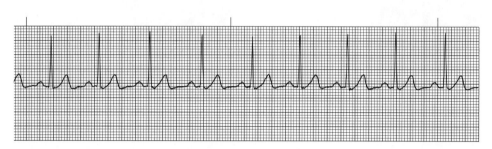

Fig. 20-3 Normal sinus rhythm. The heart rate is 80. (From Ignatavicius DD, Workman ML: *Medical-surgical nursing: critical thinking for collaborative care,* ed 5, Philadelphia, 2006, Saunders.)

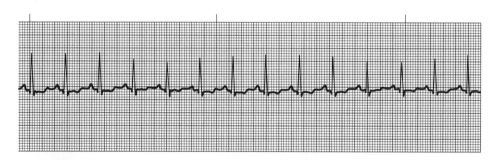

Fig. 20-4 Sinus tachycardia. The heart rate is 110. (From Ignatavicius DD, Workman ML: *Medical-surgical nursing: critical thinking for collaborative care,* ed 5, Philadelphia, 2006, Saunders.)

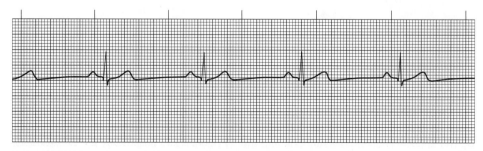

Fig. 20-5 Sinus bradycardia. The heart rate is 40. (From Atwood S and others: *Introduction to basic cardiac dysrhythmias,* ed 3, St Louis, 2003, Mosby.)

- *Premature atrial contraction (PAC)*—the SA node sends out an impulse early (Fig. 20-6).
- *Paroxysmal atrial tachycardia (PAT)*—a normal rhythm suddenly turns into tachycardia. Bursts (paroxysms) of tachycardia occur. The tachycardia stops suddenly (Fig. 20-7).

- *Atrial flutter*—impulses start in the atria at a rapid rate. The ventricles do not respond to every impulse (Fig. 20-8). There are more P waves (flutter or F waves) than QRS complexes. QRS complexes occur at regular intervals. The person's pulse is regular.

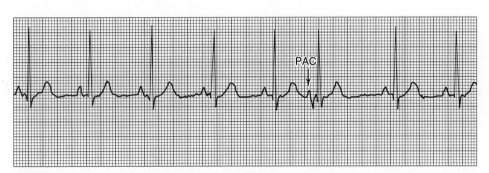

Fig. 20-6 Premature atrial contraction (PAC). (From Ignatavicius DD, Workman ML: *Medical-surgical nursing: critical thinking for collaborative care,* ed 5, Philadelphia, 2006, Saunders.)

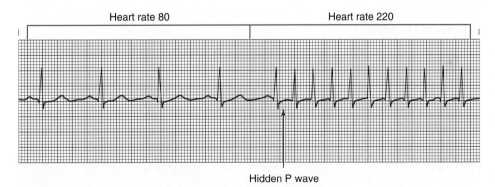

Fig. 20-7 Paroxysmal atrial tachycardia (PAT). (From Atwood S, Stanton C, Storey-Davenport J: *Introduction to basic cardiac dysrhythmias,* ed 4, St Louis, 2009, Mosby.)

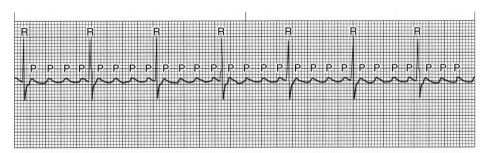

Fig. 20-8 Atrial flutter. Note the P waves (flutter or F waves). (Modified from Atwood S, Stanton C, Storey-Davenport J: *Introduction to basic cardiac dysrhythmias,* ed 4, St Louis, 2009, Mosby.)

- *Atrial fibrillation*—impulses start in the atria at multiple sites. There are no P waves. Impulses are conducted to the ventricles at irregular intervals (Fig. 20-9). QRS complexes occur at irregular intervals. Therefore the pulse is irregular. The atria quiver, not contract. Blood is not pumped from the atria to the ventricles in normal amounts. Therefore the ventricles pump inadequate amounts of blood to the rest of the body.

- *Junctional rhythms*—impulses start in the AV node. There are no P waves (Fig. 20-10). Junctional rhythms can occur at normal or slow rates.
- *Blocks in conduction pathways.* They are described by the degree of block.
  - *First-degree heart block*—the impulse takes longer to travel from the SA node to the AV node. The PR interval is longer than normal (Fig. 20-11). The rhythm is regular.

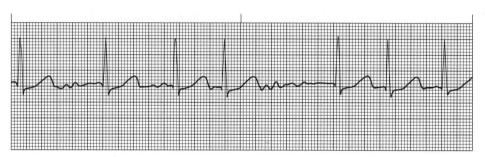

Fig. 20-9 Atrial fibrillation. No P waves occur and the rhythm is irregular. (From Atwood S, Stanton C, Storey-Davenport J: *Introduction to basic cardiac dysrhythmias,* ed 4, St Louis, 2009, Mosby.)

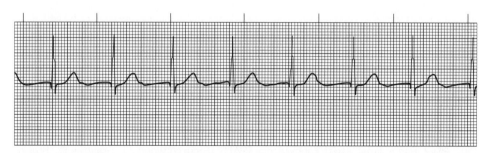

Fig. 20-10 Junctional rhythm. No P waves. (From Atwood S and others: *Introduction to basic cardiac dysrhythmias,* ed 3, St Louis, 2003, Mosby.)

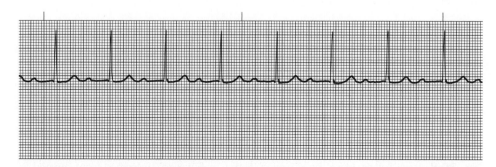

Fig. 20-11 First-degree heart block. The PR interval is 0.36 seconds. (From Ignatavicius DD, Workman ML: *Medical-surgical nursing: critical thinking for collaborative care,* ed 5, Philadelphia, 2006, Saunders.)

- *Second-degree heart block*—some impulses from the SA node do not reach the ventricles. Impulses from the SA node take longer and longer to travel through the AV node until a beat is skipped. A QRS complex does not follow a P wave (Fig. 20-12). The rhythm is irregular.
- *Third-degree heart block*—the impulse is blocked between the atria and ventricles (Fig. 20-13). The impulse cannot reach the ventricles. The ventricles must create their own impulses. P waves appear but are not related to the QRS complexes. The QRS complexes are wider than normal. The heart rate is very slow. **This is a life-threatening dysrhythmia.**
- *Ventricular dysrhythmias.* Those that develop below the bundle of His.

- *Premature ventricular contraction (PVC)*—the impulse is created in the ventricles. It occurs earlier than the next regular beat. The QRS complex is wide and bizarre (Fig. 20-14). *Unifocal PVCs* come from one *(uni)* site *(focal)*. They all look the same. *Multifocal PVCs* are created in many *(multi)* sites *(focal)* as in Figure 20-15 on p. 262. *Bigeminy* is when every second *(bi)* complex is a PVC (Fig. 20-16, p. 262). With *trigeminy*, every third *(tri)* complex is a PVC. (*Geminy* means *twin*.) Two PVCs can occur in a row (Fig. 20-17, p. 262). They can be unifocal or multifocal and are called *coupled PVCs*. A *run of ventricular tachycardia* is several PVCs in a row (Fig. 20-18, p. 262). The rhythm returns to normal. PVCs mean that the heart muscle is irritable. **PVCs are often life-threatening.**

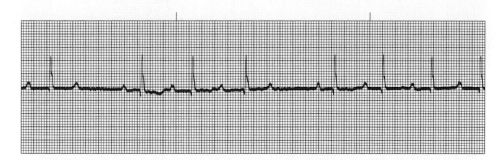

Fig. 20-12 Second-degree heart block. The PR interval gets longer until a P wave is completely blocked. (From Ignatavicius DD, Workman ML: *Medical-surgical nursing: critical thinking for collaborative care,* ed 5, Philadelphia, 2006, Saunders.)

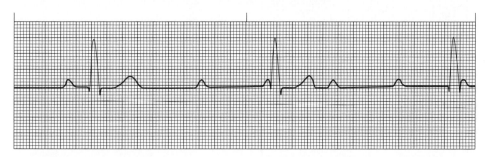

Fig. 20-13 Third-degree heart block. The atrial rate (P waves) is faster than the ventricular rate. (From Atwood S and others: *Introduction to basic cardiac dysrhythmias,* ed 3, St Louis, 2003, Mosby.)

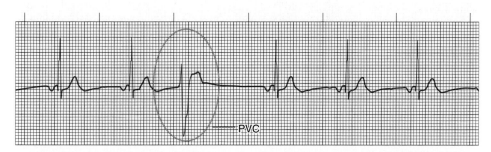

Fig. 20-14 Premature ventricular contraction (PVC). (From Atwood S, Stanton C, Storey-Davenport J: *Introduction to basic cardiac dysrhythmias,* ed 4, St Louis, 2009, Mosby.)

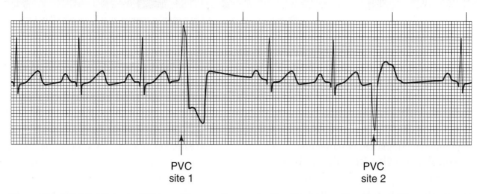

Fig. 20-15 Multifocal PVCs. (From Atwood S, Stanton C, Storey-Davenport J: *Introduction to basic cardiac dysrhythmias,* ed 4, St Louis, 2009, Mosby.)

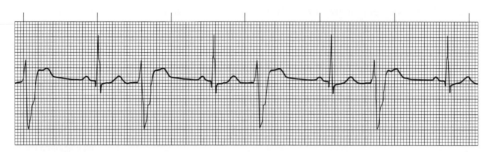

Fig. 20-16 Bigeminy. (From Atwood S and others: *Introduction to basic cardiac dysrhythmias,* ed 3, St Louis, 2003, Mosby.)

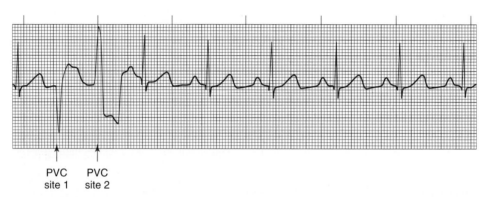

Fig. 20-17 Coupled PVCs. Two PVCs occur in a row. The PVCs are multifocal. (From Atwood S, Stanton C, Storey-Davenport J: *Introduction to basic cardiac dysrhythmias,* ed 4, St Louis, 2009, Mosby.)

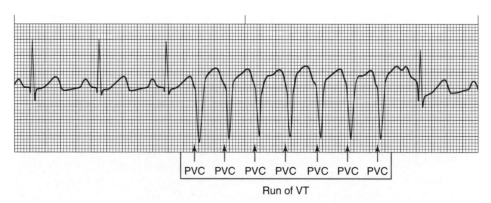

Fig. 20-18 Run of ventricular tachycardia. (From Atwood S, Stanton C, Storey-Davenport J: *Introduction to basic cardiac dysrhythmias,* ed 4, St Louis, 2009, Mosby.)

- *Ventricular tachycardia (VT)*—impulses start in the ventricles. The heart rate can range from 40 to 250 beats per minute. QRS complexes are wide and bizarre. The rhythm looks like a series of PVCs (Fig. 20-19). ***Ventricular tachycardia is life-threatening. If not corrected, it progresses to ventricular fibrillation.***

- *Ventricular fibrillation (VF or V fib)*—impulses start from multiple sites in the ventricles. P waves and QRS complexes are not present (Fig. 20-20). The ventricles quiver, not contract. ***Ventricular fibrillation is deadly. The person is in cardiac arrest.***

- *Asystole*—means no *(a)* contraction *(systole)*. No electrical activity occurs in the heart (Fig. 20-21). ***Asystole is deadly. The person is in cardiac arrest.***

Conduction system tissues are affected by calcium and sodium. An *ion* is an atom with an electrical charge. An a*tom* is the smallest part of an element. An *element* is a simple substance that cannot be broken down into another substance. Calcium and sodium are elements.

- *Calcium.* The SA and AV nodes depend on calcium ions for electrical conduction.
- *Sodium.* The atrial muscle, His-Purkinje system, and the ventricular muscle depend on sodium for contraction.

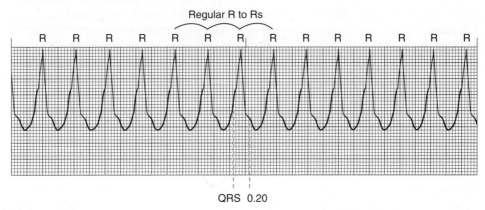

Fig. 20-19 Ventricular tachycardia (VT). [From Atwood S, Stanton C, Storey-Davenport J: *Introduction to basic cardiac dysrhythmias,* ed 4, St Louis, 2009, Mosby.]

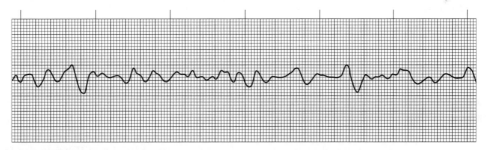

Fig. 20-20 Ventricular fibrillation—no P waves or QRS complexes. [From Atwood S, Stanton C, Storey-Davenport J: *Introduction to basic cardiac dysrhythmias,* ed 4, St Louis, 2009, Mosby.]

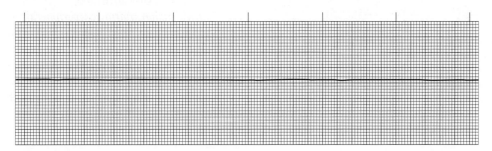

Fig. 20-21 Asystole. [From Atwood S, Stanton C, Storey-Davenport J: *Introduction to basic cardiac dysrhythmias,* ed 4, St Louis, 2009, Mosby.]

DRUG THERAPY FOR DYSRHYTHMIAS

Anti-dysrhythmic agents are drugs used to prevent or correct abnormal heart rhythms. They are complex and act in many ways. Depending on the drug, anti-dysrhythmic agents affect the heart's conduction system by:

- Inhibiting sodium ion movement. This depresses the heart muscle (myocardium).
- Prolonging or shortening the duration of electrical stimulation on the cells.
- Increasing or decreasing the time between electrical impulses.
- Slowing the conduction rate between the atria and ventricles.

The following anti-dysrhythmic agents are discussed in this chapter:

- amiodarone hydrochloride (am e o' dahr own); Cordarone (cor' dah rown)
- beta-adrenergic blocking agents
- disopyramide (die so peer' ah myd); Norpace (nor' pace)
- flecainide acetate (fleh kayn' ayd); Tambocor (tam boh' kor)
- mexiletine (mehx ihl' et een); Mexitil (mehx it' ihl)
- moricizine (mor is' ih zeen); Ethmozine (eth moh' zeen)
- procainamide hydrochloride (pro kane' ah myd); Procanbid (pro kahn' bid)
- propafenone (pro pah' fen own); Rythmol (rith' mohl)
- quinidine (kwin' i deen)

See also diltiazem (Cardizem) in Table 19-3 (Chapter 19) and digoxin (Lanoxin) in Chapter 21.

See *Delegation Guidelines: Drug Therapy for Dysrhythmias.*

DELEGATION GUIDELINES
Drug Therapy for Dysrhythmias

Some drugs used to treat dysrhythmias are given parenterally—by intramuscular or intravenous injection. Because you do not give parenteral dose forms, they are not included in this chapter. Should a nurse delegate the administration of such to you, you must:

- Remember that parenteral dosages are often very different from dosages for other routes.
- Refuse the delegation. Make sure you explain why. Do not just ignore the request. Make sure the nurse knows that you cannot give the drug and why.

---

amiodarone hydrochloride (Cordarone)

Amiodarone hydrochloride (Cordarone) slows the rate of electrical conduction. It also increases the time between contractions. The drug is given to convert (change) the following dysrhythmias to normal sinus rhythm:

- Supraventricular tachycardias—rapid arrhythmias that occur above the bundle of His
- Atrial fibrillation
- Atrial flutter
- Bradycardia-tachycardia syndromes
- Ventricular tachycardia
- Ventricular fibrillation

Assisting With the Nursing Process

When giving amiodarone (Cordarone), you assist the nurse with the nursing process.

ASSESSMENT

- Observe for dyspnea, chest pain, fatigue, edema, fainting, palpitations (the person describes palpitations as "my heart skips some beats" or "my heart is racing").
- Measure blood pressure, apical pulse (for 1 minute), and respirations.

PLANNING

Oral dose forms are 100, 200, and 400 mg tablets.

IMPLEMENTATION

- The initial adult dose is 800 to 1600 mg daily in divided doses for 1 to 3 weeks. Then a dosage of 600 to 800 mg is given for about 1 month.
- The lowest effective dose should be used, usually 400 mg.

EVALUATION

Report and record:

- *Fatigue, tremors, involuntary muscle movements, sleep problems, numbness and tingling, coordination problems, dizziness, confusion.* Many of these resolve when the dose is reduced or the drug is discontinued. Provide for safety. Remind the person to rise slowly from a supine or sitting position. Have the person sit or lie down if he or she feels faint.
- *Dyspnea on exertion, non-productive cough, chest pain with breathing.* Symptoms gradually resolve when the drug is discontinued.
- *Blurred vision, narrowed peripheral vision, halos.* Provide for safety. Remind the person not to forcefully rub his or her eyes when tearing. These symptoms resolve when the drug is discontinued.
- *Nausea, vomiting, constipation, abdominal pain, anorexia.* These are common with high dosages. They resolve with lower doses or divided doses.

- *Dysrhythmias.* The drug may cause dysrhythmias or cause existing dysrhythmias to worsen.
- *Skin reactions: rash, burning, tingling, redness, and blistering.* These are from exposure to sunlight (photo-sensitivity). The person should use sunscreens, wear long-sleeved shirts and pants, and avoid sunlamps.
- *Anorexia, nausea, vomiting, jaundice.* These may signal liver toxicity.

DRUG CLASS:
Beta-Adrenergic Blocking Agents

Beta-adrenergic blocking agents (beta blockers) are widely used as anti-dysrhythmic agents (Chapter 14). By blocking beta receptors, they block the heart's response to sympathetic nerve stimulation. Heart rate, blood pressure, and cardiac output are reduced.

See Table 14-2 (Chapter 14) for the beta blockers used to treat dysrhythmias. They are effective in converting (changing) the following dysrhythmias to normal sinus rhythm:

- Various ventricular dysrhythmias
- Sinus tachycardia
- Paroxysmal supraventricular tachycardia
- Premature ventricular contractions
- Atrial flutter when tachycardia is present
- Atrial fibrillation when tachycardia is present

Assisting With the Nursing Process

When giving beta blockers to treat dysrhythmias, you assist the nurse with the nursing process. See Chapter 14.

disopyramide (Norpace)

Disopyramide (Norpace) prolongs the stimulation on the cells and increases the time between electrical impulses. It is effective in converting (changing) the following dysrhythmias to normal sinus rhythm:

- Atrial fibrillation
- Paroxysmal supraventricular tachycardia
- Runs of ventricular tachycardia
- Ventricular tachycardia

Assisting With the Nursing Process

When giving disopyramide (Norpace), you assist the nurse with the nursing process.

ASSESSMENT
- Observe for dyspnea, chest pain, fatigue, edema, fainting, palpitations (the person describes palpitations as "my heart skips some beats" or "my heart is racing").
- Measure blood pressure, apical pulse (for 1 minute), and respirations.
- Ask about bowel elimination.
- Ask about urination.

PLANNING
Oral dose forms are:
- 100 and 150 mg capsules
- 100 and 150 extended-release capsules

IMPLEMENTATION
- The dosage depends on the person's needs. The usual adult dosage is 400 to 800 mg/day.
- The adult dosage schedule is usually 150 mg every 6 hours.

EVALUATION
Report and record:
- *Dry mouth, nose, and throat.* Provide oral hygiene. Provide ice chips or hard candy to suck on according to the care plan.
- *Bradycardia, signs of heart failure (Chapter 21).* These are signs of myocardial toxicity.
- *Difficulty starting a urine stream.* Run tap water or immerse the person's hands in water. Measure intake and output.
- *Constipation, abdominal distention, flatus.* Ask about bowel elimination and expelling gas.

flecainide acetate (Tambocor)

Flecainide acetate (Tambocor) slows the conduction rate through the atria and ventricles. It is effective in converting (changing) the following dysrhythmias to normal sinus rhythm:

- Ventricular tachycardia
- Paroxysmal supraventricular tachycardia
- Premature ventricular contractions

Assisting With the Nursing Process

When giving flecainide acetate (Tambocor), you assist the nurse with the nursing process.

ASSESSMENT
- Observe for dyspnea, chest pain, fatigue, edema, fainting, palpitations (the person describes palpitations as "my heart skips some beats" or "my heart is racing").
- Measure blood pressure, apical pulse (for 1 minute), and respirations.
- Observe for signs and symptoms of heart failure (Chapter 21).

PLANNING
Oral dose forms are 50, 100, and 150 mg tablets.

IMPLEMENTATION
- The initial adult dose is 100 mg every 12 hours. It is increased by 50 mg twice a day every 4 days.
- The usual dose is 150 mg twice a day.
- The maximum daily dose is 400 mg.

EVALUATION

Report and record:

- *Dizziness, headache, constipation, nausea.* These are mild and tend to resolve with continued therapy.
- *Vision disturbances.* Provide for safety. The person should avoid tasks that require good vision (driving, operating machines). Remind the person not to forcefully rub his or her eyes when tearing.
- *Signs and symptoms of heart failure (Chapter 21).* This drug may cause heart failure or existing heart failure to worsen.
- *Dysrhythmias.* The drug may cause dysrhythmias or cause existing dysrhythmias to worsen.

mexiletine (Mexitil)

Mexiletine (Mexitil) shortens the duration of electrical stimulation on the cells. It also increases the time between electrical impulses. It is effective in converting (changing) the following dysrhythmias to normal sinus rhythm:

- Ventricular tachycardia
- Premature ventricular contractions

Assisting With the Nursing Process

When giving mexiletine (Mexitil), you assist the nurse with the nursing process.

ASSESSMENT

- Observe for dyspnea, chest pain, fatigue, edema, fainting, palpitations (the person describes palpitations as "my heart skips some beats" or "my heart is racing").
- Measure blood pressure, apical pulse (for 1 minute), and respirations.
- Ask about gastro-intestinal (GI) symptoms.
- Observe orientation to person, time, and place.
- Observe for confusion and agitation.

PLANNING

Oral dose forms are 150, 200, and 250 mg capsules.

IMPLEMENTATION

- The usual adult dose is 200 to 400 mg every 8 hours.
- Give the drug with food or with antacids (Chapter 25) if ordered.

EVALUATION

Report and record:

- *Nausea, vomiting, indigestion.* These occur most often with higher dosages.
- *Dysrhythmias.* The drug may cause dysrhythmias or cause existing dysrhythmias to worsen.
- *Fine hand tremors, coordination problems, light-headedness, blurred vision, double vision, involuntary eye movements, difficult speech, confusion, numbness and tingling, drowsiness, seizures.* These signal that the drug has a toxic effect on the central nervous system.

- *Confusion.* Observe the person's orientation to person, time, and place. Observe for confusion. Provide for safety.

moricizine (Ethmozine)

Moricizine (Ethmozine) slows the conduction rate between the atria and ventricles. It is effective in converting (changing) ventricular dysrhythmias to normal sinus rhythm. Because it can cause other dysrhythmias, it is used when the benefits are greater than the risks.

Assisting With the Nursing Process

When giving moricizine (Ethmozine), you assist the nurse with the nursing process.

ASSESSMENT

- Observe for dyspnea, chest pain, fatigue, edema, fainting, palpitations (the person describes palpitations as "my heart skips some beats" or "my heart is racing").
- Measure blood pressure, apical pulse (for 1 minute), and respirations.
- Ask about GI symptoms.
- Observe orientation to person, time, and place.
- Observe for confusion and agitation.

PLANNING

Oral dose forms are 200, 250, and 300 mg tablets.

IMPLEMENTATION

- The initial adult dose is 200 mg every 8 hours.
- Dosages may be increased by 150 mg every 3 days.
- The usual adult dosage is between 600 and 900 mg daily.
- The drug is given in divided doses around the clock.
- Give the drug with food or milk to prevent gastric irritation.

EVALUATION

Report and record:

- *Hypotension, dizziness.* These may occur when therapy is started. They usually subside within a few days. Provide for safety. Remind the person to rise slowly from a supine or sitting position. Have the person sit or lie down if he or she feels faint.
- *Nausea.* Give the drug with food or milk.
- *Dysrhythmias.* The drug may cause dysrhythmias or cause existing dysrhythmias to worsen.
- *Euphoria (exaggerated feeling or state of physical or mental well-being), confusion.* Observe orientation to person, time, and place. Provide for safety.

procainamide hydrochloride (Procanbid)

Procainamide (Procanbid) prolongs the duration of electrical stimulation on the cells. It also increases the time between electrical impulses. It is effective in converting (changing) the following dysrhythmias to normal sinus rhythm:

- Ventricular dysrhythmias
- Supraventricular dysrhythmias
- Atrial flutter
- Atrial fibrillation

Assisting With the Nursing Process

When giving procainamide (Procanbid), you assist the nurse with the nursing process.

ASSESSMENT

- Observe for dyspnea, chest pain, fatigue, edema, fainting, palpitations (the person describes palpitations as "my heart skips some beats" or "my heart is racing").
- Measure blood pressure, apical pulse (for 1 minute), and respirations.

PLANNING

The oral dose forms are:

- 250, 375, and 500 mg capsules and tablets
- 250, 500, 750, and 1000 mg sustained-release tablets

IMPLEMENTATION

- The initial adult dose is 1 to 1.25 g. It is followed with 750 mg one hour later if the arrhythmia is still present.
- The dosage is maintained at 0.5 g to 1 g every 4 to 6 hours.
- Some persons require doses every 3 to 4 hours.
- The drug is given in divided doses around the clock.
- Give the drug with food or milk if gastric irritation occurs.

EVALUATION

Report and record:

- *Drowsiness, sedation, dizziness, hypotension.* Provide for safety. Remind the person to rise slowly from a supine or sitting position. Have the person sit or lie down if he or she feels faint. The person should avoid tasks that require alertness (driving, operating machinery).
- *Fever, chills, joint and muscle pain, skin eruptions.* These may signal changes in white blood cells.

propafenone (Rythmol)

Propafenone (Rythmol) slows the conduction rate between the atria and ventricles. It is effective in converting (changing) atrial fibrillation and ventricular dysrhythmias to normal sinus rhythm. Because it can cause other dysrhythmias, it is used when the benefits are greater than the risks.

Assisting With the Nursing Process

When giving propafenone (Rythmol), you assist the nurse with the nursing process.

ASSESSMENT

- Observe for dyspnea, chest pain, fatigue, edema, fainting, palpitations (the person describes palpitations as "my heart skips some beats" or "my heart is racing").
- Measure blood pressure, apical pulse (for 1 minute), and respirations.
- Ask about GI symptoms.

PLANNING

The oral dose forms are:

- 150, 225, and 300 mg tablets
- 225, 325, and 425 extended-release capsules

IMPLEMENTATION

- The initial adult dose is 150 mg every 8 hours.
- Every 3 to 4 days, the dosage may be increased to 225 mg every 8 hours, then 300 mg every 8 hours (900 mg daily).
- The drug is given around the clock.
- If a dose is missed, the next dose should not be doubled. (Check with the nurse. The nurse tells you what to do when a dose is missed.)

EVALUATION

Report and record:

- *Dizziness.* Provide for safety. Remind the person to rise slowly from a supine or sitting position. Have the person sit or lie down if he or she feels faint.
- *Nausea, vomiting, constipation.* Give the drug with food or milk to prevent nausea.
- *Dysrhythmias.* The drug may cause dysrhythmias or cause existing dysrhythmias to worsen.

quinidine

Quinidine shortens the duration of electrical stimulation on the cells. It also increases the time between electrical impulses. It slows the heart rate and changes a rapid, irregular pulse to a slow, regular pulse.

It is effective in converting (changing) the following dysrhythmias to normal sinus rhythm:

- Atrial flutter
- Atrial fibrillation
- Paroxysmal supraventricular tachycardia
- Premature ventricular contractions

Assisting With the Nursing Process

When giving quinidine, you assist the nurse with the nursing process.

ASSESSMENT

- Observe for dyspnea, chest pain, fatigue, edema, fainting, palpitations (the person describes palpitations as "my heart skips some beats" or "my heart is racing").
- Measure blood pressure, apical pulse (for 1 minute), and respirations.
- Ask about bowel elimination.

PLANNING

The oral dose forms are:

- quinidine sulfate:
  - 200 and 300 mg tablets
  - 300 mg sustained-release tablets
- quinidine gluconate
  - 324 mg sustained-release tablets

IMPLEMENTATION

The adult dosages are:

- quinidine sulfate:
  - 200 to 400 mg orally 3 to 5 times a day. Higher doses may be used.
  - The maximum single dose should not exceed 600 to 800 mg.
  - Give with food or milk.
- quinidine gluconate:
  - 324 to 972 mg every 8 to 12 hours

EVALUATION

Report and record:

- *Diarrhea.* This is common when therapy is started. It usually subsides. Note the frequency and consistency of stools.
- *Dizziness, faintness.* These usually subside within a few days. Provide for safety. Remind the person to rise slowly from a supine or sitting position. Have the person sit or lie down if he or she feels faint.
- *Hearing loss, headache, tinnitus (ringing in the ears), increasing mental confusion, rash, chills, fever.* These result from excess quinidine.
- *Hypotension.* This may occur if the person also takes diuretics or anti-hypertensive agents. Provide for safety. Remind the person to rise slowly from a supine or sitting position. Have the person sit or lie down if he or she feels faint.

REVIEW QUESTIONS

Circle the **BEST** answer.

1 In a normal cardiac cycle, the impulse starts in the
   a atria
   b SA node
   c AV node
   d bundle of His

2 Another term for dysrhythmia is
   a anrhythmia
   b bradyrhythmia
   c arrhythmia
   d tachyrhythmia

3 Which dysrhythmia has more P waves than QRS complexes?
   a sinus tachycardia
   b premature atrial contractions
   c atrial flutter
   d atrial fibrillation

4 Dysrhythmias that develop above the bundle of His are called
   a sinus dysrhythmias
   b premature contractions
   c junctional rhythms
   d supraventricular dysrhythmias

5 Which is life-threatening?
   a sinus bradycardia—heart rate 50
   b first-degree heart block
   c second-degree heart block
   d third-degree heart block

6 Ventricular dysrhythmias develop
   a in the SA node
   b in the AV node
   c above the bundle of His
   d below the bundle of His

7 Which of the following is *not* considered life-threatening?
   a atrial fibrillation
   b premature ventricular contractions
   c ventricular tachycardia
   d ventricular fibrillation

8 Before giving any anti-dysrhythmic drug, you should do the following *except*
   a observe for dyspnea, chest pain, and palpitations
   b observe for fatigue and fainting
   c measure blood pressure
   d measure the radial pulse and respirations

9 Before giving any anti-dysrhythmic agent, the pulse is measured
   a for 30 seconds
   b for 1 minute
   c by ECG
   d every 6 hours

10 Most anti-dysrhythmic drugs can cause
   a diarrhea
   b gastro-intestinal bleeding
   c increased urinary output
   d other dysrhythmias

11 Amiodarone hydrochloride (Cordarone) is given to
   a increase the heart rate
   b slow the heart rate
   c decrease the time between contractions
   d increase the rate of electrical conduction

12 Beta blockers are used to
   a increase the heart rate
   b slow the heart rate
   c decrease the time between contractions
   d increase the rate of electrical conduction

13 Disopyramide (Norpace) is used to
a increase the heart rate
b slow the heart rate
c decrease the time between contractions
d increase the rate of electrical conduction

14 Flecainide acetate (Tambocor) is used to
a increase the heart rate
b slow the heart rate
c decrease the time between contractions
d increase the rate of electrical conduction

15 Mexiletine (Mexitil) is used for
a atrial flutter and atrial fibrillation
b junctional rhythms
c ventricular tachycardia and premature ventricular contractions
d ventricular fibrillation and asystole

16 Moricizine (Ethmozine) is used for
a sinus rhythms
b atrial flutter and atrial fibrillation
c junctional rhythms
d ventricular dysrhythmias

17 Moricizine (Ethmozine) and procainamide hydrochloride (Procanbid) are given
a before meals
b after meals
c with food or milk
d at bedtime

18 Which of these drugs can affect urination?
a amiodarone hydrochloride (Cordarone)
b disopyramide (Norpace)
c quinidine
d propafenone (Rythmol)

19 Diarrhea is common with
a amiodarone hydrochloride (Cordarone)
b disopyramide (Norpace)
c quinidine
d propafenone (Rythmol)

Circle T if the statement is true. Circle F if the statement is false.

20 T F Areas outside the SA node can act as a pacemaker for the heart.

21 T F Dysrhythmias can occur from any part of the conduction system.

22 T F Quinidine increases the heart rate.

Answers to these questions are on p. 446.

Drugs Used to Treat Angina, Peripheral Vascular Disease, and Heart Failure

OBJECTIVES

- Define the key terms and key abbreviations used in this chapter.
- Describe the causes, signs and symptoms, and treatment of angina.
- Describe the drugs used to treat angina.
- Explain how to assist with the nursing process when giving drugs to treat angina.
- Describe the causes, signs and symptoms, and treatment of peripheral vascular disease.
- Describe the drugs used to treat peripheral vascular disease.
- Explain how to assist with the nursing process when giving drugs to treat peripheral vascular disease.
- Describe the causes, signs and symptoms, and treatment of heart failure.
- Describe the drugs used to treat heart failure.
- Explain how to assist with the nursing process when giving drugs to treat heart failure.

KEY TERMS

digitalization Giving a larger dose of digoxin for the first 24 hours, then giving the person a daily dose

fatty oxidase enzyme inhibitor A drug that reduces the oxygen needed by myocardial cells to cause muscle contractions

hemorrheologic agent A drug that prevents the clumping of red blood cells and platelets: hemorrheologic relates to the science (*logic*) of blood (*hemo*) flow (*rrheo*)

inotropic agents Drugs that stimulate the heart to increase the force of contractions

intermittent claudication A pain pattern usually described as aching, cramping, tightness, or weakness in the calves usually during walking; it is relieved with rest

platelet aggregation inhibitor A drug that prevents platelets from clumping together and causes vaso-dilation

vaso-dilators Drugs that widen blood vessels to increase blood flow

vaso-spasm A sudden contraction of a blood vessel causing vaso-constriction

KEY ABBREVIATIONS

ACE Angiotensin-converting enzyme
CAD Coronary artery disease
CHF Congestive heart failure
h Hour
MAR Medication administration record
mg Milligram
MI Myocardial infarction
mL Milliliter
PO Per os (orally)
PVD Peripheral vascular disease
q Every

Cardiovascular system disorders are leading causes of death in the United States. Many people have these disorders.

See *Delegation Guidelines: Drugs Used to Treat Angina, Peripheral Vascular Disease, and Heart Failure.*

ANGINA

The coronary arteries are in the heart. They supply the heart with blood. In coronary artery disease (CAD), the coronary arteries become hardened and narrow. One or all are affected. Therefore the heart muscle gets less blood and oxygen.

The most common cause is atherosclerosis (Chapter 18). Plaque—made up of fat, cholesterol, and other substances—collects on the arterial walls. The narrowed arteries block blood flow. Blockage may be total or partial. Blood clots also can form along the plaque and block blood flow.

The major complications of CAD are angina, myocardial infarction (MI), dysrhythmias, and sudden death. The more risk factors, the greater the chance of CAD and its complications. Risk factors are listed in Box 21-1.

Angina (pain) means *chest pain*. It is from reduced blood flow to part of the heart muscle (myocardium). It occurs when the heart needs more oxygen. Normally blood flow to the heart increases when the need for oxygen increases. Exertion, a heavy meal, stress, and excitement increase the heart's need for oxygen. So does smoking and exposure to very hot or cold temperatures. In CAD, narrowed vessels prevent increased blood flow.

Chest pain is described as a tightness, pressure, squeezing, or burning in the chest (Fig. 21-1, p. 272). Pain can occur in the shoulders, arms, neck, jaw, or back. Pain in the jaw, neck, and down one or both arms is common. The person may be pale, feel faint, and perspire. Dyspnea is common. Nausea, fatigue, and weakness may occur. Some persons complain of

BOX 21-1 **Risk Factors for Coronary Artery Disease**

RISK FACTORS THAT *CANNOT* BE CONTROLLED
- Gender—men are at greater risk than women
- Age—in men, the risk increases after age 45; in women, the risk increases after age 55
- Family history
- Race—African-Americans are at greater risk than other groups

RISK FACTORS THAT *CAN* BE CONTROLLED
- Being over-weight
- Lack of exercise
- High blood cholesterol
- Hypertension
- Smoking
- Diabetes
- Stress (anger, worry, arguing)

"gas" or indigestion. Rest often relieves symptoms in 3 to 15 minutes. Rest reduces the heart's need for oxygen. Therefore normal blood flow is achieved. Heart damage is prevented.

Things that cause angina are avoided. These include over-exertion, heavy meals and over-eating, and emotional stress. The person needs to stay indoors during cold weather or during hot, humid weather. Exercise programs are helpful. They are supervised by the doctor.

Some persons need drugs to decrease the heart's workload and relieve symptoms. Other drugs are given to prevent an MI or sudden death. Drugs also can delay the need for medical and surgical procedures that open or bypass diseased arteries (Fig. 21-2, p. 272). The goal is to increase blood flow to the heart. Doing so may prevent or lower the risk of heart attack and death.

With angina, the coronary arteries cannot deliver

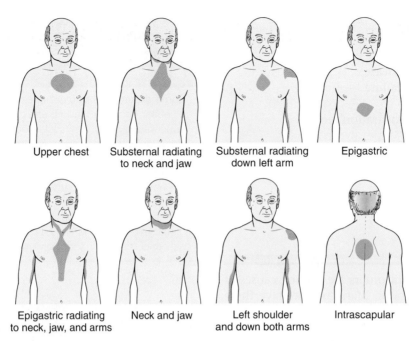

Upper chest | Substernal radiating to neck and jaw | Substernal radiating down left arm | Epigastric

Epigastric radiating to neck, jaw, and arms | Neck and jaw | Left shoulder and down both arms | Intrascapular

Fig. 21-1 *Shaded areas* show where the pain of angina is located. (From Lewis SM and others: *Medical-surgical nursing: assessment and management of clinical problems*, ed 6, St Louis, 2007, Mosby).

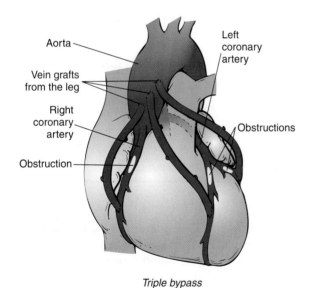

Triple bypass

Fig. 21-2 Coronary artery bypass surgery. (Modified from Thibodeau GA, Patton KT: *The human body in health and disease*, ed 4, St Louis, 2005, Mosby.)

enough oxygen to meet the heart's demands. Seven groups of drugs may be used to treat angina:

- Nitrates
- Beta-adrenergic blocking agents (beta blockers)
- Angiotensin-converting enzyme (ACE) inhibitors
- Calcium ion antagonists (calcium channel blockers)
- Statins (Chapter 18)
- Platelet-active agents (Chapter 23)
- Fatty oxidase enzyme inhibitors

DRUG CLASS: **Nitrates**

Nitrates are the oldest effective therapy for angina. They relieve angina by:

- *Relaxing peripheral vascular smooth muscles.* Arteries and veins dilate (widen). This reduces venous blood flow to the heart. It also decreases oxygen demands on the heart.
- *Dilating coronary arteries.* This enhances blood flow and myocardial oxygen supply.

Nitroglycerin is the drug of choice in the treatment of angina. Various dose forms are available to meet the person's needs. The goals of nitrate therapy are to:

- Relieve the pain of angina during an attack
- Reduce the frequency and severity of anginal attacks (prophylaxis)
- Increase activity and exercise tolerance

Assisting With the Nursing Process

When a person receives nitrates, you assist the nurse with the nursing process.

ASSESSMENT

- Ask about the severity, location, duration, intensity, and pattern of pain.
- Ask when the last dose of nitrates was taken.
- Ask if relief was obtained from the nitrate.
- Measure blood pressure.

TABLE 21-1	Nitrates					
GENERIC NAME	**BRAND NAME**	**DOSE FORMS**		**ONSET**	**DURATION**	**ADULT DOSAGE RANGE**
amyl nitrite		Inhalation: 0.3 mL ampules in a woven sack for crushing		0.5 minute	3-5 minutes	Inhalation: 1 ampule crushed in sack and placed under the person's nostrils for inhalation at time of acute attack
isosorbide dinitrate	Isordil	Sublingual tablets: 2.5, 5, 10 mg		2-3 minutes	1-3 hours	Sublingual: 2.5-10 mg for acute attack
		Oral tablets: 5, 10, 20, 30, 40 mg		30-60 minutes	4-6 hours	PO: 2.5-30 mg three or four times daily on empty stomach
		Sustained-release tablets and capsules: 40 mg		30-60 minutes	6-8 hours	PO: 20-40 mg q6-8h or 80 mg q8-12h
isosorbide mononitrate	Monoket	Oral tablets: 10 mg		30-60 minutes	NA	PO: 20 mg twice daily, 7 hours apart
	ISMO	Oral tablets: 20 mg				
	Imdur	Sustained-release tablets: 30, 60, 120 mg		3-4 hours	8-12 hours	PO: 30-240 mg once daily; do not crush or chew tablets
nitroglycerin	Nitrostat	Sublingual tablets: 0.3, 0.4, 0.6 mg		1-2 minutes	More than 30 minutes	Sublingual: 0.3-0.6 mg for prophylactic use before activity that may induce angina or at time of acute attack
	Nitrong	Oral sustained-release capsules: 2.5, 6.5, 9 mg		30-45 minutes	3-8 hours	PO: 2.5-9 mg two to four times daily for prophylaxis
	Nitro-Bid	Ointment: 2%		30 minutes	3 hours	Topical: 0.5-4 inches of ointment using special applicator q4-6h
	Nitrogard	Transmucosal: 2, 3 mg tablets		2-3 minutes	3-5 hours	Buccal: place 1-3 mg between cheek and gum q3-5h
	Nitro-Dur	Transdermal: 0.1, 0.2, 0.3, 0.4, 0.6, 0.8 mg/hour patches		30-60 minutes	Less than 24 hours	Topical: 1 patch applied for 12 hours; the person should wait 12 hours after removing old patch before applying new patch
	Nitrolingual	Translingual: 0.4 mg metered spray		2 minutes	30-60 minutes	Spray: 1-2 sprays onto or under tongue for acute attack; repeat if needed in 3-5 minutes; may be used prophylactically 5-10 minutes before exercise

PLANNING

See Table 21-1 for "Dose Forms."

IMPLEMENTATION

- See Table 21-1 for "Adult Dosage Range."
- See Box 21-2, p. 274, for the administration of nitrate dose forms.

EVALUATION

Report and record:

- *Hypotension, dizziness, nausea, flushing, and fainting.* The dosage may need adjustment.

- *Headache.* This is the most common side effect. It can range from a feeling of mild fullness in the head to an intense and severe headache. Most people develop tolerance within a few weeks. The dosage may need adjustment.

- *Tolerance (increasing dosage to attain relief).* Tolerance to nitrate dosages can develop rapidly, particularly if large doses are given often. It can appear within a few days and may be well established within a few weeks. The smallest dose for a satisfactory result should be used. To break tolerance, the doctor withdraws the drug for a short time.

BOX 21-2 **Administration of Nitrate Dose Forms**

SUBLINGUAL TABLETS

- Remind the person to sit or lie down at the first sign of an anginal attack.
- Remind the person to:
  - Place a tablet under the tongue.
  - Let the tablet dissolve.
  - Not to swallow saliva immediately.
  - Tell the nurse at once:
    - When the person takes a sublingual tablet.
    - If the person does not obtain relief of chest pain within 5 minutes. Assist the nurse as directed.
- Remind the person to tell the nursing team if he or she takes 1 or 2 tablets before activities that may cause an angina attack.
- Remind the person that sublingual tablets deteriorate within a few months.
  - The drug should produce a slight stinging or burning sensation. This means that the drug is still potent.
  - The person should have the prescription refilled every 3 months.
  - The person should discard unused tablets.
- Store nitroglycerin in the original, dark-colored glass container. Make sure the lid is tight.
- Make sure the drug is within the person's reach.
  - Home settings: The person should carry nitroglycerin at all times. It should not be carried in a pocket directly next to the person's body. Heat speeds up deterioration of the drug.
  - Health care settings: Nitroglycerin is kept at the bedside. Remind the person to tell the nursing team at once when he or she takes a nitroglycerin tablet.

SUSTAINED-RELEASE TABLETS

- Give sustained-release nitroglycerin tablets as ordered. They are usually taken on an empty stomach every 8 to 12 hours.
- Give the drug with food if gastritis develops. Check with the nurse and the MAR.

TRANSMUCOSAL TABLETS

- Place the tablet under the upper lip or buccal pouch. The drug is absorbed by the oral mucosa over 3 to 5 hours.
- Remind the person that he or she may eat, drink, and talk while the tablet is in place.
- Give the drug as ordered. The usual initial dose is 1 tablet three times a day:
  - On arising
  - After lunch
  - After the evening meal
- Do not give more than 1 tablet every 2 hours.

TRANSLINGUAL SPRAY

- *Do not use the spray where it can ignite. The spray is highly flammable.*
- Do not shake the container. Bubbles may form. They may slow the release of the drug.
- Give the spray as follows:
  - Position the person in a sitting position.
  - Hold the canister vertically so the valve head is uppermost. Hold the spray opening as close to the mouth as possible.
  - Press the button firmly to spray the dose onto or under the tongue.
  - Have the person close the mouth at once after each dose. *The spray should not be swallowed or inhaled.*
- Tell the nurse at once:
  - When the person uses a translingual spray.
  - If the person does not obtain relief of chest pain within 5 minutes. Assist the nurse as directed.

TOPICAL OINTMENT

- See Chapter 11 for applying topical ointment.
- Rotate application sites to prevent skin irritation. Do not use a site with signs of irritation.
- Close the tube tightly. Store it in a cool place according to agency policy.

TRANSDERMAL DISK

- Remember the following:
  - This dose form provides controlled release of the drug for 24 hours when applied to intact skin.
  - The dosage released depends on the surface area of the disk.
  - Therapeutic effect can be observed in about 30 minutes after application. It continues for about 30 minutes after removal.
  - The person may need sublingual nitroglycerin for anginal attacks.
- Practice hand washing before applying and after removing a patch.
- See Chapter 11 for applying a transdermal disk.
- Rotate the application site daily. The best sites are the upper chest, pelvis, and inner side of the upper arm. Avoid scars, skin-folds, and wounds.
- Remove and discard a patch that has become partly dislodged. Apply a new disk.
- Keep discarded patches out of the reach of children. Discarded patches still contain enough active drug to be dangerous to children.

DRUG CLASS:
Beta-Adrenergic Blocking Agents

Beta-adrenergic blocking agents (beta blockers) block the beta-adrenergic receptors in the heart. This prevents stimulation from norepinephrine and epinephrine (Chapter 14). Normally such stimulation would increase the heart rate and increase myocardial oxygen demands. Heart rate, oxygen demand, and blood pressure are reduced by blocking the receptors.

All beta blockers are effective in treating angina. The goals of therapy are to:
- Reduce the number of angina attacks
- Reduce nitroglycerin use
- Improve activity and exercise tolerance

Assisting With the Nursing Process

When giving beta blockers to treat angina, you assist the nurse with the nursing process.

ASSESSMENT
- Measure blood pressure in the supine and standing positions.
- Ask about respiratory signs and symptoms.
- Measure blood glucose if the person has diabetes.

PLANNING
See Chapter 14.

IMPLEMENTATION
See Chapter 14.

EVALUATION
See Chapter 14.

DRUG CLASS: Calcium Ion Antagonists

Calcium ion antagonists (calcium channel blockers) inhibit the movement of calcium ions across a cell membrane (Chapter 19). They do the following:
- Decrease myocardial oxygen demand.
- Dilate coronary arteries, which improves blood flow. This increases myocardial blood supply.
- Dilate peripheral vessels. This decreases resistance to blood flow, which reduces the heart's workload. The goals of therapy are to:
- Decrease the frequency of angina attacks
- Decrease the severity of angina attacks
- Increase activity and exercise tolerance

Assisting With the Nursing Process

When giving calcium channel blockers to treat angina, you assist the nurse with the nursing process.

ASSESSMENT
- Measure blood pressure in the supine and standing positions.
- Observe for signs and symptoms of heart failure (p. 279).

PLANNING
See Table 21-2 for "Oral Dose Forms."

IMPLEMENTATION
See Table 21-2 for "Adult Dosage Range."

EVALUATION
See Chapter 19.

TABLE 21-2	Calcium Ion Antagonists (Calcium Channel Blockers) Used to Treat Angina			
GENERIC NAME	**BRAND NAME**	**ORAL DOSE FORMS**		**ADULT DOSAGE RANGE**
amlodipine	Norvasc	Tablets: 2.5, 5, 10 mg		Initial—5 mg once daily; adjust over 7-14 days to a maximum of 10 mg/day
diltiazem	Cardizem	Tablets: 30, 60, 90, 120 mg		Initial—30 mg four times daily, gradually increasing dosage to 180-360 mg in three or four divided doses
		Tablets, extended-release: 120, 180, 240, 300, 360, 420 mg Sustained-release capsules: 60, 90, 120, 180, 240, 300 mg		Initial—120-180 mg sustained-release capsule once daily; adjust as needed after 14 days Maintenance—240-480 mg daily
bepridil	Vascor	Tablets: 200, 300 mg		Initial—200 mg daily; adjust after 10 days, depending on response Maintenance—300 mg daily Maximum—400 mg daily

Continued

TABLE 21-2	Calcium Ion Antagonists (Calcium Channel Blockers) Used to Treat Angina—cont'd		
GENERIC NAME	**BRAND NAME**	**ORAL DOSE FORMS**	**ADULT DOSAGE RANGE**
nicardipine	Cardene	Capsules: 20, 30 mg	Initial—20 mg three times daily Maximal response may require 2 weeks of therapy Allow at least 3 days between dosage adjustments Maintenance—20-40 mg three times daily
		Sustained-release capsules: 30, 45, 60 mg	Initial—30 mg twice daily Maintenance—30-60 mg twice daily
nifedipine	Procardia, Adalat	Capsules: 10, 20 mg	Initial—10 mg three times daily; adjust over 7-14 days to balance anti-anginal and hypotensive activity Maintenance—10-20 mg three times daily
		Sustained-release tablets: 30, 60, 90 mg	Sustained-release tablets are administered once daily—30-60 mg Maximum—capsules: 180 mg daily; sustained-release tablets: 120 mg daily
verapamil	Calan, Isoptin	Tablets: 40, 80, 120 mg Sustained-release tablets and capsules: 120, 180, 200, 240, 300, 360 mg	Initial—40-120 mg three times daily Maintenance—120-480 mg daily Administer with food

DRUG CLASS: Angiotensin-Converting Enzyme Inhibitors

Angiotensin-converting enzyme (ACE) inhibitors have a significant effect on the coronary arteries. By preventing vaso-constriction, the blood vessels dilate. The drugs also prevent blood clots from forming. See Chapter 19 for a discussion of ACE inhibitors.

ACE inhibitors are used to prevent MI.

Assisting With the Nursing Process

When giving ACE inhibitors to prevent MI, you assist the nurse with the nursing process.

ASSESSMENT
- Measure blood pressure in the supine and standing positions.
- Measure heart rate and rhythm for 1 minute. Use the apical pulse.
- Ask about bowel elimination.
- Ask if the person has a cough.

PLANNING
See Table 19-1 (Chapter 19) for "Oral Dose Forms."

IMPLEMENTATION
- See Table 19-1 (Chapter 19) for "Adult Dosage Range."
- Captopril (Capoten) is given twice a day 1 hour before or 2 hours after meals. All other ACE inhibitors are given once a day.

EVALUATION
See Chapter 19.

DRUG CLASS: Fatty Oxidase Enzyme Inhibitor

A **fatty oxidase enzyme inhibitor** is a drug that reduces the oxygen needed by myocardial cells to cause muscle contractions. The oxygen demand is reduced. Thus symptoms of angina are reduced.

The following drug is a fatty oxidase enzyme inhibitor:
- ranolazine (ran' ol ah zeen); Ranexa (ran' x ah)

The drug does not affect blood pressure or heart rate. It is used with a calcium channel blocker, a beta blocker, or nitrates. The goals of therapy are to:
- Decrease the frequency of angina attacks
- Decrease the severity of angina attacks
- Increase activity and exercise tolerance
- Reduce the use of nitroglycerin in anginal attacks

Assisting With the Nursing Process

When giving ranolazine (Ranexa), you assist the nurse with the nursing process.

ASSESSMENT
Ask the nurse if measurements are needed.

PLANNING
The oral dose form is 500 mg extended-release tablets.

IMPLEMENTATION

- The usual adult dose is 500 mg twice a day. It may be increased to 1000 mg twice daily.
- The drug may be taken with or without meals.
- Tablets should be swallowed whole. They should not be broken, crushed, or chewed.

EVALUATION

Report and record:

- *Dizziness, headache, constipation, nausea.* These are usually mild. The person should not drive, operate machines, or engage in activities that require mental alertness until it is known how he or she will react to the drug.

PERIPHERAL VASCULAR DISEASE

Peripheral vascular disease (PVD) involves the blood vessels in the arms and legs (extremities). They can be arterial or venous in origin.

- *Deep vein thrombosis.* This is a venous disorder. See Chapter 23.
- *Arteriosclerosis obliterans. Arterio* means *artery. Sclerosis* means *hardening. Obliterans* means *to narrow or close.* It results from atherosclerosis (Chapter 18) of the lower aorta and major arteries supplying the legs. There is gradual narrowing of the arteries with thrombus (clot) formation. Cholesterol, hypertension, smoking, and diabetes are causes. Symptoms occur when there is significant narrowing (75% or more) of the major arteries and arterioles in the legs. Blood flow is obstructed. Tissues do not get needed oxygen. The pain pattern is usually described as aching, cramping, tightness, or weakness in the calves usually during walking. It is relieved with rest. This is called **intermittent claudication.** *Intermittent* means *to come and go. Claudication* means *limping.* As the disease progresses, the person may have pain at rest, numbness, and tingling. Gangrene is a risk.
- *Raynaud's disease.* Exposure to cold or strong emotions trigger blood vessel spasms—vaso-spasms. A **vaso-spasm** is a sudden contraction of a blood vessel causing vaso-constriction. In Raynaud's disease, vaso-spasms obstruct blood flow to fingers, toes, ears, and nose. The disease is more common in women than in men. Risk factors include arterial diseases, repeated trauma (such as vibrations caused by typing, playing the piano, using air-hammers), some drugs, strong emotions, and exposure to cold. The fingers, toes, ears, or nose become white from the lack of blood flow. Then they turn blue—tiny blood vessels dilate to allow more blood to stay in the tissues. When blood flow returns, the area becomes red. Later it returns to normal color. Swelling, tingling, and painful throbbing may occur.

BOX 21-3 **Treatment of Peripheral Vascular Disease**

ARTERIOSCLEROSIS OBLITERANS
- Control of existing diseases (diabetes, hypertension, angina, high cholesterol)
- Weight control
- Daily exercise (usually walking)
- Proper foot care:
  - Feet are kept warm and dry.
  - Shoes fit properly.
- Avoiding cold
- Raising the head of the bed 12 to 16 inches
- Medical or surgical procedures to improve blood flow

RAYNAUD'S DISEASE
- Avoiding cold temperatures
- Avoiding emotional stress
- Avoiding tobacco use
- Keeping the hands and feet warm with gloves and socks
- Using foam "wrap arounds" when handling iced beverages

Attacks last from minutes to hours. As the disease progresses, the fingers become thin and tapered with smooth, shiny skin. Ulcers and gangrene may occur if an artery becomes completely blocked.

See Box 21-3 for the treatment of arteriosclerosis obliterans and Raynaud's disease. Some persons need drug therapy. The goals of treatment are to:

- Reverse disease progression
- Improve blood flow
- Provide pain relief
- Prevent skin ulcers and gangrene

DRUG CLASS: **Hemorrheologic Agent**

Hemorrheologic relates to the science *(logic)* of blood *(hemo)* flow *(rrheo).* A **hemorrheologic agent** prevents the clumping of red blood cells and platelets. Blood flow to small vessels increases. They receive more oxygen.

The following drug is a hemorrheologic agent:

- pentoxifylline (pen tox e' fi leen); Trental (tren' tahl)

Pentoxifylline (Trental) is used to treat intermittent claudication. It is used along with the measures listed in Box 21-3. The goals of therapy are to:

- Improve the blood and oxygen supply to tissues
- Reduce the frequency of pain
- Improve exercise tolerance
- Improve pulses in the legs

Assisting With the Nursing Process

When giving pentoxifylline (Trental), you assist the nurse with the nursing process.

ASSESSMENT

- Ask about nausea, vomiting, indigestion, or poor tolerance to caffeine products (coffee, tea, chocolate, colas).
- Ask about dizziness or headache.
- Ask about cardiac symptoms.
- Ask the person to rate his or her pain. Use a pain rating scale. (See Chapter 17.)

PLANNING

The oral dose form is 400 mg extended-release tablets.

IMPLEMENTATION

- The usual adult dose is 400 mg 3 times a day.
- If adverse effects occur, the dosage is reduced. Or the drug is discontinued.
- Give the drug with food or milk if directed to do so by the nurse or the MAR.

EVALUATION

Report and record:

- *Nausea, vomiting, indigestion.* These are usually mild and tend to resolve with continued therapy.
- *Dizziness, headache.* These are usually mild and tend to resolve with continued therapy. Provide for safety. Have the person sit or lie down if he or she feels faint.
- *Chest pain, dysrhythmias, shortness of breath.* These signal a cardiac event. Tell the nurse at once.
- *Nausea, tachycardia.* These may signal intolerance to other drugs or caffeine.

DRUG CLASS: Vaso-Dilators

Vaso-dilators are drugs that widen blood vessels to increase blood flow. Vaso-dilators used to treat PVD are:

- isoxsuprine hydrochloride (i sok' su preen); Vasodilan (vas o dy' lan)
- papaverine hydrochloride (pah pav' er in); Pavagen TD (pah vah' jen TD)
- phenoxybenzamine hydrochloride (fen ok se ben' zah meen); Dibenzyline (di ben' zi leen)

The goals of therapy are to:

- Improve the blood and oxygen supply to tissues
- Reduce the frequency of pain
- Improve exercise tolerance
- Improve pulses in the legs

isoxsuprine hydrochloride (Vasodilan)

Isoxsuprine (Vasodilan) causes vaso-dilation of the smooth muscles of blood vessels. It is used to treat symptoms of peripheral vascular spasm, Raynaud's disease, arteriosclerosis obliterans, and other PVDs.

Assisting With the Nursing Process

When giving isoxsuprine (Vasodilan), you assist the nurse with the nursing process.

ASSESSMENT

- Ask the person to rate his or her pain. Use a pain rating scale. (See Chapter 17.)
- Measure vital signs.

PLANNING

The oral dose forms are 10 and 20 mg tablets.

IMPLEMENTATION

The usual adult dose is 10 to 20 mg three or four times a day.

EVALUATION

Report and record:

- *Flushing, tingling, sweating, nausea, vomiting.* These tend to resolve with continued therapy.
- *Hypotension, tachycardia.* Provide for safety. Remind the person to rise slowly from a supine or sitting position. Remind the person to perform exercises to prevent blood pooling when standing or sitting in one position for a long time. Have the person sit or lie down if he or she feels faint.
- *Rash.* Tell the nurse at once. Check with the nurse before giving the next dose.
- *Nervousness, weakness.* These may develop as therapy progresses.

papaverine hydrochloride (Pavagen TD)

Papaverine hydrochloride (Pavagen TD) relaxes smooth muscles. Coronary and cerebral blood vessels dilate. The drug also inhibits premature atrial contractions, premature ventricular contractions, and ventricular dysrhythmias (Chapter 20).

Assisting With the Nursing Process

When giving papaverine hydrochloride (Pavagen TD), you assist the nurse with the nursing process.

ASSESSMENT

- Ask the person to rate his or her pain. Use a pain rating scale. (See Chapter 17.)
- Measure vital signs.

PLANNING

The oral dose form is 150 mg time-released capsules.

IMPLEMENTATION

The usual adult dose is 150 mg every 8 hours or 300 mg every 12 hours.

EVALUATION

Report and record:

- *Flushing, sweating, nausea, abdominal distress, tachycardia, dizziness, drowsiness, headache.* These are usually mild and dose related. Measure vital signs.

phenoxybenzamine hydrochloride (Dibenzyline)

Phenoxybenzamine hydrochloride (Dibenzyline) relaxes smooth muscles of blood vessels. It results in vaso-dilation and improved blood flow to peripheral tissues.

Assisting With the Nursing Process

When giving phenoxybenzamine (Dibenzyline), you assist the nurse with the nursing process.

ASSESSMENT

- Ask the person to rate his or her pain. Use a pain rating scale. (See Chapter 17.)
- Measure vital signs.

PLANNING

The oral dose form is 10 mg capsules.

IMPLEMENTATION

- The initial adult dose is 10 mg per day.
- After 4 or more days, the dose is increased 10 mg every few days to a maximum of 60 mg per day.
- Several weeks of therapy are usually required to observe the full effect.

EVALUATION

Report and record:

- *Nasal congestion, pinpoint pupils, hypotension, tachycardia.* Measure blood pressure and pulse. Provide for safety. Remind the person to rise slowly from a supine or sitting position. Remind the person to perform exercises to prevent blood pooling when standing or sitting in one position for a long time. Have the person sit or lie down if he or she feels faint.

DRUG CLASS: **Platelet Aggregation Inhibitor**

Platelets are needed for blood clotting. To aggregate means to clump. A **platelet aggregation inhibitor** prevents platelets from clumping together. It also causes vaso-dilation.

The following drug is a platelet aggregation inhibitor:

- cilostazol (sigh lo stay′ zohl); Pletal (pleh′ tahl)
  Cilostazol (Pletal) is used in the treatment of intermittent claudication. It is used along with the measures listed in Box 21-3. The goals of therapy are to:
- Improve the blood and oxygen supply to tissues
- Reduce the frequency of pain
- Improve exercise tolerance
- Improve pulses in the legs

Assisting With the Nursing Process

When giving cilostazol (Pletal), you assist the nurse with the nursing process.

ASSESSMENT

- Ask about dizziness and headache.
- Ask the person to rate his or her pain. Use a pain rating scale. (See Chapter 17.)
- Ask about cardiac symptoms.

PLANNING

The oral dose forms are 50 and 100 mg tablets.

IMPLEMENTATION

- The usual adult dose is 100 mg two times a day.
- The dose is given 30 minutes before or 2 hours after breakfast and dinner.
- Symptom relief may start within 2 to 4 weeks. It may take 12 weeks for the full effect.

EVALUATION

Report and record:

- *Indigestion, diarrhea.* These are usually mild and tend to resolve with continued therapy.
- *Dizziness, headache.* These are usually mild and tend to resolve with continued therapy. Provide for safety. Remind the person to rise slowly from a supine or sitting position. Have the person sit or lie down if he or she feels faint.
- *Chest pain, palpitations, dysrhythmias, shortness of breath.* These signal a cardiac event. Tell the nurse at once.

HEART FAILURE

Heart failure or congestive heart failure (CHF) occurs when the heart is weakened and cannot pump normally. Blood backs up. Tissue congestion occurs.

When the left side of the heart cannot pump blood normally, blood backs up into the lungs. Respiratory congestion occurs. The person has dyspnea, increased sputum, cough, and gurgling sounds in the lungs. Also, the rest of the body does not get enough blood. Signs and symptoms occur from the effects on other organs. Poor blood flow to the brain causes confusion, dizziness, and fainting. The kidneys produce less urine. The skin is pale. Blood pressure falls.

When the right side of the heart cannot pump blood normally, blood backs up into the venous system. Feet and ankles swell. Neck veins bulge. Liver congestion affects liver function. The abdomen becomes congested with fluid. The right side of the heart pumps less blood to the lungs. Normal blood flow does not occur from the lungs to the left side of the heart. The left side has less blood to pump to the body. As with left-sided heart failure, organs receive less blood. The signs and symptoms occur as described for when the left side fails.

A very severe form of heart failure is *pulmonary edema* (fluid in the lungs). It is an emergency. The person can die.

A damaged or weakened heart usually causes heart failure. CAD, MI, hypertension, age, diabetes, and dysrhythmias (Chapter 20) are common causes. So are damaged heart valves and kidney disease. Treatment involves the cause of the heart failure. Drug therapy is common. The goals of therapy are to:

- Reduce signs and symptoms
- Increase exercise tolerance
- Prolong life

DRUGS USED TO TREAT HEART FAILURE

Heart failure is treated with a combination of vasodilator, inotropic, and diuretic therapy. If failure is acute, most drugs are given intravenously.

- Vaso-dilators widen blood vessels. This reduces the heart's workload. Tissues receive more blood and oxygen. Vaso-dilators also reduce the amount of blood returning to the heart. This decreases lung congestion. The person can breathe more easily.
- Inotropic (in oh troh' pik) agents stimulate the heart to increase the force of contractions. This increases cardiac output (the amount of blood pumped with each heartbeat). Digitalis glycosides are inotropic agents.
- Diuretics are given to increase sodium and water excretion (Chapter 22). This relieves congestion and the heart's workload.

DRUG CLASS: Digitalis Glycosides

Digitalis glycosides are among the oldest agents used to treat heart failure. The only digitalis glycoside currently available for use in the United States is:

- digoxin (di joks' in); Lanoxin (lah noks' in)

Digoxin (Lanoxin) increases the force of heart muscle contraction. It also slows the heart rate. The heart is able to fill and empty more completely. This improves circulation. With improved circulation, swelling in the lungs and tissues is reduced. Heart size returns to normal. Edema lessens because of improved circulation to the kidneys.

The drug is used to treat heart failure that does not respond to diuretics, beta blockers, and ACE inhibitors. It may be used to treat dysrhythmias—atrial fibrillation, atrial flutter, and paroxysmal tachycardia.

Digitalization is giving a larger dose of digoxin for the first 24 hours. Then the person is given a daily dose.

Assisting With the Nursing Process

When giving digoxin (Lanoxin), you assist the nurse with the nursing process.

ASSESSMENT

- Observe for dyspnea, chest pain, fatigue, edema, fainting, palpitations (the person describes palpitations as "my heart skips some beats" or "my heart is racing").
- Measure vital signs: blood pressure, the apical pulse for 1 minute, and respirations.
- Measure daily weight.
- Measure intake and output.

PLANNING

Adult oral dose forms are:

- 0.125 and 0.25 mg tablets
- 0.05, 0.1, and 0.2 mg gelcaps

IMPLEMENTATION

- The adult digitalizing dose is 0.25 to 0.5 mg. It is followed by 0.125 mg every 6 hours until adequate digitalization is achieved.
- The maintenance dose is 0.125 to 0.25 mg daily. Some people need 0.375 to 0.5 mg daily.
- *Measure the apical pulse for 1 minute before giving the drug.* Follow agency policy for withholding the drug. Usually the drug is not given if the pulse is less than 60 or greater than 100 beats per minute.
- The drug is given in very small amounts. If you are allowed to do dose calculations, have a nurse check your calculation. If a pharmacist or nurse did the dose calculation, ask another nurse to check the calculation.
- Give the drug after meals to reduce stomach irritation.

EVALUATION

Report and record:

- *Signs and symptoms of digoxin toxicity.* See Box 21-4.
- *Nausea, vomiting, diarrhea, excessive urinary output.* The person is at risk for low serum potassium levels (hypokalemia).

DRUG CLASS: Angiotensin-Converting Enzyme Inhibitors

Angiotensin-converting enzyme (ACE) inhibitors are discussed in Chapter 19. They are useful in the treatment of heart failure because they:

- Prevent vaso-constriction. Blood pressure is reduced.
- Inhibit aldosterone secretion. Blood volume is reduced.

Assisting With the Nursing Process

See Chapter 19.

BOX 21-4   Signs and Symptoms of Digoxin Toxicity

- Bradycardia
- Tachycardia
- Anorexia
- Nausea
- Vomiting
- Diarrhea
- Fatigue: extreme
- Weakness: arm and leg
- Nightmares
- Agitation
- Listlessness
- Hallucinations
- Vision problems: hazy or blurred vision, problems reading, problems seeing red and green

---

DRUG CLASS: **Beta-Adrenergic Blocking Agents**

Beta-adrenergic blocking agents (beta blockers) are discussed in Chapters 14 and 19. The are useful in the treatment of heart failure because they:

- Lower the heart rate
- Reduce cardiac output
- Lower blood pressure
- Prevent sodium and water retention by blocking renin release

Assisting With the Nursing Process

See Chapter 19.

REVIEW QUESTIONS

Circle the **BEST** answer.

1 Nitrates relieve angina by
  a dilating the coronary arteries
  b lowering the heart rate
  c lowering blood pressure
  d increasing oxygen use

2 Which is the *most* common side effect from nitrates?
  a dizziness   c fainting
  b flushing   d headache

3 Tell the nurse at once after the person takes
  a 1 dose of sublingual nitroglycerin
  b 2 doses of sublingual nitroglycerin
  c 3 doses of sublingual nitroglycerin
  d 4 doses of sublingual nitroglycerin

4 Sustained-released nitroglycerin tablets are taken
  a in the morning before breakfast
  b on an empty stomach every 8 to 12 hours
  c with meals
  d at bedtime

5 The application sites for transdermal disks are rotated
  a daily   c every other day
  b every 8 hours   d weekly

6 A transdermal nitroglycerin disk is dislodged. What should you do?
  a Remove the disk and apply a new one.
  b Re-apply the disk.
  c Leave the disk as is until the next ordered dose.
  d Tape the disk in place.

7 Beta blockers are used to treat angina because they
  a dilate coronary arteries
  b reduce oxygen demands
  c raise blood pressure
  d prevent the clumping of platelets

8 Before giving a beta blocker for angina, you need to measure the person's
  a weight
  b intake and output
  c blood pressure in the supine and standing positions
  d the apical pulse for 30 seconds

9 Calcium channel blockers are used in the treatment of angina. They do the following *except*
  a decrease myocardial oxygen demand
  b dilate the coronary arteries
  c dilate peripheral vessels
  d prevent the clumping of platelets

10 ACE inhibitors are used to prevent
  a CAD   c MI
  b PVD   d peripheral vascular disease

11 Before giving a drug for peripheral vascular disease, you should ask the person
  a to void
  b to rate his or her pain
  c if you can take the apical pulse for 1 minute
  d what application site he or she prefers

Continued

REVIEW QUESTIONS—cont'd

12 Besides dilating blood vessels, ACE inhibitors prevent
   a peripheral vascular disease
   b blood clots
   c atherosclerosis
   d vaso-dilation

13 Intermittent claudication occurs with
   a deep vein thrombosis
   b arteriosclerosis obliterans
   c Raynaud's disease
   d heart failure

14 Pentoxifylline (Trental) is used to treat intermittent claudication. The drug
   a prevents the clumping of red blood cells and platelets
   b reduces oxygen needs
   c dilates blood vessels
   d constricts blood vessels

15 A person taking pentoxifylline (Trental) complains of chest pain and shortness of breath. What should you do?
   a Tell the nurse at once.
   b Have the person take a nitroglycerin tablet.
   c Measure blood pressure in the supine and standing positions.
   d Have the person rest.

16 Which is *not* a vaso-dilator?
   a digoxin (Lanoxin)
   b isoxsuprine (Vasodilan)
   c papaverine hydrochloride (Pavagen TD)
   d phenoxybenzamine (Dibenzyline)

17 A platelet aggregation inhibitor prevents
   a platelet production
   b platelets from clumping
   c the destruction of platelets
   d platelets from splitting

18 Digoxin (Lanoxin) is used in the treatment of heart failure. It
   a prevents vaso-constriction
   b promotes sodium excretion
   c increases the force of heart muscle contraction
   d decreases blood flow to the kidneys

19 The maintenance dose of digoxin (Lanoxin) is usually
   a 0.125 to 0.25 mg daily
   b 0.25 to 0.5 mg daily
   c 1.25 to 2.5 mg daily
   d 2.5 to 5 mg daily

20 ACE inhibitors are used in the treatment of heart failure because they
   a reduce blood pressure and blood volume
   b increase sodium and water retention
   c lower the heart rate
   d increase cardiac output

21 Beta blockers are used in the treatment of heart failure. They do the following *except*
   a reduce blood pressure
   b increase sodium and water retention
   c lower the heart rate
   d reduce cardiac output

Circle T if the statement is true. Circle F if the statement is false.

22 T F Sublingual nitroglycerin should produce a slight stinging or burning sensation.

23 T F Sublingual nitroglycerin is stored in a clear container.

24 T F Sublingual nitroglycerin should be kept within the person's reach.

25 T F The person can eat, drink, and talk with a transmucosal tablet in place.

26 T F Translingual nitroglycerin spray is highly flammable.

27 T F Vaso-dilators are used to treat peripheral vascular disease.

28 T F Pentoxifylline (Trental) should be given with caffeine products.

29 T F Before giving digoxin (Lanoxin) you need to measure the apical pulse for 1 minute.

30 T F Diuretics are used in the treatment of heart failure.

Answers to these questions are on p. 446.

22

Drugs Used for Diuresis

OBJECTIVES

- Define the key terms and key abbreviations used in this chapter.
- Identify the causes of excess fluid in the body.
- Describe the drugs that promote diuresis.
- Explain how to assist with the nursing process when giving drugs to promote diuresis.

KEY TERMS

ascites The abnormal accumulation of fluid in the peritoneal cavity

diuresis The increased formation and excretion of urine; *dia* means *through*, *ur* means *urine*

diuretic A drug that promotes the formation and excretion of urine

KEY ABBREVIATIONS

mg Milligram
mL Milliliter

Diuresis means the increased formation and excretion of urine. (*Dia* means *through. Ur* means *urine.*) A **diuretic** is a drug that promotes the formation and excretion of urine. Diuretics increase the flow of urine. Their purpose is to increase the loss of water from the body. They do so by increasing the excretion of sodium.

Diuretics are used in the treatment of hypertension and heart failure. Diuretics also are used in the treatment of cerebral edema, glaucoma, and liver disease. Ascites may occur with liver disease. **Ascites** is the abnormal accumulation of fluid in the peritoneal cavity (Fig. 22-1). The peritoneum is a two-layer membrane that lines the abdomen. The peritoneal cavity is the space between the layers.

See Box 22-1 for a review of the urinary system.

See *Delegation Guidelines: Drugs Used for Diuresis.*

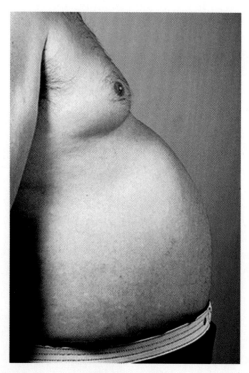

Fig. 22-1 Ascites. (From Lewis and others: *Medical-surgical nursing: assessment and management of clinical problems,* ed 7, St Louis, 2007, Mosby.)

DELEGATION GUIDELINES
Drugs Used for Diuresis

Some drugs used for diuresis are given parenterally—by intramuscular or intravenous injection. Because you do not give parenteral dose forms, they are not included in this chapter. Should a nurse delegate the administration of such to you, you must:

* Remember that parenteral dosages are often very different from dosages for other routes.
* Refuse the delegation. Make sure you explain why. Do not just ignore the request. Make sure the nurse knows that you cannot give the drug and why.

BOX 22-1 The Urinary System: Body Structure and Function

The urinary system (Fig. 22-2):
* Removes waste products from the blood
* Maintains water balance within the body

The *kidneys* are two bean-shaped organs in the upper abdomen. They lie against the back muscles on each side of the spine. They are protected by the lower edge of the rib cage.

Each kidney has over a million tiny *nephrons* (Fig. 22-3). Each nephron is the basic working unit of the kidney. Each nephron has a *convoluted tubule*, which is a tiny coiled tubule. Each convoluted tubule has a *Bowman's capsule* at one end. The capsule partly surrounds a cluster of capillaries called a *glomerulus*. Blood passes through the glomerulus and is filtered by the capillaries. The fluid part of the blood is squeezed into the Bowman's capsule. The fluid then passes into the tubule. Most of the water and other needed substances are re-absorbed by the blood. The rest of the fluid and the waste products form *urine* in the tubule. Urine flows through the tubule to a *collecting tubule*. All collecting tubules drain into the *renal pelvis* in the kidney.

A tube, called the *ureter,* is attached to the renal pelvis of the kidney. Each ureter is about 10 to 12 inches long. The ureters carry urine from the kidneys to the *bladder.* The bladder is a hollow, muscular sac. It lies toward the front in the lower part of the abdominal cavity.

Urine is stored in the bladder until the need to urinate is felt. This usually occurs when there is about a half pint (250 mL) of urine in the bladder. Urine passes from the bladder through the *urethra.* The opening at the end of the urethra is the *meatus.* Urine passes from the body through the meatus. Urine is a clear, yellowish fluid.

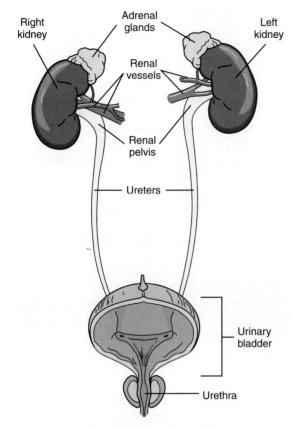

Fig. 22-2 Urinary system.

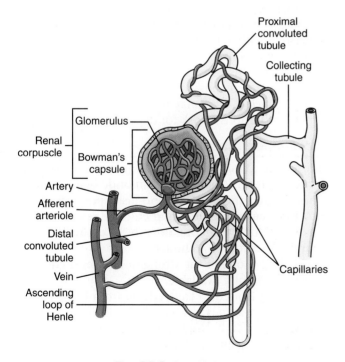

Fig. 22-3 A nephron.

DRUG CLASS: **Loop Diuretics**

The *loop of Henle* is the U-shaped part of a renal tubule (see Fig. 22-3). It has a thin descending limb and a thick ascending limb. Loop diuretics inhibit the re-absorption of sodium and chloride from the ascending loop of Henle.

The following are loop diuretics:
- bumetanide (bu met' an eyd); Bumex (bu' mex)
- ethacrynic acid (eth ah krin' ik); Edecrin (eh' deh krin)
- furosemide (fuhr oh' sah myd); Lasix (lay' siks)
- torsemide (tohr sah' myd); Demadex (dehm' ah dex)

The goals of therapy are to:
- Promote diuresis
- Reduce edema
- Improve symptoms related to excess fluid in tissues

bumetanide (Bumex)

Bumetanide (Bumex) is a strong diuretic. The drug inhibits sodium and chloride re-absorption in the ascending loop of Henle. It also increases blood flow into the glomeruli.

Diuretic activity begins 30 to 60 minutes after administration. It peaks within 1 to 2 hours and lasts 4 to 6 hours.

The drug is used to treat edema from heart failure and liver and kidney diseases.

Assisting With the Nursing Process

When giving bumetanide (Bumex), you assist the nurse with the nursing process.

ASSESSMENT
- Measure vital signs.
- Measure weight daily.
- Measure intake and output.
- Observe alertness and orientation to person, time, and place.
- Observe for confusion.
- Observe muscle strength.
- Observe for tremors.
- Ask about muscle cramps.
- Ask about nausea.
- Measure blood glucose if the person has diabetes.

PLANNING

The oral dose forms are 0.5, 1, and 2 mg tablets.

IMPLEMENTATION

- The initial adult dose is 0.5 to 2 mg given as a single, daily dose.
- Additional doses may be given at 4- to 5-hour intervals.
- The maximum daily dose is 10 mg.
- Give the drug with food or milk to reduce stomach irritation.
- Give the drug before mid-afternoon. This prevents nocturia.

EVALUATION

Report and record:

- *Oral irritation, dry mouth.* Give oral hygiene as directed by the nurse and the care plan. The nurse may allow the person to suck on ice chips or hard candy.
- *Orthostatic hypotension, dizziness, weakness, fainting.* Blood pressure is measured daily in the supine and standing positions. Provide for safety. Remind the person to rise slowly from a supine or sitting position. Have the person sit or lie down if he or she feels faint.
- *Stomach irritation, abdominal pain.* Give the drug with food or milk.
- *Changes in alertness and orientation to person, time, and place; confusion; muscle cramps; nausea.* These may signal dehydration or electrolyte imbalance (potassium, sodium, and chloride).

ethacrynic acid (Edecrin)

Ethacrynic acid (Edecrin) inhibits sodium and chloride re-absorption in the ascending loop of Henle. Diuretic activity begins within 30 minutes. It peaks in about 2 hours and lasts 6 to 8 hours.

The drug is used to treat edema from heart failure, liver disease, kidney disease, and cancer.

Assisting With the Nursing Process

When giving ethacrynic acid (Edecrin), you assist the nurse with the nursing process.

ASSESSMENT

- Measure vital signs.
- Measure weight daily.
- Measure intake and output.
- Observe alertness and orientation to person, time, and place.

- Observe for confusion.
- Observe muscle strength.
- Observe for tremors.
- Ask about muscle cramps.
- Ask about nausea.
- Measure blood glucose if the person has diabetes.

PLANNING

The oral dose forms are 25 and 50 mg tablets.

IMPLEMENTATION

- The initial adult dose is 50 to 100 mg. It is followed by 50 to 200 mg daily.
- The maximum daily dose is 400 mg daily.
- Give the drug with food or milk to reduce stomach irritation.
- Give the drug before mid-afternoon. This prevents nocturia.

EVALUATION

Report and record:

- *Orthostatic hypotension, dizziness, weakness, fainting.* Blood pressure is measured daily in the supine and standing positions. Provide for safety. Remind the person to rise slowly from a supine or sitting position. Have the person sit or lie down if he or she feels faint.
- *Changes in alertness and orientation to person, time, and place; confusion; muscle cramps; nausea.* These may signal dehydration or electrolyte imbalance (potassium, sodium, and chloride).
- *"Coffee ground" vomitus; dark, tarry stools.* These signal gastro-intestinal bleeding.
- *Changes in hearing and balance, deafness, tinnitus.* Persons with impaired kidney function may have these symptoms.
- *Diarrhea.* This may become severe. Dehydration and electrolyte imbalance are risks.
- *Hyperglycemia.* This may occur in persons with diabetes or persons at risk for diabetes.

furosemide (Lasix)

Furosemide (Lasix) acts on the ascending loop of Henle to prevent sodium and chloride re-absorption. It also acts on the proximal and distal portions of the tubule to prevent sodium and chloride re-absorption. Maximum effect from oral dose forms occurs in 1 to 2 hours. It lasts for 4 to 6 hours.

The drug is one of the strongest and most effective diuretics currently available.

The drug is used to treat edema from heart failure and liver and kidney diseases. It is also used to treat hypertension. It is used alone or with other anti-hypertensive agents.

Assisting With the Nursing Process

When giving furosemide (Lasix), you assist the nurse with the nursing process.

ASSESSMENT

- Measure vital signs.
- Measure weight daily.
- Measure intake and output.
- Observe alertness and orientation to person, time, and place.
- Observe for confusion.
- Observe muscle strength.
- Observe for tremors.
- Ask about muscle cramps.
- Ask about nausea.
- Measure blood glucose if the person has diabetes.
- Observe for signs of hearing loss.

PLANNING

The oral dose forms are:

- 20, 40, and 80 mg tablets
- 10 mg/mL and 40 mg/5 mL oral solution

IMPLEMENTATION

- *Persons allergic to sulfonamides* (Chapter 34) *may also be allergic to furosemide (Lasix).*
- The adult dose is 20 to 80 mg given as a single dose.
- If a second dose is needed, it is given 6 to 8 hours later.
- The dose is increased 20 to 40 mg per day.
- The drug is usually given in the morning.
- Give the drug with food or milk to reduce stomach irritation.

EVALUATION

Report and record:

- *Oral irritation, dry mouth.* Give oral hygiene as directed by the nurse and the care plan. The nurse may allow the person to suck on ice chips or hard candy.
- *Orthostatic hypotension, dizziness, weakness, fainting.* Blood pressure is measured daily in the supine and standing positions. Provide for safety. Remind the person to rise slowly from a supine or sitting position. Have the person sit or lie down if he or she feels faint.
- *Changes in alertness and orientation to person, time, and place; confusion; muscle cramps; nausea.* These may signal dehydration or electrolyte imbalance (potassium, sodium, and chloride).
- *Hyperglycemia.* This may occur in persons with diabetes or persons at risk for diabetes.
- *Hives, rash, itching.* These may signal an allergic reaction. Tell the nurse at once. Do not give the next dose unless approved by the nurse.

torsemide (Demadex)

Torsemide (Demadex) acts on the ascending loop of Henle to prevent sodium and chloride re-absorption. Maximum effect from oral dose forms occurs in 1 to 2 hours. It lasts for 6 to 8 hours.

The drug is used to treat edema from heart failure and liver and kidney diseases. It is also used to treat hypertension. It is used alone or with other antihypertensive agents.

Assisting With the Nursing Process

When giving torsemide (Demadex), you assist the nurse with the nursing process.

ASSESSMENT

- Measure vital signs.
- Measure weight daily.
- Measure intake and output.
- Observe alertness and orientation to person, time, and place.
- Observe for confusion.
- Observe muscle strength.
- Observe for tremors.
- Ask about muscle cramps.
- Ask about nausea.
- Measure blood glucose if the person has diabetes.
- Observe for signs of hearing loss.

PLANNING

The oral dose forms are 5, 10, 20, and 100 mg tablets.

IMPLEMENTATION

- *Persons allergic to sulfonamides* (Chapter 34) *may also be allergic to torsemide (Demadex).*
- The initial adult dose is 5 to 20 mg once daily.
- The dose may be doubled until the desired response is achieved.

EVALUATION

Report and record:

- *Oral irritation, dry mouth.* Give oral hygiene as directed by the nurse and the care plan. The nurse may allow the person to suck on ice chips or hard candy.
- *Orthostatic hypotension, dizziness, weakness, fainting.* Blood pressure is measured daily in the supine and standing positions. Provide for safety. Remind the person to rise slowly from a supine or sitting position. Have the person sit or lie down if he or she feels faint.
- *Changes in alertness and orientation to person, time, and place; confusion; muscle cramps; nausea.* These may signal dehydration or electrolyte imbalance (potassium, sodium, and chloride).
- *Hyperglycemia.* This may occur in persons with diabetes or persons at risk for diabetes.
- *Hives, rash, itching.* These may signal an allergic reaction. Tell the nurse at once. Do not give the next dose unless approved by the nurse.

DRUG CLASS: **Thiazide Diuretics**

Thiazide diuretics act on the distal tubules to block the re-absorption of sodium and chloride. The sodium and chloride that are not re-absorbed take water with them. This results in diuresis.

Thiazides are used in the treatment of edema from:
- Heart failure
- Kidney disease
- Liver disease
- Pregnancy
- Obesity
- Pre-menstrual syndrome
- The administration of cortico-steroids (Chapter 28)

Thiazides also have anti-hypertensive effects. They cause vaso-dilation of peripheral arterioles.

The goals of therapy are to:
- Promote diuresis
- Reduce edema
- Improve symptoms related to excess fluid in tissues
- Reduce blood pressure

Assisting With the Nursing Process

When giving thiazides, you assist the nurse with the nursing process.

ASSESSMENT
- Measure vital signs.
- Measure weight daily.
- Measure intake and output.
- Observe alertness and orientation to person, time, and place.
- Observe for confusion.
- Observe muscle strength.
- Observe for tremors.
- Ask about muscle cramps.
- Ask about nausea.
- Measure blood glucose if the person has diabetes.
- Observe for signs of hearing loss.

PLANNING
See Tables 22-1 and 22-2 for "Oral Dose Forms."

IMPLEMENTATION
- See Tables 22-1 and 22-2 for "Adult Dosage Range."
- Give the drug before mid-afternoon. This prevents nocturia.
- For hypertension: most of the diuretics listed are given in divided doses.
- For edema: most of the diuretics listed are given in single daily doses.

TABLE 22-1 Thiazide Diuretic Products

GENERIC NAME	BRAND NAME	ORAL DOSE FORMS	ADULT DOSAGE RANGE
bendroflumethiazide	Naturetin	Tablets: 5, 10 mg	2.5-15 mg
chlorothiazide	Diuril	Tablets: 250, 500 mg Oral suspension: 250 mg/5 mL	1000-2000 mg
hydrochlorothiazide	Esidrix, HydroDiuril, Oretic	Tablets: 25, 50, 100 mg Capsules: 12.5 mg Solution: 50 mg/5 mL	12.5-100 mg
hydroflumethiazide		Tablets: 50 mg	25-100 mg
methyclothiazide	Enduron	Tablets: 2.5, 5 mg	2.5-5 mg
polythiazide		Tablets: 1, 2, 4, mg	1-4 mg

TABLE 22-2 Thiazide-Related Diuretics

GENERIC NAME	BRAND NAME	ORAL DOSE FORMS	ADULT DOSAGE RANGE
chlorthalidone	Hygroton, Thalitone	Tablets: 15, 25, 50, 100 mg	50-200 mg
indapamide	Lozol	Tablets: 1.25, 2.5 mg	2.5-5 mg
metolazone	Zaroxolyn, Mykrox	Tablets: 0.5, 2.5, 5, 10 mg	2.5-10 mg

EVALUATION

Report and record:

- *Orthostatic hypotension, dizziness, weakness, fainting.* Blood pressure is measured daily in the supine and standing positions. Provide for safety. Remind the person to rise slowly from a supine or sitting position. Have the person sit or lie down if he or she feels faint.
- *Stomach irritation, nausea, vomiting, constipation.* Give the drug with food or milk if stomach irritation occurs.
- *Changes in alertness and orientation to person, time, and place; confusion; muscle cramps; nausea.* These may signal dehydration or electrolyte imbalance (potassium, sodium, and chloride).
- *Hyperglycemia.* This may occur in persons with diabetes or persons at risk for diabetes.
- *Hives, rash, itching.* These may signal an allergic reaction. Tell the nurse at once. Do not give the next dose unless approved by the nurse.

DRUG CLASS:
Potassium-Sparing Diuretics

Potassium-sparing diuretics excrete sodium but retain potassium. The following are potassium-sparing diuretics:

- amiloride (ah mihl′ or eyd); Midamor (my′ da mor)
- spironolactone (spy ro no lak′ tone); Aldactone (al dak′ tone)
- triamterene (try am′ ter een); Dyrenium (dy reen′ ee um)

amiloride (Midamor)

Amiloride (Midamor) acts on the distal renal tubule to retain potassium and excrete sodium. Diuresis is mild. The drug has weak anti-hypertensive effects.

The drug is used with other diuretics to treat hypertension or heart failure. The goals of therapy are to:

- Reduce edema
- Improve symptoms related to excess fluid in tissues

Assisting With the Nursing Process

When giving amiloride (Midamor), you assist the nurse with the nursing process.

ASSESSMENT

- Measure vital signs.
- Measure weight daily.
- Measure intake and output.
- Observe alertness and orientation to person, time, and place.
- Observe for confusion.
- Observe muscle strength.
- Observe for tremors.

- Ask about muscle cramps.
- Ask about nausea.

PLANNING

The oral dose form is 5 mg tablets.

IMPLEMENTATION

- The initial adult dose is 5 mg daily.
- Dosages may be increased by 5 mg to achieve a maximum daily dose of 20 mg.
- Give the drug with food or milk to reduce stomach irritation.
- Give the drug before mid-afternoon. This prevents nocturia.

EVALUATION

Report and record:

- *Anorexia, nausea, vomiting, flatulence.* These should be mild if the drug is given with food.
- *Headache.* Measure blood pressure.
- *Changes in alertness and orientation to person, time, and place; confusion; muscle cramps; nausea.* These may signal dehydration or electrolyte imbalance (potassium, sodium, and chloride).

spironolactone (Aldactone)

Spironolactone (Aldactone) blocks the sodium-retaining properties of aldosterone (Chapter 19). It blocks potassium and magnesium excretion caused by aldosterone. Sodium and water are excreted.

The drug is useful in relieving edema and ascites that do not respond to the usual diuretics. The drug may be given with other diuretics. The goals of therapy are to:

- Reduce edema
- Improve symptoms related to excess fluid in tissues
- Improve symptoms from heart failure

Assisting With the Nursing Process

When giving spironolactone (Aldactone), you assist the nurse with the nursing process.

ASSESSMENT

- Measure vital signs.
- Measure weight daily.
- Measure intake and output.
- Observe alertness and orientation to person, time, and place.
- Observe for confusion.
- Observe muscle strength.
- Observe for tremors.
- Ask about muscle cramps.
- Ask about nausea.

PLANNING

The oral dose forms are 25, 50, and 100 mg tablets.

IMPLEMENTATION

- The initial adult dose is 50 to 100 mg daily.
- The maintenance dose is usually 100 to 200 mg daily. Some persons need up to 400 mg daily.

- Give the drug with food or milk to reduce stomach irritation.
- Give the drug before mid-afternoon. This prevents nocturia.

EVALUATION

Report and record:

- *Confusion.* Provide for safety.
- *Headache.* Measure blood pressure.
- *Diarrhea.* Note the number and consistency of stools.
- *Changes in alertness and orientation to person, time, and place; confusion; muscle cramps; nausea.* These may signal dehydration or electrolyte imbalance (potassium, sodium, and chloride).
- *Breasts may enlarge in men; breast tenderness and menstrual irregularities in women.* These reverse when therapy is discontinued.

triamterene (Dyrenium)

Triamterene (Dyrenium) is a mild diuretic. It blocks the exchange of potassium for sodium in the distal tubules. Potassium is retained. Sodium and water are excreted through the urine.

The drug is used with potassium-excreting diuretics—thiazides and loop diuretics. The goals of therapy are to:

- Cause diuresis
- Improve symptoms related to excess fluid in tissues

Assisting With the Nursing Process

When giving triamterene (Dyrenium), you assist the nurse with the nursing process.

ASSESSMENT

- Measure vital signs.
- Measure weight daily.
- Measure intake and output.

- Observe alertness and orientation to person, time, and place.
- Observe for confusion.
- Observe muscle strength.
- Observe for tremors.
- Ask about muscle cramps.
- Ask about nausea.

PLANNING

The oral dose forms are 50 and 100 mg tablets.

IMPLEMENTATION

The adult dose is 50 to 150 mg two times a day.

EVALUATION

Report and record:

- *Changes in alertness and orientation to person, time, and place; confusion; muscle cramps; nausea.* These may signal dehydration or electrolyte imbalance (potassium, sodium, and chloride).
- *Hives, rash, itching.* These may signal an allergic reaction. Tell the nurse at once. Do not give the next dose unless approved by the nurse.

DRUG CLASS:
Combination Diuretic Products

Low potassium (hypokalemia) is a common problem with thiazide diuretics. Several products contain a potassium-sparing diuretic with a thiazide diuretic (Table 22-3). The goal is to promote diuresis and antihypertensive effects while maintaining normal potassium levels.

Persons receiving a combination product are at risk for side effects from each of the drugs in the product. High potassium and low sodium levels have been reported.

TABLE 22-3 Combination Diuretics		
GENERIC NAME	BRAND NAME	ADULT DOSAGE RANGE
spironolactone 25 mg, hydrochlorothiazide 25 mg	Aldactazide	1-8 tablets daily
spironolactone 50 mg, hydrochlorothiazide 50 mg	Aldactazide	1-4 tablets daily
triamterene 37.5 mg, hydrochlorothiazide 25 mg	Dyazide	1 or 2 capsules twice daily after meals
triamterene 37.5 mg, hydrochlorothiazide 25 mg	Maxzide-25	1 or 2 tablets daily after meals
triamterene 75 mg, hydrochlorothiazide 50 mg	Maxzide	1 tablet daily
amiloride 5 mg, hydrochlorothiazide 50 mg	Moduretic	1 or 2 tablets daily with meals

REVIEW QUESTIONS

Circle the **BEST** answer.

1 Diuretics increase water loss from the body by
a increasing sodium excretion
b increasing sodium retention
c decreasing potassium excretion
d increasing potassium retention

2 Ascites occurs from
a kidney disease
b liver disease
c cerebral edema
d hypertension

3 Loop diuretics inhibit the re-absorption of
a sodium
b potassium
c aldosterone
d renin

4 Which is *not* a loop diuretic?
a furosemide (Lasix)
b ethacrynic acid (Edecrin)
c bumetanide (Bumex)
d chlorthalidone (Hygroton)

5 Which is *not* a thiazide diuretic?
a chlorothiazide (Diuril)
b hydrochlorothiazide (HydroDiuril)
c methyclothiazide (Enduron)
d spironolactone (Aldactone)

6 The effects of loop diuretics last about
a 30 minutes
b 1 hour
c 4 hours
d 6 hours

7 Which diuretics are used in the treatment of obesity, pregnancy, and pre-menstrual syndrome?
a loop diuretics
b thiazide diuretics
c potassium-sparing diuretics
d combination diuretic products

8 Diuretics are given
a at 0500
b before lunch
c before mid-afternoon
d at bedtime

9 Which may signal dehydration and electrolyte imbalance from diuretics?
a stomach irritation
b changes in alertness and confusion
c dry mouth
d orthostatic hypotension

10 Potassium-sparing diuretics
a retain potassium
b excrete potassium
c retain sodium
d excrete aldosterone

11 Which is *not* a potassium-sparing diuretic?
a amiloride (Midamor)
b spironolactone (Aldactone)
c triamterene (Dyrenium)
d spironolactone, hydrochlorothiazide (Aldactazide)

12 Which is a combination diuretic?
a Dyazide
b Lozol
c Naqua
d Oretic

Answers to these questions are on p. 446.

23

Drugs Used to Treat Thrombo-Embolic Diseases

OBJECTIVES

- Define the key terms and key abbreviations listed in this chapter.
- Describe thrombo-embolic diseases.
- Describe the drugs used to treat thrombo-embolic diseases.
- Explain how to assist with the nursing process when giving drugs to treat thrombo-embolic diseases.

KEY TERMS

anti-coagulants Drugs that prevent arterial and venous thrombi; "blood thinners"

anti-platelet agents See "platelet inhibitors"

embolus A small part of a thrombus that breaks off and travels through the vascular system until it lodges in a blood vessel

infarction A local area of tissue death

ischemia A decreased supply of oxygenated blood to a body part

platelet inhibitors Drugs that prevent platelet aggregation (clumping); anti-platelet agents

thrombosis The process of clot formation

thrombo-embolic diseases Diseases associated with abnormal clotting within blood vessels

thrombus A blood clot

KEY ABBREVIATIONS

GI Gastro-intestinal
IV Intravenous
mg Milligram
MI Myocardial infarction
TED hose Thrombo-embolic disease hose
TIA Transient ischemic attack

Thrombosis is the process of clot formation. A **thrombus** is a blood clot (Fig. 23-1, *A*). An **embolus** is a small part of a thrombus that breaks off and travels through the vascular system until it lodges in a blood vessel (Fig. 23-1, *B*). Pulmonary embolism and cerebral embolism are examples. An embolus causes ischemia or infarction to the area below the obstruction:

- **Ischemia** is a decreased supply of oxygenated blood to a body part. The person has pain. Involved organs and tissues cannot function properly.
- **Infarction** is a local area of tissue death (Fig. 23-2).

Diseases associated with abnormal clotting within blood vessels are known as **thrombo-embolic diseases.** Major causes of thrombosis are:

- Immobility with venous stasis (slowed blood flow through a vein)
- Surgery and the post-operative period
- Leg trauma
- Heart failure
- Vaso-spasm
- Cancer—lung, prostate, stomach, and pancreas
- Pregnancy
- Contraceptive agents (Chapter 29)
- Heredity

Diseases caused by clotting within blood vessels are major causes of death. They include:

- Deep vein thrombosis
- Myocardial infarction (MI)
- Dysrhythmias with clot formation
- Coronary artery spasm leading to clot formation
- See Box 23-1 on p. 294 for the methods used to treat thrombo-embolic disease.

See *Delegation Guidelines: Drugs Used to Treat Thrombo-Embolic Disorders* on p. 295.

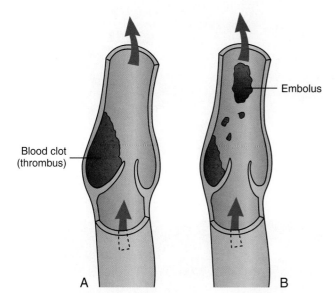

Fig. 23-1 A, A blood clot is attached to the wall of a vein. The arrow shows the direction of blood flow. **B,** Part of the thrombus breaks off and becomes an embolus. The embolus travels in the bloodstream until it lodges in a distant vessel.

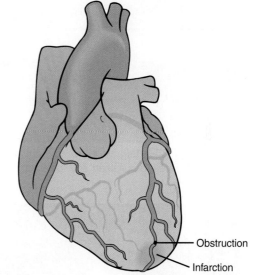

Fig. 23-2 Myocardial infarction. (Modified from Lewis SM and others: *Medical-surgical nursing: assessment and management of clinical problems*, ed 7, St Louis, 2007, Mosby.)

BOX 23-1 Treatment of Thrombo-Embolic Diseases

PREVENTION
- Leg exercises (Fig. 23-3).
- Leg elevation.
- Early ambulation after surgery.
- Turning and repositioning at least every 2 hours.
- No standing or sitting for prolonged periods.
- Thrombo-embolic disease hose (TED hose). See Figure 23-4.
- Sequential compression device (Fig. 23-5). This device is wrapped around the leg and is secured in place with Velcro. The device is attached to a pump. The pump inflates the device with air. This promotes venous blood flow to the heart by causing pressure on the veins. Then the pump deflates the device. After deflation, the device is inflated again. The inflation and deflation sequence is repeated as ordered by the doctor.

PROCEDURES TO RE-OPEN THE BLOOD VESSEL
- *Thrombolytic agents. Thrombo* means *clot. Lytic* means *to produce decomposition.* Thrombolytic agents are used to dissolve the clot.
- *Angioplasty. Angio* means *blood vessel. Plasty* means *to mold.* A balloon-tipped catheter is inserted into a coronary artery. The balloon is repeatedly inflated and deflated to stretch and open the artery.
- *Stents.* A *stent* is a wire-mesh tube inserted after angioplasty. It is placed to keep obstructed areas open. The stent stays in the artery.
- *Coronary artery bypass graft* (Fig. 23-6). A leg vein or an artery from the chest or wrist is used to bypass the obstructed area. This is commonly known as "bypass surgery."

DRUG THERAPY
- Platelet inhibitors.
- Anti-coagulants (p. 297).

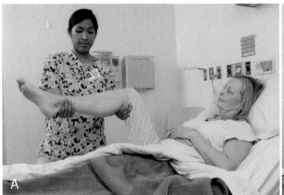
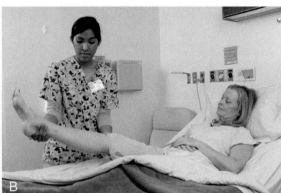

Fig. 23-3 Leg exercises to stimulate circulation. **A,** The knee is flexed and then extended. **B,** The leg is raised and lowered.

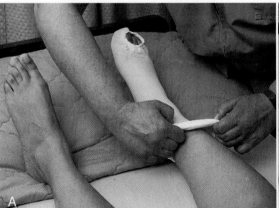
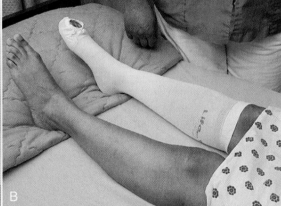

Fig. 23-4 Applying TED hose. **A,** The stocking is slipped over the toes, foot, and heel. **B,** The stocking turns right side out as it is pulled up over the leg.

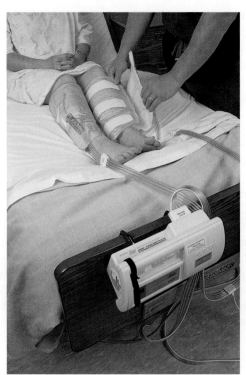

Fig. 23-5 Sequential compression device. (From deWit SC: *Fundamental concepts and skills for nursing,* ed 2, Philadelphia, 2005, Saunders.)

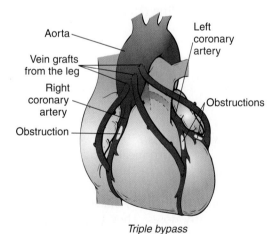

Triple bypass

Fig. 23-6 Coronary artery bypass graft. (Modified from Thibodeau GA, Patton KT: *The human body in health and disease,* ed 4, St Louis, 2005, Mosby.)

DELEGATION GUIDELINES
Drugs Used to Treat
Thrombo-Embolic Disorders

Some drugs used to treat thrombo-embolic disorders are given parenterally—by subcutaneous or intravenous injection. Because you do not give parenteral dose forms, they are not included in this chapter. Should a nurse delegate the administration of such to you, you must:

- Remember that parenteral dosages are often very different from dosages for other routes.
- Refuse the delegation. Make sure you explain why. Do not just ignore the request. Make sure the nurse knows that you cannot give the drug and why.

DRUG CLASS: **Platelet Inhibitors**

Platelet inhibitors also are called **anti-platelet agents.** They prevent platelet aggregation (clumping). They are used to reduce arterial clot formation. The following are platelet inhibitors:

- aspirin (as' per in)
- dipyridamole (dye per id' a mole); Persantine (per sahn' teen)
- clopidogrel (clo pid' oh grel); Plavix (plah' vix)
- ticlopidine (ty cloh' ped een); Ticlid (ty' clid)

aspirin

Aspirin is used to relieve pain, fever, and inflammation (Chapter 17). It also inhibits platelet clumping and prolongs bleeding time. The platelet loses its ability to clump and form clots for the duration of its life-time. Platelets live 7 to 10 days.

Aspirin is used to reduce the risk of MI in persons with a previous MI or persons who have angina (Chapter 21). It also is used to reduce the risk of re-current transient ischemic attacks and stroke caused by blood clots.

- *Transient ischemic attack (TIA). Transient* means temporary or short-term. *Ischemic* means to hold back *(ischein)* blood *(hemic).* Blood supply to the brain is interrupted for a short time. Sometimes a TIA occurs before a stroke.
- *Stroke.* Stroke is a disease that affects the arteries that supply blood to the brain. It occurs when a blood clot blocks blood flow to the brain. Another cause is when a blood vessel in the brain bursts. Bleeding occurs in the brain (cerebral hemorrhage). Brain cells in the affected area do not get enough oxygen and nutrients. Brain cells die. Brain damage occurs. Functions controlled by that part of the brain are lost.

The goals of therapy are to:

- Reduce the frequency of TIA
- Reduce the frequency of stroke
- Reduce the frequency of MI

Assisting With the Nursing Process

When giving aspirin, you assist the nurse with the nursing process.

ASSESSMENT

- Observe alertness and orientation to person, time, and place.
- Observe the person's balance.
- Observe the person's hearing.
- Observe hand strength.
- Test stools for occult blood.

PLANNING

See Table 17-2 (Chapter 17).

IMPLEMENTATION

- To prevent blood clots, the oral adult dose is usually 81 to 325 mg daily.
- Larger doses may be given. They are usually divided into 325 mg in 2, 3, or 4 doses daily.
- The dose depends on the person's history of clot formation and other drugs the person is taking.
- Give the drug with meals to prevent stomach irritation.

EVALUATION

See Chapter 17.

dipyridamole (Persantine)

Dipyridamole (Persantine) prevents excessive blood clotting. It is used with other drugs to reduce the risk of blood clots after heart valve replacement.

Assisting With the Nursing Process

When giving dipyridamole (Persantine), you assist the nurse with the nursing process.

ASSESSMENT

Measure vital signs.

PLANNING

The oral dose forms are 25, 50, and 75 mg tablets.

IMPLEMENTATION

The usual adult dose is 75 to 100 mg four times a day with warfarin. Or 75 mg is given 3 or 4 times a day with aspirin.

EVALUATION

Report and record:

- *Dizziness, abdominal distress*. These tend to resolve with continued therapy. Observe for orthostatic hypotension. Measure blood pressure in the supine and standing positions. Provide for safety. Remind the person to rise slowly from a supine or sitting position. Have the person sit or lie down if he or she feels faint.

clopidogrel (Plavix)

Clopidogrel (Plavix) helps prevent harmful blood clots. It is used to prevent strokes and MIs in persons at risk for such problems.

Assisting With the Nursing Process

When giving clopidogrel (Plavix), you assist the nurse with the nursing process.

ASSESSMENT

- Measure vital signs.
- Ask about gastro-intestinal (GI) symptoms.

PLANNING

The oral dose form is 75 mg tablets.

IMPLEMENTATION

- The adult dose is 75 mg once a day.
- The drug is given with food or on an empty stomach.

EVALUATION

Report and record:

- *Nausea, vomiting, anorexia, diarrhea*. These tend to occur with early doses. They tend to resolve with continued therapy over the next 2 weeks. Give the drug with food.
- *Sore throat, fever, fatigue*. These may signal changes in white blood cells.
- *Bleeding*. This includes nosebleeds, easy bruising, bright red or "coffee ground" emesis, blood in the urine (hematuria), dark tarry stools.

ticlopidine (Ticlid)

Ticlopidine (Ticlid) prevents excessive blood clotting. It is used to prevent stroke in persons with a history of stroke or who are at risk for a stroke.

Assisting With the Nursing Process

When giving ticlopidine (Ticlid), you assist the nurse with the nursing process.

ASSESSMENT

- Measure vital signs.
- Ask about GI symptoms.

PLANNING

The oral dose form is 250 mg tablets.

IMPLEMENTATION

- The usual adult dose is 250 mg two times a day.
- The drug is given with meals.

EVALUATION

Report and record:

- *Nausea, vomiting, anorexia, diarrhea*. These tend to occur with early doses. They tend to resolve with continued therapy over the next 2 weeks. Give the drug with food.
- *Sore throat, fever, fatigue*. These may signal changes in white blood cells.
- *Bleeding*. This includes nosebleeds, easy bruising, bright red or "coffee ground" emesis, blood in the urine (hematuria), dark tarry stools.

DRUG CLASS: **Anti-Coagulants**

Anti-coagulants are used to prevent arterial and venous thrombi. They are often called "blood thinners." The intent is to prevent blood clots from forming or growing larger. They cannot dissolve an existing clot.

Common anti-coagulant drugs are:
- heparin (hep' ahr in). *Heparin is only given subcutaneously and intravenously (IV). You do not give subcutaneous or IV drugs.*
- warfarin (war' fah rin); Coumadin (koo' mah din).

warfarin (Coumadin)

Warfarin (Coumadin) is a very strong anti-coagulant. It inhibits the activity of vitamin K. Vitamin K is needed for blood clotting. The drug is used to prevent:
- Venous thrombosis
- Embolism associated with atrial fibrillation
- Embolism associated with heart valve replacement
- Pulmonary embolism
- MI

Assisting With the Nursing Process

When giving warfarin (Coumadin), you assist the nurse with the nursing process.

ASSESSMENT
- Measure vital signs.
- Check for bleeding. This includes nosebleeds, bleeding gums, bruises, bright red or "coffee ground" emesis, blood in the urine (hematuria), dark tarry stools.
- Ask about GI symptoms.

PLANNING
The oral dose forms are 1, 2, 2.5, 3, 4, 5, 6, 7.5, and 10 mg tablets.

IMPLEMENTATION
- Give the dose only if the nurse instructs you to do so. The nurse checks laboratory prothrombin times before the drug is given.
- The oral dose is usually 10 mg daily for 2 to 4 days.
- The maintenance dose is usually 2 to 10 mg daily.

EVALUATION
Report and record:
- *Bleeding.* This includes nosebleeds, bleeding gums, easy bruising, bright red or "coffee ground" emesis, blood in the urine (hematuria), dark tarry stools.
- *Low blood pressure; rapid pulse; cold, clammy skin; faintness, changes in alertness.* These may signal internal bleeding.

REVIEW QUESTIONS

Circle the **BEST** answer.

1 A blood clot is called
 a ischemia
 b an embolus
 c thrombosis
 d a thrombus

2 A part of a blood clot breaks off and travels in the vascular system. This is called
 a ischemia
 b an embolus
 c thrombosis
 d a thrombus

3 Aspirin is
 a a platelet inhibitor
 b a thrombolytic agent
 c an anti-coagulant
 d a blood thinner

4 Aspirin is used to reduce the frequency of the following *except*
 a TIA
 b MI
 c stroke
 d dysrhythmias

5 Aspirin is given
 a before meals
 b with meals
 c after meals
 d at bedtime

6 Dipyridamole (Persantine) is used after
 a stroke
 b MI
 c heart valve replacement
 d coronary artery bypass surgery

7 Dipyridamole (Persantine) is given with
 a diuretics
 b warfarin (Coumadin)
 c clopidogrel (Plavix)
 d ticlopidine (Ticlid)

8 Clopidogrel (Plavix) is given to prevent
 a stroke and MI
 b angina
 c dysrhythmias
 d heart failure

Continued

REVIEW QUESTIONS—cont'd

9 The adult dose of clopidogrel (Plavix) is
   a 75 mg
   b 80 mg
   c 100 mg
   d 250 mg

10 Ticlopidine (Ticlid) is used to prevent
   a stroke
   b MI
   c angina
   d dysrhythmias

11 Anti-coagulant drugs
   a dissolve clots
   b destroy clots
   c prevent new clots
   d prevent dysrhythmias

12 Coumadin inhibits
   a red blood cell formation
   b vitamin K activity
   c vitamin C activity
   d platelet formation

Circle T if the statement is true. Circle F if the statement is false.

13 T F A person is receiving aspirin. You need to observe for bleeding.

14 T F A person is receiving dipyridamole (Persantine). You need to observe for orthostatic hypotension.

15 T F A person is receiving clopidogrel (Plavix). You need to observe for bleeding.

16 T F Clopidogrel (Plavix) is given with food or on an empty stomach.

17 T F Ticlopidine (Ticlid) is given on an empty stomach.

18 T F You can give heparin.

19 T F Anti-coagulants are often called "blood thinners."

20 T F The nurse tells you when to give warfarin (Coumadin).

Answers to these questions are on p. 446.

24

Drugs Used to Treat Respiratory Diseases

OBJECTIVES

- Define the key terms and key abbreviations used in this chapter.
- Describe the common respiratory diseases.
- Describe the drugs used to treat upper respiratory diseases.
- Explain how to assist with the nursing process when giving drugs to treat upper respiratory diseases.
- Describe the drugs used to treat lower respiratory diseases.
- Explain how to assist with the nursing process when giving drugs to treat lower respiratory diseases.

KEY TERMS

antihistamines Drugs that compete with released histamine for receptor sites in the arterioles, capillaries, and glands in mucous membranes

antitussives Drugs that suppress the cough center in the brain; cough suppressants

broncho-dilators Drugs that relax the smooth muscles of the tracheo-bronchial tree

cilia Small hair-like structures that project outward from the surfaces of some cells

cough suppressants See "antitussives"

decongestants Drugs that cause vaso-constriction of the nasal mucosa

expectorants Drugs that liquify mucus to promote the ejection of mucus from the lungs and tracheo-bronchial tree

histamine A substance released in response to allergic reactions and tissue damage from trauma or infection

intra-nasal Within (*intra*) the nose (*nasal*)

mucolytic agents Drugs that reduce the stickiness and thickness of pulmonary secretions

rhinitis medicamentosa Drug-induced congestion

rhinorrhea Nasal discharge (*rhino* means *nose*; *rrhea* means *discharge*); runny nose

tracheo-bronchial tree The trachea, bronchi, and bronchioles

KEY ABBREVIATIONS

CO₂ Carbon dioxide
COPD Chronic obstructive pulmonary disease
g Gram
GI Gastro-intestinal
h Hour
kg Kilogram
mcg Microgram
mg Milligram
mL Milliliter
O₂ Oxygen
PO Per os (orally)
q Every

The respiratory system is a series of airways that start with the nose and mouth and end at the alveoli in the lungs. See Box 24-1 for a review of the respiratory system. The respiratory system is divided into the:

- Upper respiratory tract—the nose, sinuses, nasopharynx, pharynx, tonsils, eustachian tubes, and larynx (Fig. 24-2).
- Lower respiratory tract—larynx, trachea, bronchi, bronchioles, and alveoli (Fig. 24-3, p. 302).
- See Box 24-2 on pp. 302-303 for common respiratory disorders.

See *Delegation Guidelines: Drugs Used to Treat Respiratory Diseases*, p. 302.

BOX 24-1 The Respiratory System: Structure and Function

The respiratory system (Fig. 24-1) brings oxygen into the lungs and removes carbon dioxide. Air enters the body through the *nose*. The nose and its structure serve two functions: olfactory and respiratory.

- Olfactory (smell). The olfactory region is in the upper part of each nostril. Olfactory cells contain microscopic hairs that react to odors in the air. The hairs stimulate the olfactory cells. Those cells send signals to the brain where the sense of smell is processed.
- Respiratory. The nose warms, humidifies (adds water), and filters inhaled air. Both nasal passages have folds of skin called *turbinates*. Because they consist of folds, the turbinates increase the amount of nasal tissue. Turbinate tissue contains many, many blood vessels. The turbinates are lined with membranes. Blood circulating through these membranes warms and humidifies inhaled air.

Particles in the inhaled air are filtered. Large hairs at the nostril entrances remove large particles. Turbinates and the narrow nasal passages cause turbulence of airflow as air passes with each inhalation. All nose surfaces are coated with a thin layer of mucus. The mucus is secreted by mucous glands *(goblet cells)*. Because of the turbulent airflow, particles are "thrown" against the walls of the nasal passages. The particles become trapped in the mucous secretions.

Cells lining the back two-thirds of the nasal passages contain cilia. Cilia are small hair-like structures that project outward from the surfaces of some cells. The cilia sweep the particulate matter back toward the naso-pharynx and pharynx. Once in the pharynx, the particulate matter is expectorated or swallowed. Warming, humidifying, and filtering continue as the air passes into the trachea, bronchi, and bronchioles.

The autonomic nervous system controls the nasal structures. Cholinergic stimulation causes vaso-dilation. Blood vessels lining the nasal mucous membranes dilate (widen). When cholinergic fibers in the secretory glands are stimulated, serous and mucous secretions are produced. Sympathetic stimulation causes vaso-constriction.

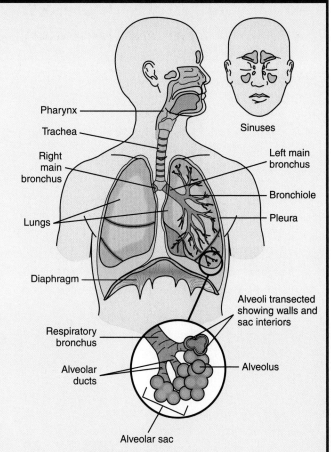

Fig. 24-1 Respiratory system.

The *sinuses* are hollow air-filled cavities. They are in the cranial bones on both sides and behind the nose. There are eight sinuses—four on each side. The sinuses are lined with the same mucous membranes and cilia as those of the upper respiratory tract. The sinuses are connected to the nasal passages by ducts. They drain into the nasal cavity.

BOX 24-1 **The Respiratory System: Structure and Function—cont'd**

The *tonsils* are on each side of the pharynx. The tonsils are lymph tissue. They are located in an area where mucus filled with particulate matter collects from ciliary action in the naso-pharynx. The particulate matter includes virus particles and bacteria. The lymph tissue is thought to play a role in immune defense mechanisms of the upper airway.

Sneezing is a reflex the body uses to clear the nasal passages of particulate matter. The sneeze reflex starts by irritation of the nasal membranes caused by the particulate matter.

The air then passes into the *pharynx* (throat). It is a tube-shaped passageway for air and food. Air passes from the pharynx into the *larynx* (voice box). A piece of cartilage, the *epiglottis,* acts like a lid over the larynx. The epiglottis prevents food from entering the airway during swallowing. During inhalation the epiglottis lifts up to let air pass over the larynx. Air passes from the larynx into the *trachea* (windpipe).

The trachea divides at its lower end into the *right bronchus* and the *left bronchus.* Each bronchus enters a lung. Upon entering the lungs, the bronchi divide many times into smaller branches. The smaller branches are called *bronchioles.* Eventually the bronchioles subdivide. They end up in tiny one-celled air sacs called *alveoli.*

Alveoli look like small clusters of grapes. They are supplied by capillaries. Oxygen (O_2) and carbon dioxide (CO_2) are exchanged between the alveoli and capillaries. Blood in the capillaries picks up O_2 from the alveoli. Then the blood is returned to the left side of the heart and pumped to the rest of the body. Alveoli pick up CO_2 from the capillaries for exhalation.

The lungs are spongy tissues. They are filled with alveoli, blood vessels, and nerves. Each lung is divided into lobes. The right lung has three lobes; the left lung has two. The lungs are separated from the abdominal cavity by a muscle called the *diaphragm.*

Each lung is covered by a two-layered sac called the *pleura.* One layer is attached to the lung and the other to the chest wall. The pleura secretes a very thin fluid that fills the space between the layers. The fluid prevents the layers from rubbing together during inhalation and exhalation. A bony framework made up of the ribs, sternum, and vertebrae protects the lungs.

Respiratory tract fluids come from glands that line the respiratory tract: mucous glands (goblet cells) and serous glands:

- Goblet cells produce a gel-like mucus that forms a thin layer over the inner surfaces of the **tracheo-bronchial tree**—trachea, bronchi, and bronchioles. Mucus secretion is caused by exposure to irritants—smoke, airborne particles, bacteria.
- Serous glands are controlled by the cholinergic nervous system (Chapter 14). When stimulated, the glands secrete a watery fluid to the interior surface of the tracheo-bronchial tree.

Mucous secretions from the goblet cells and water secretions from the serous cells combine to form respiratory tract fluid. Normally the fluid forms a protective layer over the tracheo-bronchial tree. Foreign bodies (smoke, bacteria, and so on) are caught in the fluid. They are swept upward by cilia that line the bronchi and trachea to the larynx. They are removed by the cough reflex.

The expectorated (coughed up) matter contains pulmonary mucous secretions, foreign particles (smoke, bacteria), and cells from the airway lining. The coughed-up matter is commonly called *sputum* and *phlegm.*

The respiratory fluid can become thick and sticky and form mucous plugs (see Fig. 24-2). Causes are:

- Too much mucus is secreted as a result of chronic irritation
- Cilia are destroyed by chronic smoke inhalation
- Dehydration dries the mucus
- Anti-cholinergic agents inhibit water secretions from the serous glands (drying effect)

Thick mucous plugs are hard to remove by coughing. Microbes can grow in the lower respiratory tract. This causes more mucous secretions. Pneumonia can develop from trapped bacteria.

Smooth muscles of the tracheo-bronchial tree are controlled by the autonomic nervous system (parasympathetic and sympathetic systems).

- Stimulation of cholinergic (parasympathetic) fibers causes bronchial constriction and increased mucus secretion.
- Stimulation of adrenergic (sympathetic) fibers causes dilation of the bronchi and bronchioles. Mucus secretion decreases.

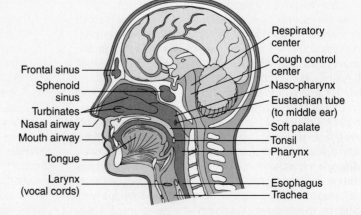

Fig. 24-2 The upper respiratory tract.

Frontal sinus
Sphenoid sinus
Turbinates
Nasal airway
Mouth airway
Tongue
Larynx (vocal cords)

Respiratory center
Cough control center
Naso-pharynx
Eustachian tube (to middle ear)
Soft palate
Tonsil
Pharynx
Esophagus
Trachea

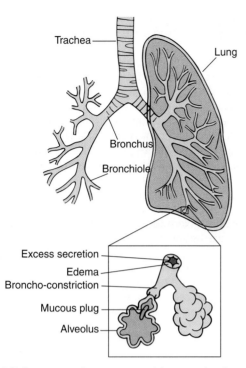

Fig. 24-3 Lower respiratory tract. Mucous plug formed in alveoli.

BOX 24-2 Common Respiratory Disorders

THE UPPER RESPIRATORY TRACT

Rhinitis. Rhin means *nose.* Itis means *inflammation.* Rhinitis is inflammation of the mucous membranes of the nose. Signs and symptoms are sneezing, nasal discharge, and nasal congestion. Rhinitis can be acute or chronic. The most common causes of acute rhinitis are the common cold, bacterial infection, a foreign body, and drug-induced congestion (rhinitis medicamentosa). Common causes of chronic rhinitis are allergies, non-allergic rhinitis, chronic sinusitis, and a deviated septum (broken nose, fractured nose).

Common cold. The common cold is a viral infection of the upper respiratory tissues. It usually occurs in mid-winter, the spring, and in early fall. Viruses are spread from person to person by direct contact and sneezing. Early symptoms are a clear, watery nasal discharge and sneezing. Nasal congestion quickly follows. Over the next 48 hours, the discharge becomes cloudy and thicker. Other symptoms include coughing, a "scratchy" or mildly sore throat, and hoarseness. Headache, malaise, fever, and chills may occur. Some persons have a fever. Symptoms should subside over 5 to 7 days. Sinusitis and otitis media (middle ear infection) are possible complications.

Allergic rhinitis. This is inflammation of the mucous membranes of the nose caused by an allergic reaction. After exposure to an allergen, the person develops antibodies to the antigen. Common allergens are pollens, grasses, and house dust mites. When a person inhales the allergen, an antigen-antibody reaction occurs. This causes inflammation and swelling of the nasal passages. A major cause of symptoms is the release of histamine during the antigen-antibody reaction. Histamine is a substance released in response to allergic reactions and tissue damage from trauma or infection. Histamine is stored in most body tissues. When histamine is released in the area of tissue damage or the site of an antigen-antibody reaction, these reactions take place:

- Arterioles and capillaries in the region dilate. This allows increased blood flow to the area causing redness.
- Capillaries allow fluid to leak into extracellular spaces. This causes:
  - Edema (congestion) of nasal mucous membranes and turbinates.
  - The release of nasal and bronchial secretions. These result in nasal discharge (rhinorrhea). *Rhino* means *nose;* rrhea means *discharge.* Rhinorrhea is commonly called "runny nose." Watery eyes also occur.
- Itching of the palate, eyes, and ears.

Large amounts of histamine are released in a severe allergic reaction. Hypotension results from extensive dilation of the arterioles. Edema is severe. The skin becomes flushed with severe itching. Constriction and spasm of bronchiole tubes cause dyspnea. Large amounts of pulmonary and gastric secretions are released.

BOX 24-2 Common Respiratory Disorders—cont'd

Rhinitis medicamentosa. This is inflammation *(itis)* of the mucous membranes of the nose *(rhin)* caused by a drug *(medica)*. The drug causes excess vaso-constriction and irritation of the nasal membranes. When the vaso-constrictor effect wears off, swelling and congestion re-appear. The nose feels more stuffy and congested than before treatment. More frequent use of the topical decongestant is needed to relieve the nasal passage of swelling and obstruction.

THE LOWER RESPIRATORY TRACT

Chronic obstructive pulmonary disease. Three disorders are grouped under chronic obstructive pulmonary disease (COPD). They interfere with O_2 and CO_2 exchange in the lungs. They obstruct airflow. COPD affects the airways and alveoli. Less air gets into the lungs; less air goes out of the lungs.

- ***Chronic bronchitis.*** Chronic bronchitis occurs after repeated episodes of bronchitis. *Bronchitis* means inflammation *(itis)* of the bronchi *(bronch)*. Smoking is the major cause. Infection, air pollution, and industrial dusts are risk factors. *Smoker's cough* in the morning is often the first symptom. At first the cough is dry. Over time, the person coughs up mucus. Mucus may contain pus. The cough becomes more frequent. The person has difficulty breathing and tires easily. Mucus and inflamed breathing passages obstruct airflow into the lungs. The body cannot get normal amounts of oxygen. The person must stop smoking. Oxygen therapy and breathing exercises are often ordered. Respiratory tract infections are prevented. If one occurs, the person needs prompt treatment.

- ***Emphysema.*** In emphysema, the alveoli enlarge. They become less elastic. They do not expand and shrink normally with breathing in and out. As a result, some air is trapped in the alveoli when exhaling. Trapped air is not exhaled. Over time, more alveoli are involved. O_2 and CO_2 exchange cannot occur in affected alveoli. As more air is trapped in the lungs, the person develops a *barrel chest* (Fig. 24-4). Smoking is the most common cause. Air pollution and industrial dusts are risk factors. The person has shortness of breath and a cough. At first, shortness of breath occurs with exertion. Over time, it occurs at rest. Sputum may contain pus. Fatigue is common. The person works hard to breathe in and out. And the body does not get enough oxygen. Breathing is easier when the person sits upright and slightly forward. The person must stop smoking. Respiratory therapy, breathing exercises, oxygen, and drug therapy are ordered.

- ***Asthma.*** The airway becomes inflamed and narrow. Extra mucus is produced. Dyspnea results. Wheezing and coughing are common. So are pain and tightening in the chest. Symptoms are mild to severe. Asthma usually is triggered by allergies. Other triggers include air pollutants and irritants, smoking and second-hand smoke, respiratory infections, exertion, and cold air. Sudden attacks *(asthma attacks)* can occur. There is shortness of breath, wheezing, coughing, rapid pulse, sweating, and cyanosis. The person gasps for air and is very frightened. Fear makes the attack worse. Asthma is treated with drugs.

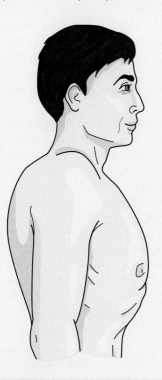

Fig. 24-4 Barrel chest from emphysema.

DRUG THERAPY FOR UPPER RESPIRATORY DISEASES

Antihistamines are the drugs of choice for allergic rhinitis. They are given orally and distributed throughout the body. Therefore they reduce the symptoms of nasal itching, sneezing, rhinorrhea, tearing, and itchy eyes. Antihistamines do not reduce nasal congestion.

Decongestants cause vaso-constriction of the nasal mucosa. This greatly reduces nasal congestion.

Anti-inflammatory agents (p. 306) are given intranasally. They are used to treat nasal symptoms caused by mild to moderate allergic rhinitis. They are not used to treat cold symptoms. Cold symptoms start to resolve before the anti-inflammatory agents become effective.

DRUG CLASS: Sympathomimetic Decongestants

Sympathomimetic nasal decongestants stimulate the alpha-adrenergic receptors of the nasal mucous membranes. This causes vaso-constriction. Blood flow is reduced in the swollen nasal area. Turbinates and mucous membranes shrink. Sinus drainage is promoted. Feelings of stuffiness and obstruction are relieved.

Decongestants are the drugs of choice for relieving congestion from rhinitis and the common cold. To treat allergic rhinitis, decongestants are often given with antihistamines to:
* Reduce nasal congestion
* Reduce sedation caused by many antihistamines

Oral and topical dose forms are available (Table 24-1). Topical dose forms are nasal sprays or drops. Topical drugs have no systemic effects. And they do not relieve other symptoms. They can cause rhinitis medicamentosa.

Nasal decongestants provide temporary symptom relief. At first stuffiness is relieved. Rhinitis medicamentosa is a risk from misuse. Always follow label directions.

Drugs in this class can stimulate receptors in other body sites. Caution is needed when oral drugs are taken by persons who have hypertension, hyperthyroidism, diabetes, heart disease, glaucoma, and prostate enlargement.

The goals of therapy are to:
* Reduce nasal congestion
* Ease breathing

Assisting With the Nursing Process

When a person takes nasal decongestants, you assist the nurse with the nursing process.

ASSESSMENT
Measure vital signs.

PLANNING
See Table 24-1 for "Dose Forms."

IMPLEMENTATION
* See Table 24-1 for "Adult Dosage Range."
* See Chapter 12 for how to apply topical nose medications.

EVALUATION
Report and record:
* *Burning or stinging of the nasal membranes.* A weaker solution may be needed.
* *Hypertension.* This may occur from excessive use. Measure blood pressure.

DRUG CLASS: Antihistamines

Antihistamines compete with released histamine for receptor sites in the arterioles, capillaries, and glands in mucous membranes. Antihistamines do not prevent histamine release. They reduce the symptoms of an allergic reaction if the amount of antihistamine is greater than the amount of histamine. Therefore, antihistamines are more effective if taken:
* Before histamine is released
* When symptoms first appear

Antihistamines are the drugs of choice for the treatment of allergic rhinitis and conjunctivitis. The *conjunctiva* is the mucous membrane lining the inner surfaces of the eyelids and outer part of the sclera. *Conjunctivitis* is the inflammation of the conjunctiva. It is caused by bacterial or viral infections, allergies, or environmental factors. Signs and symptoms include red eyelids, itching, thick discharge, and sticky eyelids in the morning.

The drugs reduce rhinorrhea, tearing, eye itching, and sneezing. They do not stop nasal congestion. They are best taken on a schedule for allergies. They are more effective if taken before exposure to the allergen. For example, they are taken 45 to 60 minutes before going outside during the pollen season.

All antihistamines have anti-cholinergic side effects:
* Dilation of the pupil with increased intraocular pressure in persons with glaucoma
* Dry, thick secretions of the mouth, nose, throat, and bronchi
* Decreased secretions and motility of the gastrointestinal (GI) tract
* Increased heart rate
* Decreased sweating

Therefore, persons with asthma, prostate enlargement, or glaucoma should take antihistamines only with medical supervision.

The goals of therapy are to reduce the signs and symptoms from allergic rhinitis.

Assisting With the Nursing Process

When a person takes nasal decongestants, you assist the nurse with the nursing process.

ASSESSMENT

- Observe for nasal congestion.
- Measure intake and output.

PLANNING

See Table 24-2 for "Dose Forms."

IMPLEMENTATION

- See Table 24-2 for "Adult Dosage Range."
- See Table 24-2 for "Maximum Daily Dose."

TABLE 24-1 Nasal Decongestants

GENERIC NAME	BRAND NAME	DOSE FORMS	ADULT DOSAGE RANGE
ephedrine	Pretz-D	Solution: 0.25%	Nasal: 2 or 3 drops two or three times daily
epinephrine	Adrenalin	Solution: 0.1%	Nasal: 1 or 2 drops in each nostril q4-6h
naphazoline	Privine	Solution: 0.05%	Nasal: 2 or 3 drops or sprays no more than q3h (drops) or q4-6h (spray)
oxymetazoline	Afrin, Duration	Solution: 0.05%	Nasal: 2 or 3 drops or sprays of 0.05% solution twice daily
phenylephrine	Neo-Synephrine, Sinex	Solution: 0.125%, 0.25%, 0.5%, 1%	Nasal: 0.25% q3-4h
pseudoephedrine	Sudafed, Efidac/24	Tablets or capsules: 15, 30, 60, 120, 240 mg Liquid: 15, 30 mg/5 mL Drops: 7.5 mg/0.8 mL	PO: 60 mg q6h; do not exceed 240 mg/24 hours
tetrahydrozoline	Tyzine	Solution: 0.05%, 0.1%	Nasal: 2-4 drops of 0.1% solution q4-6h
xylometazoline	Otrivin	Solution: 0.05%, 0.1%	Nasal: 2 or 3 sprays q8-10h

TABLE 24-2 Antihistamines*

GENERIC NAME	BRAND NAME	DOSE FORMS	ADULT DOSAGE RANGE	MAXIMUM DAILY DOSE (mg)
azelastine	Astelin	Nasal spray	2 sprays per nostril twice daily	—
cetirizine	Zyrtec	Tablets, syrup	5-10 mg once daily	20
chlorpheniramine maleate	Chlor-Trimeton	Tablets, capsules, syrup	4 mg three to six times daily	24
clemastine fumarate	Tavist	Tablets, syrup	1.34-2.68 mg twice daily	8.04
cyproheptadine hydrochloride		Tablets, syrup	4 mg three times daily	32
desloratidine	Clarinex	Tablets, syrup	5 mg once daily	5
diphenhydramine hydrochloride	Benadryl, AllerMax	Capsules, tablets, syrup, elixir	25-50 mg three or four times daily	300
fexofenadine	Allegra	Tablets	60 mg twice daily	180
ipratropium	Atrovent	Nasal spray	2 sprays per nostril two or three times daily	—
loratadine	Claritin	Tablets, syrup	10 mg daily	10
promethazine hydrochloride†	Phenergan	Tablets, syrup, suppository	12.5-25 mg three or four times daily	100

* Many of these antihistamines are also available in combination with decongestants.

† Promethazine is a phenothiazine with antihistaminic properties.

EVALUATION

Report and record:

- *Sedation, cognitive impairment, memory problems, co-ordination problems.* Sedation is the most common side effect from antihistamines. Tolerance may develop over time. Provide for safety. People working around machines, driving a car, pouring and giving drugs, or performing other duties that require mental alertness should not take these drugs while working.

- *Drying effects.* Observe the person's cough and sputum production. Because of drying effects, antihistamines may impair expectoration.

- *Blurred vision; constipation; urinary retention; mouth, throat, and nose dryness.* These are caused by the drying effects of antihistamines. The nurse may allow the person to chew gum or suck on ice chips or hard candy. Provide for safety if the person has blurred vision. Follow the care plan for constipation.

DRUG CLASS: Respiratory Anti-Inflammatory Agents

Anti-inflammatory agents used to treat upper respiratory diseases are:

- intra-nasal cortico-steroids
- cromolyn sodium (kro' mo lin); Nasalcrom (nay zal krom')

intra-nasal cortico-steroids

Intra-nasal means within *(intra)* the nose *(nasal)*. Cortico-steroids (Chapter 28) are given to reduce inflammation. Persons with allergic rhinitis who do not respond to other drugs may be given cortico-steroids to relieve allergy symptoms.

Intra-nasal cortico-steroids control nasal symptoms associated with mild to moderate allergic rhinitis. They are used for short courses of therapy for acute seasonal allergies.

The goals of therapy are to reduce:
- Rhinorrhea
- Rhinitis
- Itching
- Sneezing

Assisting With the Nursing Process

When a person takes intra-nasal cortico-steroids, you assist the nurse with the nursing process.

ASSESSMENT

Observe for nasal congestion.

PLANNING

See Table 24-3 for "Dose Forms."

TABLE 24-3 Intra-Nasal Cortico-Steroids			
GENERIC NAME	**BRAND NAME**	**DOSE FORMS**	**ADULT DOSAGE RANGE**
beclomethasone dipropionate, monohydrate	Beconase AQ	Nasal spray: 180 doses/canister	1 or 2 sprays (42-84 mcg) in each nostril twice daily
budesonide	Rhinocort Aqua	Nasal aerosol: 120 doses/canister	2 inhalations (64 mcg) in each nostril morning and evening
flunisolide	Nasarel	Nasal spray: 200 doses/bottle	2 sprays (58 mcg) in each nostril twice daily; maximum daily dose is 8 sprays (464 mcg) in 24 hours
fluticasone	Flonase	Nasal spray: 120 doses/bottle	2 sprays (100 mcg) in each nostril once daily
mometasone	Nasonex	Nasal spray: 120 doses/bottle	2 sprays (100 mcg) in each nostril once daily
triamcinolone	Nasacort AQ	Nasal spray: 30 and 120 doses/bottle	2 sprays (110 mcg) in each nostril once daily; maximum daily dose is 4 sprays in 24 hours
	Nasacort HFA	Nasal aerosol: 100 doses/canister	

IMPLEMENTATION

- See Table 24-3 for "Adult Dosage Range."
- Full therapeutic effect requires regular use. It is usually evident within a few days. Some persons require up to 3 weeks for maximum benefit.
- Advise the person to clear nasal passages of secretions before a topical application.
- A decongestant may be ordered for use right before a topical cortico-steroid. This promotes adequate penetration.
- See Chapter 12 for how to apply topical nose medications.

EVALUATION

Report and record:

- *Nasal burning.* This is usually mild and tends to resolve with continued therapy.

cromolyn sodium (Nasalcrom)

Cromolyn sodium (Nasalcrom) is an anti-inflammatory agent. It inhibits the release of histamine and other substances of inflammation. To be effective, it must be used before the body receives a stimulus to release histamine.

Cromolyn sodium (Nasalcrom) is used with other drugs that prevent the release of histamine. It does not relieve nasal congestion. An antihistamine or nasal decongestant may be needed when treatment is started. A 2- to 4-week course of therapy is usually needed for a clinical response. Treatment is continued only if there is a decrease in symptoms.

The goals of therapy are to reduce:

- Rhinorrhea
- Itching
- Sneezing

Assisting With the Nursing Process

When a person takes cromolyn sodium (Nasalcrom), you assist the nurse with the nursing process.

ASSESSMENT

Observe for nasal congestion.

PLANNING

Dose forms are:

- Nasal spray: 40 mg/mL in 13 mL (gives 100 sprays) and 26 mL (gives 200 sprays)
- Aerosol spray: 800 mcg from an 8.1 g container (112 metered sprays) and 14.2 g container (200 metered sprays)
- Oral concentrate: 100 mg/5 mL

IMPLEMENTATION

- The adult dose is 1 spray in each nostril 3 or 4 times daily at regular intervals. Maximum dose is 6 sprays in each nostril daily.
- Full therapeutic effect requires regular use. It is usually evident within 2 to 4 weeks.

- Advise the person to clear nasal passages of secretions before a topical application.
- See Chapter 12 for how to apply topical nose medications.

EVALUATION

Report and record:

- *Nasal irritation—sneezing, itching, burning, stuffiness.* Tolerance usually develops.

DRUG THERAPY FOR LOWER RESPIRATORY DISEASES

Lower respiratory diseases are treated with:

- **Expectorants**—drugs that liquify mucus to promote the ejection of mucus from the lungs and tracheo-bronchial tree. They stimulate the secretion of natural fluids from the serous glands. The flow of serous fluids helps liquify thick mucous plugs that may narrow bronchioles. Ciliary action and coughing then expel the phlegm from the respiratory system. Expectorants are used to treat non-productive cough, bronchitis, and pneumonia.
- **Antitussives (cough suppressants)**—drugs that suppress the cough center in the brain. They are used when a person has a dry, hacking, non-productive cough. The cough is not stopped completely. However, these agents should decrease the frequency and suppress severe spasms that affect sleep.
- **Broncho-dilators**—drugs that relax the smooth muscles of the tracheo-bronchial tree. Bronchiole and alveolar ducts open, which decreases the resistance to airflow. These agents are used in the treatment of COPD.
- Anti-inflammatory agents—drugs that reduce inflammation. They are used for asthma. Cortico-steroids are the most effective. They are commonly given by inhalation. The drug is placed at the site of inflammation with few side effects. Some persons with asthma require short term systemic steroid treatment (Chapter 28).
- **Mucolytic agents**—drugs that reduce the stickiness and thickness of pulmonary secretions. They act directly on mucous plugs to cause them to dissolve. This eases the removal of secretions by cough, postural drainage, and suction. These agents are used to treat acute and chronic respiratory disorders, before and after bronchoscopy, after chest surgery, and as part of tracheostomy care. Mucomyst (acetylcysteine) is often given by nebulizer (Fig. 24-5, p. 308). A *nebulizer* is a device that produces a fine spray. See *Delegation Guidelines: Drug Therapy for Lower Respiratory Diseases*, p. 308.

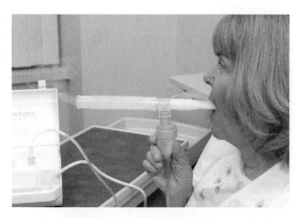

Fig. 24-5 Nebulizer. [From Perry AG, Potter PA: *Clinical skills and nursing techniques*, ed 6, St Louis, 2006, Mosby.]

DELEGATION GUIDELINES
Drug Therapy for Lower Respiratory Diseases

Many states and agencies do not let MA-Cs give drugs by nebulizer. If allowed to do so, make sure you receive the necessary education and training. Also make sure that a nurse is available to supervise your work.

DRUG CLASS: Expectorants

The following expectorants are used to treat lower respiratory diseases:
- guaifenesin (gwi feh' neh sin); Robitussin (row bih tus' sin)
- potassium iodide (SSKI)

guaifenesin (Robitussin)

Guaifenesin (Robitussin) is an expectorant that enhances the output of respiratory tract fluid. The increased flow of secretions decreases mucus thickness and promotes ciliary action. Ciliary action and coughing expel the phlegm out of the respiratory system.

The drug is used to relieve a dry, non-productive cough and to remove mucous plugs. The drug is often used with broncho-dilators, decongestants, antihistamines, or antitussive agents to make a non-productive cough productive.

The goal of therapy is to reduce the frequency of non-productive cough.

Assisting With the Nursing Process

When a person takes guaifenesin (Robitussin), you assist the nurse with the nursing process.

ASSESSMENT
Note the person's cough:
- Is it productive or non-productive?
- What is the color, consistency, amount, and appearance of sputum?

PLANNING
Oral dose forms are:
- 100, 200, 400, and 600 mg tablets
- 200 mg capsules
- 100 and 200 mg/5 mL liquid

IMPLEMENTATION
- The adult dose is 100 to 400 mg every 4 to 6 hours.
- The dose should not exceed 2400 mg per day.
- The person should drink eight to twelve 8-ounce glasses of water daily.

EVALUATION
Report and record:
- *GI upset, nausea, vomiting.* These side effects are rare.

potassium iodide (SSKI)

Potassium iodide (SSKI) stimulates increased secretion from the bronchial glands. This decreases the thickness of mucous plugs. It is easier for the person to cough up dry, hardened plugs blocking the bronchial tubes.

The drug is used in the treatment of COPD when thick mucus is present. It is often used with other drugs to remove mucus.

The goals of therapy are to:
- Reduce the thickness of mucus
- Allow a more productive cough to remove phlegm

Assisting With the Nursing Process

When a person takes potassium iodide (SSKI), you assist the nurse with the nursing process.

ASSESSMENT
Note the person's cough:
- Is it productive or non-productive?
- What is the color, consistency, amount, and appearance of sputum?

PLANNING
Oral dose forms are:
- Solution: 1 g/mL in 30, 240, and 480 mL containers
- Syrup: 325 mg/5 mL in 480 mL containers

IMPLEMENTATION
The adult dosage is:
- Solution: 0.3 mL (300 mg) to 0.6 mL (600 mg) diluted in one glassful of water, fruit juice, or milk 3 or 4 times daily.
- Syrup: 5 to 10 mL three times daily. Give with food or milk to lessen gastric irritation.
- The person should drink eight to twelve 8-ounce glasses of water daily.

EVALUATION

Report and record:

- *Nausea, vomiting, diarrhea.* These are usually mild. Give with food or milk to lessen gastric irritation.

DRUG CLASS: Antitussives

Antitussives (cough suppressants) depress the cough center in the brain. Codeine is an effective cough suppressant. Low-dose, short-term use for a cough should not produce addiction. Dependence may develop after long-term use.

The goal of therapy is to reduce the frequency of a non-productive cough.

Assisting With the Nursing Process

When a person takes antitussives, you assist the nurse with the nursing process.

ASSESSMENT

Note the person's cough:

- Is it productive or non-productive?
- What is the color, consistency, amount, and appearance of sputum?

PLANNING

- See Table 24-4 for "Oral Dose Forms."

IMPLEMENTATION

See Table 24-4 for "Adult Oral Dosage Range."

- Benzonatate (Tessalon Perles) must be swallowed whole. The drug numbs the tongue if chewed or crushed. This creates a choking hazard.

EVALUATION

Report and record:

- *Drowsiness, sedation.* Provide for safety. Remind the person to use caution when performing tasks that require alertness.
- *Constipation.* Codeine is the most constipating of the antitussives. Give stool softeners as ordered. Follow the care plan for fluid intake.

DRUG CLASS: Beta-Adrenergic Broncho-Dilating Agents

Beta-adrenergic broncho-dilating agents relax the smooth muscles of the tracheo-bronchial tree. This opens airways to greater amounts of air. These drugs are used to reverse airway constriction caused by acute and chronic asthma, bronchitis, and emphysema.

The drugs have many side effects. This is because they also stimulate receptors in the heart, blood vessels, uterus, and gastro-intestinal, urinary, and central nervous systems. Those given by inhalation usually have fewer side effects. With inhalation, the drug is placed at the site of action. Lower doses are used.

The goals of therapy are to:

- Ease breathing
- Reduce wheezing

Assisting With the Nursing Process

When giving a person beta-adrenergic broncho-dilating agents, you assist the nurse with the nursing process.

ASSESSMENT

- Measure vital signs.
- Note the pulse rate and rhythm.
- Observe for confusion and orientation to person, time, and place.

PLANNING

See Table 24-5, p. 310, for "Dose Forms."

IMPLEMENTATION

- See Table 24-5, p. 310, for "Adult Dosage Range."
- The person waits at least 10 minutes between inhalations. This allows the drug to dilate the bronchioles. The second dose can be inhaled more deeply into the lungs.
- Follow the manufacturer's instructions.

TABLE 24-4 Antitussive Agents

GENERIC NAME	BRAND NAME	ORAL DOSE FORMS	ADULT ORAL DOSAGE RANGE
benzonatate	Tessalon Perles	Capsules: 100, 200 mg	100-200 mg three times daily
codeine*		Tablets: 15, 30, 60 mg Solution: 10, 15 mg/5 mL	10-20 mg q4-6h
dextromethorphan	Robitussin CoughGels, Delsym, Benylin Adult	Lozenges: 5, 7.5, 10, 15 mg Syrup: 7.5, 10 mg/5 mL Liquid: 5, 7.5, 10, 15 mg/5 mL Gelcaps: 15, 30 mg Oral suspension, extended-release: 300 mg/5 mL	10-30 mg q4-8h; do not exceed 60-120 mg/24 hours 10 mL q12h; do not exceed 20 mL/24 hours
diphenhydramine	Diphen, Tusstat	Syrup: 12.5 mg/5 mL Capsules and tablets: 25, 50 mg	25 mg q4h; do not exceed 150 mg/24 hours
hydrocodone bitartrate* and homatropine methylbromide	Hycodan	Tablets: 5 mg Syrup: 5 mg/5 mL	5 mg q4-6h

*Often an ingredient in combination antitussive products. A controlled substance. May be habit-forming.

TABLE 24-5 Broncho-Dilators

GENERIC NAME	BRAND NAME	DOSE FORMS	ADULT DOSAGE RANGE
BETA-ADRENERGIC AGONISTS			
albuterol	Proventil, Ventolin, Volmax	Tablets: 2, 4 mg Aerosol: 90 mcg Syrup: 2 mg/5 mL Tablets, extended-release: 4, 8 mg Solution for inhalation	PO: 2-4 mg three or four times daily Inhale: two inhalations q4-6h See manufacturer's recommendations
bitolterol	Tornalate	Solution for inhalation	See manufacturer's recommendations
ephedrine		Capsules: 25 mg	25-50 mg q3-4h
epinephrine	Primatene Mist	Nebulization: 1:100 Aerosol: 0.2 mg	See manufacturer's recommendations
formoterol	Foradil	Inhaler capsule: 12 mcg	Inhale: using aerolizer inhaler, 1 capsule q12h
isoetharine		Solution for inhalation: 1%	See manufacturer's recommendations
levalbuterol	Xopenex Xopenex HFA	Solution for inhalation Aerosol: 45 mcg/puff	See manufacturer's recommendations Inhale: 1-2 inhalations q4-6h
metaproterenol	Alupent	Aerosol: 0.65 mg/puff Nebulization: 0.4%, 0.6%, 5%	See manufacturer's recommendations
pirbuterol	Maxair	Aerosol: 0.2 mg/puff	Inhale: 1-2 inhalations q4-6h
salmeterol	Serevent Diskus	Inhalation powder: 50 mcg	Inhale: 1 inhalation q12h
terbutaline	Brethine	Tablets: 2.5, 5 mg	5 mg q6h
XANTHINE-DERIVATIVES			
aminophylline		Tablets: 100, 200 mg Liquid: 105 mg/5 mL Suppositories: 250, 500 mg	See manufacturer's recommendations
dyphylline	Dilor, Lufyllin	Tablets: 200, 400 mg Elixir: 100, 160 mg/15 mL	15 mg/kg five times daily
oxtriphylline		Tablets: 100, 200 mg Elixir: 100 mg/5 mL	200 mg four times daily
theophylline	Bronkodyl, Elixophyllin, Theolair, others	Capsules: 100, 200, 250 mg Elixir: 80 mg/15 mL Syrup: 80, 150 mg/15 mL Solution (oral): 80 mg/15 mL Tablets, extended-release: 100, 200, 300, 400, 450, 600 mg Capsules, extended-release: 100, 125, 200, 250, 260, 300 mg	9-20 mg/kg/24 hours in four divided doses

EVALUATION

Report and record:

- *Tachycardia, palpitations.* These are dose related. Measure heart rate and note the rhythm. Report an increase of 20 beats or more per minute after a treatment. Report dysrhythmias and palpitations.
- *Tremors.* The dosage may need adjustment.
- *Nervousness, anxiety, restlessness, headache.*
- *Nausea, vomiting.* Give the drug with food and a full glass of water.
- *Dizziness.* Provide for safety.

DRUG CLASS: **Anti-Cholinergic Broncho-Dilating Agents**

The anti-cholinergic broncho-dilating agents used to treat lower respiratory diseases are:
- ipratropium bromide (ihp rah trop' eum); Atrovent (at' roh vent) and Atrovent HFA
- tiotropium bromide (ti oh trop' eum); Spiriva (spy ree' vah)

ipratropium bromide (Atrovent and Atrovent HFA)

Ipratropium bromide (Atrovent and Atrovent HFA) act on the bronchial smooth muscle. They produce broncho-dilation.

These drugs are used for long-term treatment of broncho-spasm associated with COPD. They may be used with beta-adrenergic broncho-dilators in persons with asthma. The initial effect is seen within the first few minutes after inhalation. Maximum effects are seen in 1 to 2 hours. Broncho-dilation lasts for 4 to 6 hours with usual dosages.

Nasal spray is used to relieve rhinorrhea from allergic and non-allergic rhinitis and the common cold. It does not relieve nasal congestion, sneezing, or post-nasal drip from these conditions.

The goals of therapy are to:
- Ease breathing (metered-dose inhaler)
- Reduce rhinorrhea (nasal spray)

Assisting With the Nursing Process

When a person takes ipratropium bromide (Atrovent and Atrovent HFA), you assist the nurse with the nursing process.

ASSESSMENT

Measure vital signs.

PLANNING

- Aerosol canister: 18 mcg/metered dose inhaler (200 inhalations)
- Nasal spray pumps:
  - 0.03% (21 mcg/spray) (30 mL)
  - 0.06% (42 mcg/spray) (15 mL)

IMPLEMENTATION

- Inhalation:
  - The usual dose is 2 inhalations (36 mcg) four times a day.
  - Additional inhalations may be taken as required.
  - Total dosage should not exceed 12 inhalations in 24 hours.
- Nasal spray:
  - Allergic and non-allergic rhinitis—2 sprays (42 mcg) of a 0.3% solution in each nostril 2 or 3 times a day
  - Common cold—2 sprays (84 mcg) of 0.6% solution in each nostril 3 or 4 times a day
- See Chapter 12 for how to give inhaled drugs.

EVALUATION

Report and record:
- *Mouth dryness, throat irritation.* These are usually mild and tend to resolve with continued therapy. Provide oral hygiene. The nurse may allow the person to suck on ice chips or hard candy.
- *Tachycardia, urinary retention, worsening of respiratory symptoms.*

tiotropium bromide (Spiriva)

Tiotropium bromide (Spiriva) is given by dry powder inhalation. It causes bronchial smooth muscles to relax, resulting in broncho-dilation.

The drug is used as a once-daily broncho-dilator to treat broncho-spasm associated with COPD. The broncho-dilating effect does not happen at once. Therefore the drug is used for maintenance treatment.

The goal of therapy is easier breathing with less effort.

Assisting With the Nursing Process

When giving a person tiotropium bromide (Spiriva), you assist the nurse with the nursing process.

ASSESSMENT

Measure vital signs.

PLANNING

The inhalation dose form is 18 mcg capsules for use in a supplied HandiHaler.

IMPLEMENTATION

- The usual dose is 1 capsule daily given through the HandiHaler.
- See Chapter 12 for giving inhaled drugs.

EVALUATION

Report and record:
- *Mouth dryness, throat irritation.* These are usually mild and tend to resolve with continued therapy. Provide oral hygiene. The nurse may allow the person to suck on ice chips or hard candy.
- *Tachycardia, urinary retention, worsening of respiratory symptoms.*

DRUG CLASS: Xanthine-Derivative Broncho-Dilating Agents

Xanthine-derivative broncho-dilating agents also are called xanthine-derivatives. They act directly on the smooth muscle of the tracheo-bronchial tree to dilate the bronchi. This increases airflow in and out of the alveoli.

These drugs are used with sympathomimetic broncho-dilators to reverse airway constriction caused by COPD. The goal of therapy is easier breathing with less effort.

Assisting With the Nursing Process

When giving a person xanthine-derivatives, you assist the nurse with the nursing process.

ASSESSMENT

- Measure vital signs.
- Note heart rate and rhythm.
- Observe orientation to person, time, and place.
- Observe for anxiety and nervousness.

PLANNING

See Table 24-5 for "Dose Forms."

IMPLEMENTATION

See Table 24-5, p. 310, for "Adult Dosage Range."

EVALUATION

Report and record:

- *Nausea, vomiting, epigastric pain, abdominal cramps.* These occur from irritation caused by the stimulation of gastric acid secretion. Give the drug with food or milk.
- *Tachycardia, palpitations.* These are usually dose related. Measure heart rate and note the rhythm.
- *Tremors.* A dosage adjustment may be needed.
- *Nervousness, anxiety, restlessness, headache.* Observe for changes in mental status.

DRUG CLASS: Respiratory Anti-Inflammatory Agents

Cortico-steroids are given to reduce inflammation (Chapter 28). They are highly effective in treating COPD. They:

- Relax smooth muscles
- Enhance the effect of beta-adrenergic bronchodilators
- Inhibit inflammatory responses that may cause broncho-constriction

These agents may be added to a drug therapy program if the person does not respond to other bronchodilators. The goal of therapy is easier breathing with less effort.

TABLE 24-6 Inhalant Cortico-Steroids

GENERIC NAME	BRAND NAME	INHALANT DOSE FORMS	ADULT DOSAGE RANGE
INHALANT CORTICO-STEROIDS			
beclomethasone dipropionate	QVAR	Aerosol: 40 and 80 mcg/dose; 100 doses/inhaler	One or two inhalations (40 to 80 mcg) three to four times daily; maximum of 640 mcg daily
budesonide phosphate	Pulmicort Turbuhaler	Aerosol: 200 doses/inhaler	One or two inhalations twice daily; maximum four inhalations twice daily
flunisolide	AeroBid	Aerosol: 100 doses/inhaler	Two inhalations (500 mcg) twice daily; do not exceed 2 mg (eight inhalations) daily
fluticasone	Flovent HFA	Aerosol: 44, 110, 220 mcg/dose	100-250 mcg twice daily; maximum 500 mcg twice daily
	Flovent Diskus	Powder: 50, 100, 250 mcg	
	Flovent Rotadisk	Powder: 50, 100, 250 mcg	
mometasone furoate	Asmanex Twisthaler	Powder: 220 mcg/dose	One or two inhalations once daily; maximum of two doses daily
triamcinolone acetonide	Azmacort	Aerosol: 240 doses/inhaler	Two inhalations (200 mcg) three to four times daily; do not exceed 1600 mcg (16 inhalations) daily
INHALANT CORTICO-STEROID BETA-ADRENERGIC BRONCHO-DILATOR			
fluticasone-salmeterol	Advair Diskus	Powder 100 mcg fluticasone/ 50 mcg salmeterol 250 mcg fluticasone/ 50 mcg salmeterol 500 mcg fluticasone/ 50 mcg salmeterol	One inhalation twice daily for maintenance therapy on a regularly scheduled basis; not for acute bronchospasm

Assisting With the Nursing Process

When a person uses inhalant cortico-steroids, you assist the nurse with the nursing process.

ASSESSMENT

Observe the mouth for signs and symptoms of infection.

PLANNING

See Table 24-6 for "Inhalant Dose Forms."

IMPLEMENTATION

- See Table 24-6 for "Adult Dosage Range."
- Full therapeutic effect requires regular use. It is usually evident within a few days. Some persons require up to 4 weeks for maximum benefit.
- Persons receiving broncho-dilators by inhalation should use them before the cortico-steroid inhalant. Doing so enhances penetration of the cortico-steroid into the bronchial tree. Wait several minutes before the cortico-steroid is inhaled. This allows time for the broncho-dilator to relax the smooth muscle.

EVALUATION

Report and record:

- *Hoarseness, dry mouth.* These are usually mild and tend to resolve with continued therapy.
- *Signs and symptoms of a mouth infection.* Provide oral hygiene. Follow the care plan for using a mouthwash.

DRUG CLASS: Anti-Leukotriene Agents

Inflammatory cells are in the membrane lining the airway. A series of chemical reactions occur when the inflammatory cells are triggered by irritants. Such irritants include smoke, allergens, and viruses. One reaction is the release of leukotrienes. *Leukotrienes* are substances in white blood cells. White blood cells are called *leukocytes.* (*Leuko* means *white. Cyte* means *cell.*) Leukotrienes produce allergic and inflammatory reactions similar to histamine. They produce many of the signs and symptoms of asthma (see Box 24-2).

The following are anti-leukotriene agents:

- montelukast (mon teh lu' cast); Singular (sing' yu lair')
- zafirlukast (zaf ihr' lu cast); Accolate (ak' oh late)

montelukast (Singulair)

Montelukast (Singulair) competes for the receptor sites that trigger symptoms of asthma. It has been shown to reduce:

- Broncho-constriction
- Daytime asthma symptoms
- Night-time awakening

The goal of therapy is fewer episodes of acute asthma symptoms.

Assisting With the Nursing Process

When giving a person montelukast (Singulair), you assist the nurse with the nursing process.

ASSESSMENT

Measure vital signs.

PLANNING

Oral dose forms are:

- 5 and 10 mg tablets
- 4 mg chewable tablets
- 4 mg granules

IMPLEMENTATION

The adult dose is 10 mg taken once daily in the evening.

EVALUATION

Report and record:

- *Headache, nausea, indigestion.* These are usually mild and resolve with continued therapy. Give the drug with food or milk to lessen discomfort.

zafirlukast (Accolate)

Zafirlukast (Accolate) competes for the receptor sites that trigger symptoms of asthma. It has been shown to reduce:

- Broncho-constriction
- Daytime asthma symptoms
- Night-time awakening

The goal of therapy is fewer episodes of acute asthma symptoms.

Assisting With the Nursing Process

When giving a person zafirlukast (Accolate), you assist the nurse with the nursing process.

ASSESSMENT

Measure vital signs.

PLANNING

The oral dose form is 20 mg tablets.

IMPLEMENTATION

The adult dose is 20 mg two times a day.

EVALUATION

Report and record:

- *Headache, nausea.* These are usually mild and resolve with continued therapy. Give the drug with food or milk to lessen discomfort.

REVIEW QUESTIONS

Circle the **BEST** answer.

1 Which are the drugs of choice for allergic rhinitis?
a antihistamines
b anti-inflammatory agents
c antitussives
d decongestants

2 Decongestants cause
a vaso-dilation of the nasal mucosa
b vaso-constriction of the nasal mucosa
c vaso-dilation of the tracheo-bronchial tree
d vaso-constriction of the tracheo-bronchial tree

3 Decongestants are used to treat the following *except*
a allergic rhinitis
b asthma
c the common cold
d rhinitis

4 Decongestants are often used with antihistamines to
a liquify secretions
b ease breathing
c reduce sedation
d reduce inflammation

5 Topical dose forms of nasal decongestants
a are drops or sprays
b have systemic side effects
c relieve other symptoms
d prevent rhinitis medicamentosa

6 Which is a nasal decongestant?
a Benadryl
b Chlor-Trimeton
c Phenergan
d Sudafed

7 These statements are about antihistamines. Which is *false?*
a They prevent histamine release.
b They are more effective if taken before histamine is released.
c They are more effective if taken when symptoms first appear.
d Sedation is the most common side effect.

8 Antihistamines are the drugs of choice for the treatment of
a the common cold
b rhinitis
c allergic rhinitis
d rhinitis medicamentosa

9 Antihistamines cause
a diarrhea
b decreased heart rate
c increased sweating
d dry, thick secretions of the mouth, nose, throat, and bronchi

10 Intra-nasal cortico-steroids are given to
a liquify secretions
b ease breathing
c reduce sedation
d reduce inflammation

11 Intra-nasal cortico-steroids are given to treat
a the common cold
b emphysema
c allergic rhinitis
d rhinitis medicamentosa

12 Intra-nasal cortico-steroids are given to reduce the following *except*
a nasal burning
b itching
c rhinorrhea
d sneezing

13 Cromolyn sodium (Nasalcrom)
a competes for histamine receptor sites
b prevents the release of histamine
c relieves nasal congestion
d increases rhinorrhea

14 Cromolyn sodium (Nasalcrom) is sprayed into each nostril
a as needed
b once daily
c at bedtime
d 3 or 4 times a day at regular intervals

15 Which liquify mucus?
a anti-inflammatory agents
b antitussives
c broncho-dilators
d expectorants

16 Which are cough suppressants?
a anti-inflammatory agents
b antitussives
c broncho-dilators
d expectorants

17 Guaifenesin (Robitussin) and potassium iodide (SSKI) are
a anti-inflammatory agents
b antitussives
c broncho-dilators
d expectorants

18 Broncho-dilators are given to
a promote a productive cough
b ease breathing
c liquify secretions
d dry secretions

REVIEW QUESTIONS—cont'd

19 When ipratropium bromide (Atrovent) is given by metered-dose inhaler, the goal of therapy is to
  a prevent COPD
  b reduce rhinorrhea
  c relieve symptoms of allergic rhinitis
  d ease breathing

20 The total dosage of ipratropium bromide (Atrovent) in 24 hours should not exceed
  a 4 inhalations
  b 8 inhalations
  c 12 inhalations
  d 16 inhalations

21 Tiotropium bromide (Spiriva) is
  a a tablet taken orally
  b a dry powder taken with an inhaler
  c a nasal spray
  d an aerosol

22 Which is *not* a xanthine-derivative broncho-dilator?
  a aminophylline
  b terbutaline (Brethine)
  c dyphylline (Dilor)
  d theophylline (Theolair)

23 These statements are about montelukast (Singulair). Which is *false*?
  a It is an anti-leukotriene.
  b It is used to treat asthma.
  c It is inhaled.
  d The dose is taken once a day in the evening.

Circle T if the statement is true. Circle F if the statement is false.

24 T F Antihistamines reduce nasal congestion.

25 T F Anti-inflammatory agents are given to treat the common cold.

26 T F A nasal decongestant and an intra-nasal cortico-steroid are ordered. The nasal decongestant is taken first.

27 T F Cromolyn sodium (Nasalcrom) is an intra-nasal cortico-steroid.

28 T F Codeine is an antitussive.

29 T F Antitussives can cause drowsiness.

30 T F When given orally, broncho-dilators can cause systemic side effects. Tachycardia, tremors, and nervousness are examples.

31 T F Persons taking inhalant cortico-steroids need good oral hygiene.

32 T F A broncho-dilator inhalant and a cortico-steroid inhalant are ordered. The cortico-steroid is taken first.

Answers to these questions are given on p. 446.

Drugs Used to Treat Gastro-Esophageal Reflux and Peptic Ulcer Diseases

OBJECTIVES

- Define the key terms and key abbreviations used in this chapter.
- Describe gastro-esophageal reflux disease.
- Describe peptic ulcer disease.
- Describe the drugs used to treat gastro-esophageal reflux disease and peptic ulcer disease.
- Explain how to assist with the nursing process when drugs are used to treat gastro-esophageal reflux disease and peptic ulcer disease.

KEY TERMS

antacids Drugs that buffer, neutralize, or absorb hydrochloric acid in the stomach; *ant* means *against, acid* means *sour*

antagonist A drug that has the opposite action of another drug or competes for the same receptor sites

anti-spasmodic agents Drugs that have an anti-cholinergic action and prevent acetylcholine from attaching to cholinergic receptors in the GI tract

coating agents Drugs that form a substance that adheres to the crater of an ulcer

gastro-intestinal prostaglandins Drugs that inhibit gastric acid secretion

histamine A substance released in response to allergic reactions and tissue damage from trauma or infection

histamine (H_2)-receptor antagonists Drugs that block the action of histamine; histamine blockers

peptic Pertains to digestion or the enzymes and secretions needed for digestion

peptic ulcer An ulcer in the stomach, duodenum, or other part of the GI system exposed to gastric juices

prokinetic agents Drugs that stimulate movement or motility

Continued

KEY TERMS—cont'd

proton pump inhibitors Drugs that inhibit the gastric acid pump of the parietal cells

ulcer A shallow or deep crater-like sore of a mucous membrane

KEY ABBREVIATIONS

g Gram
GERD Gastro-esophageal reflux disease
GI Gastro-intestinal
MAR Medication administration record
mcg Microgram
mg Milligram
mL Milliliter
NSAID Non-steroidal anti-inflammatory drug
PPI Proton pump inhibitor
PUD Peptic ulcer disease

Gastro-esophageal reflux disease (GERD) is a common stomach disorder. With peptic ulcer disease (PUD), there are ulcerations in the gastro-intestinal (GI) tract. See Box 25-1. See Box 25-2 on p. 318.

The goals of drug therapy for GERD and PUD are to:
- Relieve symptoms
- Promote healing
- Prevent recurrence

See *Delegation Guidelines: Drugs Used to Treat Gastro-Esophageal Reflux and Peptic Ulcer Diseases*, p. 318.

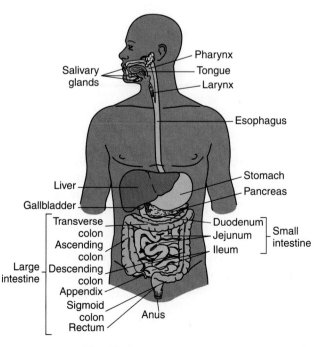

Fig. 25-1 Digestive system.

The digestive system breaks down food physically and chemically so it can be absorbed for use by the cells. This process is called *digestion*. The digestive system is also called the *gastro-intestinal (GI) system*. The system also removes solid wastes from the body.

The digestive system involves the *alimentary canal (GI tract)* and the accessory organs of digestion (Fig. 25-1). The alimentary canal is a long tube. It extends from the mouth to the anus. Its major parts are the mouth, pharynx, esophagus, stomach, small intestine, and large intestine. Accessory organs are the teeth, tongue, salivary glands, liver, gallbladder, and pancreas.

Digestion begins in the *mouth*. The mouth also is called the *oral cavity*. It receives food and prepares it for digestion. Using chewing motions, the *teeth* cut, chop, and grind food into small particles for digestion and swallowing. The *tongue* aids in chewing and swallowing. Taste buds on the tongue's surface contain nerve endings. Taste buds allow sweet, sour, bitter, and salty tastes to be sensed. *Salivary glands* in the mouth secrete *saliva*. Saliva moistens food particles to ease swallowing and begin digestion. During swallowing, the tongue pushes food into the *pharynx*.

The *pharynx* (throat) is a muscular tube. Swallowing continues as the pharynx contracts. Contraction of the pharynx pushes food into the *esophagus*. The esophagus is a muscular tube about 10 inches long. It extends from the pharynx to the *stomach*. Involuntary muscle contractions called *peristalsis* move food down the esophagus through the alimentary canal.

The stomach is a muscular, pouch-like sac. It is in the upper left part of the abdominal cavity. Strong stomach muscles stir and churn food to break it up into even smaller particles. A mucous membrane lines the stomach. It contains glands that secrete *gastric juices*. Food is mixed and churned with the gastric juices to form a semi-liquid substance called *chyme*. Through peristalsis, the chyme is pushed from the stomach into the small intestine. The *duodenum* is the first part of the small intestine.

BOX 25-2   **Gastro-Esophageal Reflux and Peptic Ulcer Diseases**

Gastro-esophageal reflux disease (GERD). Gastro-esophageal reflux disease is a disease in which stomach contents flow back *(reflux)* from the stomach *(gastro)* into the esophagus *(esophageal)*. It is commonly called heartburn, acid indigestion, and sour stomach.

The stomach contents contain acid. The acid can cause irritation and inflammation of the lining of the esophagus. This is called *esophagitis* (inflammation *[itis]* of the esophagus).

Heartburn is the most common symptom of GERD. Heartburn is a burning sensation in the chest and sometimes the throat. The person may have a sour taste in the back of the mouth. Occasional heartburn is not a problem. If it occurs more than twice a week, the person may have GERD. Besides heartburn, other signs and symptoms of GERD include:
- Chest pain, often when lying down
- Hoarseness in the morning
- Dysphagia
- Choking sensation
- Feeling like food is stuck in the throat
- Feeling like the throat is tight
- Dry cough
- Sore throat
- Bad breath

Risk factors for GERD include being over-weight, alcohol use, pregnancy, and smoking. A weakened lower esophagus and hiatal hernia are risks. With hiatal hernia, the upper part of the stomach is above the diaphragm. Large meals and lying down after eating can cause gastric reflux. So can certain foods—citrus fruits, chocolate, caffeine drinks, fried and fatty foods, garlic, onions, spicy foods, tomato-based foods (pasta sauce, chili, pizza).

Most cases of GERD pass quickly with only mild discomfort. Frequent or prolonged bouts of acid reflux cause inflammation, tissue erosion, and ulcerations in the lower esophagus.

The doctor may order drugs to prevent stomach acid production. Some drugs promote emptying of the stomach. Surgery may be needed if drugs and life-style changes do not work. Life-style changes include:
- No smoking
- Not drinking alcohol
- Losing weight
- Eating small meals
- Wearing loose belts and loose-fitting clothes
- Not lying down for 3 hours after meals
- Raising the head of the bed 6 to 8 inches. Blocks of cement or wood are placed under the legs at the head of the bed.

Peptic ulcer disease (PUD). Peptic pertains to digestion or the enzymes and secretions needed for digestion. (*Peptic* means *to digest.*) An ulcer is a shallow or deep crater-like sore of a mucous membrane. A peptic ulcer is an ulcer in the stomach, duodenum, or other part of the GI system exposed to gastric juices.

PUD results from an imbalance between acidic stomach contents and the body's normal defense barriers that protect the stomach wall. Ulcers occur in the stomach (gastric ulcer) and duodenum (duodenal ulcer).

Often the only symptom is epigastric pain. It is described as burning, gnawing, or aching. The pain is most often noted when the stomach is empty—at night or between meals. It is relieved by food or antacids. Other symptoms include bloating, nausea, vomiting, and anorexia.

Ulcers appear to be caused by:
- Over-secretion of hydrochloric acid
- Injury to the mucosal barrier
- Infection of the mucosal wall
  Risk factors include:
- A family history of PUD
- Stress
- Cigarette smoking
- Non-steroidal anti-inflammatory drugs (NSAIDs) (Chapter 17)
- Spicy foods
- Alcohol

DELEGATION GUIDELINES
Drugs Used to Treat Gastro-Esophageal Reflux and Peptic Ulcer Diseases

Some drugs used to treat GERD and PUD are given parenterally—by subcutaneous, intramuscular, or intravenous injection. Because you do not give parenteral dose forms, they are not included in this chapter. Should a nurse delegate the administration of such to you, you must:
- Remember that parenteral dosages are often very different from dosages for other routes.
- Refuse the delegation. Make sure you explain why. Do not just ignore the request. Make sure the nurse knows that you cannot give the drug and why.

DRUG CLASS: **Antacids**

Antacids are drugs that buffer, neutralize, or absorb hydrochloric acid in the stomach. (*Ant* means *against. Acid* means *sour.*) The pH of hydrochloric acid is 1 or 2. Antacids raise the pH to 3 or 4. The gastric juice loses its corrosive effect.

Assisting With the Nursing Process

When giving a person antacids, you assist the nurse with the nursing process.

ASSESSMENT
- Ask about constipation or diarrhea.
- Measure blood pressure if the person has hypertension. Some antacids are high in sodium.
- Observe for edema and signs and symptoms of heart failure (Chapter 21). Some antacids are high in sodium.
- Observe for "coffee ground" vomitus and bloody or tarry stools. These signal GI bleeding.
- Ask the person to describe the onset, duration, and location of pain or discomfort.

PLANNING
See Table 25-1 for "Dose Forms."

IMPLEMENTATION
- Follow directions on the MAR and product container.
- Give other drugs 1 hour before or 2 hours after giving antacids.

EVALUATION
Report and record:
- *Chalky taste.* This is a common problem. The brand or flavor may need to be changed. The form may need to be changed from liquid to tablets.
- *Diarrhea, constipation.* Some products cause diarrhea. Others cause constipation. The drug order may alternate products.

TABLE 25-1 Commonly Used Antacids	
PRODUCT	DOSE FORMS
Aludrox	Tablets, suspension
Di-Gel	Tablets, liquid
Gelusil	Tablets
Maalox TC	Suspension
Maalox Extra Strength	Suspension
Mylanta	Tablets, suspension
Mylanta Double Strength	Suspension
Mylanta Supreme	Liquid
Phillips' Milk of Magnesia	Tablets, suspension
Riopan	Tablets, suspension
Riopan Plus	Tablets, suspension
Titralac	Tablets, suspension
Tums	Tablets

DRUG CLASS: Histamine (H_2)-Receptor Antagonists

Histamine is a substance released in response to allergic reactions and tissue damage from trauma or infection. An **antagonist** is a drug that has the opposite action of another drug or competes for the same receptor sites.

Histamine causes an increase in the secretion of gastric juices. **Histamine (H_2)-receptor antagonists** block the action of histamine. They bind to the H_2 receptor. This results in decreased amounts of gastric juices. The pH of stomach contents rises. (The pH is less acidic.) Histamine (H_2)-receptor antagonists are also called *histamine blockers.*

These drugs are used to treat GERD, duodenal ulcers, and stress ulcers in critically ill persons. A *stress ulcer* is a gastric or duodenal ulcer that develops in persons under severe stress. For example, a severe burn can cause a stress ulcer.

Assisting With the Nursing Process
When giving a person a histamine blocker, you assist the nurse with the nursing process.

ASSESSMENT
Observe for confusion and orientation to person, time, and place.

PLANNING
See Table 25-2 on p. 320 for "Oral Dose Forms."

IMPLEMENTATION
- See Table 25-2 on p. 320 for "Adult Dosage Range."
- Give the drug with food or milk as directed by the nurse and MAR.
- Give antacids (if ordered) 1 hour before or 2 hours after a histamine blocker.

EVALUATION
Report and record:
- *Dizziness, headache, sleepiness.* These are usually mild and resolve with continued therapy. Provide for safety. Remind the person to use caution when driving or using machines.
- *Diarrhea, constipation.* Give drugs as ordered for diarrhea or constipation. Follow the care plan for fluid intake and diet.
- *Confusion, slurred speech, disorientation, hallucinations.* These may occur in persons with liver or kidney diseases and in persons over 50 years of age. They resolve over 3 or 4 days after therapy is discontinued. Provide for safety.
- *Anorexia, nausea, vomiting, jaundice.* These may signal liver toxicity.

TABLE 25-2 Histamine (H₂)-Receptor Antagonists			
GENERIC NAME	**BRAND NAME**	**ORAL DOSE FORMS**	**ADULT DOSAGE RANGE**
cimetidine	Tagamet, Tagamet HB	Tablets: 200, 300, 400, 800 mg Suspension: 300 mg/5 mL	Duodenal and gastric ulcers—800-1600 mg at bedtime, 400 mg twice daily, or 300 mg four times daily GERD—800 mg twice daily or 400 mg four times daily
famotidine	Pepcid, Pepcid AC	Tablets: 10, 20, 40 mg Tablets, chewable: 10 mg Suspension: 40 mg/5 mL	Duodenal and gastric ulcers—40 mg once daily at bedtime or 20 mg twice daily GERD—20 mg twice daily
nizatidine	Axid	Capsules: 150, 300 mg Tablets: 75 mg Oral solution: 15 mg/mL	Duodenal and gastric ulcers—300 mg at bedtime or 150 mg twice daily GERD—150 mg twice daily
ranitidine	Zantac; Zantac 75, 150	Tablets: 75, 150, 300 mg Efferdose tablets: 150 mg Syrup: 15 mg/mL	Duodenal and gastric ulcers—300 mg at bedtime or 150 mg twice daily GERD—150 mg twice daily

DRUG CLASS:
Gastro-Intestinal Prostaglandins

Prostaglandins are fatty acids. They are normally present in the GI tract. They inhibit gastric juice secretion—gastric acid and pepsin. This protects the stomach and duodenal lining from ulcers. **Gastro-intestinal prostaglandins** inhibit gastric acid secretion. The following drug is a gastro-intestinal prostaglandin:

• misoprostol (mis oh pros' tohl); Cytotec (site' oh tech)

The drug is used to prevent and treat gastric ulcers caused by NSAIDs and aspirin (Chapter 17).

Assisting With the Nursing Process

When giving a person misoprostol (Cytotec), you assist the nurse with the nursing process.

ASSESSMENT
Ask about diarrhea.
PLANNING
The oral dose forms are 100 and 200 mcg tablets.
IMPLEMENTATION
■ The adult dose is 100 to 200 mcg tablets 4 times a day.
■ Give the drug with food during NSAID therapy.
EVALUATION
Report and record:
■ *Diarrhea.* This is dose related. It usually develops after about 2 weeks of therapy. It often resolves after about 8 days. It may be lessened by giving the drug with meals and at bedtime. Follow the care plan for fluid intake and diet.

DRUG CLASS: **Proton Pump Inhibitors**

Parietal cells in the stomach secrete gastric acid (hydrochloric acid). **Proton pump inhibitors** (PPIs) inhibit the gastric acid pump of the parietal cells. Thus they block gastric acid production.

PPIs are used to treat severe esophagitis (inflammation of the esophagus), GERD, and gastric and duodenal ulcers. They may be used with antibiotics if infection is the cause of PUD.

Assisting With the Nursing Process

When giving PPIs, you assist the nurse with the nursing process.

ASSESSMENT
Ask about diarrhea.
PLANNING
See Table 25-3 for "Oral Dose Forms."
IMPLEMENTATION
■ See Table 25-3 for "Adult Dosage Range."
■ Capsules and tablets should be swallowed whole. They should not be opened, crushed, or chewed.
EVALUATION
Report and record:
■ *Diarrhea, headache, muscle pain, fatigue.* These are usually mild. Follow the care plan for fluid intake and diet.
■ *Rash.* This may signal an allergic reaction. Do not give the next dose unless approved by the nurse.

TABLE 25-3 Proton Pump Inhibitors			
GENERIC NAME	**BRAND NAME**	**ORAL DOSE FORMS**	**ADULT DOSAGE RANGE**
esomeprazole	Nexium	Capsules: 20, 40 mg	Initial—20-40 mg once daily for 4 to 8 weeks Maintenance—20 mg daily
lansoprazole	Prevacid	Capsules: 15, 30 mg Tablets: 15, 30 mg Granules for oral suspension: 15, 30 mg	Initial—15-30 mg once daily 30 minutes before a meal for 4 weeks Maintenance—15 mg once daily Maximum—30 mg once daily before a meal
omeprazole	Prilosec	Capsules: 10, 20, 40 mg Tablets: 20 mg Powder for oral suspension: 20, 40 mg	Initial—20 mg once daily for 4 weeks Maintenance—20 mg daily Maximum—120 mg three times daily for Zollinger-Ellison syndrome (A rare disorder causing pancreatic and duo- denal tumors and gastric and duodenal ulcers.)
pantoprazole	Protonix	Tablets: 20, 40 mg	Initial—40 mg once daily for 8 weeks Maintenance—40 mg daily
rabeprazole	Aciphex	Tablets: 20 mg	Initial—20 mg daily after morning meal for up to 4 weeks Maintenance—20 mg once daily Maximum—60 mg twice daily

DRUG CLASS: **Coating Agents**

Coating agents form a substance that adheres to the crater of an ulcer. The agent protects the ulcer from gastric juices. It does not inhibit gastric secretions or change gastric pH. The following coating agent is used to treat duodenal ulcers:

- sucralfate (sook rahl′ fate); Carafate (kair′ ah fate)

Assisting With the Nursing Process

When giving a person sucralfate (Carafate), you assist the nurse with the nursing process.

ASSESSMENT

Ask about constipation.

PLANNING

The oral dose forms are:

- 1 g tablets
- 1 g/10 mL suspension

IMPLEMENTATION

- The adult dose is 1 tablet one hour before each meal and at bedtime.
- The drug is given on an empty stomach.
- Antacids (if ordered) are given at least 30 minutes before sucralfate (Carafate).

EVALUATION

Report and record:

- *Constipation.* This is usually mild and tends to re-solve with continued therapy. Follow the care plan for fluid intake and diet.

- *Dry mouth.* Provide oral hygiene. This is usually mild and tends to resolve with continued therapy. The nurse may allow the person to suck on ice chips or hard candy.
- *Dizziness.* This is usually mild and tends to resolve with continued therapy. Provide for safety.

DRUG CLASS: **Prokinetic Agents**

Prokinetic agents are drugs that stimulate move-ment or motility. *Pro* means *forward. Kinetic* means *motion* or *movement.* The following is a prokinetic agent that is a gastric stimulant:

- metoclopramide (met oh klo′ prah myd); Reglan (reg′ lan)

The drug is used to:

- Lower esophageal sphincter pressure. This reduces acid reflux.
- Increase stomach contractions. This empties the stomach faster.
- Relax the pyloric valve. This allows stomach con-tents to empty into the duodenum faster.
- Increase GI peristalsis. This increases the rate of stomach emptying. It also moves chyme and feces faster through the intestinal tract.
- Prevent vomiting during cancer therapy.

Assisting With the Nursing Process

When giving a person metoclopramide (Reglan), you assist the nurse with the nursing process.

ASSESSMENT

- Observe for GI bleeding.
- Ask about abdominal pain or discomfort.
- Observe for restlessness, involuntary movements, facial grimacing, abnormal tongue movements.
- Measure blood glucose if the person has diabetes.

PLANNING

The oral dose forms are:

- 5 and 10 mg tablets
- 5 mg/5 mL syrup

IMPLEMENTATION

The adult oral dose is 10 mg thirty minutes before meals and at bedtime.

EVALUATION

Report and record:

- *Drowsiness, fatigue, lethargy, dizziness, nausea.* These are usually mild and tend to resolve with continued therapy. Provide for safety. Remind the person to use caution when driving or using machines.
- *Restlessness, involuntary movements, facial grimacing, abnormal tongue movements.* Provide for safety.

DRUG CLASS: Anti-Spasmodic Agents

The GI tract is controlled by the cholinergic branch of the autonomic nervous systems (Chapter 14). *Cholinergic fibers* are nerve endings that release acetylcholine (a neurotransmitter). Nerve endings that release acetylcholine are called *cholinergic fibers.* Cholinergic fibers stimulate the GI tract to:

- Secrete saliva and gastric juices
- Move stomach and intestinal contents through the GI tract (peristalsis)

Agents that block or inhibit cholinergic activity are called *anti-cholinergic agents.* **Anti-spasmodic agents** have an anti-cholinergic action. They prevent acetylcholine from attaching to cholinergic receptors in the GI tract. This results in decreased gastric juices and decreased GI motility.

Cholinergic fibers are throughout the body. They are not selective to the GI tract. Therefore the effects of anti-spasmodics are seen throughout the body:

- Reduced perspiration
- Reduced oral and bronchial secretions
- Dilated pupils
- Blurred vision

- Constipation
- Urinary hesitancy or retention
- Tachycardia and palpitations
- Orthostatic hypotension
- Mental confusion
- Delusions
- Nightmares
- Euphoria
- Paranoia
- Hallucinations

Assisting With the Nursing Process

When giving anti-spasmodics, you assist the nurse with the nursing process.

ASSESSMENT

- Observe for confusion, depression, nightmares, and hallucinations.
- Measure blood pressure and the apical heart rate for 1 minute. Note if the rhythm is regular or irregular.
- Measure intake and output.

PLANNING

See Table 25-4 for "Oral Dose Forms."

IMPLEMENTATION

See Table 25-4 for "Initial Adult Dosage Range."

EVALUATION

Report and record:

- *Blurred vision.* Provide for safety.
- *Constipation, urinary retention.* Follow the care plan for fluid intake and diet. Give stool softeners as ordered (Chapter 26).
- *Dryness of the mouth, nose, and throat.* Provide oral hygiene. The nurse may allow the person to chew gum or suck on ice chips or hard candy.
- *Confusion, depression, nightmares, hallucinations.* Provide for safety.
- *Orthostatic hypotension.* This side effect is generally mild when it occurs. Dizziness and weakness may occur when the drug is started. Blood pressure is measured daily in the supine and standing positions. Provide for safety. Remind the person to rise slowly from a supine or sitting position. Have the person sit or lie down if he or she feels faint.
- *Palpitations, dysrhythmias.* Measure the apical heart rate for 1 minute. Note if the rhythm is regular or irregular.

TABLE 25-4 Anti-Spasmodic Agents			
GENERIC NAME	**BRAND NAME**	**ORAL DOSE FORMS**	**INITIAL ADULT DOSAGE RANGE**
atropine	Atropine Sulfate	Tablets: 0.4 mg	0.4-0.6 mg
dicyclomine	Bentyl, Di-Spaz, Bentylol	Tablets: 20 mg Capsules: 10, 20 mg Syrup: 10 mg/5 mL	20-40 mg three or four times daily
glycopyrrolate	Robinul	Tablets: 1, 2 mg	1 mg two or three times daily
mepenzolate	Cantil	Tablets: 25 mg	25-50 mg four times daily
methscopolamine	Pamine	Tablets: 2.5, 5 mg	2.5 mg 30 min before meals and 2.5-5 mg at bedtime
propantheline	Pro-Banthine	Tablets: 7.5, 15 mg	15 mg before meals and 30 mg at bedtime
scopolamine	Scopace	Tablets: 0.4 mg	0.4 to 0.8 mg

REVIEW QUESTIONS

Circle the **BEST** answer.

1 Antacids
   a form a substance that adheres to the crater of an ulcer
   b stimulate GI movement and motility
   c block the action of histamine
   d buffer, neutralize, or absorb hydrochloric acid in the stomach

2 A person has other drugs ordered. The drugs are given
   a with the antacids
   b 30 minutes before the antacids
   c 30 minutes after the antacids
   d 1 hour before or 2 hours after the antacids

3 Antacids can cause
   a diarrhea or constipation
   b orthostatic hypotension
   c tachycardia
   d blurred vision

4 An antacid is high in sodium. You should observe for signs and symptoms of
   a heart failure   c asthma
   b diabetes   d urinary retention

5 Histamine (H_2)-receptor antagonists result in
   a decreased amounts of gastric juices
   b a low pH of stomach contents
   c increased GI motility
   d decreased GI motility

6 Histamine (H_2)-receptor antagonists are given
   a with food or milk
   b on an empty stomach
   c with antacids
   d after meals

7 Which is a (H_2)-receptor antagonist?
   a Tagamet
   b Maalox
   c Mylanta
   d Phillips' Milk of Magnesia

8 Gastro-intestinal prostaglandins
   a form a substance that adheres to the crater of an ulcer
   b stimulate GI movement and motility
   c block the action of histamine
   d inhibit gastric acid secretion

9 Which is a gastro-intestinal prostaglandin?
   a Di-Gel
   b cimetidine
   c Cytotec
   d Carafate

10 Which is *not* a proton pump inhibitor?
   a Pepcid AC
   b Nexium
   c Prilosec
   d Prevacid

Continued

REVIEW QUESTIONS

11 When giving a proton pump inhibitor, the dose form
  a should be swallowed whole
  b can be opened
  c can be crushed
  d can be chewed

12 Coating agents can cause
  a diarrhea
  b heartburn
  c constipation
  d urinary retention

13 Metoclopramide (Reglan) is given
  a 30 minutes before meals and at bedtime
  b with food or milk
  c on an empty stomach
  d after meals

14 The effects of anti-spasmodic agents occur
  a in the esophagus
  b in the stomach
  c in the intestines
  d throughout the body

15 Anti-spasmodic agents result in
  a decreased gastric juices and decreased GI motility
  b increased gastric juices and increased GI motility
  c decreased amounts of histamine
  d increased amounts of histamine

16 Which is an anti-spasmodic agent?
  a Aciphex
  b Atropine sulfate
  c Riopan
  d Zantac

17 Which can cause a chalky taste in the mouth?
  a antacids
  b coating agents
  c anti-spasmodics
  d gastro-intestinal prostaglandins

18 Which can cause mental disturbances?
  a antacids
  b coating agents
  c anti-spasmodics
  d gastro-intestinal prostaglandins

Answers to these questions are on p. 446.

26

Drugs Used to Treat Nausea, Vomiting, Constipation, and Diarrhea

OBJECTIVES

- Define the key terms and key abbreviations used in this chapter.
- Describe nausea, vomiting, constipation, and diarrhea.
- Describe the drugs used to control nausea and vomiting.
- Explain how to assist with the nursing process when giving drugs to control nausea and vomiting.
- Describe the drugs used to control constipation.
- Explain how to assist with the nursing process when giving drugs to control constipation.
- Describe the drugs used to control diarrhea.
- Explain how to assist with the nursing process when giving drugs to control diarrhea.

KEY TERMS

anti-diarrheals Drugs that relieve the symptoms of diarrhea

anti-emetics Drugs used to treat nausea and vomiting

constipation The passage of a hard, dry stool

diarrhea The frequent passage of liquid stools

emesis Vomiting, vomitus

fecal impaction The prolonged retention and build-up of feces in the rectum

griping Severe and spasm-like pain in the abdomen caused by an intestinal disorder; gripping

laxatives Substances that cause evacuation of the bowel; *laxare* means *to loosen*

nausea The sensation of abdominal discomfort that may lead to the urge or need to vomit

retching The involuntary, labored, spasmodic contractions of the abdominal and respiratory muscles without vomitus; "dry heaves"

vomiting Expelling stomach contents through the mouth; emesis

vomitus The food and fluids expelled from the stomach through the mouth; emesis

KEY ABBREVIATIONS

GI Gastro-intestinal
h Hour
MAR Medication administration record
mg Milligram
MI Myocardial infarction
mL Milliliter
PO Per os (orally)
q Every
VC Vomiting center

Nausea is the sensation of abdominal discomfort that may lead to the urge or need to vomit. **Vomiting (emesis)** means expelling stomach contents through the mouth. It signals illness or injury. **Vomitus (emesis)** is the food and fluids expelled from the stomach through the mouth.

Nausea may occur without vomiting. Sudden vomiting may occur without prior nausea. However, nausea and vomiting often occur together.

Retching is the involuntary, labored, spasmodic contractions of the abdominal and respiratory muscles without vomitus. It is commonly called the "dry heaves."

Nausea and vomiting can occur with almost any illness. See Box 26-1 for the structures involved in vomiting. See Box 26-2 for the common causes of nausea and vomiting.

Constipation is the passage of a hard, dry stool. The person usually strains to have a bowel movement. Stools are large or marble-size. Large stools cause pain as they pass through the anus. Constipation occurs when feces move slowly through the bowel. This allows more time for water absorption. Common causes of constipation include:

- A low-fiber diet
- Ignoring the urge to defecate
- Decreased fluid intake
- Inactivity
- Drugs
- Aging
- Certain diseases

Dietary changes, fluids, and activity prevent or relieve constipation. So do drugs and enemas.

If not relieved, constipation can lead to fecal impaction. **Fecal impaction** is the prolonged retention and buildup of feces in the rectum. Feces are hard or putty-like. The person cannot defecate. More water is absorbed from the already hard feces. Liquid feces pass around the hardened fecal mass in the rectum. The liquid feces seep from the anus.

BOX 26-1 Structures Involved in Vomiting

The structures involved in vomiting are shown in Figure 26-1. The vomiting center (VC) is located in the medulla of the brain. It coordinates the vomiting reflex. Nerves from sensory receptors in the pharynx, stomach, intestines, and other tissues connect directly with the VC through the vagus and splanchnic nerves. The nerves produce vomiting when stimulated.

The VC also responds to stimuli from other tissues—cerebral cortex, vestibular apparatus of the inner ear, and blood. These stimuli travel to the chemo-receptor trigger zone in the medulla. This activates the VC to induce vomiting.

When the VC is stimulated, nerve impulses are sent to the salivary, vaso-motor, and respiratory centers. The vomiting reflex begins with a sudden deep inspiration that increases abdominal pressure. Abdominal muscles contract. The soft palate rises and the epiglottis closes. This prevents aspirating vomitus into the lungs. The pyloric sphincter contracts and the cardiac sphincter and esophagus relax. Stomach contents are expelled. Saliva increases to aid expulsion. Pallor, sweating, and tachycardia also occur with vomiting.

BOX 26-2 Common Causes of Nausea and Vomiting

- Chemotherapy
- Drug therapy
- Emotional disturbances
- GI disorders (Gastritis and liver, gallbladder, and pancreatic diseases are examples.)
- Infection
- Mental illness
- Motion sickness
- Over-eating
- Pain
- Pregnancy
- Radiation therapy
- Stomach irritation by certain foods or liquids
- Surgical procedures
- Unpleasant sights and odors

Diarrhea is the frequent passage of liquid stools. Feces move through the intestines rapidly. This reduces the time for fluid absorption. The need to defecate is urgent. Some people cannot get to a bathroom in time. Abdominal cramping, nausea, and vomiting may occur.

Unpleasant stimuli
from environment
(e.g., sight, smell,
emotional shock)
Cortical input
Disturbances of
balance (e.g.,
motion sickness)
Direct input from
drugs, toxins,
metabolites, etc.
carried by blood
Vestibular
apparatus
Vestibular input
Throat, epiglottis,
etc.
Efferent fibers (vagal)
mediating vomiting reflex
Input from sensory
receptors in stomach
and intestines carried
by afferent fibers
Stomach
Chemo-receptor
trigger zone (CTZ)
Vomiting center

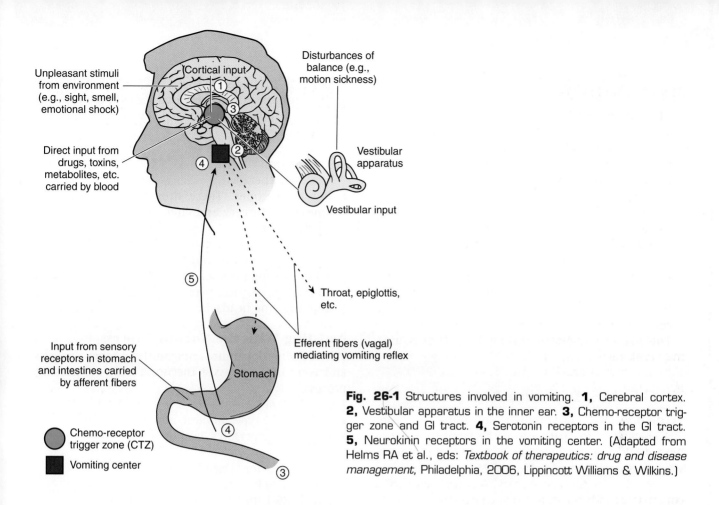

Fig. 26-1 Structures involved in vomiting. **1,** Cerebral cortex. **2,** Vestibular apparatus in the inner ear. **3,** Chemo-receptor trigger zone and GI tract. **4,** Serotonin receptors in the GI tract. **5,** Neurokinin receptors in the vomiting center. (Adapted from Helms RA et al., eds: *Textbook of therapeutics: drug and disease management,* Philadelphia, 2006, Lippincott Williams & Wilkins.)

FOCUS ON OLDER PERSONS

Drugs Used to Treat Nausea, Vomiting, Constipation, and Diarrhea

Older persons are at risk for dehydration from diarrhea. The amount of body water decreases with aging. Many diseases common in older persons affect body fluids. So do many drugs. Report signs of diarrhea at once. Ask the nurse to observe the stool. Death is a risk when dehydration is not recognized and treated.

DELEGATION GUIDELINES

Drugs Used to Treat Nausea, Vomiting, Constipation, and Diarrhea

Some drugs used to treat nausea, vomiting, constipation, and diarrhea are given parenterally—by intramuscular or intravenous injection. Because you do not give parenteral dose forms, they are not included in this chapter. Should a nurse delegate the administration of such to you, you must:

- Remember that parenteral dosages are often very different from dosages for other routes.
- Refuse the delegation. Make sure you explain why. Do not just ignore the request. Make sure the nurse knows that you cannot give the drug and why.

Causes of diarrhea include infections, some drugs, irritating foods, and microbes in food and water. Diet and drugs are ordered to reduce peristalsis.

Fluid lost through diarrhea needs to be replaced. Otherwise, dehydration occurs. The person has pale or flushed skin, dry skin, and a coated tongue. The urine is dark and scant in amount (oliguria). Thirst, weakness, dizziness, and confusion also occur. Falling blood pressure and increased pulse and respirations are serious signs. Death can occur. The nursing process is used to meet the person's fluid needs. In severe cases, the doctor may order intravenous fluids and drugs to control diarrhea.

Microbes can cause diarrhea. Preventing the spread of infection is important. Always follow Standard Precautions and the Bloodborne Pathogen Standard (Appendix C) when in contact with stools.

See *Focus on Older Persons: Drugs Used to Treat Nausea, Vomiting, Constipation, and Diarrhea.*

See *Delegation Guidelines: Drugs Used to Treat Nausea, Vomiting, Constipation, and Diarrhea.*

DRUG THERAPY FOR NAUSEA AND VOMITING

Control of vomiting is important to:
- Relieve the distress caused by vomiting
- Prevent aspiration of stomach contents into the lungs
- Prevent dehydration
- Prevent electrolyte imbalance

Treatment is directed at the cause (see Box 26-2). Treatment measures may involve non-drug measures and drugs. **Anti-emetics** are drugs used to treat nausea and vomiting. They are generally more effective if given before the onset of nausea. Most anti-emetics do one of the following:
- Suppress the action of the vomiting center
- Inhibit impulses going to or from the vomiting center

The goal of anti-emetic therapy is relief of nausea and vomiting.

DRUG CLASS: **Dopamine Antagonists**

Dopamine antagonists inhibit dopamine receptors that are part of the pathway to the vomiting center. Dopamine receptors in other parts of the brain are blocked. See Chapters 14, 15, and 25.

Drugs in this class are the:
- Phenothiazines. They are used for mild to moderate nausea and vomiting associated with:
  - Anesthesia
  - Surgery
  - Radiation therapy
  - Chemotherapy
- Butyrophenones. These drugs are used as anti-emetics in surgery and chemotherapy. Sedation is a side effect.
- Metoclopramide (Reglan). This drug also acts on receptors in the gastro-intestinal (GI) tract. It is useful in treating nausea and vomiting associated with GI cancers, gastritis, peptic ulcer, radiation sickness, and migraine headache.

Assisting With the Nursing Process

When giving dopamine antagonists to relieve nausea and vomiting, you assist the nurse with the nursing process.

ASSESSMENT
- Observe the type, amount, and frequency of emesis.
- Observe the person's level of alertness.

PLANNING

See Table 26-1 for "Dose Forms."

IMPLEMENTATION

See Table 26-1 for "Adult Dosage Range."

EVALUATION
- See Chapter 15 for phenothiazines.
- See Chapter 15 for haloperidol (Haldol).
- See Chapter 25 for metoclopramide (Reglan).

TABLE 26-1 Anti-Emetic Agents				
GENERIC NAME	**BRAND NAME**	**DOSE FORMS**	**ADULT DOSAGE RANGE**	**COMMENTS**
DOPAMINE ANTAGONISTS				
Phenothiazines				**Comments for All Phenothiazines**
chlorpromazine	Thorazine	Tablets: 10, 25, 50, 100, 200 mg	PO: 10-25 mg q4-6h	Phenothiazines may suppress the cough reflex.
		Syrup: 10 mg/5 mL		Ensure that the person does not aspirate vomitus.
		Concentrate: 100 mg/mL		Use with caution in persons with undiagnosed vomiting. Phenothiazines can mask signs of toxicity of other drugs or mask symptoms of other diseases, such as brain tumor, Reye syndrome, or intestinal obstruction.
		Suppositories: 100 mg	Rectal: 50-100 mg q6-8h	Use with extreme caution in persons with seizure disorders.

TABLE 26-1 Anti-Emetic Agents—cont'd

GENERIC NAME	BRAND NAME	DOSE FORMS	ADULT DOSAGE RANGE	COMMENTS
DOPAMINE ANTAGONISTS—cont'd				
Phenothiazines, cont'd				
perphenazine	Perphenazine	Tablets: 2, 4, 8, 16 mg	4 mg q4-6h	
prochlorperazine	Compazine	Tablets: 5, 10 mg Capsules: 10, 15 mg Syrup: 5 mg/mL Suppositories: 2.5, 5, 25 mg	PO: 5-10 mg q6-8h Rectal: 25 mg twice daily	
Butyrophenones				
haloperidol (see Chapter 15)	Haldol			See comments for phenothi- azines on p. 328.
metoclopramide (Chapter 25)	Reglan			
trimethobenzamide	Tigan	Capsules: 300 mg Suppositories: 100, 200 mg	PO: 300 mg three or four times daily Rectal: 200 mg three or four times daily	
SEROTONIN ANTAGONISTS				
dolasetron	Anzemet	Tablets: 50, 100 mg	100 mg within 1 hour before chemotherapy; 100 mg 2 hours before surgery	Recommended for prevention of nausea and vomiting as- sociated with cancer chemo- therapy and post-operative nausea and vomiting.
granisetron	Kytril	Tablets: 1 mg Liquid: 1 mg/5 mL	1 mg up to 1 hour before chemo- therapy, followed by a second dose 12 hours later; or 2 mg once daily	Recommended for prevention of nausea and vomiting as- sociated with cancer che- motherapy, post-operative nausea and vomiting, and nausea and vomiting associ- ated with radiation therapy.
ondansetron	Zofran	Tablets: 4, 8, 24 mg Tablets, orally disinte- grating: 4, 8 mg Liquid: 4 mg/5 mL	8 mg 30 minutes before chemo- therapy, followed by 8 mg 8 hours later	Recommended for prevention of nausea and vomiting asso- ciated with cancer chemo- therapy and post-operative nausea and vomiting.
ANTI-CHOLINERGIC AGENTS USED FOR MOTION SICKNESS				
cyclizine	Marezine	Tablets: 50 mg	50 mg, repeated in 4-6 hours; do not exceed 200 mg daily	May suppress cough reflex. Ensure that the person does not aspirate vomitus. Must be administered 30-45 minutes before travel.
dimenhydrinate	Dramamine	Tablets: 50 mg Liquid: 12.5 mg/4 mL, 15.6 mg/5 mL	50-100 mg q4-6h; do not ex- ceed 400 mg in 24 hours	Will cause sedation. Beware of operating machinery.
diphenhydramine	Benadryl, Diphenhist	Tablets: 25, 50 mg Capsules: 25, 50 mg Elixir: 12.5 mg/5 mL Liquid: 6.25, 12.5 mg/5 mL	25-50 mg three or four times daily	

Continued

TABLE 26-1	Anti-Emetic Agents—cont'd				
GENERIC NAME	**BRAND NAME**	**DOSE FORMS**	**ADULT DOSAGE RANGE**	**COMMENTS**	
ANTI-CHOLINERGIC AGENTS USED FOR MOTION SICKNESS—cont'd					
hydroxyzine	Atarax, Vistaril	Tablets: 10, 25, 50, 100 mg Capsules: 25, 50, 100 mg Syrup: 10 mg/5 mL Suspension: 25 mg/5 mL Liquid: 10 mg/5 mL	25-100 mg three or four times daily		
meclizine	Antivert	Tablets: 12.5, 25, 50 mg Capsules: 25 mg	25-50 mg; may be repeated every 24 hours		
scopolamine, transdermal	Transderm-Scop	Transdermal patch: Delivers 1.5 mg over 3 days	Patch: Apply to skin behind the ear at least 4 hours before anti-emetic effect is required. Replace in 3 days if continued therapy is required.	*Do not cut patches.*	
CORTICO-STEROIDS					
dexamethasone	Decadron	Tablets: 0.25, 0.5, 0.75, 1, 1.5, 2, 4, 6 mg Elixir: 0.5 mg/5 mL Liquid: 1 mg/mL, 0.5 mg/5 mL	4-25 mg q4-6h for 1-2 days	Recommended for prevention of nausea and vomiting associated with chemotherapy.	
BENZODIAZEPINES					
lorazepam	Ativan	Tablets: 0.5, 1, 2 mg Liquid: 2 mg/mL	1-4 mg q4-6h	Recommended for prevention of nausea and vomiting associated with chemotherapy.	
NEUROKININ-1 RECEPTOR INHIBITOR					
aprepitant	Emend	Capsules: 40, 80, 125 mg	125 mg 1 hour before chemotherapy on day 1; 80 mg daily in the morning of days 2 and 3 40 mg 3 hours before anesthesia	Recommended for prevention of acute and delayed nausea and vomiting associated with initial and repeat courses of highly nauseating chemotherapy. Given to prevent post-operative nausea.	

DRUG CLASS: **Serotonin Antagonists**

Serotonin antagonists block receptors in the medulla and GI tract that cause nausea and vomiting. They are used to treat emesis associated with:

- Chemotherapy
- Radiation therapy
- Post-operative nausea and vomiting

Assisting With the Nursing Process

When giving serotonin antagonists to relieve nausea and vomiting, you assist the nurse with the nursing process.

ASSESSMENT

- Observe the type, amount, and frequency of emesis.
- Observe the person's level of alertness.

PLANNING

See Table 26-1 for "Dose Forms."

IMPLEMENTATION

See Table 26-1 for "Adult Dosage Range."

EVALUATION

Report and record:

- *Headache, diarrhea, constipation.* These are usually mild.
- *Sedation.* Provide for safety.

DRUG CLASS: **Anti-Cholinergic Agents**

Motion sickness is thought to result from stimulation of structures in the inner ear. The stimuli are transmitted to areas near the vomiting center. Excess acetylcholine is present. Anti-cholinergic agents are used to counter-balance the excessive amounts of acetylcholine present.

Assisting With the Nursing Process

When giving anti-cholinergic agents to relieve nausea and vomiting, you assist the nurse with the nursing process.

ASSESSMENT

- Observe the type, amount, and frequency of emesis.
- Observe the person's level of alertness.

PLANNING

See Table 26-1 for "Dose Forms."

IMPLEMENTATION

See Table 26-1 for "Adult Dosage Range."

EVALUATION

See Chapter 14.

DRUG CLASS: **Cortico-Steroids**

Cortico-steroids used for nausea and vomiting are effective alone or when used with other anti-emetics. They may help the person accept and control emesis because of these actions:

- Mood elevation
- Increased appetite
- A sense of well-being

Assisting With the Nursing Process

When giving cortico-steroids to relieve nausea and vomiting, you assist the nurse with the nursing process.

ASSESSMENT

- Observe the type, amount, and frequency of emesis.
- Observe the person's level of alertness.

PLANNING

See Table 26-1 for "Dose Forms."

IMPLEMENTATION

See Table 26-1 for "Adult Dosage Range."

EVALUATION

Side effects do not occur often. Because only a few doses are given, the usual complications from long-term cortico-steroid therapy do not occur (Chapter 28).

DRUG CLASS: **Benzodiazepines**

Benzodiazepines act as anti-emetics through a combination of effects. They do the following:

- Cause sedation
- Reduce anxiety
- Depress the vomiting center
- Have an amnesic effect (memory loss)

Benzodiazepines are effective in reducing the frequency of nausea and vomiting. They also reduce the anxiety associated with chemotherapy.

Assisting With the Nursing Process

When giving benzodiazepines to relieve nausea and vomiting, you assist the nurse with the nursing process.

ASSESSMENT

- Observe the type, amount, and frequency of emesis.
- Observe the person's level of alertness.

PLANNING

See Table 26-1 for "Dose Forms."

IMPLEMENTATION

See Table 26-1 for "Adult Dosage Range."

EVALUATION

See Chapter 15.

DRUG CLASS: **Neurokinin-1 Receptor Inhibitor**

Another anti-emetic is used to prevent nausea and vomiting associated with chemotherapy and anesthesia:

- aprepitant (a prep' eh tant); Emend (e mend')

The drug blocks the actions of substances that cause nausea and vomiting. It is used with a cortico-steroid and a serotonin antagonist.

Assisting With the Nursing Process

When giving aprepitant (Emend) to relieve nausea and vomiting, you assist the nurse with the nursing process.

ASSESSMENT

Observe the type, amount, and frequency of emesis.

PLANNING

See Table 26-1 for "Dose Forms."

IMPLEMENTATION

See Table 26-1 for "Adult Dosage Range."

EVALUATION

Report and record:

- *Tiredness, nausea, hiccups, constipation, diarrhea, loss of appetite, headache, hair loss.* The drug is taken for up to 3 days. Therefore side effects are short-lived and rarely troublesome.

DRUG THERAPY FOR CONSTIPATION AND DIARRHEA

Laxatives are substances that cause evacuation of the bowel. (*Laxare* means *to loosen*). Anti-diarrheals are drugs that relieve the symptoms of diarrhea.

DRUG CLASS: **Laxatives**

Types of laxatives are:

- Stimulant laxatives—act directly on the intestine. They cause an irritation that promotes peristalsis and evacuation.
  - Oral agents act within 6 to 10 hours.
  - Rectal agents act within 60 to 90 minutes.
- Saline laxatives—draw water into the intestine from surrounding tissues. The extra water affects stool consistency and distends the bowel. Peristalsis increases. These agents usually act within 1 to 3 hours.
- Lubricant laxatives—contain oils. They lubricate the intestinal wall and soften feces. This allows smooth passage of feces. Onset of action is often 6 to 8 hours but may be up to 48 hours. Peristalsis does not appear to increase. They are sometimes used to prevent constipation in persons who should not strain during defecation. Examples are persons recovering from myocardial infarction (MI) or abdominal surgery.
- Bulk-producing laxatives—are given with a full glass of water. The drug causes water to be retained in the feces. This increases bulk. The increased bulk stimulates peristalsis. Onset of action is usually 12 to 24 hours or as long as 72 hours.
- Fecal softeners—draw water into the feces. This softens feces. These agents do not stimulate peristalsis. It may take 72 hours for a soft bowel movement. These agents are often called *wetting agents* and *stool softeners*. They often are used to prevent constipation or straining to have a bowel movement. For example, they may be ordered for persons after an MI or abdominal surgery.
- Bulk-forming laxatives—soften and increase fecal mass. They also are used to control certain types of diarrhea. They control diarrhea by absorbing the irritating substance. The substance is removed from the bowel with defecation. These agents are dispersed into a glass of water or juice for administration.
- Stimulant and saline laxatives—these are a combination of stimulant and saline laxatives. They are used to relieve acute constipation. They are routinely used as bowel preparations to remove gas and feces before x-ray exams of the kidneys, intestine, or gallbladder.

The goals of laxative therapy are:

- Relief from abdominal discomfort
- Passage of bowel contents within a few hours of administration

Assisting With the Nursing Process

When giving laxatives, you assist the nurse with the nursing process.

ASSESSMENT

- Ask about the person's bowel elimination pattern.
- Ask the person to describe any abdominal pain.

PLANNING

See Table 26-2.

TABLE 26-2 Laxatives

PRODUCT	STIMULANT	SALINE	BULK-FORMING	LUBRICANT	FECAL SOFTENER	OTHER
Citrate of Magnesia		X				
Colace					X	
Colyte						X
Correctol	X					
Dulcolax	X					
Ex-Lax	X					
Fiber Con			X			
Go-LYTELY						X
Haley's M-O		X		X		
Metamucil			X			
Modane	X					
Peri-Colace	X			X		
Phillips' Milk of Magnesia		X				
Phospho-Soda			X			
Surfak					X	
X-Prep	X					

IMPLEMENTATION
- Follow directions on the MAR and container.
- Give adequate water with bulk-forming agents. Without enough water, they can cause esophageal, gastric, intestinal, or rectal obstruction.

EVALUATION
Report and record:
- *Griping (gripping), abdominal discomfort.* **Griping** *(gripping)* is a severe and spasm-like pain in the abdomen caused by an intestinal disorder. Griping and abdominal discomfort result from excessive bowel stimulation.
- *Abdominal tenderness, pain, bleeding, vomiting, diarrhea, abdominal distention.* No bowel movement or having only a small stool may signal an impaction. Or they may signal an *acute abdomen.* This is a serious problem that may require surgery.

DRUG CLASS: **Anti-Diarrheal Agents**

The two types of anti-diarrheal agents are:
- Local acting agents—absorb excess water to cause a formed stool. They absorb irritants or bacteria causing the diarrhea.
- Systemic agents—act through the nervous system to reduce peristalsis and GI motility. The intestinal lining can absorb nutrients, water, and electrolytes. This leaves formed feces in the colon. Because GI motility is reduced, toxins remain in the GI tract longer. This can cause further irritation.

Anti-diarrheal agents are usually ordered:
- When diarrhea is of sudden onset, has lasted more than 2 or 3 days, and is causing significant fluid loss
- When persons with inflammatory bowel disease develop diarrhea
- Post-operatively for diarrhea after GI surgery

The goal of therapy is relief from diarrhea and its discomforts.

Assisting With the Nursing Process

When giving anti-diarrheal agents, you assist the nurse with the nursing process.

ASSESSMENT
- Ask about the person's bowel elimination pattern.
- Ask the person to describe any abdominal pain.

PLANNING
See Table 26-3 for "Oral Dose Forms."

IMPLEMENTATION
- See Table 26-3 for "Adult Dosage."
- Follow directions on the MAR and container.
- Give adequate water with bulk-forming agents. Without enough water, they can cause esophageal, gastric, intestinal, or rectal obstruction.

EVALUATION
Report and record:
- *Abdominal distention, nausea, constipation.* These may result from the excessive use of local agents.
- *Prolonged or worsening diarrhea.* Toxins may be present.

TABLE 26-3 Anti-Diarrheal Agents				
GENERIC NAME	**BRAND NAME**	**ORAL DOSE FORMS**	**ADULT DOSAGE**	**COMMENTS**
SYSTEMIC ACTION				
difenoxin with atropine	Motofen	Tablets: 1 mg difenoxin with 0.025 mg atropine	Two tablets, then one tablet each loose stool. Do not exceed eight tablets in 24 hours	Inhibits peristalsis. Atropine added to minimize potential over-dose or abuse. May cause drowsiness or dizziness; use caution in performing tasks requiring alertness
diphenoxylate with atropine	Lomotil, Lomanate	Tablets: 2.5 mg diphenoxylate with 0.025 mg atropine. Liquid: 2.5 mg diphenoxylate, with 0.025 mg atropine per 5 mL	5 mg four times daily	Inhibits peristalsis. Atropine added to minimize potential over-dose or abuse. May cause drowsiness or dizziness; use caution in performing tasks requiring alertness

TABLE 26-3	Anti-Diarrheal Agents—cont'd			
GENERIC NAME	**BRAND NAME**	**ORAL DOSE FORMS**	**ADULT DOSAGE**	**COMMENTS**
loperamide	Imodium, Imodium A-D, Pepto Diarrhea Control	Tablets: 2 mg Capsules: 2 mg Liquid: 1 mg/5 mL; 1 mg/mL	4 mg initially, followed by 2 mg after each unformed movement. Do not exceed 16 mg/day.	Inhibits peristalsis Used in acute, non-specific diarrhea and to reduce the volume of discharge from ileostomy
opium	Paregoric	Liquid	5-10 mL four times daily	Inhibits peristalsis and pain of diarrhea; 5 mL of liquid = 2 mg morphine Schedule III—may be habit-forming
LOCAL ACTION *Lactobacillus acidophilus*	Lactinex	Capsules, granules, tablets	Two to four tablets or capsules two to four times daily, with milk Granules: One packet added to cereal, fruit juice, milk three or four times daily	Bacteria used to recolonize the gastro-intestinal tract in an attempt to treat chronic diarrhea Do not use in acute diarrhea
bismuth subsalicylate	Pepto-Bismol Kaopectate	Tablets, suspension	30 mL or two tablets chewed every 30-60 minutes up to eight doses	Used as adsorbent

REVIEW QUESTIONS

Circle the BEST answer.

1 Emesis means
   a diarrhea
   b constipation
   c retching or griping
   d vomiting or vomitus

2 Drugs that cause bowel evacuation are called
   a anti-diarrheals
   b anti-emetics
   c laxatives
   d enemas

3 Which is a phenothiazine used to control vomiting?
   a prochlorperazine (Compazine)
   b haloperidol (Haldol)
   c trimethobenzamide (Tigan)
   d dimenhydrinate (Dramamine)

4 Which is often used to control motion sickness?
   a prochlorperazine (Compazine)
   b haloperidol (Haldol)
   c trimethobenzamide (Tigan)
   d dimenhydrinate (Dramamine)

5 Benzodiazepines are used to prevent nausea and vomiting from chemotherapy because they also
   a control diarrhea
   b reduce anxiety
   c improve alertness
   d improve memory

6 Stimulant laxatives
   a cause an irritation that promotes peristalsis
   b draw water into the intestine
   c contain oils
   d draw water into the feces

7 These statements are about lubricant laxatives. Which is *false?*
   a They lubricate the intestinal wall.
   b They soften feces.
   c They may act within 6 to 8 hours.
   d They increase the fecal mass in the bowel.

Continued

REVIEW QUESTIONS—cont'd

8 Which are often ordered to prevent straining during a bowel movement?
   a stimulant laxatives
   b saline laxatives
   c fecal softeners
   d bulk-forming laxatives

9 Which is *not* a laxative?
   a Colace
   b Correctol
   c Dulcolax
   d Lomotil

10 A local-acting anti-diarrheal agent
   a reduces peristalsis
   b reduces GI motility
   c absorbs excess water to cause a formed stool
   d allows the toxin to remain in the intestine

11 Which is *not* an anti-diarrheal agent?
   a Imodium
   b Kaopectate
   c Haley's M-O
   d Pepto-Bismol

Circle **T** if the statement is true. Circle **F** if the statement is false.

12 T F Some drugs used to control nausea and vomiting cause sedation.

13 T F Cortico-steroids are sometimes used to treat constipation.

14 T F Phillips' Milk of Magnesia is a bulk-forming laxative.

15 T F Metamucil is a saline laxative.

Answers to these questions are on p. 447.

27

Drugs Used to Treat Diabetes and Thyroid Diseases

OBJECTIVES

- Define the key terms and key abbreviations used in this chapter.
- Describe diabetes.
- Describe the drugs used to control diabetes.
- Explain how to assist with the nursing process when giving drugs to control diabetes.
- Describe hypothyroidism and hyperthyroidism.
- Describe the drugs used to treat thyroid diseases.
- Explain how to assist with the nursing process when giving drugs to treat thyroid diseases.

KEY TERMS

anti-diabetic agents Drugs used to prevent or relieve the symptoms of diabetes

anti-thyroid agents Drugs used to suppress the production of thyroid hormones

cretinism Congenital hypothyroidism

diabetes A disorder in which the body cannot produce or use insulin properly

hyperglycemia High *(hyper)* sugar *(glyc)* in the blood *(emia)*

hyperthyroidism The disease that occurs from the excess *(hyper)* production of the thyroid hormones

hypoglycemia Low *(hypo)* sugar *(glyc)* in the blood *(emia)*

hypo-glycemic agents Drugs that lower *(hypo)* the blood *(emic)* glucose *(glyc)* level

hypothyroidism The disease that results from inadequate *(hypo)* thyroid hormone production

insulin A hormone produced by the pancreas; it is needed for glucose to enter skeletal muscles, heart muscle, and fat

lactic acid A product of glucose metabolism

lactic acidosis A build-up of lactic acid in the blood

myxedema Hypothyroidism that occurs during adult life

thyroid replacement hormones Drugs that replace thyroid hormones in the treatment of hypothyroidism

KEY ABBREVIATIONS

F Fahrenheit
g Gram
GI Gastro-intestinal
mcg Microgram
mg Milligram
mL Milliliter
T₃ Tri-iodothyronine
T₄ Thyroxine
TSH Thyroid-stimulating hormone
TZD Thiazolidinedione

The endocrine system is made up of glands (Fig. 27-1). The endocrine glands secrete hormones that affect other organs and glands. The pancreas and thyroid gland are part of the endocrine system. Diabetes is the most common endocrine disorder (Box 27-1). It involves the pancreas. Hyperthyroidism and hypothyroidism are thyroid disorders (Box 27-2).

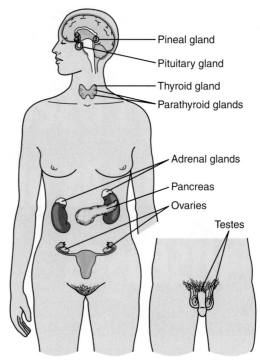

Fig. 27-1 Endocrine system.

BOX 27-1 Diabetes

Diabetes is a disorder in which the body cannot produce or use insulin properly. Insulin is needed for glucose to move from the blood into the cells. The cells need glucose for energy. The pancreas secretes insulin. Without enough insulin, sugar builds up in the blood. Blood glucose (sugar) is high. Cells do not have enough sugar for energy and cannot function.

Three types of diabetes are:
- *Type 1*—occurs most often in children, teenagers, and young adults. The pancreas produces little or no insulin. Onset is rapid.
- *Type 2*—can occur at any age, even during childhood. Persons over 45 years of age are at risk. Being overweight, lack of exercise, and hypertension are risk factors. The pancreas secretes insulin. However, the body cannot use it well. Onset is slow. Infections are frequent. Wounds heal slowly. Gum disease is common.
- *Gestational diabetes*—develops during pregnancy. (*Gestare* means *to bear.*) It usually goes away after the baby is born. The mother is at risk for type 2 diabetes later in life.

Risk factors include a family history of the disease. For type 1, whites are at greater risk than non-whites. Type 2 is more common in older and over-weight persons. These ethnic groups are at risk for type 2:
- African-Americans
- Native Americans
- Hispanics

Signs and symptoms of diabetes are:
- Being very thirsty
- Urinating often
- Feeling very hungry or tired
- Losing weight without trying
- Having sores that heal slowly
- Having dry, itchy skin
- Losing feeling or tingling in the feet
- Having blurred vision

Diabetes must be controlled to prevent complications. They include blindness, renal failure, nerve damage, and damage to the gums and teeth. Heart and blood vessel diseases are serious problems. They can lead to stroke, heart attack, and slow healing. Foot and leg wounds and ulcers can lead to infection and gangrene. Sometimes amputation is necessary.

Type 1 is treated with daily insulin therapy (p. 340), healthy eating, and exercise. Type 2 is treated with healthy eating and exercise. Many persons with type 2 take oral drugs. Some need insulin. Over-weight persons need to lose weight. Types 1 and 2 involve controlling blood pressure, cholesterol, and the risk factors for coronary artery disease.

The person's blood sugar level can fall too low or go too high. Blood glucose is monitored daily or 3 or 4 times a day for:
- **Hypoglycemia** means low *(hypo)* sugar *(glyc)* in the blood *(emia)*.
- **Hyperglycemia** means high *(hyper)* sugar *(glyc)* in the blood *(emia)*.

See Table 27-1 for the causes, signs, and symptoms of hypoglycemia and hyperglycemia. Both can lead to death if not corrected. You must call for the nurse at once.

TABLE 27-1 Hypoglycemia and Hyperglycemia		
	CAUSES	**SIGNS AND SYMPTOMS**
Hypoglycemia (low blood sugar)	Too much insulin or diabetic drugs Omitting or missing a meal Delayed meal Eating too little food Increased exercise Vomiting Drinking alcohol	Hunger Fatigue; weakness Trembling; shakiness Sweating Headache Dizziness Faintness Pulse: rapid Blood pressure: low Respirations: rapid and shallow Motions: clumsy and jerky Tingling around the mouth Confusion Vision: changes in Skin: cold and clammy Convulsions Unconsciousness
Hyperglycemia (high blood sugar)	Undiagnosed diabetes Not enough insulin or diabetic drugs Eating too much food Too little exercise Emotional stress Infection or sickness	Weakness Drowsiness Thirst Dry mouth (very) Hunger Urination: frequent Cramps: leg Face: flushed Breath odor: sweet Respirations: slow, deep, and labored Pulse: rapid, weak Blood pressure: low Skin: dry Vision: blurred Headache Nausea and vomiting Convulsions Coma

BOX 27-2 Thyroid Diseases

The anterior pituitary gland secretes thyroid-stimulating hormone (TSH). TSH stimulates the thyroid gland to release the hormones:
- Tri-iodothyronine (T_3)
- Thyroxine (T_4)

The thyroid hormones regulate metabolism. Imbalances in thyroid hormone production may interfere with:
- Growth and development
- Carbohydrate, protein, and fat metabolism
- Temperature regulation
- Cardiovascular function
- Lactation (producing and secreting breast milk)
- Reproduction

The goal of therapy for thyroid diseases is to return the person to a normal thyroid state.

Continued

BOX 27-2 Thyroid Diseases—cont'd

HYPOTHYROIDISM

Hypothyroidism is the result of inadequate *(hypo)* thyroid hormone production. Myxedema is hypothyroidism that occurs during adult life. The onset of symptoms is usually mild and vague. They include:

- Slowness in motion, speech, and mental processes
- Lethargy—dullness, prolonged sleepiness, drowsiness, sluggishness
- Physical activity levels: low
- Appetite: decreased
- Weight gain
- Constipation
- Cold: being unable to tolerate
- Weakness
- Fatigue: easy
- Body temperature: low
- Skin: dry, coarse, and thick
- Face: puffy
- Blood pressure: low
- Heart rate: low
- Anemia
- Cholesterol levels: high
- Infection: susceptibility to

One cause of myxedema is the excessive use of anti-thyroid drugs. Such drugs are used to treat hyperthyroidism. Other causes include radiation exposure, thyroid surgery, and acute or chronic thyroiditis.

Congenital hypothyroidism is called cretinism. It occurs when a child is born without a thyroid gland. Or the thyroid gland is hypo-active.

Hypothyroidism is treated with thyroid hormones.

HYPERTHYROIDISM

Hyperthyroidism occurs from the excess *(hyper)* production of the thyroid hormones. Signs and symptoms are:

- Pulse: rapid, bounding (even during sleep)
- Palpitations
- Dysrhythmias
- Nervousness
- Agitation: easy
- Tremors
- Fever: low-grade
- Weight loss
- Appetite: increased
- Insomnia
- Heat: being unable to tolerate
- Skin: warm, flushed, moist
- Sweating: increased
- Edema around the eye
- Amenorrhea (no *[a]* menstruation *[menorrhea]*)
- Dyspnea with minor exertion
- Hoarseness
- Speech: rapid
- Infection: susceptibility to

Causes of hyperthyroidism include thyroid cancer and tumors of the pituitary gland. Over-doses of thyroid hormones, thyroiditis, and goiter are other causes. Goiter is an enlarged thyroid gland.

Hyperthyroidism is treated with surgery, radio-active iodine, and anti-thyroid drugs.

DRUG THERAPY FOR DIABETES

Insulin is required to control type 1 diabetes. If not controlled with diet and exercise, oral agents are used to treat type 2 diabetes. Many persons with type 2 diabetes need insulin:

- If it is not controlled with other measures (see Box 27-1).
- During increased physical and psychological stress. Surgery, infection, and pregnancy are examples.

The goals of treatment for diabetes are:

- Normal blood glucose levels
- Fewer long-term complications from poorly controlled diabetes

DRUG CLASS: Insulin

Insulin is a hormone produced by the pancreas. Insulin is needed for glucose to enter skeletal muscles, heart muscle, and fat. It also is needed for protein and lipid metabolism.

The pancreas secretes insulin at a steady rate. It is released in greater amounts when the blood glucose rises, such as after a meal. Insulin deficiency reduces the rate of glucose transport into cells. This results in hyperglycemia.

See *Delegation Guidelines: Drug Class: Insulin.*

See *Promoting Safety and Comfort: Drug Class: Insulin.*

DELEGATION GUIDELINES
Drug Class: Insulin

Insulin is given parenterally—by subcutaneous or intravenous injection. Because you do not give parenteral dose forms, you do not give insulin. Should a nurse delegate the administration of insulin to you, you must:

- Refuse the delegation. Make sure you explain why. Do not just ignore the request. Make sure the nurse knows that you cannot give the drug and why.

  Some states allow MA-Cs to give insulin by the subcutaneous route or by inhalation. Exubera (ex uh bear′ ah) is an insulin inhalation powder. If you are allowed to give subcutaneous or inhaled insulin, make sure that:

- You receive the necessary education about the drug and the dose form.
- You receive the necessary education and training to perform the skill correctly.
- A nurse is available to supervise you.
- A nurse is available to monitor how the drug affects the person.

PROMOTING SAFETY AND COMFORT
Drug Class: Insulin

SAFETY

Insulin should not be allowed to freeze or be heated above 98° F. Therefore insulin is stored in the refrigerator. Once opened, an insulin bottle is discarded in 30 days. After 30 days, the contents may not be sterile. If not sterile, microbes can grow in the bottle. Pre-filled insulin syringes are stored vertically with the needle up. They are stored for up to 30 days.

Having cold insulin injected is uncomfortable. Therefore the agency may keep insulin at room temperature (68° to 75° F). Insulin loses potency if kept above room temperature.

For most refrigerated insulins, the bottle or syringe is gently rolled between the hands (not shaken) to warm and re-mix the insulin. Label directions must be followed.

Assisting With the Nursing Process

When a person receives insulin, you assist with the assessment and evaluation steps of the nursing process. If allowed to give insulin, you also assist with the planning and implementation steps. To assist the nurse, you need to understand the onset, peak, and duration for the type of insulin used (Table 27-2).

- *Onset*—the time required for the insulin to have an initial effect or action
- *Peak*—when the insulin will have the greatest effect
- *Duration*—the length of time that the insulin is active in the body

Knowing the onset, peak, and duration helps you to know when a person is at risk for hypo- or hyperglycemia.

ASSESSMENT

- Measure blood glucose.
- Note the person's activity level.
- Note when and what the person eats.

EVALUATION

Report and record:

- *Signs and symptoms of hypoglycemia.* See Table 27-1. These are more likely to occur when the insulin reaches its peak.
- *Signs and symptoms of hyperglycemia.* See Table 27-1.
- *Itching, swelling, redness at the injection site.* These signal an allergic reaction. Tell the nurse at once. If allowed to give insulin, do not give the next dose unless approved by the nurse.

TABLE 27-2	Forms of Insulin					
TYPE OF INSULIN	**STRENGTH (UNITS/mL)**	**ONSET (HOURS)**	**PEAK (HOURS)**	**DURATION* (HOURS)**	**HYPERGLYCEMIA†**	**HYPOGLYCEMIA†**
RAPID-ACTING INSULIN **Insulin Analog Injection**						
Novolog (aspart)	100	0.2-0.33	1-3	3-5	After lunch (3)	Within 1-3 hours
Humalog (lispro)	100	0.2-0.33	0.5-2.5	3-6.5	After lunch (3)	Within 1-3 hours
Apidra (glulisine)	100	0.2-0.33	0.5-1.5	1-2.5	After lunch (3)	Within 1-3 hours

*The times listed are averages based on a newly diagnosed diabetic patient or resident. Factors modifying these times include patient or resident variation, site and route of administration, and dosage.
†Most often occurs when insulin is administered (1) at bedtime the previous night; (2) before breakfast the previous day; (3) before breakfast the same day.

Continued

TABLE 27-2 Forms of Insulin—cont'd

TYPE OF INSULIN	STRENGTH (UNITS/mL)	ONSET (HOURS)	PEAK (HOURS)	DURATION* (HOURS)	HYPERGLYCEMIA†	HYPOGLYCEMIA†
SHORT-ACTING INSULIN **Insulin Injection**						
Humulin R (human)	100, 500	0.5-4	2.5-5	5-10	Early AM (1)	Before lunch (3)
Novolin R (human)	100	0.5	2.5-5	8	Early AM	Before lunch
INTERMEDIATE-ACTING INSULIN **Isophane Insulin Suspension (NPH)**						
Humulin N (human)	100	1-4	4-12	16-28	Before lunch (2)	3 PM to supper (3)
Novolin N (human)	100	1.5	4-12	24	Before lunch	3 PM to supper
Isophane Insulin Suspension and Insulin Injection						
Humulin 50/50 (human)	100	0.5	4-8	24	Before lunch	3 PM to supper
Humulin 70/30 (human)	100	0.5	4-12	24	Before lunch	3 PM to supper
Novolin 70/30 (human)	100	0.5	2-12	24	Before lunch	3 PM to supper
Lispro Protamine Suspension and Lispro Injection						
Humalog Mix 75/25	100	0.25-0.5	0.5-1.5	12-24		3 PM to supper
Novolog Mix 70/30	100	0.2-0.33	2.4	24		3 PM to supper
Insulin Zinc Suspension						
Lente Iletin II	100	1-1.5	8-12	24	Before lunch	3 PM to supper
Novolin L (human)	100	1-4	7-15	20-28	Before lunch	3 PM to supper
LONG-ACTING INSULIN						
Lantus (glargine)	100	1.1	—‡	24	Mid-AM to mid-PM (1)	—‡
Levemir (detemir)	100	1	—‡	Up to 24	Mid-AM to mid-PM (1)	—‡

*The times listed are averages based on a newly diagnosed diabetic patient or resident. Factors modifying these times include patient or resident variation, site and route of administration, and dosage.

†Most often occurs when insulin is administered (1) at bedtime the previous night; (2) before breakfast the previous day; (3) before breakfast the same day.

‡No pronounced peak activity.

DRUG CLASS: Biguanide Oral Anti-Diabetic Agents

Anti-diabetic agents prevent or relieve the symptoms of diabetes. The following is a biguanide oral anti-diabetic agent:

• metformin (met for' mihn); Glucophage (glue' ko fagh)

Metformin (Glucophage) decreases the amount of glucose produced by the liver. It also decreases the amount of glucose absorbed by the small intestine. By improving insulin sensitivity, more glucose enters skeletal muscle cells and fat cells.

The drug is used alone or with other oral anti-diabetic agents.

Assisting With the Nursing Process

When giving metformin (Glucophage), you assist the nurse with the nursing process.

ASSESSMENT

- Measure blood glucose.
- Note the person's activity level.
- Note when and what the person eats.

PLANNING

The oral dose forms are:

- 500, 850, and 1000 mg tablets
- 500 and 750 mg extended-release tablets
- 500 mg/5 mL oral solution

IMPLEMENTATION

Adult dosages are:

- The initial dose is 500 mg twice daily with the morning and evening meals.

- The dosage is increased by adding 500 mg to the daily dose each week, up to 2000 or 2500 mg daily.
- Most persons need at least 1500 mg daily for the desired effect.
- At dosages of 2000 mg and more, one of the following is ordered:
  - The drug is given 3 times a day: 1000 mg with breakfast, 500 mg with lunch, 1000 mg with dinner.
  - 850 mg is given 3 times a day with breakfast, lunch, and dinner.

EVALUATION

Report and record:

- *Nausea, vomiting, anorexia, abdominal cramps, flatulence.* These are usually mild and tend to resolve with continued therapy. Taking the drug with meals helps reduce these side effects.
- *Malaise, muscle pains, respiratory distress, hypotension.* These signal a build-up of lactic acid in the blood **(lactic acidosis). Lactic acid** is a product of glucose metabolism.

DRUG CLASS: Sulfonylurea Oral Hypo-Glycemic Agents

Hypo-glycemic agents are drugs that lower *(hypo)* the blood *(emic)* glucose *(glyc)* level. Sulfonylureas lower blood glucose by stimulating the release of insulin from the pancreas. They also reduce the amount of sugar produced and metabolized by the liver.

These drugs are used when the pancreas can still secrete insulin. Hypoglycemia may result if too much insulin is produced.

Assisting With the Nursing Process

When giving sulfonylureas, you assist the nurse with the nursing process.

ASSESSMENT

- Measure blood glucose.
- Note the person's activity level.
- Note when and what the person eats.

PLANNING

See Table 27-3 for "Oral Dose Forms."

IMPLEMENTATION

- The "first generation" drugs were first produced over 30 years ago. The newer "second generation" drugs are used more often.
- See Table 27-3 for:
  - "Initial Adult Dose"
  - "Adult Dosage Range"
  - "Duration"

EVALUATION

Report and record:

- *Nausea, vomiting, anorexia, abdominal cramps.* These are mild and tend to resolve with continued therapy.
- *Signs and symptoms of hypoglycemia.* See Table 27-1.
- *Anorexia, nausea, vomiting, jaundice.* These may signal liver toxicity.
- *Sore throat, fever, jaundice, weakness.* These may signal changes in red blood cells and white blood cells.
- *Rash, itching.* These may signal an allergic reaction. Tell the nurse at once. Do not give the next dose unless approved by the nurse.

TABLE 27-3 Sulfonylurea Oral Hypo-Glycemic Agents

GENERIC NAME	BRAND NAME	ORAL DOSE FORMS	INITIAL ADULT DOSAGE	ADULT DOSAGE RANGE	DURATION* (HOURS)
FIRST GENERATION					
acetohexamide		Tablets: 250, 500 mg	0.5 g daily	0.25-1.5 g daily	12-18
chlorpropamide	Diabinese	Tablets: 100, 250 mg	100 mg daily	100-750 mg daily	24-72
tolazamide	Tolinase	Tablets: 100, 250, 500 mg	100 mg daily	0.1-1 g daily	12-16
tolbutamide	Orinase	Tablets: 500 mg	1 g twice daily	0.25-3 g daily	6-12
SECOND GENERATION					
glimepiride	Amaryl	Tablets: 1, 2, 4 mg	1-2 mg daily	1-8 mg daily	24
glipizide	Glucotrol	Tablets: 5, 10 mg	2.5-5 mg daily	15-40 mg daily	10-24
glipizide XL	Glucotrol XL	Extended-release 2.5, 5, 10 mg	5 mg daily	5-20 mg daily	24
glyburide	Glynase, Micronase	Prestabs: 1.5, 3, 6 mg Tablets: 1.25, 2.5, 5 mg	1.5-3 mg daily 2.5-5 mg daily	0.75-12 mg daily 1.25-20 mg daily	24 24

*The times listed are averages based on a newly diagnosed diabetic patient or resident. Factors modifying these times include patient or resident variation and dosage.

TABLE 27-4	Meglitinide Oral Hypo-Glycemic Agents				
GENERIC NAME	**BRAND NAME**	**ORAL DOSE FORMS**	**DAILY ADULT DOSE**	**MAXIMUM DAILY DOSE**
repaglinide	Prandin	Tablets: 0.5, 1, 2 mg	Initial—0.5 to 2 mg before each meal	16
nateglinide	Starlix	Tablets: 60, 120 mg	Initial—60 to 120 mg before each meal	360

DRUG CLASS: Meglitinide Oral Hypo-Glycemic Agents

Meglitinide oral hypo-glycemic agents stimulate the pancreas to release insulin.

These drugs are used when the pancreas can still secrete insulin. They may cause hypoglycemia if too much insulin is produced.

These drugs are used alone or with metformin (Glucophage). Meglitinides have a short duration of action. This reduces the risk of hypoglycemia.

Assisting With the Nursing Process

When giving meglitinides, you assist the nurse with the nursing process.

ASSESSMENT
- Measure blood glucose.
- Note the person's activity level.
- Note when and what the person eats.

PLANNING
See Table 27-4 for "Oral Dose Forms."

IMPLEMENTATION
- See Table 27-4 for "Daily Adult Dose" and "Maximum Daily Dose."
- The dose is given 1 minute to 30 minutes before meals.
- Doses are taken 2, 3, or 4 times daily in response to changing meal times.
- The person should skip a dose if a meal is skipped. This reduces the risk of hypoglycemia.

EVALUATION
Report and record:
- *Signs and symptoms of hypoglycemia.* See Table 27-1.

DRUG CLASS: Thiazolidinedione Oral Anti-Diabetic Agents

Thiazolidinedione (TZD) oral anti-diabetic agents make muscle and fat cells more sensitive to insulin. This lowers blood glucose levels. TZDs also may decrease the amount of glucose produced and released by the liver.

These drugs are used when the pancreas can still secrete insulin.

Assisting With the Nursing Process

When giving TZDs, you assist the nurse with the nursing process.

ASSESSMENT
- Measure blood glucose.
- Note the person's activity level.
- Note when and what the person eats.

PLANNING
See Table 27-5 for "Oral Dose Forms."

IMPLEMENTATION
See Table 27-5 for "Daily Adult Dose" and "Maximum Daily Dose."

EVALUATION
Report and record:
- *Nausea, vomiting, anorexia, abdominal cramps.* These are usually mild and tend to resolve with continued therapy.
- *Signs and symptoms of hypoglycemia.* See Table 27-1.
- *Anorexia, nausea, vomiting, jaundice.* These may signal liver toxicity.
- *Weight gain.* Weight gain of a few pounds is common. However, it may signal edema.

DRUG CLASS: Alpha-Glucosidase Inhibitor Agents

The following are alpha-glucosidase inhibitors:
- acarbose (a' kar bohs); Precose (pre' kohs)
- miglitol (mig' lih tohl); Glyset (gly' set)

acarbose (Precose)

The drug inhibits a pancreatic enzyme and a GI enzyme used to digest sugars. This results in delayed glucose absorption and lowers hyperglycemia after eating.

The drug does not cause hypoglycemia. It may be used with other oral anti-diabetic drugs to lower blood glucose.

Assisting With the Nursing Process

When giving acarbose (Precose), you assist the nurse with the nursing process.

ASSESSMENT
- Measure blood glucose.
- Note the person's activity level.
- Note when and what the person eats.

TABLE 27-5 Thiazolidinedione Oral Hypo-Glycemic Agents				
GENERIC NAME	**BRAND NAME**	**ORAL DOSE FORMS**	**DAILY DOSE**	**MAXIMUM DAILY DOSE (mg)**
pioglitazone	Actos	Tablets: 15, 30, 45 mg	Initial—15-30 mg once daily	45
rosiglitazone	Avandia	Tablets: 2, 4, 8 mg	Initial—2 mg twice daily or 4 mg once daily	8

PLANNING

The oral dose forms are 25, 50, and 100 mg tablets.

IMPLEMENTATION

- The initial adult oral dose is 25 mg three times a day. The dose is given at the start of each main meal.
- The dosage is adjusted at 4 to 8 week intervals based on blood glucose levels.
- The maintenance dosage is 50 to 100 mg three times a day.

EVALUATION

Report and record:

- *Abdominal cramps, diarrhea, flatulence.* These are usually mild and tend to resolve with continued therapy.
- *Signs and symptoms of hypoglycemia.* See Table 27-1. Monitor for hypoglycemia if the drug is taken with other anti-diabetic agents.
- *Anorexia, nausea, vomiting, jaundice.* These may signal liver toxicity.

miglitol (Glyset)

The drug inhibits a pancreatic enzyme and a GI enzyme used to digest sugars. This results in delayed glucose absorption and lower hyperglycemia after eating.

The drug does not cause hypoglycemia. It may be used with other oral anti-diabetic drugs to lower blood glucose.

Assisting With the Nursing Process

When giving miglitol (Glyset), you assist the nurse with the nursing process.

ASSESSMENT

- Measure blood glucose.
- Note the person's activity level.
- Note when and what the person eats.

PLANNING

The oral dose forms are 25, 50, and 100 mg tablets.

IMPLEMENTATION

- The initial adult oral dose is 25 mg three times a day. The dose is given at the start (first bite) of each main meal.
- The dosage is adjusted at 4 to 8 week intervals based on blood glucose levels.

- The maintenance dosage is 50 to 100 mg three times a day.
- The maximum dosage is 100 mg three times a day.

EVALUATION

Report and record:

- *Abdominal cramps, diarrhea, flatulence.* These are usually mild and tend to resolve with continued therapy.
- *Signs and symptoms of hypoglycemia.* See Table 27-1. Monitor for hypoglycemia if the drug is taken with other anti-diabetic agents.

DRUG THERAPY FOR THYROID DISEASES

Two classes of drugs are used to treat thyroid diseases:

- **Thyroid replacement hormones**—replace thyroid hormones. These are used in the treatment of hypothyroidism.
- **Anti-thyroid agents**—suppress the production of thyroid hormones.

See *Delegation Guidelines: Drug Therapy for Thyroid Diseases.*

DRUG CLASS: **Thyroid Replacement Hormones**

Hypothyroidism is treated by replacing the thyroid hormones—T_3 and T_4. Thyroxine (T_4) is partially metabolized into T_3. Therapy with thyroxine (T_4) replaces both T_3 and T_4.

DELEGATION GUIDELINES
Drug Therapy for Thyroid Diseases

Some drugs used to treat thyroid diseases are given parenterally. Because you do not give parenteral dose forms, they are not included in this chapter. Should a nurse delegate the administration of such to you, you must:

- Remember that parenteral dosages are often very different from dosages for other routes.
- Refuse the delegation. Make sure you explain why. Do not just ignore the request. Make sure the nurse knows that you cannot give the drug and why.

TABLE 27-6	Thyroid Hormones			
GENERIC NAME	**BRAND NAME**	**ORAL DOSE FORMS**	**COMPOSITION**	**ADULT DOSAGE RANGE**
levothyroxine	Synthroid Levoxyl	Tablets: 0.025, 0.05, 0.075, 0.088, 0.1, 0.112, 0.125, 0.137, 0.15, 0.175, 0.2, 0.3 mg	Thyroxine (T_4)	Initial—0.025 mg daily Maintenance—0.1 to 0.2 mg daily
liothyronine	Cytomel	Tablets: 5, 25, 50 mcg	Liothyronine (T_3)	Initial—25 mcg daily; Maintenance—25 to 75 mcg daily
liotrix	Thyrolar-$1/4$ Thyrolar-$1/2$ Thyrolar-1 Thyrolar-2 Thyrolar-3	Tablets: 12.5/3.1 mcg Tablets: 25/6.25 mcg Tablets: 50/12.5 mcg Tablets: 100/25 mcg Tablets: 150/37.5 mcg	$T_4:T_3 = 4:1$	Maintenance—$1/4$ or $1/2$ adjusted as needed at 2 week intervals
thyroid, USP	—	Tablets: 16, 32, 65, 98, 130, 195, 260, 325 mg Capsules: 65, 130, 195, 325 mg Tablets, extended-release: 32, 65, 130 mg	Unpredictable $T_4:T_3$ ratio	Maintenance—65-195 mg daily

Assisting With the Nursing Process

When giving thyroid replacement hormones, you assist the nurse with the nursing process.

ASSESSMENT

- Measure vital signs. Use the apical site to measure heart rate.
- Ask about bowel elimination.
- Measure weight.
- Observe for signs and symptoms of hyperthyroidism (see Box 27-2).

PLANNING

See Table 27-6 for "Oral Dose Forms."

IMPLEMENTATION

See Table 27-6 for "Adult Dosage Range."

EVALUATION

Report and record:

- *Signs and symptoms of hyperthyroidism.* See Box 27-2.

DRUG CLASS: Anti-Thyroid Drugs

Anti-thyroid drugs block the formation of T_3 and T_4 in the thyroid gland. They do not destroy any T_3 and T_4 already produced. Once therapy is started, it usually takes a few days to 3 weeks before symptoms improve.

The following are anti-thyroid drugs:

- propylthiouracil (pro pil thy o you' rah sil); PTU, Propacil (pro' pa sil)
- methimazole (meth im' ah zohl); Tapazole (tap' ah zoal)

Assisting With the Nursing Process

When giving anti-thyroid drugs, you assist the nurse with the nursing process.

ASSESSMENT

- Measure vital signs.
- Measure weight.
- Observe for signs and symptoms of hypothyroidism (see Box 27-2).

PLANNING

The oral dose forms are:

- propylthiouracil (PTU, Propacil): 50 and 100 mg tablets
- methimazole (Tapazole): 5 and 10 mg tablets

IMPLEMENTATION

- propylthiouracil (PTU, Propacil):
  - The initial adult dose is 100 to 150 mg every 6 to 8 hours.
  - The dosage ranges up to 900 mg daily.
  - The maintenance dose is 50 mg two or three times a day.
- methimazole (Tapazole):
  - The initial adult dose is 5 to 20 mg every 8 hours.
  - The maintenance dose is 5 to 15 mg daily.

EVALUATION

Report and record:

- *Rash, itching.* These often occur during the first 2 weeks of therapy. They usually resolve without treatment.
- *Headache, salivary gland and lymph node enlargement, loss of taste.* These are usually mild and tend to resolve with continued therapy.
- *Sore throat, fever, jaundice.* These may signal problems with blood cell production.
- *Anorexia, nausea, vomiting, jaundice.* These may signal liver toxicity.
- *Decreased urine output, bloody or smoky-colored urine.* These may signal kidney toxicity.

REVIEW QUESTIONS

Circle the **BEST** answer.

1 Insulin is a hormone produced by the
   a adrenal glands
   b pancreas
   c pituitary gland
   d thyroid gland

2 Blood glucose is higher
   a before meals
   b after meals
   c at bedtime
   d before breakfast

3 Insulin is given
   a orally or by inhalation
   b by subcutaneous or intramuscular injection
   c by intramuscular or intravenous injection
   d by subcutaneous or intravenous injection

4 Insulin is usually stored
   a in the freezer
   b in the refrigerator
   c at room temperatures above 75° F
   d for up to 45 days

5 To re-mix insulin, the nurse
   a shakes the bottle or syringe 3 times
   b shakes the bottle or syringe 6 times
   c turns the bottle or syringe upside down
   d gently rolls the bottle or syringe between the hands

6 An insulin reaches its peak in 4 to 8 hours. This is when the insulin
   a has its initial action
   b has its greatest effect
   c remains active in the body
   d must be discarded

7 A person received insulin. You assist the nurse by observing for
   a hypoglycemia
   b hyperglycemia
   c hypothyroidism
   d hyperthyroidism

8 Metformin (Glucophage) is
   a a form of insulin
   b an oral anti-diabetic agent
   c a hypo-glycemic agent
   d a first generation sulfonylurea

9 The initial doses of metformin (Glucophage) are given
   a before each meal
   b with the morning and evening meals
   c after each meal
   d on awakening and at bedtime

10 Sulfonylurea agents lower blood glucose by
   a decreasing the amount of glucose produced by the liver
   b sensitizing muscle and fat cells to insulin
   c stimulating the release of insulin
   d inhibiting enzymes used to digest sugars

11 Which is *not* a sulfonylurea?
   a glimepiride (Amaryl)
   b glipizide (Glucotrol)
   c glyburide (Glynase)
   d repaglinide (Prandin)

12 Meglitinides are given
   a 1 hour before meals
   b 1 hour after meals
   c 1 to 30 minutes before meals
   d 1 to 30 minutes after meals

13 Which is a thiazolidinedione?
   a rosiglitazone (Avandia)
   b chlorpropamide (Diabinese)
   c tolbutamide (Orinase)
   d nateglinide (Starlix)

14 Acarbose (Precose) is given
   a 30 minutes before meals
   b 30 minutes after meals
   c within 1 to 30 minutes of a meal
   d at the start of each meal

15 Acarbose (Precose) and miglitol (Glyset)
   a decrease the amount of glucose produced by the liver
   b sensitize muscle and fat cells to insulin
   c stimulate the release of insulin
   d inhibit enzymes used to digest sugars

16 A person is receiving a thyroid replacement hormone. You need to observe for
   a hypoglycemia
   b hyperglycemia
   c hypothyroidism
   d hyperthyroidism

17 Which is a *not* a thyroid replacement hormone?
   a liothyronine (Cytomel)
   b levothyroxine (Synthroid)
   c methimazole (Tapazole)
   d liotrix (Thyrolar)

Circle **T** if the statement is true. Circle **F** if the statement is false.

18 T F Insulin is always used to treat type 1 diabetes.

19 T F Insulin is never used to treat type 2 diabetes.

20 T F Anti-thyroid drugs are used to treat myxedema.

Answers to these questions are on p. 447

28

Cortico-Steroids and Gonadal Hormones

OBJECTIVES

- Define the key terms and key abbreviations used in this chapter.
- Identify the purposes and uses of cortico-steroids.
- Identify the cortico-steroid preparations.
- Explain how to assist with the nursing process when giving cortico-steroids.
- Identify the purposes and uses of gonadal hormones.
- Identify the estrogen preparations.
- Explain how to assist with the nursing process when giving estrogens.
- Identify the progestin preparations.
- Explain how to assist with the nursing process when giving progestins.
- Identify the androgen preparations.
- Explain how to assist with the nursing process when giving androgens.

KEY TERMS

androgens Steroid hormones that produce masculine effects

cortico-steroids Hormones secreted by the adrenal cortex of the adrenal glands

endometriosis A condition *(osis)* in which the tissue that lines *(endo)* the inside of the uterus *(metri)* grows outside the uterus

estrogen The female hormone

eunuchism A condition in which the male lacks male hormones

gluco-corticoids Hormones that regulate carbohydrate, protein, and fat metabolism; they have anti-inflammatory, anti-allergenic, and immuno-suppressant activity

gonads The reproductive glands

hypogonadism A condition in which the body does not produce enough *(hypo)* testosterone

mineralo-corticoids Hormones that maintain fluid and electrolyte balance

progesterone The hormone associated with body changes that favor pregnancy and lactation

testosterone The male hormone

KEY ABBREVIATIONS

g Gram
mg Milligram
PO Per os (orally)

Cortico-steroids are hormones secreted by the adrenal cortex of the adrenal glands (see Fig. 27-1 in Chapter 27).

- The mineralo-corticoids maintain fluid and electrolyte balance. They are used to treat adrenal insufficiency caused by hypo-function of the pituitary or adrenal glands (Addison's disease).
- The gluco-corticoids regulate carbohydrate, protein, and fat metabolism. They have anti-inflammatory, anti-allergenic, and immuno-suppressant activity.

The gonads are the reproductive glands: the testes of the male and the ovaries of the female (see Fig. 27-1 in Chapter 27). The testes produce sperm and testosterone (the male hormone). Testosterone controls the development of the male sex organs. It also controls the development of male secondary sex characteristics—voice, hair distribution, male body form. Androgens are other steroid hormones that produce masculine effects.

The ovaries produce estrogen and progesterone. These hormones stimulate development of the female sex organs. They influence breast development, voice quality, and the broader pelvis of the female body. Estrogen is the female hormone. It is responsible for most of the changes. Progesterone is the hormone needed for body changes that favor pregnancy and lactation.

See *Delegation Guidelines: Cortico-Steroids and Gonadal Hormones.*

DRUG CLASS: Mineralo-Corticoids

The following is a mineralo-corticoid:

- fludrocortisone (flu droh kort' ih sown); Florinef (flohr' in ehf)

The drug is a mineralo-corticoid with gluco-corticoid effects. It affects fluid and electrolyte balance by causing:

- Sodium and water retention
- Potassium and hydrogen excretion

The drug is used with gluco-corticoids. The goals of therapy are to:

- Control blood pressure
- Restore fluid and electrolyte balance

Assisting With the Nursing Process

When giving mineralo-corticoids, you assist the nurse with the nursing process.

DELEGATION GUIDELINES
Cortico-Steroids and Gonadal Hormones

Some cortico-steroids and gonadal hormones are given parenterally—by intramuscular or intravenous injection. Because you do not give parenteral dose forms, they are not included in this chapter. Should a nurse delegate the administration of such to you, you must:

- Remember that parenteral dosages are often very different from dosages for other routes.
- Refuse the delegation. Make sure you explain why. Do not just ignore the request. Make sure the nurse knows that you cannot give the drug and why.

ASSESSMENT

- Measure vital signs.
- Measure weight.
- Measure intake and output.
- Observe for signs and symptoms of infection. Cortico-steroid therapy may mask signs and symptoms of infection.
- Observe level of alertness and orientation to person, time, and place.
- Test stools for occult blood.

PLANNING

The oral dose form is 0.1 mg tablets.

IMPLEMENTATION

The adult dose is 0.1 mg daily.

EVALUATION

See "Drug Class: Gluco-Corticoids."

DRUG CLASS: Gluco-Corticoids

Gluco-corticoids are given for their anti-inflammatory, anti-allergenic, and immuno-suppressant effects. They relieve symptoms of inflammation, but do not cure disease. These drugs are used in the treatment of:

- Some cancers
- Organ transplants
- Auto-immune diseases
- Rheumatoid arthritis
- Allergy signs and symptoms
- Shock
- Nausea and vomiting from chemotherapy
The goals of treatment are to:
- Reduce pain and inflammation
- Minimize shock and hasten recovery
- Reduce nausea and vomiting from chemotherapy

TABLE 28-1　Cortico-Steroid Preparations

GENERIC NAME	BRAND NAME	DOSE FORMS
alclometasone	Aclovate	Cream, ointment
amcinonide	Cyclocort	Cream, ointment, lotion
betamethasone	Celestone, Valisone, Diprosone, Luxiq, others	Tablets, syrup, cream, ointment, lotion, aerosol, gel, foam, powder
clobetasol	Temovate, Embeline E	Cream, ointment, scalp application, lotion
clocortolone	Cloderm	Cream
cortisone	Cortisone	Tablets
desonide	Tridesilon, DesOwen	Cream, ointment, lotion
desoximetasone	Topicort	Cream, ointment, gel
dexamethasone	Decadron, Dexone, Hexadrol, Decaspray	Cream, aerosol, tablets, elixir
diflorasone	Florone, Maxiflor, Psorcon E	Cream, ointment
fludrocortisone	Florinef	Tablets
fluocinolone	Synalar, Flurosyn	Cream, ointment, solution, shampoo, oil
fluocinonide	Lidex	Cream, ointment, gel, solution
flurandrenolide	Cordran	Cream, ointment, tape, lotion
fluticasone	Cutivate	Cream, ointment
halcinonide	Halog, Halog E	Cream, ointment, solution
halobetasol	Ultravate	Cream, ointment
hydrocortisone	Cortef, Solu-Cortef, Hydrocortone	Cream, ointment, tablets, enema, gel, lotion, suppositories, oral suspension, spray
methylprednisolone	Solu-Medrol, Depo-Medrol, Medrol	Tablets, powder
mometasone	Elocon, Asmanex, Nasonex	Cream, ointment, lotion, spray, inhalant
prednicarbate	Dermatop E	Cream, ointment
prednisolone	Prelone	Tablets, syrup, suspension, solution
prednisone	Deltasone, Orasone	Tablets, solution
triamcinolone	Aristocort, Kenalog, Nasacort HFA	Cream, ointment, lotion, tablets, syrup, aerosol, paste, inhalant, spray

Assisting With the Nursing Process

When giving gluco-corticoids, you assist the nurse with the nursing process.

ASSESSMENT
- Measure vital signs.
- Measure weight.
- Measure intake and output.
- Observe for signs and symptoms of infection. Cortico-steroid therapy may mask signs and symptoms of infection.
- Observe level of alertness and orientation to person, time, and place.
- Test stools for occult blood.

PLANNING
See Table 28-1 for "Dose Forms."

IMPLEMENTATION
- Persons taking these drugs for at least 1 week must not abruptly stop therapy. Otherwise, the following may occur:
  - Fever
  - Malaise and fatigue
  - Weakness
  - Anorexia
  - Nausea
  - Dizziness
  - Hypotension
  - Fainting
  - Dyspnea
  - Hypoglycemia
  - Muscle and joint pain
  - Return of the disease process

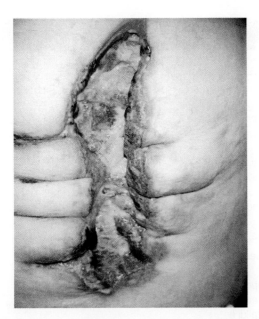

Fig. 28-1 Wound dehiscence. (Courtesy Kinetic Concepts, Inc. [KCI] Licensing, Inc., San Antonio, Tex.)

- Follow the manufacturer's instructions to apply topical dose forms.
- Alternate-day therapy may be used for chronic conditions.
  - Some cortico-steroids are given between 0600 and 0900 on alternate days.
  - Give oral dose forms with meals to lessen stomach irritation.

EVALUATION
Many side effects are related to dosage and duration of therapy. Report and record:

- *Changes in alertness and orientation to person, time, and place; confusion; muscle cramps; nausea.* These may signal electrolyte imbalance (potassium, sodium, and chloride).
- *Sore throat, fever, malaise, nausea, vomiting, and other signs and symptoms of infection.* Cortico-steroid therapy may mask signs and symptoms of infection.
- *Behavior changes.* Psychotic behaviors (Chapter 15) are more likely in persons with a history of mental health problems.
- *Signs and symptoms of hypoglycemia.* See Chapter 27.
- *Signs and symptoms of peptic ulcer.* See Chapter 25.
- *Vision problems.* These drugs may cause cataracts.
- *Delayed wound healing.* Observe surgical patients for signs of dehiscence (Fig. 28-1). Dehiscence is the separation of wound layers.

DRUG CLASS: **Estrogens**

Estrogens are used:
- To relieve the hot flash symptoms of menopause
- For contraception

- For hormone replacement therapy after surgical removal of the ovaries
- As part of the treatment for osteoporosis
- To treat severe acne in females
- To slow the progress of advanced prostate cancers
- To slow the progress of some types of breast cancer

Assisting With the Nursing Process
When giving estrogen, you assist the nurse with the nursing process.
ASSESSMENT
- Measure vital signs.
- Measure weight.
PLANNING
See Table 28-2 on pp. 352-353 for "Dose Forms."
IMPLEMENTATION
See Table 28-2 on pp. 352-353 for "Adult Doses."
EVALUATION
Report and record:
- *Weight gain, edema, breast tenderness, nausea.* These tend to be mild and resolve with continued therapy.
- *Hypertension, signs and symptoms of hyperglycemia (Chapter 27), break-through uterine bleeding, signs and symptoms of thrombo-embolic diseases (Chapter 23).* These are complications of estrogen therapy.

DRUG CLASS: **Progestins**

Progesterone and the progestins inhibit ovulation. They are used to treat amenorrhea (no menstruation), break-through uterine bleeding, and endometriosis. **Endometriosis** is a condition *(osis)* in which the tissue that lines *(endo)* the inside of the uterus *(metri)* grows outside the uterus. Usually the tissue grows on organs in the pelvic and abdominal areas. Symptoms include painful (often severe) menstrual cramps, lower back and pelvic pain, heavy menstrual periods, spotting between periods, and pain during or after sex.

The progestins may be used with estrogens as contraceptives (Chapter 29). The goals of progestin therapy are:
- Contraception
- Relief of endometriosis symptoms
- Hormone balance to relieve amenorrhea or abnormal uterine bleeding

Assisting With the Nursing Process
When giving progestins, you assist the nurse with the nursing process.
ASSESSMENT
- Measure vital signs.
- Measure weight.
PLANNING
See Table 28-3 on p. 353 for "Dose Forms."
IMPLEMENTATION
See Table 28-3 on p. 353 for "Adult Doses."

TABLE 28-2 Estrogens

GENERIC NAME	BRAND NAME	DOSE FORMS	USES	ADULT DOSES
Conjugated estrogen	Premarin	Tablets: 0.3, 0.45, 0.625, 0.9, 1.25 mg	Menopause	PO: 0.625-1.25 mg daily cyclically*
			Female hypogonadism	PO: 0.3-0.625 mg daily for 20 days, followed by 10 days off
			Ovarian failure or post-oophorectomy	PO: 1.25 mg daily cyclically*
			Osteoporosis prevention	PO: 0.625 mg daily cyclically*
			Breast carcinoma	PO: 10 mg three times daily
			Prostatic carcinoma	PO: 1.25-2.5 mg three times daily
		Cream: 0.625 mg/g	Atrophic vaginitis	Intra-vaginal: 0.5 to 2 g daily
Esterified estrogen	Menest	Tablets: 0.3, 0.625, 1.25, 2.5 mg	Menopause, atrophic vaginitis	0.3-1.25 mg daily cyclically*
			Female hypogonadism, post-oophorectomy, ovarian failure	1.25-7.5 mg daily cyclically*
			Breast carcinoma	10 mg three times daily
			Prostatic carcinoma	1.25-2.5 mg three times daily
estradiol	Estrace	Tablets: 0.45, 0.5, 1, 1.5, 1.8, 2 mg	Menopause, atrophic vaginitis, hypogonadism, post-oophorectomy, ovarian failure	PO: 1-2 mg daily cyclically*
			Prostatic carcinoma	PO: 1-2 mg three times daily
			Breast carcinoma	PO: 10 mg three times daily
	Vivelle	Transdermal patch: 0.014, 0.025, 0.0375, 0.05, 0.06, 0.075, 0.1 mg	Menopause Female hypogonadism Primary ovarian failure Atrophic vaginitis Post-oophorectomy Prevention of osteoporosis	Transdermal system: A patch should be placed on a clean, dry area of the skin on the trunk (usually abdomen or buttock) twice weekly on a cyclic schedule (3 weeks of therapy followed by 1 week without). Rotate application site; interval of 1 week between uses of same site.
	Estrasorb	Topical emulsion: 4.35 mg/pouch	Menopause	Topical: Apply contents of 1 pouch to left leg and 1 pouch to right leg daily. Rub from upper thigh area to ankles. Allow to dry. Wash hands with soap and water. If uterus is intact, progestin should also be taken to prevent endometrial cancer.
	Estrogel	Topical gel: 0.06% in tube or pump	Menopause; vaginal atrophy	Topical: Apply contents of 1 applicator or 1 pump daily to 1 arm, spreading from wrist to upper arm on all sides. Allow to dry. Wash hands with soap and water. If uterus is intact, progestin should also be taken to prevent endometrial cancer. Alcohol gel is flammable until dry; avoid fire, flame, or smoking until dry.

*Cyclically = 3 weeks of daily estrogen followed by 1 week off.

TABLE 28-2	Estrogens—cont'd			
GENERIC NAME	**BRAND NAME**	**DOSE FORMS**	**USES**	**ADULT DOSES**
estropipate	Ogen	Tablets: 0.75, 1.5, 3, 6 mg	Menopause Female hypogonadism, post-oophorectomy, ovarian failure	PO: 0.625-6 mg daily cyclically* PO: 1.25-9 mg daily cyclically*
		Cream: 1.5 mg/g	Osteoporosis prevention Atrophic vaginitis	0.75 mg daily cyclically* Intra-vaginal: 2 to 4 g daily

*Cyclically = 3 weeks of daily estrogen followed by 1 week off.

TABLE 28-3	Progestins			
GENERIC NAME	**BRAND NAME**	**DOSE FORMS**	**USES**	**ADULT DOSES**
medroxyprogesterone	Provera, Amen, Curretab	Tablets: 2.5, 5, 10 mg	Secondary amenorrhea Abnormal uterine bleeding	5-10 mg daily for 5-10 days 5-10 mg daily for 5-10 days, beginning on the 16th or 21st day of the menstrual cycle
norethindrone	Aygestin	Tablets: 5 mg	Amenorrhea, abnormal uterine bleeding Endometriosis	2.5-10 mg starting with the 20th and ending on the 25th day of the menstrual cycle 5 mg for 2 weeks; increase in increments of 2.5 mg/day every 2 weeks until 15 mg/day is reached
norgestrel	Ovrette	Tablets: 0.075 mg	Oral contraceptive	1 tablet daily
progesterone	Progesterone	Vaginal gel 4%, 8%	Amenorrhea, functional uterine bleeding	

EVALUATION

Report and record:

- *Weight gain, edema, nausea, vomiting, diarrhea, tiredness, oily scalp, acne.* These tend to be mild and resolve with continued therapy.
- *Break-through uterine bleeding, amenorrhea, continuing headache, jaundice, depression.* These are complications of progestin therapy.
- *Pregnancy.* Birth defects are possible.

DRUG CLASS: **Androgens**

Androgens are used to treat:

- **Hypogonadism**—a condition in which the body does not produce enough *(hypo)* testosterone (the male hormone secreted from the male sex gland). This affects the development of the male sex organs and growth and development.

- **Eunuchism**—a condition in which the male lacks male hormones. The testicles were destroyed or removed. If this occurs before puberty, secondary sex characteristics do not develop.
- Androgen deficiency—lower than normal amounts of testosterone.
- Breast cancer in post-menopausal women. The goal is to suppress cancer growth and reduce discomfort.

Assisting With the Nursing Process

When giving androgens, you assist the nurse with the nursing process.

ASSESSMENT
- Measure vital signs.
- Measure weight.
- Measure blood glucose. Androgens may cause hypoglycemia in persons with diabetes.

PLANNING
See Table 28-4 for "Dose Forms."

IMPLEMENTATION
See Table 28-4 for "Adult Doses."

EVALUATION
Report and record:
- *Stomach irritation.* Give the drug with food or milk.
- *Changes in alertness and orientation to person, time, and place; confusion; muscle cramps; nausea; edema.* These may signal electrolyte imbalance (potassium, sodium, and chloride).
- *Women: masculine characteristics such as deepening voice, hoarseness, growth of facial hair, menstrual irregularities.* These may not reverse when therapy is discontinued.
- *Men: excessive sexual stimulation, priapism (prolonged or constant penis erection), breast enlargement.* These signal androgen overdose.
- *Nausea, vomiting, constipation, poor muscle tone, lethargy.* These signal hypercalcemia—high *(hyper)* blood *(emia)* calcium *(calc)* levels.
- *Anorexia, nausea, vomiting, jaundice.* These may signal liver toxicity.

TABLE 28-4 Androgens

GENERIC NAME	BRAND NAME	DOSE FORMS	USES	ADULT DOSES
SHORT-ACTING				
testosterone gel	AndroGel 1%, Testim	Topical gel 1%	Hypogonadism	Open one or more hormone packets (depending on dosage), squeeze entire contents onto palm of hand, and apply to clean, dry, intact skin of shoulders, upper arms, and abdomen. Allow to dry prior to dressing. Wash hands with soap and water. Do not apply to genitals.
testosterone USP in gel base	Androderm Transdermal System; Testoderm TTS	Transdermal patch: 12.5, 25 mg	Androgen deficiency	1-3 patches applied on hips, abdomen, thighs, or buttocks nightly for 24 hours; replace every 24 hours; do not apply to scrotum.
	Testoderm	Transdermal patch: 4, 6 mg	Androgen deficiency	Shave scrotal area. Apply a 4 or 6 mg patch to the scrotum once daily at about the same time each day. Apply to clean, dry skin. Do not apply to other skin surfaces. The drug is poorly absorbed from other tissues.

TABLE 28-4 Androgens—cont'd

GENERIC NAME	BRAND NAME	DOSE FORMS	USES	ADULT DOSES
ORAL PRODUCTS				
testosterone	Striant	Buccal system: 30 mg	Hypogonadism	1 buccal system applied to the gum above the incisor tooth every 12 hours. Alternate with opposite side for each new dose. When applying, hold the rounded surface against the gum for 30 seconds to ensure adhesion. Do not chew or swallow.
methyltestosterone	Methitest, Test-red, Virilon	Tablets: 10, 25 mg Capsules: 10 mg Buccal tablets: 10 mg	Eunuchism Cryptorchidism Breast carcinoma	10-40 mg daily 30 mg daily 50-200 mg daily
fluoxymesterone	Halotestin	Tablets: 2, 5, 10 mg	Male hypogonadism Female breast carcinoma	5-20 mg daily 10-40 mg daily

REVIEW QUESTIONS

Circle the **BEST** answer.

1 Which maintain fluid and electrolyte balance?
a androgens
b estrogens
c gluco-corticoids
d mineralo-corticoids

2 Which have anti-inflammatory, anti-allergenic, and immuno-suppressant activity?
a androgens
b estrogens
c testosterone
d mineralo-corticoids

3 Testosterone is produced by the
a adrenal glands
b gonads
c ovaries
d testes

4 Fludrocortisone (Florinef) is
a an androgen
b an estrogen
c a gluco-corticoid
d a mineralo-corticoid

5 Fludrocortisone (Florinef) is used to
a control blood pressure
b relieve inflammation
c treat nausea and vomiting from chemotherapy
d prevent conception

6 Oral gluco-corticoids are given
a before meals
b with meals
c after meals
d at bedtime

7 Which is *not* a cortico-steroid?
a triamcinolone (Aristocort)
b dexamethasone (Decadron)
c conjugated estrogen (Premarin)
d methylprednisolone (Solu-Medrol)

8 Cortico-steroids may cause signs and symptoms of
a electrolyte imbalance
b masculine characteristics
c infection and inflammation
d allergies

9 A person has a history of mental health problems. Behavior changes may occur when taking
a cortico-steroids
b estrogens
c progestins
d androgens

Continued

REVIEW QUESTIONS

10 Estrogens may be used in the treatment of the following *except*
   a endometriosis
   b menopause
   c advanced prostate cancers
   d some types of breast cancer

11 Which is a progestin?
   a estradiol (Estrace)
   b esterified estrogen (Menest)
   c estropipate (Ogen)
   d medroxyprogesterone (Provera)

12 Progestins are used for the following *except*
   a breast cancer in post-menopausal women
   b contraception
   c endometriosis
   d abnormal uterine bleeding

13 Male hormones are lacking because the testes were removed. This is called
   a androgen deficiency
   b eunuchism
   c hypogonadism
   d priapism

14 Which is an androgen?
   a medroxyprogesterone (Amen)
   b fluocinonide (Lidex)
   c methyltestosterone (Methitest)
   d estradiol (Vivelle)

Circle T if the statement is true. Circle F if the statement is false.

15 T F Cortico-steroids are secreted by the cerebral cortex.

16 T F Estrogen and progesterone are female hormones.

17 T F Many cortico-steroids are applied topically.

18 T F Thrombo-embolic disease is a complication of estrogen therapy.

Answers to these questions are on p. 447.

29

Drugs Used in Men's and Women's Health

OBJECTIVES

- Define the key terms and key abbreviations used in this chapter.
- Describe the sexually transmitted diseases.
- Identify the drugs used to treat sexually transmitted diseases.
- Describe the various types of contraceptives.
- Explain how to assist with the nursing process when contraceptives are taken.
- Identify the purposes for using drugs in obstetrics.
- Explain benign prostatic hyperplasia.
- Identify the drugs used to treat benign prostatic hyperplasia.
- Explain how to assist with the nursing process when giving drugs to treat benign prostatic hyperplasia.
- Explain erectile dysfunction.
- Explain how to assist with the nursing-process when drugs to treat erectile dysfunction are taken.

KEY TERMS

contraception The processes or methods used to prevent *(contra)* pregnancy

erectile dysfunction (ED) The inability of the male to have an erection; impotence

impotence See "erectile dysfunction"

leukorrhea An abnormal whitish *(leuko)* vaginal discharge *(rrhea)*

oral contraceptives Birth control pills

priapism A prolonged or constant erection

KEY ABBREVIATIONS

BPH Benign prostatic hyperplasia
ED Erectile dysfunction
MAR Medication administration record
mg Milligram
STD Sexually transmitted disease
TURP Trans-urethral resection of the prostate

Drug therapy for men's and women's health involves treating genital infections and sexually transmitted diseases (STDs). Many women use contraceptives for birth control. Drugs also are used in obstetrics. Some men require treatment of prostatic hyperplasia or erectile dysfunction.

DRUG THERAPY FOR LEUKORRHEA AND GENITAL INFECTIONS

Having vaginal secretions is normal. Excessive discharge is abnormal. **Leukorrhea** is an abnormal whitish *(leuko)* vaginal discharge *(rrhea)*. A symptom of an underlying disorder, it can occur at any age. The most common cause is an infection.

STDs are described in Table 29-1. See Table 29-2 for drugs used to treat genital infections. Also see Chapter 34.

DRUGS USED FOR CONTRACEPTION

Contraception means the process or methods used to prevent *(contra)* pregnancy. **Oral contraceptives** (birth control pills) are the most common form of birth control in the United States. The goal of contraceptive therapy is to prevent pregnancy.

See Box 29-1 on p. 360 for a review of menstruation and fertilization.

TABLE 29-1 Sexually Transmitted Diseases		
DISEASE	**SIGNS AND SYMPTOMS**	**TREATMENT**
Herpes	Painful, blister-like sores on or near the genitals, mouth, or anus The sores may have a watery discharge Pain, itching, burning, and tingling in the affected area Vaginal discharge Pain during urination or intercourse Fever Swollen glands	No known cure Anti-viral drugs
Gonorrhea	Burning and pain on urination Urinary frequency and urgency Genital discharge (vagina, urethra, rectum)	Antibiotic drugs
Chlamydia	May not show symptoms Discharge from the penis or vagina Burning or pain on urination Testicular pain or swelling Vaginal bleeding Rectal inflammation and/or discharge Pain during intercourse Diarrhea Nausea Abdominal pain Fever	Antibiotic drugs
Trichomoniasis (occurs in women; men are carriers)	No symptoms in men Frothy, thick, foul-smelling, yellow vaginal discharge Genital itching and irritation Burning and pain on urination Genital swelling	Metronidazole
Syphilis	*Stage 1:* 10 to 90 days after exposure • Painless sores (chancres) on the penis, in the vagina, or on the genitalia; the chancre may also be on the lips, inside of the mouth, or anywhere on the body	Penicillin and other antibiotic drugs

TABLE 29-1	Sexually Transmitted Diseases—cont'd	
DISEASE	**SIGNS AND SYMPTOMS**	**TREATMENT**
Syphilis—cont'd	*Stage 2*: About 3 to 6 weeks after the sores • General fatigue, loss of appetite, nausea, fever, headache, rash, swollen glands, sore throat, bone and joint pain, hair loss, lesions on the lips and genitalia • Symptoms may come and go for many years *Stage 3*: 3 to 15 years after infection • Central nervous system damage (including paralysis), heart damage, blindness, liver damage, mental health problems, death	

TABLE 29-2	Causative Organisms and Products Used to Treat Genital Infections	
CAUSATIVE ORGANISM	**GENERIC NAME**	**BRAND NAME**
VAGINITIS		
Candida albicans (fungus)	butoconazole vaginal cream	Gynazolel; Mycelex-3
	clotrimazole vaginal cream, vaginal tablets	Gyne-Lotrimin, Mycelex-7
	fluconazole oral tablets	Diflucan
	miconazole vaginal cream, suppositories	Monistat
	terconazole vaginal cream, suppositories	Terazol 7, Terazol 3
	tioconazole vaginal ointment	Vagistat
Trichomonas vaginalis (protozoa)	metronidazole oral tablets	Flagyl
	tinidazole oral tablets	Tindamax
Gardnerella vaginalis (bacteria)	metronidazole oral tablets, vaginal gel	Flagyl; MetroGel-Vaginal
	clindamycin vaginal cream	Cleocin
GONORRHEA		
Neisseria gonorrhea (bacteria)	ceftriaxone	Rocephin
	cefixime	Suprax
SYPHILIS		
Treponema pallidum (spirochete)	penicillin G, benzathine	Bicillin C-R
	tetracycline	Tetracycline
	doxycycline	Vibramycin
	azithromycin	Zithromax
GENITAL HERPES		
Herpes simplex genitalis (virus)	acyclovir oral capsules	Zovirax
	famciclovir oral tablets	Famvir
	valacyclovir oral tablets	Valtrex
CHLAMYDIA		
Chlamydia trachomatis (chlamydia)	doxycycline	Vibramycin
	erythromycin	Erythromycin
	azithromycin	Zithromax
	ofloxacin	Floxin
	levofloxacin	Levaquin

From Centers for Disease Control and Prevention: Sexually transmitted diseases treatment guidelines, *MMWR* 2006:55 (No. RR-11), 2006; and Centers for Disease Control and Prevention: Updated recommended treatment of gonococcal infections and associated conditions—United States, April 2007.

BOX 29-1 Menstruation and Fertilization

Menstruation. The endometrium is rich in blood to nourish the cell that grows into a fetus. If pregnancy does not occur, the endometrium breaks up. It is discharged from the body through the vagina. This process is called *menstruation*. Menstruation occurs about every 28 days. Therefore it is called the *menstrual cycle (period)*.

The first day of the menstrual cycle begins with menstruation. Blood flows from the uterus through the vaginal opening. Menstrual flow usually lasts 3 to 7 days. Ovulation occurs during the next phase. An ovum matures in an ovary and is released. Ovulation usually occurs on or about day 14 of the cycle.

Meanwhile, estrogen and progesterone (the female hormones) are secreted by the ovaries. These hormones cause the endometrium to thicken for pregnancy. If pregnancy does not occur, the hormones decrease in amount. This causes the blood supply to the endometrium to decrease. The endometrium breaks up. It is discharged through the vagina. Another menstrual cycle begins.

Fertilization. To reproduce, a male sex cell (sperm) must unite with a female sex cell (ovum). The uniting of the sperm and ovum into one cell is called *fertilization*. A sperm has 23 chromosomes. An ovum has 23 chromosomes. The fertilized cell has 46 chromosomes.

During intercourse, millions of sperm are deposited into the vagina. Sperm travel up the cervix, through the uterus, and into the fallopian tubes (Fig. 29-1). If a sperm and an ovum unite in a fallopian tube, fertilization results. Pregnancy occurs. The fertilized cell travels down the fallopian tube to the uterus. After a short time, the fertilized cell implants in the thick endometrium and grows during pregnancy.

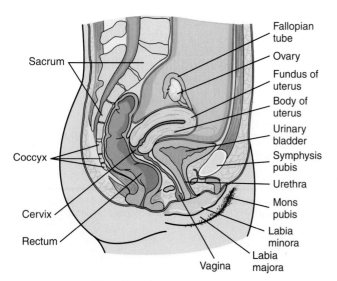

Fig. 29-1 Female reproductive system.

DRUG CLASS: Oral Contraceptives

Oral contraceptives prevent ovulation. The two types of oral contraceptives are:

- The combination pill. It contains both estrogen and progestin. These pills are packaged with 28 tablets. The last 7 tablets contain iron but no hormones. The package has 28 tablets so there is no break in the daily routine of taking a pill. The three types of combination pills are:
  - Mono-phasic. They contain a fixed amount of estrogen and progestin given daily for 21 days. The first dose is taken on day 5 of the menstrual cycle.
  - Bi-phasic. They contain a fixed dose of estrogen and a progestin dose on days 1 to 10 that is lower than the dose on days 11 to 21 of the menstrual cycle.
  - Tri-phasic. They have varying amounts of hormones to provide the lowest doses necessary to prevent conception.
- The mini-pill. It contains only progestin. All 28 tablets contain an active hormone.

Levonorgestrel/ethinyl estradiol (lee' voe nor jess trel/eth' in il ess tra dye' ole) (Seasonale) is a new combination oral contraceptive. The woman has only 4 menstrual periods each year—one each season. The drug contains estrogen and progestin in lower doses than other combination oral contraceptives. The package has 84 active tablets and 7 that contain no hormones. Active tablets are taken for 84 days, and then the other 7 are taken. One tablet is taken daily.

Assisting With the Nursing Process

When giving oral contraceptives, you assist the nurse with the nursing process.

ASSESSMENT
- Measure weight.
- Measure blood pressure in the supine and sitting positions.

PLANNING
See Box 29-2.

IMPLEMENTATION
- Combination pills: The first pill is taken on the first Sunday after the period begins. One pill is taken daily at the same time until the pack is gone.
  - 21-day pack—wait 1 week and start a new pack on Sunday.
  - 28-day pack—start a new pack the day after finishing a pack.
- Mini-pills: The first pill is taken on the first day of the period.
- Another form of birth control is needed the first month.
- One pill is taken daily at the same time of day until the pack is gone.
- Follow the nurse's directions for missed doses.

BOX 29-2 Oral Contraceptives

MONO-PHASIC ORAL CONTRACEPTIVES
Alesse
Apri
Aviane
Brevicon
Cryselle
Demulen 1/35
Demulen 1/50
Desogen
Junel Fe 15/35 E
Junel Fe 1/20
Lessina
Levlen
Levlite
Levora
Loestrin-21 1/20
Loestrin-21 1.5/30
Loestrin Fe 1/20
Loestrin Fe 1.5/30
Low-Ogestrel
Lo/Ovral
Lutera
Microgestin Fe
Modicon
MonoNessa
Necon 0.5/35
Necon 1/35
Necon 1/50
Nordette
Norinyl 1 + 35
Norinyl 1 + 50
Nortrel 0.5/35
Nortrel 1/35
Ogestrel
Ortho-Cept
Ortho-Cyclen
Ortho-Novum 1/35
Ortho-Novum 1/150
Ovcon-35
Ovcon-50
Ovral
Portia

Seasonale
Solia
Sprintec
Yasmin
Zovia 1/35 E
Zovia 1/50 E

BI-PHASIC ORAL CONTRACEPTIVES
Kariva
Mircette
Necon
Ortho Novum

TRI-PHASIC ORAL CONTRACEPTIVES
Aranelle
Cesia
Cyclessa
Enpresse
Estrostep 21
Estrostep Fe
Leena
Necon 7/7/7
Ortho-Novum 7/7/7
Ortho Tri-Cyclen
Tri-Levlen
TriNessa
Tri-Norinyl
Triphasil
Triprevifem
Tri-Sprintec
Trivora-28
Velivet

PROGESTIN-ONLY CONTRACEPTIVES
Camila
Errin
Jolivette
Ortho-Micronor
Nora-BE
Nor-QD
Ovrette

EVALUATION

Report and record:

- *Nausea, weight gain, spotting, changed menstrual flow, missed periods, depression, mood changes, headaches, and brown pigmentation on the forehead, cheeks, and nose.* These are common side effects. A prescription change is needed if they do not resolve after 3 months.
- *Vaginal discharge, break-through bleeding, yeast infection.* A prescription change and other drugs may be needed.
- *Blurred vision, severe headaches, dizziness, leg pain, chest pain, shortness of breath, acute abdominal pain.* These may signal serious complications.

DRUG CLASS:
Transdermal Contraceptive

The following is a transdermal contraceptive:
- norelgestromin-ethinyl estradiol transdermal system (nor ehl ges' troh min); Ortho Evra

The drug contains estrogen and progestin to inhibit ovulation. Cervical mucus becomes thick. This inhibits sperm from traveling up the cervix to the uterus and fallopian tubes. The hormones also change the endometrial wall. This impairs implantation of a fertilized ovum.

Assisting With the Nursing Process

When applying a transdermal contraceptive, you assist the nurse with the nursing process.

ASSESSMENT

Measure blood pressure in the supine and sitting positions.

PLANNING

The dose form is a transdermal patch.

IMPLEMENTATION

- Apply a new patch on the same day of the week. This day is called "patch change day."
- Apply a patch to clean, dry, intact, healthy skin. Do not apply the patch to an irritated area.
- The patch sites are the buttock, abdomen, upper outer arm, or upper torso. Do not apply a patch on a breast. Avoid areas where tight clothing can rub the patch.
- Do not apply makeup, powder, lotion, or cream to the skin or patch area. The patch may not adhere properly. Hormone absorption may be impaired.
- One of the following methods is used:
  - First day start. Apply the first patch during the first 24 hours of the menstrual period. Note the day of the week. This becomes "patch change day."
  - Sunday start. Apply the first patch on the first Sunday after menstruation begins. This becomes "patch change day."
- Follow the nurse's directions if a patch is loose or comes off.
- Another form of birth control is needed the first 7 days of the first menstrual cycle.

EVALUATION

Report and record:

- *Nausea, weight gain, spotting, changed menstrual flow, missed periods, depression, mood changes, headaches, and brown pigmentation on the forehead, cheeks, and nose.* These are common side effects. A prescription change is needed if they do not resolve after 3 months.
- *Vaginal discharge, break-through bleeding, yeast infection.* A prescription change and other drugs may be needed.
- *Blurred vision, severe headaches, dizziness, leg pain, chest pain, shortness of breath, acute abdominal pain.* These may signal serious complications.

DRUGS USED IN OBSTETRICS

Obstetrics is the branch of medicine concerned with the care of women during pregnancy, labor, and childbirth and for the first 6 to 8 weeks after birth. Drugs are used in obstetrics to:

- Induce labor
- Control bleeding after delivery
- Maintain uterine firmness after delivery
- Induce therapeutic abortion
- Prevent premature labor
- Prevent seizure activity
- Promote ovulation
- Prevent mother-child blood incompatibilities in future pregnancies

Some of the drugs used in obstetrics are listed in Table 29-3.

See *Delegation Guidelines: Drugs Used in Obstetrics.*

TABLE 29-3 Drugs Used in Obstetrics

GENERIC NAME	BRAND NAME	DOSE FORMS	ADULT DOSAGE RANGE	USES
dinoprostone	Prostin E$_2$	Vaginal suppository: 20 mg		Start and continue cervical ripening at term
	Cervidil	Vaginal insert: 10 mg		Expel uterine contents
ergonovine maleate	Ergotrate Maleate	Tablets: 0.2 mg	0.2 mg every 6 to 8 hours after delivery for up to 1 week	Stimulate uterine contractions post-partum to control bleeding and maintain uterine firmness
methylergonovine maleate	Methergine	Tablets: 0.2 mg	0.2 mg every 6 to 8 hours after delivery for up to 1 week	Stimulate uterine contractions post-partum to control bleeding and maintain uterine firmness
clomiphene citrate	Clomid	Tablets: 50 mg	50 mg daily for 5 days (first course; follow the MAR for second and third courses)	Induce ovulation in women who are not ovulating

DELEGATION GUIDELINES
Drugs Used in Obstetrics

Drugs used in obstetrics must be given carefully to protect the health of the mother and fetus. If allowed to give such drugs, you need to learn more about them. Ask for the necessary education and supervision.

Some drugs are given parenterally—by intramuscular or intravenous injection. Because you do not give parenteral dose forms, they are not included in this chapter. Should a nurse delegate the administration of such to you, you must:
* Remember that parenteral dosages are often very different from dosages for other routes.
* Refuse the delegation. Make sure you explain why. Do not just ignore the request. Make sure the nurse knows that you cannot give the drug and why.

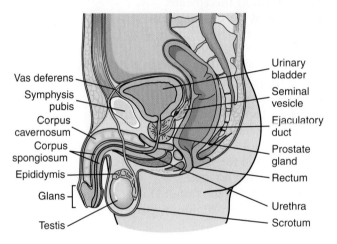

Fig. 29-2 Male reproductive system.

Vas deferens
Symphysis pubis
Corpus cavernosum
Corpus spongiosum
Epididymis
Glans
Testis

Urinary bladder
Seminal vesicle
Ejaculatory duct
Prostate gland
Rectum
Urethra
Scrotum

DRUG THERAPY FOR BENIGN PROSTATIC HYPERPLASIA

The prostate is a gland in men. It lies in front of the rectum and just below the bladder (Fig. 29-2). The prostate also surrounds the urethra. In young men, the prostate is about the size of a walnut. The prostate grows larger (enlarges) as the man grows older. This is called benign prostatic hyperplasia (BPH). *(Benign* means *non-malignant. Hyper* means *excessive. Plasia* means *formation* or *development.)* Benign prostatic hypertrophy is another name for enlarged prostate. *(Trophy* means *growth.)*

Usually BPH does not cause problems until after age 50. Most men in their 60s, 70s, and 80s have some symptoms of BPH.

BPH causes urinary problems. The enlarged prostate presses against the urethra. This obstructs urine flow through the urethra. Bladder function is gradually lost. These problems are common:
* A weak urine stream
* Frequent voidings of small amounts of urine
* Urgency and leaking or dribbling of urine
* Frequent urination at night
* Urinary retention

Treatment depends on the extent of the problem. For mild BPH, the doctor may order drugs. Drugs can shrink the prostate or stop its growth. Some microwave and laser treatments destroy the excess prostate tissue.

Trans-urethral resection of the prostate (TURP) is a common surgical procedure. A lighted scope is inserted through the penis. The scope has a wire loop. The doctor uses the loop to cut tissue and seal blood vessels. The removed tissue is flushed out of the bladder at the end of the surgery. A special catheter is inserted and left in place for a few days. Flushing fluid enters the bladder through the catheter. Urine and the flushing fluid flow out of the bladder through the same catheter. Some bleeding and blood clots are normal.

DRUG CLASS: Alpha-1 Adrenergic Blocking Agents

The following alpha-1 adrenergic blocking agents are used to treat BPH:
* alfuzosin (al fuse oh' sin); Uroxatral (uhr ox' ah tral)
* tamsulosin (tam suhl oh' sin); Flomax (floh' max)

These drugs block alpha-1 receptors on the prostate gland and certain areas of the bladder neck. Muscles relax, allowing greater urine flow.

The drugs are used to treat mild to moderate urinary obstruction in men with BPH. The goals of therapy are to:
* Reduce symptoms of BPH
* Improve urine flow

Assisting With the Nursing Process

When giving alpha-1 adrenergic blocking agents to treat BPH, you assist the nurse with the nursing process.

ASSESSMENT

Measure blood pressure in the supine and standing positions.

PLANNING
* alfuzosin (Uroxatral): the dose form is 10 mg extended-release tablets.
* tamsulosin (Flomax): the dose form is 0.4 mg capsules.

IMPLEMENTATION
* alfuzosin (Uroxatral):
    * A 10 mg tablet is given at once after the same meal each day.
    * Tablets should not be chewed or crushed.

- tamsulosin (Flomax):
    - A 0.4 mg capsule is given about 30 minutes after the same meal each day.
    - The dosage may be increased to 0.8 mg daily after 2 to 4 weeks of therapy if needed to control symptoms.

EVALUATION

Report and record:

- *Drowsiness, headache, dizziness, weakness, lethargy.* These tend to be self-limiting. Provide for safety.
- *Dizziness, tachycardia, fainting.* These may develop 15 to 90 minutes after the first dose. Give the drug with food to avoid these symptoms. Have the person lie down if they occur. Provide for safety.

DRUG CLASS: Anti-Androgen Agents

The following anti-androgen agents are used to treat BPH:

- dutasteride (du tas' ter ide); Avodart (av'oh dart)
- finasteride (fin as' ter ide); Proscar (pro' scar)

These drugs reduce the cell growth associated with BPH. The goals of therapy are to:

- Reduce BPH symptoms
- Improve urine flow
- Reduce the need for surgery

Assisting With the Nursing Process

When giving drugs to treat BPH, you assist the nurse with the nursing process.

ASSESSMENT

Ask the nurse what to observe and report.

PLANNING

- dutasteride (Avodart): the dose form is 0.5 mg capsules.
- finasteride (Proscar): the dose form is 5 mg tablets.

IMPLEMENTATION

- dutasteride (Avodart): a 0.5 mg capsule is given once a day with or without food.
- finasteride (Proscar): a 5 mg tablet is given once a day with or without food.

EVALUATION

Report and record:

- *Complaints of impotence, decreased sexual drive, decreased volume of ejaculate.* These tend to be self-limiting.

DRUG THERAPY FOR ERECTILE DYSFUNCTION

Erectile dysfunction (ED) or **impotence** is the inability of the male to have an erection. Diabetes, spinal cord injuries, and multiple sclerosis are causes. So are prostate problems and alcoholism. Heart and circulatory disorders, drug abuse, and psychological factors are other causes. Some drugs for high blood pressure cause impotence. So do other drugs. Some drugs treat impotence.

DRUG CLASS: Phospho-Diesterase Inhibitors

Drugs in this class result in smooth muscle relaxation. This allows blood to fill the erectile tissue in the penis during sexual stimulation. An erection results that can last an hour or so.

The goals of therapy are:

- Improved erectile function
- Sexual satisfaction in men with ED

Assisting With the Nursing Process

When drugs are used to treat ED, you assist the nurse with the nursing process.

ASSESSMENT

Measure vital signs.

PLANNING

See Table 29-4 for "Oral Dose Forms."

IMPLEMENTATION

- See Table 29-4 for "Adult Dosage Range."
- A dose is taken 30 minutes to 4 hours before sexual activity.

EVALUATION

Report and record:

- *Headache, flushing of the face and neck.* These tend to be self-limiting.
- *Color (blue or green) vision impairment.* The dosage may need to be reduced.
- *Hypotension, dizziness, angina.* The person should lie down and stop sexual activity. The person should not take nitroglycerin for angina.
- *Priapism.* **Priapism** is a prolonged or constant erection. Medical attention is needed if this lasts longer than 4 hours.

TABLE 29-4 Drugs Used for Erectile Dysfunction

GENERIC NAME	BRAND NAME	ORAL DOSE FORMS	ADULT DOSAGE RANGE
sildenafil	Viagra	Tablets: 25, 50, 100 mg	Initial: 50 mg Maximum: 100 mg/24 hours
tadalafil	Cialis	Tablets: 5, 10, 20 mg	Initial: 10 mg Maximum: 20 mg/24 hours
vardenafil	Levitra	Tablets: 2.5, 5, 10, 20 mg	Initial: 10 mg Maximum: 20 mg/24 hours

REVIEW QUESTIONS

Circle the **BEST** answer.

1 Contraceptives are used to
  a prevent pregnancy
  b treat benign prostatic hyperplasia
  c treat erectile dysfunction
  d prevent leukorrhea

2 Combination oral contraceptives contain
  a estrogen only
  b progestin only
  c estrogen and progestin
  d progestin and testosterone

3 Combination oral contraceptives are packaged with 28 tablets. The last 7 contain
  a estrogen
  b progestin
  c testosterone
  d no hormones

4 Mini-pill oral contraceptives are packaged with 28 tablets. All tablets contain only
  a estrogen
  b progestin
  c testosterone
  d no hormones

5 Which oral contraceptive results in 4 periods in one year?
  a mono-phasic
  b bi-phasic
  c tri-phasic
  d Seasonale

6 The following are side effects from contraceptives. Which may signal a serious complication?
  a weight gain
  b leg pain
  c vaginal discharge
  d break-through bleeding

7 A transdermal contraceptive patch can be applied to the following areas *except*
  a the breast   c the abdomen
  b a buttock   d the upper outer arm

8 Drugs are used in obstetrics for the following reasons *except*
  a to induce labor
  b to control bleeding after delivery
  c to prevent premature labor
  d to change the mother's blood type

9 Tamsulosin (Flomax) is used to treat benign prostatic hyperplasia. It
  a causes muscles to relax so blood can fill erectile tissue
  b causes muscles to relax to allow greater urine flow
  c reduces cell growth
  d inhibits estrogen secretion

10 When giving alfuzosin (Uroxatral) and tamsulosin (Flomax), the dose form
  a can be chewed or crushed
  b is given after the same meal each day
  c is given at bedtime
  d is changed on "change day"

11 Which drug is *not* used to treat erectile dysfunction?
  a tadalafil (Cialis)   c finasteride (Proscar)
  b vardenafil (Levitra)   d sildenafil (Viagra)

Circle **T** if the statement is true. Circle **F** if the statement is false.

12 T F Angina is experienced after taking a drug for erectile dysfunction. Nitroglycerin tablets should be taken.

13 T F Priapism is another term for erectile dysfunction.

14 T F Drugs for impotence are taken 30 minutes to 4 hours before sexual activity.

Answers to these questions are on p. 447.

Drugs Used to Treat Urinary System Disorders

30

OBJECTIVES

- Define the key terms and key abbreviations used in this chapter.
- Describe urinary tract infections.
- Describe over-active bladder syndrome.
- Describe the drugs used to treat urinary tract infections.
- Explain how to assist with the nursing process when giving drugs to treat urinary tract infections.
- Describe the drugs used to treat over-active bladder syndrome.
- Explain how to assist with the nursing process when giving drugs to treat over-active bladder syndrome.

KEY TERMS

cystitis Inflammation *(itis)* of the bladder *(cyst)*

healthcare-associated infection (HAI) An infection that develops in a person cared for in any setting where health care is given; the infection is related to receiving health care

over-active bladder (OAB) A syndrome characterized by urinary frequency, urgency, and incontinence; urge syndrome or urgency/frequency syndrome

prostatitis Inflammation *(itis)* of the prostate *(prostat)*

pyelonephritis Inflammation *(itis)* of the kidney *(nephr)* pelvis *(pyelo)*

urethritis Inflammation *(itis)* of the urethra *(urethr)*

urinary anti-microbial agents Substances that have an antiseptic effect on urine and the urinary tract

KEY ABBREVIATIONS

g Gram
GI Gastro-intestinal
HAI Healthcare-associated infection
mg Milligram
mL Milliliter
OAB Over-active bladder
UTI Urinary tract infection

Urinary tract infections (UTIs) are common. Infection in one area can involve the entire system. Microbes can enter the system through the urethra. Catheterization, urological exams, intercourse, poor perineal hygiene, immobility, and poor fluid intake are common causes. UTI is a common healthcare-associated infection. A **healthcare-associated infection (HAI)** is an infection that develops in a person cared for in any setting where health care is given. The infection is related to receiving health care.

Women are at high risk for UTIs. Microbes can easily enter the short female urethra. Prostate gland secretions help protect men from UTIs. However, an enlarged prostate increases the risk of UTI in older men (Chapter 29).

Older persons are at high risk for UTIs. Incomplete bladder emptying, perineal soiling from fecal incontinence, poor fluid intake, and poor nutrition increase the risk of UTI in older men and women.

UTIs include:

• **Cystitis**—inflammation *(itis)* of the bladder *(cyst)*
• **Pyelonephritis**—inflammation *(itis)* of the kidney *(nephr)* pelvis *(pyelo)*
• **Prostatitis**—inflammation *(itis)* of the prostate *(prostat)*

• **Urethritis**—inflammation *(itis)* of the urethra *(urethr)*

Over-active bladder (OAB) is another urinary disorder. It also is known as urge syndrome and urgency/frequency syndrome. The major symptoms of OAB are urinary:

• Frequency—the need to void 8 or more times a day. Nocturia is common (the need to void at night).
• Urgency—a sudden, compelling desire to pass urine that is hard to ignore.
• Incontinence—the inability to control urine from passing from the bladder.

For a review of the urinary system, see Box 30-1.

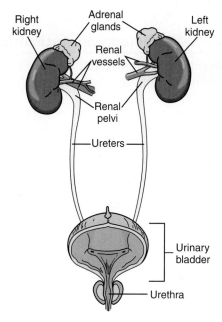

Fig. 30-1 Urinary system.

BOX 30-1 **The Urinary System: Body Structure and Function**

The digestive system rids the body of solid wastes. The lungs rid the body of carbon dioxide. Water and other substances leave the body through sweat. There are other waste products in the blood from cells burning food for energy. The urinary system (Fig. 30-1):

• Removes waste products from the blood
• Maintains water balance within the body

The *kidneys* are two bean-shaped organs in the upper abdomen. They lie against the back muscles on each side of the spine. They are protected by the lower edge of the rib cage.

Each kidney has over a million tiny *nephrons* (Chapter 22). Each nephron is the basic working unit of the kidney. Each nephron has a *convoluted tubule*, which is a tiny coiled tubule. Each convoluted tubule has a *Bowman's capsule* at one end. The capsule partly surrounds a cluster of capillaries called a *glomerulus*. Blood passes through the glomerulus and is filtered by the capillaries.

The fluid part of the blood is squeezed into the Bowman's capsule. The fluid then passes into the tubule. Most of the water and other needed substances are re-absorbed by the blood. The rest of the fluid and the waste products form *urine* in the tubule. Urine flows through the tubule to a *collecting tubule*. All collecting tubules drain into the *renal pelvis* in the kidney.

A tube, called the *ureter*, is attached to the renal pelvis of the kidney. Each ureter is about 10 to 12 inches long. The ureters carry urine from the kidneys to the *bladder*. The bladder is a hollow, muscular sac. It lies toward the front in the lower part of the abdominal cavity.

Urine is stored in the bladder until the need to urinate is felt. This usually occurs when there is about a half pint (250 mL) of urine in the bladder. Urine passes from the bladder through the *urethra*. The opening at the end of the urethra is the *meatus*. Urine passes from the body through the meatus. Urine is a clear, yellowish fluid.

DRUG THERAPY FOR URINARY TRACT INFECTIONS

Urinary anti-microbial agents are substances that have an antiseptic effect on urine and the urinary tract. The drug ordered depends on the pathogen causing the infection. Besides the drugs described in this chapter, other antibiotics are used to treat UTIs. They are described in Chapter 34.

The person should have a fluid intake of 2000 mL daily. The length of treatment depends on many factors:

- If the infection is acute, chronic, or re-current
- The pathogen
- The drug ordered

DRUG CLASS: Fosfomycin Antibiotics

The following is a fosfomycin antibiotic:

- fosfomycin (fos foh my' sin); Monurol (mohn' urh ol)

The drug affects the cell walls of bacteria. It also reduces the ability of bacteria to adhere to the urinary tract.

The drug is used as a single dose to treat uncomplicated acute cystitis in women. The goal of therapy is to resolve the UTI.

Assisting With the Nursing Process

When giving fosfomycin (Monurol), you assist the nurse with the nursing process.

ASSESSMENT

- Note the amount, color, clarity, and odor of urine.
- Ask about urgency, burning, pain, or other problems.
- Measure vital signs.
- Ask about gastro-intestinal (GI) complaints.

PLANNING

The dose form is 3 g packets of granules.

IMPLEMENTATION

- Pour the entire contents of a single-dose packet of granules into 90 to 120 mL (3 to 4 ounces) of water. Stir to dissolve. Do not use hot water.
- Have the person take the drug at once after the granules dissolve in water.
- The drug may be taken with or without food.
- The drug must be mixed with water. It is not taken in its dry form.

EVALUATION

Report and record:

- *Nausea, diarrhea, abdominal cramps, flatulence.* These are mild and tend to resolve without the need for therapy.
- *Perineal burning, dysuria.* Burning with voiding may be due to the infection. Symptoms should improve in 2 to 3 days after taking the drug.

DRUG CLASS: Quinolone Antibiotics

Quinolone antibiotics prevent bacteria from reproducing. They are effective in treating initial and re-current UTIs. The goal of therapy is to resolve the UTI.

Assisting With the Nursing Process

When giving quinolone antibiotics, you assist the nurse with the nursing process.

ASSESSMENT

- Note the amount, color, clarity, and odor of urine.
- Ask about urgency, burning, pain, or other problems.
- Measure vital signs.
- Ask about GI complaints.
- Ask about vision problems—color perception, problems focusing, double vision.

PLANNING

See Table 30-1 for "Oral Dose Forms."

IMPLEMENTATION

See Table 30-1 for "Adult Dosage Range."

TABLE 30-1 Quinolone Urinary Antibiotics			
GENERIC NAME	**BRAND NAME**	**ORAL DOSE FORMS**	**ADULT DOSAGE RANGE**
nalidixic acid	NegGram	Tablets: 500 mg	1 g four times daily for 7 to 14 days. Take with meals.
norfloxacin	Noroxin	Tablets: 400 mg	400 mg twice daily for 7 to 10 days. Take 1 hour before or 2 hours after meals with a large glass of fluid. Do not exceed 800 mg daily.

EVALUATION

Report and record:

- *Nausea, diarrhea, abdominal cramps, flatulence.* These are mild and tend to resolve with continued therapy.
- *Drowsiness, headache, dizziness.* These are mild and tend to resolve with continued therapy. Provide for safety.
- *Visual problems—color perception, problems focusing, double vision.* These may occur shortly after each dose is given during the first few days. Provide for safety.
- *Photo-sensitivity.* This is sensitivity to sunlight and ultra-violet light (sunlamps, tanning beds). The person should avoid exposure to sunlight, sunlamps, and tanning beds. He or she should apply a sunscreen and wear long-sleeved garments, a hat, and sunglasses when outdoors. Sunburn needs medical attention.
- *Hematuria (blood in the urine).* The person should drink eight to twelve 8-ounce glasses of water daily.
- *Itching, rash, hives, perineal burning.* These may signal an allergic reaction. Tell the nurse at once. Do not give the next dose unless approved by the nurse.
- *Headache, ringing in the ears (tinnitus), dizziness, tingling sensation, photo-sensitivity.* These require medical attention.

DRUG CLASS: Other Urinary Anti-Bacterial Agents

The following anti-bacterial agents also are used to treat UTIs:

- methenamine mandelate (meth en' a meen man del' ate); Mandelamine (man del' ah min)
- nitrofurantoin (ny tro fuhr' an toe in); Macrodantin (mak ro dan' tin) and Furadantin (fuhr ah dan' tin)

methenamine mandelate (Mandelamine)

The drug suppresses the growth and multiplication of bacteria that may cause re-current infection. It is used in persons susceptible to chronic, re-current UTIs.

Assisting With the Nursing Process

When giving methenamine mandelate (Mandelamine), you assist the nurse with the nursing process.

ASSESSMENT

- Note the amount, color, clarity, and odor of urine.
- Ask about urgency, burning, pain, or other problems.
- Measure vital signs.

PLANNING

The oral dose forms are 500 mg and 1 g enteric-coated tablets.

IMPLEMENTATION

- The adult dosage is 1 g four times daily—with meals and at bedtime.
- Give the drug with food to lessen GI symptoms.
- Do not crush the tablets.

EVALUATION

Report and record:

- *Nausea, vomiting, belching.* These are mild and tend to resolve with continued therapy.
- *Hives, itching, rash.* These may signal an allergic reaction. Do not give the next dose unless approved by the nurse.
- *Bladder irritation, dysuria, frequency.* These may signal another UTI.

nitrofurantoin (Macrodantin and Furadantin)

These drugs interfere with several bacterial enzyme systems. They are not effective against microbes in blood or tissues outside the urinary tract.

Assisting With the Nursing Process

When giving nitrofurantoin (Macrodantin and Furadantin), you assist the nurse with the nursing process.

ASSESSMENT

- Note the amount, color, clarity, and odor of urine.
- Ask about urgency, burning, pain, or other problems.
- Measure vital signs.
- Ask about GI complaints.
- Ask about numbness or tingling in the extremities.

PLANNING

The oral dose forms are:

- 25, 50, and 100 mg capsules
- 25 mg/5 mL suspension

IMPLEMENTATION

- The adult oral dosage is 50 to 100 mg four times a day for 10 to 14 days.
- Give the drug with food or milk to reduce GI side effects.
- The drug is given every 6 hours to maintain adequate urine concentrations.

EVALUATION

Report and record:

- *Nausea, vomiting, anorexia.* Give the drug with food or milk to reduce GI irritation.
- *Rust brown to yellow-colored urine.* This is harmless.
- *Dyspnea, chills, rash, itching.* These signal an allergic reaction. Tell the nurse at once. Do not give the next dose unless approved by the nurse.
- *Numbness and tingling in the extremities.* The drug needs to be discontinued.
- *Dysuria, foul-smelling urine, fever.* These signal a second infection.

DRUG THERAPY FOR OVER-ACTIVE BLADDER

Anti-cholinergic drugs are the treatment of choice for OAB. They also are known as urinary anti-spasmodic agents. They relax the outer muscle layer of the bladder. Involuntary bladder contractions decrease. The bladder can hold more urine. Urinary frequency and urgency are reduced. The desire to void is delayed.

The goals of therapy are to:

* Decrease frequency by increasing the amount voided
* Decrease urgency
* Reduce incidents of incontinence

Cholinergic receptors are throughout the body (Chapter 14). Therefore anti-cholinergic agents can lead to dry mouth, blurred vision, constipation, confusion, and sedation.

Assisting With the Nursing Process

When giving anti-cholinergic agents to control OAB, you assist the nurse with the nursing process.

ASSESSMENT

* Note the amount, color, clarity, and odor of urine.
* Ask about urgency, burning, pain, or other problems.
* Measure vital signs.

PLANNING

See Table 30-2 for "Dose Forms."

IMPLEMENTATION

See Table 30-2 for "Adult Dosage Range."

EVALUATION

Report and record:

* *Dry mouth, urinary hesitancy, urinary retention.* These are usually dose related. They may respond to a lower dosage. The nurse may allow the person to chew gum or suck on ice chips or hard candy.
* *Constipation, bloating.* Follow the care plan for diet and fluid intake.
* *Blurred vision.* The person should not drive or operate machinery. Provide for safety.

TABLE 30-2 Urinary Anti-Cholinergic Agents			
GENERIC NAME	**BRAND NAME**	**DOSE FORMS**	**ADULT DOSAGE RANGE**
darifenacin	Enablex	Tablets: 7.5 and 15 mg	Initial dose: 7.5 mg once daily. Based on individual response, the dose may be increased to 15 mg once daily as early as 2 weeks after starting therapy. May be taken without regard to food.
oxybutynin	Ditropan	Tablets: 5 mg Syrup: 5 mg/5 mL	Initial dose: 5 mg (tablets or syrup) 2 or 3 times/day. Maximum dose: 20 mg daily.
	Ditropan XL	Extended-release tablets: 5, 10, and 15 mg	Initial dose: 5 mg once daily. Dosage may be adjusted at weekly intervals in 5 mg increments. Maximum dose: 30 mg daily. May be administered with or without food and must be swallowed whole with the aid of liquids. Do not crush or chew.
	Oxytrol	Transdermal patch: 36 mg (3.9 mg/day release)	Initial dose: Apply one patch every 3 to 4 days to dry, intact skin on the abdomen, hip, or buttock. Select a new application site with each new patch to avoid reapplication to the same site within 7 days.
solifenacin	Vesicare	Extended-release tablets: 5 and 10 mg	Initial dose: 5 mg once daily. If well tolerated, the dose may be increased to 10 mg once daily. May be taken without regard to food.
tolterodine	Detrol	Tablets: 1 and 2 mg	Initial dose: 1-2 mg twice daily based on individual response and tolerance.
	Detrol LA	Extended-release capsules: 2 and 4 mg	Initial dose: 2-4 mg once daily taken with liquids and swallowed whole.
trospium	Sanctura	Tablets: 20 mg	Initial dose: 20 mg twice daily at least 1 hour before meals on an empty stomach. For persons with reduced kidney function, the recommended dose is 20 mg once daily at bedtime.

REVIEW QUESTIONS

Circle the BEST answer.

1 Cystitis is an inflammation of the
   a bladder
   b kidney pelvis
   c prostate
   d urethra

2 Which does *not* occur in over-active bladder syndrome?
   a urgency
   b frequency
   c incontinence
   d diuresis

3 Which is given as a single dose to treat cystitis?
   a norfloxacin (Noroxin)
   b nitrofurantoin (Furadantin)
   c fosfomycin (Monurol)
   d nalidixic acid (NegGram)

4 Which is a quinolone urinary antibiotic?
   a nitrofurantoin (Macrodantin)
   b trospium (Sanctura)
   c fosfomycin (Monurol)
   d nalidixic acid (NegGram)

5 The dose form of fosfomycin (Monurol) is 3 g packets of granules. To give the drug, you
   a dissolve the granules in 90 to 120 mL of cool water
   b give the drug right before the granules fully dissolve
   c give the drug in its dry form
   d mix the granules with hot food

6 Nitrofurantoin (Macrodantin or Furadantin) is given
   a to treat over-active bladder
   b before meals
   c every 6 hours
   d dissolved in water

7 To be effective, nitrofurantoin (Macrodantin or Furadantin) is given
   a in one dose
   b for 7 to 10 days
   c for 7 to 14 days
   d for 10 to 14 days

8 The following are given to control over-active bladder *except*
   a tolterodine (Detrol)
   b darifenacin (Enablex)
   c norfloxacin (Noroxin)
   d solifenacin (Vesicare)

9 Drugs given for over-active bladder syndrome can cause
   a numbness and tingling in the arms and legs
   b rust brown to yellow-colored urine
   c dry mouth, constipation, and blurred vision
   d hematuria and nocturia

Circle T if the statement is true. Circle F if the statement is false.

10 T F Women are at high risk for urinary tract infections.

11 T F Over-active bladder syndrome is treated with urinary anti-microbial agents.

12 T F The methenamine mandelate (Mandelamine) dose form is enteric-coated tablets. You can crush the tablets.

Answers to these questions are given on p. 447.

31

Drugs Used to Treat Eye Disorders

OBJECTIVES

- Define the key terms and key abbreviations used in this chapter.
- Describe the common eye disorders.
- Describe the drugs used to treat eye disorders.
- Explain how to assist with the nursing process when giving drugs to treat eye disorders.

KEY TERMS

miosis Narrowing of the pupil

mydriasis Dilation of the pupil

osmotic agents Drugs that cause fluid to be drawn from outside of the vascular system into the blood

KEY ABBREVIATIONS

g Gram
GI Gastro-intestinal
IOP Intra-ocular pressure
kg Kilogram
mg Milligram
mL Milliliter
PO Per os (orally)

The structures and functions of the eye are reviewed in Box 31-1. For common eye disorders, see Box 31-2, p. 374. To safely give topical ophthalmic agents, see Chapter 12. Also follow these rules:

- Do not use more than one drop (unless otherwise ordered). The eye can only hold a small amount of fluid.
- Wait at least 5 minutes if more than one drug is ordered. This prevents:
  - The second drug from washing away the first drug
  - The second drug from diluting the first drug
- Apply drops before ointments.
- Wait a few hours to apply drops after applying an ointment.
- Provide for safety after applying ointments. They may blur vision.
- Know the standard colors for ophthalmic labels and bottle caps:
  - Anti-infectives—brown or tan
  - Beta-adrenergic blocking agents—yellow, blue, or both
  - Miotics—green
  - Mydriatics and cycloplegics—red (*Cycloplegics* paralyze the ciliary muscle of the eye. They are used for eye exams.)
  - Non-steroidal anti-inflammatory agents—gray
  See *Delegation Guidelines: Drugs Used to Treat Eye Disorders,* p. 374.

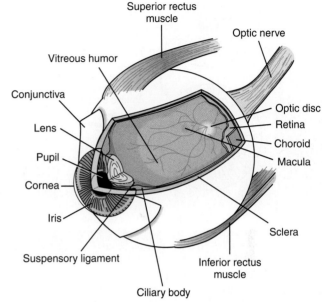

Fig. 31-1 The eye.

BOX 31-1 The Eye: Structures and Functions

Receptors for vision are in the *eyes* (Fig. 31-1). The eye is easily injured. Bones of the skull, eyelids and eyelashes, and tears protect the eyes from injury. The eye has three layers:

- The *sclera*, the white of the eye, is the outer layer. It is made of tough connective tissue.
- The *choroid* is the second layer. Blood vessels, the *ciliary muscle*, and the *iris* make up the choroid. The iris gives the eye its color. The opening in the middle of the iris is the *pupil*. Pupil size varies with the amount of light entering the eye (Fig. 31-2, p. 374). The pupil constricts (narrows) in bright light. Narrowing of the pupil is called **miosis** (*to become less*). The pupil dilates (widens) in dim or dark places. Dilation of the pupil is called **mydriasis** (*hot mass*).

- The *retina* is the inner layer. It has receptors for vision and the nerve fibers of the *optic nerve*.

Light enters the eye through the *cornea*. It is the transparent part of the outer layer that lies over the eye. Light rays pass to the *lens*, which lies behind the pupil. The light is then reflected to the retina. Light is carried to the brain by the optic nerve.

The *aqueous chamber* separates the cornea from the lens. The chamber is filled with a fluid called *aqueous humor*. The fluid helps the cornea keep its shape and position. The *vitreous humor* is behind the lens. It is a gelatin-like substance that supports the retina and maintains the eye's shape.

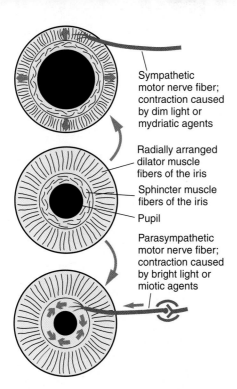

Sympathetic motor nerve fiber; contraction caused by dim light or mydriatic agents

Radially arranged dilator muscle fibers of the iris

Sphincter muscle fibers of the iris

Pupil

Parasympathetic motor nerve fiber; contraction caused by bright light or miotic agents

Fig. 31-2 Effect of light or ophthalmic agents on the iris of the eye.

BOX 31-2 Eye Disorders

GLAUCOMA

Glaucoma results in damage to the optic nerve. The eye produces a fluid that nourishes certain structures in the eye. The fluid normally drains from the eye (Fig. 31-3, *A*). When the fluid cannot drain properly (Fig. 31-3, *B*), fluid builds up in the eye. This causes pressure on the optic nerve—intra-ocular pressure (IOP). The optic nerve is damaged. Vision loss with eventual blindness occurs.

Glaucoma can develop in one or both eyes. Onset is sudden or gradual. Peripheral vision (side vision) is lost. The person sees through a tunnel (Fig. 31-4). Other signs and symptoms vary. They include blurred vision and halos around lights. With sudden onset, the person has severe eye pain, nausea, and vomiting.

Risk Factors. Glaucoma is a leading cause of vision loss in the United States. Persons at risk include:

• African-Americans over 40 years of age
• Everyone over 60 years of age
• Those with a family history of the disease
• Those who have diabetes, high blood pressure, or heart disease
• Those who have eye diseases or eye injuries
• Those who have had eye surgery

Treatment. Glaucoma has no cure. Prior damage cannot be reversed. Drugs and surgery can control glaucoma and prevent further damage to the optic nerve.

CATARACTS

Cataract is a clouding of the lens in the eye (Fig. 31-5, p. 376). Normally the lens is clear. *Cataract* comes from the Greek word that means *waterfall*. Trying to see is like looking through a waterfall. A cataract can occur in one or both eyes. Signs and symptoms include:

• Cloudy, blurry, or dimmed vision (Fig. 31-6, p. 376).

• Colors seem faded. Blues and purples are hard to see.
• Sensitivity to light and glares.
• Poor vision at night.
• Halos around lights.
• Double vision in one eye.

Risk Factors. Most cataracts are caused by aging. By age 80, more than 50% of all Americans have a cataract or have had cataract surgery. Diabetes, smoking, alcohol use, and prolonged exposure to sunlight are risk factors. So is a family history of cataracts.

Treatment. Surgery is the only treatment. Surgery is done when the cataract starts to interfere with daily activities. Driving, reading, and watching TV are examples.

Surgery involves removing the lens. Then a plastic lens is implanted. Vision improves after surgery. Post-operative care includes the following:

• Keep the eye shield or patch in place as directed. Some doctors allow the shield or patch off during the day if eyeglasses are worn. The shield or patch is worn for sleep, including naps.
• Follow measures for persons who are visually impaired or blind when an eye shield or patch is worn. The person may have vision loss in the other eye.
• Remind the person not to rub or press the affected eye.
• Do not let the person bend at the waist, pick up objects from the floor, or lift heavy objects. Assist the person with putting on socks or hose and footwear.
• Do not bump the eye.
• Do not shower or shampoo the person without a doctor's order.
• Place the overbed table and the bedside stand on the un-operative side.
• Place the signal light within reach.

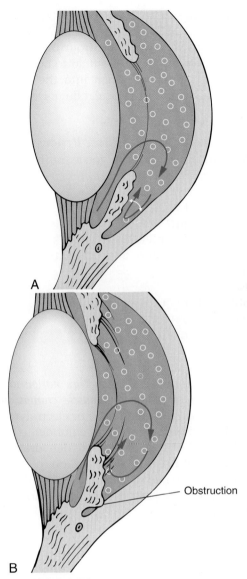

Fig. 31-3 A, Fluid drains normally from the eye. **B,** Flow of fluid from the eye is obstructed.

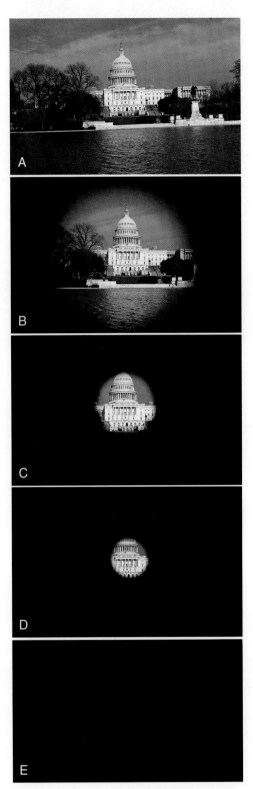

Fig. 31-4 Vision loss from glaucoma. **A,** Normal vision. **B,** Loss of peripheral vision begins. **C, D,** and **E,** Vision loss continues, with eventual blindness.

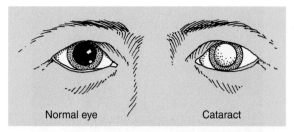

Fig. 31-5 One eye is normal. The other has a cataract. (From Phipps WJ and others: *Medical-surgical nursing: concepts and clinical practice*, ed 5, St Louis, 1995, Mosby.)

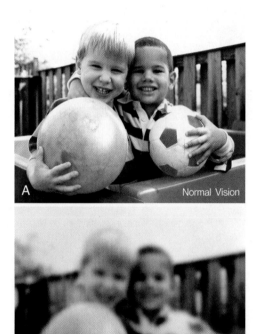

Fig. 31-6 Vision loss from a cataract. **A,** Normal vision. **B,** Scene viewed with a cataract. (From National Eye Institute: *Cataract: what you should know*, National Institutes of Health, Bethesda, Md.)

DRUG THERAPY FOR GLAUCOMA

Several drug classes are used to treat glaucoma. The goals of therapy are to:
* Reduce intra-ocular pressure (IOP)
* Prevent further blindness

DRUG CLASS: **Osmotic Agents**

Osmosis means to move fluid from one area to another. **Osmotic agents** cause fluid to be drawn from outside of the vascular system into the blood. This lowers the amount of intra-ocular fluid. Decreased IOP results.

Assisting With the Nursing Process

When giving osmotic agents, you assist the nurse with the nursing process.

ASSESSMENT
* Measure vital signs.
* Measure weight.
* Measure intake and output.
* Observe for alertness and orientation to person, time, and place.

PLANNING
See Table 31-1 for "Oral Dose Forms."

IMPLEMENTATION
See Table 31-1 for "Adult Dosage."

EVALUATION
Report and record:
* *Thirst; changes in alertness and orientation to person, time, and place; confusion; muscle cramps; nausea.* These may signal dehydration or electrolyte imbalance (potassium, sodium, and chloride).
* *Headache.* This signals cerebral dehydration. The person is kept in the supine position.
* *Edema and signs and symptoms of heart failure (Chapter 21).* These are caused by fluid moving into the blood stream.

DRUG CLASS: **Carbonic Anhydrase Inhibitors**

These agents inhibit carbonic anhydrase—an enzyme. Inhibiting the enzyme causes decreased production of aqueous humor. IOP lowers.

Assisting With the Nursing Process

When giving carbonic anhydrase inhibitors, you assist the nurse with the nursing process.

ASSESSMENT
* Measure vital signs.
* Measure weight.
* Measure intake and output.
* Observe for alertness and orientation to person, time, and place.
* Ask about gastro-intestinal (GI) signs and symptoms.

PLANNING
See Table 31-2 for "Dose Forms."

TABLE 31-1	Osmotic Agents			
GENERIC NAME	**BRAND NAME**	**ORAL DOSE FORMS**	**ADULT DOSAGE**	**COMMENTS**
glycerin	Osmoglyn	50% solution	1-2 g/kg	An oral osmotic agent for reducing intra-ocular pressure Administer 60-90 minutes before surgery Use with caution in diabetic patients; monitor for hyperglycemia
isosorbide	Ismotic	100 g in 220 mL solution (45%)	1.5 g/kg (range: 1-3 g/kg) two to four times daily	An oral osmotic agent for reducing intra-ocular pressure Onset of action is 30 minutes; duration is 5-6 hours With repeated doses, monitor fluids and electrolytes The solution will taste better if poured over cracked ice and sipped

TABLE 31-2	Carbonic Anhydrase Inhibitors		
GENERIC NAME	**BRAND NAME**	**DOSE FORMS**	**ADULT DOSAGE RANGE**
acetazolamide	Diamox	Tablets: 125, 250 mg Capsules: 500 mg	250 mg to 1 g every 24 hours
brinzolamide	Azopt	Ophthalmic solution: 1% in 2.5, 5, 10, and 15 mL dropper bottles	Intra-ocular: 1 drop in affected eye(s) three times daily; if more than one ophthalmic agent is to be administered in the same eye, separate the administration by at least 10 minutes
dorzolamide	Trusopt	Ophthalmic solution: 2% in 5 and 10 mL dropper bottles	Intra-ocular: 1 drop in affected eye(s) three times daily; if more than one ophthalmic agent is to be administered in the same eye, separate the administration by at least 10 minutes
methazolamide		Tablets: 25, 50 mg	50 to 100 mg, two or three times daily

IMPLEMENTATION

- See Table 31-2 for "Adult Dosage Range."
- Remove contact lenses for topical dose forms.
- Do not give the drug if the person is allergic to sulfonamide antibiotics (Chapter 34).
- Give oral dose forms with food or milk to lessen stomach irritation.

EVALUATION

Report and record:

- *Thirst; changes in alertness and orientation to person, time, and place; confusion; muscle cramps; nausea.* These may signal dehydration or electrolyte imbalance (potassium, sodium, and chloride).

- *Signs and symptoms of allergic reaction to sulfonamide antibiotics.* See Chapter 34. Tell the nurse at once. Do not give the next dose unless approved by the nurse.
- *Confusion.* Provide for safety.
- *Drowsiness.* This is usually mild and tends to resolve with continued therapy. Provide for safety.

DRUG CLASS: **Cholinergic Agents**

Cholinergic agents produce strong contractions of the iris (miosis). They also produce muscle contractions that allow the eye to adjust to distances. The drugs lower IOP in persons with glaucoma by permitting the out-flow of aqueous humor. They also reverse pupil dilation after eye surgery or eye exams.

TABLE 31-3	Cholinergic Agents			
GENERIC NAME	**BRAND NAME**	**TOPICAL DOSE FORMS**	**ADULT DOSAGE**	**COMMENTS**
carbachol, topical	Isopto-Carbachol, Carboptic	0.75%, 1.5%, 2.25%, and 3% solutions	1-2 drops into eye two to four times daily	Miotic action lasts 4-8 hours May be particularly useful in persons resistant to pilocarpine
pilocarpine	Isopto-Carpine, Pilocar, Akarpine, Pilopine HS	0.25%, 0.5%, 1%, 2%, 3%, 4%, 5%, 6%, 8%, 10% solutions; 4% gel	1-2 drops up to six times daily; 0.5%-4% solutions used most frequently	Safest, most commonly used miotic for glaucoma Also used to reverse mydriasis after eye examination Onset is 15 minutes to 1 hour; lasts for 2-3 hours

Assisting With the Nursing Process

When giving cholinergic agents, you assist the nurse with the nursing process.

ASSESSMENT

Measure vital signs.

PLANNING

See Table 31-3 for "Topical Dose Forms."

IMPLEMENTATION

See Table 31-3 for "Adult Dosage."

EVALUATION

Report and record:

- *Problems adjusting to changes in light, problems seeing at night, blurred vision.* Provide for safety. The person should not drive or perform dangerous tasks in poor light.
- *Eye irritation, eye redness, headache.* These are usually mild and tend to resolve with continued therapy.
- *Pain, discomfort.* These may occur in bright light.
- *Sweating, increased saliva, abdominal discomfort, diarrhea, broncho-spasm, tremors, hypotension, dysrhythmias, bradycardia.* These signal that the person is receiving too much of a cholinergic agent.

DRUG CLASS: Cholinesterase Inhibitors

The following is a cholinesterase inhibitor:

- echothiophate iodide (ek oh thi' oh fate); Phospholine Iodide (fos' foe lean)

Cholinesterase is an enzyme that destroys acetylcholine. Cholinesterase inhibitors prevent the metabolism of acetylcholine within the eye. Cholinergic activity increases. This results in decreased IOP and miosis (pupil constriction).

Assisting With the Nursing Process

When giving echothiophate iodide (Phospholine Iodide), you assist the nurse with the nursing process.

ASSESSMENT

Measure vital signs.

PLANNING

The topical dose form is a 0.125% solution.

IMPLEMENTATION

One drop is instilled 1 or 2 times a day.

EVALUATION

Report and record:

- *Problems adjusting to changes in light, problems seeing at night, blurred vision.* Provide for safety. The person should not drive or perform dangerous tasks in poor light.
- *Eye irritation, eye redness, headache.* These are usually mild and tend to resolve with continued therapy.
- *Sweating, increased saliva, vomiting, abdominal discomfort, diarrhea, urinary incontinence, dyspnea, broncho-spasm, tremors, hypotension, dysrhythmias, bradycardia.* These signal that the person is receiving too much of a cholinergic agent.

DRUG CLASS: Adrenergic Agents

Adrenergic agents are used for eye disorders because they cause:

- Pupil dilation
- Increased out-flow of aqueous humor
- Vaso-constriction
- Relaxation of the ciliary muscle
- A decrease in the formation of aqueous humor
  The goals of therapy are to:
- Dilate the pupils (mydriasis) for eye exams
- Reduce IOP
- Reduce redness of the eyes from irritation

TABLE 31-4   Adrenergic Agents

GENERIC NAME	BRAND NAME	TOPICAL DOSE FORMS	ADULT DOSAGE	COMMENTS
apraclonidine	Iopidine	0.5%, 1% solutions	1 drop 1 hour before surgery	Used to control intra-ocular pressure after laser surgery
brimonidine	Alphagan P	0.1%, 0.15%, 0.2% solutions	1 drop every 8 hours in affected eye(s)	An alpha-2 adrenergic agent used to lower intra-ocular pressure in open-angle glaucoma or ocular hypertension
dipivefrin hydrochloride	Propine	0.1% solutions	1 drop every 12 hours	This drug has no activity itself but is metabolized to epinephrine; used because it can penetrate the anterior chamber more readily than epinephrine and is less irritating
naphazoline hydrochloride	Vasoclear, Allerest, Naphcon, Albalon Liquifilm	0.012%, 0.02%, 0.03%, 0.1% solutions	1-2 drops every 3-4 hours	Used as a topical vaso-constrictor
phenylephrine	Prefrin, Mydfrin	0.12%, 2.5%, 10% solutions	1-2 drops two or three times daily	0.12% used as a decongestant for minor eye irritation; 2.5% and 10% solutions used for pupil dilation in uveitis, open-angle glaucoma, and diagnostic procedures
tetrahydrozoline hydrochloride	Murine Plus, Optigene 3	0.05% solutions	1-2 drops two or three times daily	Used as a topical vaso-constrictor

Assisting With the Nursing Process

When giving adrenergic agents in the treatment of eye disorders, you assist the nurse with the nursing process.

ASSESSMENT

Measure vital signs.

PLANNING

See Table 31-4 for "Topical Dose Forms."

IMPLEMENTATION

See Table 31-4 for "Adult Dosage."

EVALUATION

Report and record:

- *Sensitivity to bright light.* When pupils are dilated, excess amounts of light enter the eyes. This causes squinting. Sunglasses help reduce brightness. Provide for safety. The person should not drive or perform dangerous tasks in poor light.
- *Eye irritation, tearing.* These tend to be mild and resolve with continued therapy.
- *Palpitations, tachycardia, dysrhythmias, hypertension, faintness, trembling, sweating.* These signal over-dose or excessive amounts of an adrenergic agent.

DRUG CLASS:
Beta-Adrenergic Blocking Agents

Beta-adrenergic blocking agents are used to reduce elevated IOP. These agents are thought to reduce the production of aqueous humor.

Assisting With the Nursing Process

When giving beta-adrenergic blocking agents in the treatment of IOP, you assist the nurse with the nursing process.

ASSESSMENT

Measure vital signs.

PLANNING

See Table 31-5, p. 380, for "Topical Dose Forms."

IMPLEMENTATION

See Table 31-5, p. 380, for "Initial Adult Dosage."

EVALUATION

Report and record:

- *Eye irritation, tearing.* These tend to be mild and resolve with continued therapy.
- *Bradycardia, dysrhythmias, hypotension, faintness, broncho-spasm.* The dosage may need adjustment.

TABLE 31-5	Beta-Adrenergic Blocking Agents			
GENERIC NAME	**BRAND NAME**	**TOPICAL DOSE FORMS**	**INITIAL ADULT DOSAGE**	**COMMENTS**
betaxolol hydrochloride	Betoptic	0.25%, 0.5% solutions in 2.5, 5, 10, and 15 mL dropper bottles	1 drop twice daily	A beta-1 blocking agent; onset in 30 minutes, duration is 12 hours; several weeks of therapy may be required to determine optimal dosage
carteolol	Ocupress	1% solution in 5, 10, 15 mL dropper bottles	1 drop twice daily	A beta-1, 2 blocking agent; duration is up to 12 hours
levobunolol hydrochloride	Betagan	0.25% and 0.5% solutions in 5, 10, and 15 mL dropper bottles	1 drop once or twice daily	A beta-1, 2 blocking agent; onset within 60 minutes, duration is up to 24 hours
metipranolol	OptiPranolol	0.3% solution in 5 and 10 mL dropper bottles	1 drop twice daily in affected eye(s)	A beta-1, 2 blocking agent; onset within 30 minutes, duration is 12-24 hours
timolol maleate	Timoptic	0.25%, 0.5% solutions in 5, 10, and 15 mL dropper bottles 0.25%, 0.5% solutions, gel forming	1 drop of 0.25% solution twice daily 1 drop of solution once daily	A beta-1, 2 blocking agent; onset within 30 minutes, duration is up to 24 hours Gel may be used once daily

TABLE 31-6	Prostaglandin Agonists			
GENERIC NAME	**BRAND NAME**	**TOPICAL DOSE FORMS**	**ADULT DOSAGE RANGE**	**COMMENTS**
bimatoprost	Lumigan	0.03% solution in 2.5 and 5 mL dropper bottles	1 drop in each affected eye in the evening	Do not exceed dosage because it may reduce IOP-lowering effect
latanoprost	Xalatan	0.005% solution in 2.5 mL dropper bottle	1 drop in each affected eye in the evening	Do not exceed dosage because it may reduce IOP-lowering effect
travoprost	Travatan	0.004% solution in 2.5 mL dropper bottle	1 drop in each affected eye in the evening	Do not exceed dosage because it may reduce IOP-lowering effect

DRUG CLASS: Prostaglandin Agonists

Prostaglandin agonists reduce IOP by increasing the out-flow of aqueous humor. They are used to reduce IOP in persons with glaucoma who have not responded well to other IOP-lowering agents.

Assisting With the Nursing Process

When giving prostaglandin agonists in the treatment of IOP, you assist the nurse with the nursing process.

ASSESSMENT

Measure vital signs.

PLANNING

See Table 31-6 for "Topical Dose Forms."

IMPLEMENTATION

See Table 31-6 for "Adult Dosage Range."

EVALUATION

Report and record:

- *Eye irritation, burning and stinging, tearing.* These tend to be mild and resolve with continued therapy.
- *Changes in eye color.* Eye color may gradually change. The amount of brown pigment in the eye may increase. This may take several months to years and is likely permanent. Eyelids may develop color changes. Eyelashes may increase in growth.

TABLE 31-7 Anti-Cholinergic Agents

GENERIC NAME	BRAND NAME	TOPICAL DOSE FORMS	ADULT DOSAGE	COMMENTS
atropine sulfate	Isopto-Atropine	1% ointment; 0.5%, 1%, 2% solutions	Uveitis: 1-2 drops up to three times daily	Onset of mydriasis and cyclo-plegia (paralysis of ciliary muscles) is 30-40 minutes; duration is 7-12 days
cyclopentolate hydrochloride	Cyclogyl, AK-Pentolate	0.5%, 1%, 2% solutions	Refraction: 1 drop followed by an-other drop in 5-10 minutes	For mydriasis and cycloplegia (paralysis of ciliary muscles), necessary for diagnostic pro-cedures 1-2 drops of 1%-2% pilocar-pine allows full recovery within 3-6 hours
homatropine hydrobromide	Isopto-Homatropine	2%, 5% solutions	Uveitis: 1-2 drops every 3-4 hours	Onset of mydriasis and cyclo-plegia (paralysis of ciliary muscles) is 40-60 minutes; duration is 1-3 days
scopolamine hydrobromide	Isopto-Hyoscine	0.25% solution	Uveitis: 1-2 drops up to three times daily	Onset of mydriasis and cyclo-plegia (paralysis of ciliary muscles) is 20-30 minutes; duration is 3-7 days
tropicamide	Mydriacyl	0.5%, 1% solutions	Refraction: 1 or 2 drops, repeated in 5 minutes	Onset of mydriasis and cyclo-plegia (paralysis of ciliary muscles) is 20-40 minutes; duration is 6 hours

OTHER OPHTHALMIC AGENTS

Other drug classes are used to treat eye disorders. They are:

- Anti-cholinergic agents
- Anti-fungal agents
- Anti-viral agents
- Anti-bacterial agents
- Cortico-steroids
- Ophthalmic anti-inflammatory agents
- Antihistamines
- Anti-allergic agents
- Artificial tear solutions

DRUG CLASS: Anti-Cholinergic Agents

Anti-cholinergic agents cause relaxation of certain eye muscles. As a result the pupils dilate. This allows:

- Examination of the interior of the eye
- Resting of the eye during *uveitis*—inflammation of the uveal tract (middle coat of the eye)
- Measurement of lens strength for eyeglasses (refraction)

Assisting With the Nursing Process

When giving anti-cholinergic agents in the treatment of IOP, you assist the nurse with the nursing process.

ASSESSMENT

Measure vital signs.

PLANNING

See Table 31-7 for "Topical Dose Forms."

IMPLEMENTATION
See Table 31-7, p. 381, for "Adult Dosage."
EVALUATION
Report and record:

- *Sensitivity to bright light.* When pupils are dilated, excess amounts of light enter the eyes. This causes squinting. Sunglasses help reduce brightness. Provide for safety. The person should not drive or perform dangerous tasks in poor light.
- *Eye irritation, tearing.* These tend to be mild and resolve with continued therapy.
- *Flushing, dry skin, dry mouth, blurred vision, tachycardia, dysrhythmias, urinary hesitancy and retention, vaso-dilation, constipation.* These signal overdose or excessive administration of an anti-cholinergic agent.

DRUG CLASS: **Anti-Fungal Agents**

The following is an anti-fungal agent used to treat fungal infections of the eye:

- natamycin (na tah my' sin); Natacyn (na' tah sin)

Assisting With the Nursing Process
When giving natamycin (Natacyn), you assist the nurse with the nursing process.
ASSESSMENT

- Ask about eye symptoms.
- Ask about the amount and type of visual impairment.

PLANNING
The topical dose form is a 5% suspension.
IMPLEMENTATION

- One drop in the eye at 1- or 2-hour intervals for the first 3 to 4 days.
- The dosage may be reduced to 1 drop every 3 to 4 hours.
- Therapy is continued for 14 to 21 days.

EVALUATION
Report and record:

- *Sensitivity to bright light.* When pupils are dilated, excess amounts of light enter the eyes. This causes squinting. Sunglasses help reduce brightness. Provide for safety. The person should not drive or perform dangerous tasks in poor light.
- *Blurred vision, tearing, redness.* These are usually mild and tend to resolve with continued therapy. Provide for safety. Remind the person not to forcefully rub his or her eyes when tearing.
- *Eye pain.* The person needs medical attention.
- *Worsening of symptoms.* The person needs medical attention if symptoms worsen or do not improve after several days.

DRUG CLASS: **Anti-Viral Agents**

Ophthalmic anti-viral agents inhibit the virus from reproducing. They are used to treat herpes infections of the eye. The following agent is given topically:

- trifluridine (trye flure' i deen); Viroptic (ver op' tic)

Assisting With the Nursing Process
When giving trifluridine (Viroptic), you assist the nurse with the nursing process.
ASSESSMENT

- Ask about eye symptoms.
- Ask about the amount and type of visual impairment.

PLANNING
The topical dose form is 1% solution in 7.5 mL.
IMPLEMENTATION

- 1 drop onto the cornea of the affected eye every 2 hours while awake.
- Dosage should not exceed 9 drops daily.
- Continue for 7 more days after healing to prevent recurrence—1 drop every 4 hours (at least 5 drops daily).
- Store in the refrigerator.

EVALUATION
Report and record:

- *Visual haze, tearing, redness, burning.* These are usually mild and tend to resolve with continued therapy. Provide for safety. Remind the person not to forcefully rub his or her eyes when tearing.
- *Sensitivity to bright light.* When pupils are dilated, excess amounts of light enter the eyes. This causes squinting. Sunglasses help reduce brightness. Provide for safety. The person should not drive or perform dangerous tasks in poor light.
- *Allergic reactions.* The person needs medical attention.

DRUG CLASS: **Ophthalmic Antibiotics**

Ophthalmic antibiotics are used to treat superficial eye infections. Prolonged or frequent use of topical antibiotics should be avoided because of these risks:

- Hyper-sensitivity reactions
- The development of resistant organisms, including fungi
See Table 31-8.

TABLE 31-8   Ophthalmic Antibiotics

ANTIBIOTIC	BRAND NAME	DOSE FORMS
bacitracin	Bacitracin Ophthalmic	Ointment
chloramphenicol	Chloromycetin Ophthalmic	Drops, ointment
ciprofloxacin	Ciloxan	Drops, ointment
erythromycin	Ilotycin Ophthalmic	Ointment
gentamicin	Garamycin Ophthalmic	Drops, ointment
levofloxacin	Quixin, Iquix	Drops
ofloxacin	Ocuflox	Drops
polymyxin B	Polymyxin B Sulfate	Drops
sulfacetamide	Cetamide, Ocusulf-10	Drops, ointment
tobramycin	Tobrex Ophthalmic	Drops, ointment
COMBINATIONS		
trimethoprim/Polymyxin B	Polytrim Ophthalmic	Drops
neomycin/Polymyxin B/Bacitracin	Neosporin Ophthalmic	Ointment
neomycin/Polymyxin B/Gramicidin	AK-Spore Solution	Drops

TABLE 31-9   Cortico-Steroids

GENERIC NAME	BRAND NAME	DOSE FORMS
dexamethasone	Decadron Maxidex	Ointment Suspension
fluorometholone	FML	Suspension
loteprednol	Lotemax	Suspension
medrysone	HMS	Suspension
prednisolone	Econopred Plus Inflamase Mild	Suspension Solution
rimexolone	Vexol	Suspension

DRUG CLASS: **Cortico-Steroids**

Cortico-steroids are used for allergic reactions of the eye. They also are used for other acute non-infectious inflammatory conditions of the eye. Prolonged therapy may cause glaucoma and cataracts.

See Table 31-9.

DRUG CLASS: **Ophthalmic Anti-Inflammatory Agents**

The following ophthalmic anti-inflammatory agents are used before and after cataract surgery:

- flurbiprofen (Ocufen)—1 drop in the eye every 30 minutes beginning 2 hours before surgery. A total of 4 drops are given.
- suprofen (Profenal)—2 drops in the eye 3 hours, 2 hours, and 1 hour before surgery.
- diclofenac (Voltaren)—1 drop in the eye 4 times a day beginning 24 hours after surgery. The drug is continued for 2 weeks.

The following drug is used to relieve eye itching from seasonal allergies:

- ketorolac (Acular)—1 drop in each eye 4 times a day.

TABLE 31-10	Ophthalmic Antihistamines		
GENERIC NAME	**BRAND NAME**	**TOPICAL DOSE FORMS**	**ADULT DOSAGE**
azelastine	Optivar	Solution: 0.5 mg/mL in 6 mL dropper bottle	Instill 1 drop in each affected eye twice daily
emedastine	Emadine	Solution: 0.05% in 5 mL dropper bottle	Instill 1 drop in each eye up to four times daily
epinastine	Elestat	Solution: 0.05% in 8 and 12 mL dropper bottles	Instill 1 drop in each eye two times daily
ketotifen	Zaditor	Solution: 0.025% in 5 and 7.5 mL dropper bottles	Instill 1 drop in each eye every 8-12 hours
olopatadine	Patanol	Solution: 0.1% in 5 mL dropper bottle	Instill 1 or 2 drops in each affected eye two times daily at an interval of 6 to 8 hours
	Olopatadine	Solution: 0.2% in 2.5 mL dropper bottle	Instill one drop in each affected eye once daily

DRUG CLASS: **Antihistamines**

Antihistamines are used to relieve the signs and symptoms associated with allergic conjunctivitis. They also prevent itching. For best results, they should be instilled before exposure to allergens. See Table 31-10.

DRUG CLASS: **Anti-Allergic Agents**

Anti-allergic agents inhibit the release of histamine. These agents are used to treat allergic eye disorders:
* cromolyn (Crolom, Opticrom)—1 or 2 drops in each eye 4 to 6 times a day at regular intervals
* lodoxamide (Alomide)—1 or 2 drops in each affected eye 4 times a day
* pemirolast (Alamast)—1 or 2 drops in each affected eye 4 times a day
* nedocromil (Alocril)—1 or 2 drops in each eye twice a day at regular intervals

DRUG CLASS: **Artificial Tear Solutions**

Artificial tear solutions are like natural eye secretions. They lubricate dry eyes. They may be used as lubricants for artificial eyes.

The dosage is 1 to 3 drops in each eye 3 or 4 times a day as needed. Product names include:
* Isopto Plain
* Teargen
* Tears Naturale
* Murine
* Liquifilm Tears

REVIEW QUESTIONS

Circle the BEST answer.

1 Two types of eye drops are ordered. You apply the first type. How long should you wait before applying the second type?
a at least 5 minutes   b 30 minutes
c 1 hour   d a few hours

2 A person has glaucoma. The goal of drug therapy is to
a prevent infection
b reduce intra-ocular pressure
c reverse blindness
d restore normal vision

3 Osmotic agents are used in the treatment of glaucoma to
a prevent infection
b reduce intra-ocular pressure
c reverse blindness
d restore normal vision

4 A person is given osmotic agents to treat glaucoma. You should observe for signs and symptoms of
a heart failure   b psychosis
c blood clots   d asthma

5 Acetazolamide (Diamox) is used to treat glaucoma because it
a prevents infection
b reduces intra-ocular pressure
c reverses blindness
d restores normal vision

6 Cholinergic agents are used to treat glaucoma because they
a prevent infection
b reduce intra-ocular pressure
c reverse blindness
d restore normal vision

7 Which is a cholinergic agent used to treat glaucoma?
a brinzolamide (Azopt)
b tetrahydrozoline hydrochloride (Murine Plus)
c pilocarpine (Pilocar)
d dipivefrin hydrochloride (Propine)

8 Cholinergic agents and cholinesterase inhibitors may cause
a increased intra-ocular pressure
b infection
c problems seeing at night
d kidney failure

9 Adrenergic agents
a dilate the pupils
b increase intra-ocular pressure
c cause problems seeing at night
d cause heart failure

10 Beta-adrenergic blocking agents
a decrease intra-ocular pressure
b increase intra-ocular pressure
c dilate the pupils
d constrict the pupils

11 Which is a beta-adrenergic blocking agent?
a bimatoprost (Lumigan)
b tetrahydrozoline hydrochloride (Murine Plus)
c carteolol (Ocupress)
d natamycin (Natacyn)

12 Prostaglandin agonists
a decrease intra-ocular pressure
b increase intra-ocular pressure
c dilate the pupils
d constrict the pupils

13 Anti-cholinergic agents
a decrease intra-ocular pressure
b increase intra-ocular pressure
c dilate the pupils
d constrict the pupils

14 Anti-cholinergic agents
a lubricate the eyes
b prevent infection
c cause problems seeing at night
d cause sensitivity to bright light

15 Cortico-steroids are used
a to increase intra-ocular pressure
b to decrease intra-ocular pressure
c before and after cataract surgery
d to treat allergic reactions of the eye

16 Which is an anti-inflammatory agent used in the treatment of eye disorders?
a bacitracin (Bacitracin Ophthalmic)
b dexamethasone (Decadron)
c emedastine (Emadine)
d flurbiprofen (Ocufen)

17 Which is *not* an anti-allergic agent?
a ketorolac (Acular)
b pemirolast (Alamast)
c nedocromil (Alocril)
d lodoxamide (Alomide)

18 Artificial tears are used to
a treat allergies
b dilate the pupils
c constrict the pupils
d lubricate the eyes

Circle T if the statement is true. Circle F if the statement is false.

19 T F   Ointments are applied before eye drops.

20 T F   Eye ointments may blur vision.

21 T F   Ophthalmic labels and bottle caps are color coded.

22 T F   Murine is an artificial tear solution.

Answers to these questions are on p. 447.

32

Drugs Used in the Treatment of Cancer

OBJECTIVES

- Define the key terms used in this chapter.
- Explain the difference between benign tumors and cancer.
- Identify cancer risk factors.
- Identify the signs and symptoms of cancer.
- Explain the common cancer treatments.
- Identify the agents used for chemotherapy.
- Identify the common side effects of chemotherapy.

KEY TERMS

alopecia Hair loss

benign tumor A tumor that does not spread to other body parts; it can grow to a large size

cancer Malignant tumor

malignant tumor A tumor that invades and destroys nearby tissue and can spread to other body parts; cancer

metastasis The spread of cancer to other body parts

stomatitis Inflammation *(itis)* of the mouth *(stomat)*

tumor A new growth of abnormal cells; tumors are benign or malignant

Cells reproduce for tissue growth and repair. Cells divide in an orderly way. Sometimes cell division and growth are out of control. A mass or clump of cells develops. This new growth of abnormal cells is called a **tumor.** Tumors are benign or malignant (Fig. 32-1):

- **Malignant tumors (cancer)** invade and destroy nearby tissue (Fig. 32-2). They can spread to other body parts. They may be life-threatening. Sometimes they grow back after removal.
- **Benign tumors** do not spread to other body parts. They can grow to a large size, but rarely threaten life. They usually do not grow back when removed.

Metastasis is the spread of cancer to other body parts (Fig. 32-3, p. 388). Cancer cells break off the tumor and travel to other body parts. New tumors grow in other body parts. This occurs if cancer is not treated and controlled.

Cancer can occur almost anywhere. Common sites are the skin, lung and bronchus, colon and rectum, breast, prostate, uterus, ovary, urinary bladder, kidney, mouth and pharynx, pancreas, and thyroid gland (Fig. 32-4, p. 388). Cancer is the second leading cause of death in the United States.

Certain factors increase the risk of cancer. The National Cancer Institute describes these risk factors:

- *Growing older.* Cancer occurs in all age groups. However, most cancers occur in persons over 65 years of age.
- *Tobacco.* This includes using tobacco (smoking, snuff, and chewing tobacco) and being around tobacco (second-hand smoke). This risk can be avoided.

- *Sunlight.* Sun, sunlamps, and tanning booths cause early aging of the skin and skin damage. These can lead to skin cancer. Time in the sun should be limited. Sunlamps and tanning booths should be avoided.
- *Ionizing radiation.* This can cause cell damage that leads to cancer. X-rays are one source. So is radon gas that forms in the soil and some rocks. People who work in mines are at risk for radon exposure. Radon is found in homes in some parts of the country. Radioactive fallout is another source. It can come from nuclear power plant accidents. It also can come from the production, testing, or use of atomic weapons.
- *Certain chemicals and other substances.* Painters, construction workers, and those in the chemical industry are at risk. Household substances also carry risks—paint, pesticides, used engine oil, and other chemicals.
- *Some viruses and bacteria.* Being infected with certain viruses increases the risk of the following cancers—cervical, liver, lymphoma, leukemia, Kaposi's sarcoma (a cancer associated with acquired immunodeficiency syndrome—AIDS), stomach.
- *Certain hormones.* Hormone replacement therapy for menopause may increase the risk of breast cancer. Diethylstilbestrol (DES), a form of estrogen, was given to some pregnant women between the early 1940s and 1971. Women who took the drug are at risk for breast cancer. Their daughters are at risk for a certain type of cervical cancer.
- *Family history of cancer.* Certain cancers tend to occur in families. They include melanoma and cancers of the breast, ovary, prostate, and colon.

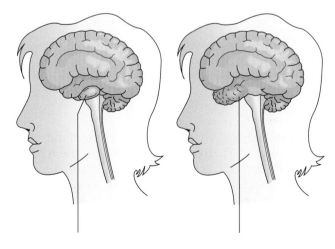

A   Benign tumor   B   Malignant tumor

Fig. 32-1 Tumors. **A,** A benign tumor grows within a local area. **B,** A malignant tumor invades other tissues.

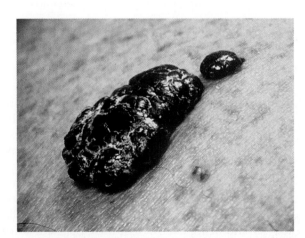

Fig. 32-2 Malignant tumor on the skin. (From Belcher AE: *Cancer nursing,* St Louis, 1992, Mosby.)

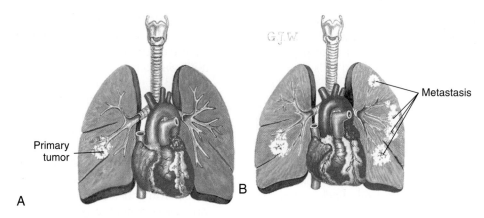

Fig. 32-3 A, Tumor in the lung. **B,** Tumor has metastasized to the other lung. (Modified from Belcher AE: *Cancer nursing*, St Louis, 1992, Mosby.)

Leading Sites of New Cancer Cases and Deaths—2008 Estimates

Estimated New Cases*

Male	Female
Prostate 186,320 (25%)	Breast 182,460 (26%)
Lung & bronchus 114,690 (15%)	Lung & bronchus 100,330 (14%)
Colon & rectum 77,250 (10%)	Colon & rectum 71,560 (10%)
Urinary bladder 50,051 (7%)	Uterine corpus 40,100 (6%)
Non-Hodgkin lymphoma 35,450 (5%)	Non-Hodgkin lymphoma 30,670 (4%)
Melanoma of the skin 34,950 (5%)	Melanoma of the skin 27,530 (4%)
Kidney & renal pelvis 33,130 (4%)	Thyroid 28,410 (4%)
Oral cavity & pharynx 25,310 (3%)	Ovary 21,650 (3%)
Leukemia 25,180 (3%)	Kidney & renal pelvis 21,260 (3%)
Pancreas 18,770 (3%)	Leukemia 19,090 (3%)
All sites 745,180 (100%)	All sites 692,000 (100%)

Estimated Deaths

Male	Female
Lung & bronchus 90,810 (31%)	Lung & bronchus 71,030 (26%)
Prostate 28,660 (10%)	Breast 40,480 (15%)
Colon & rectum 24,260 (8%)	Colon & rectum 25,700 (9%)
Pancreas 17,500 (6%)	Pancreas 16,790 (6%)
Liver & intrahepatic bile duct 12,570 (4%)	Ovary 15,520 (6%)
Leukemia 12,460 (4%)	Non-Hodgkin lymphoma 9,370 (3%)
Esophagus 11,250 (4%)	Leukemia 9,250 (3%)
Urinary bladder 9,950 (3%)	Uterine corpus 7,470 (3%)
Non-Hodgkin lymphoma 9,790 (3%)	Liver & intrahepatic bile duct 5,840 (2%)
Kidney & renal pelvis 8,100 (3%)	Brain & other nervous system 5,650 (2%)
All sites 294,120 (100%)	All sites 271,530 (100%)

*Excludes basal and squamous cell skin cancers and in situ carcinoma except urinary bladder.

Fig. 32-4 Leading sites of new cancer cases and deaths—2008 estimates. (American Cancer Society. Cancer Facts & Figures 2008. Atlanta, American Cancer Society, Inc.)

- *Alcohol.* The risk of certain cancers increases with more than two drinks a day. Such cancers are of the mouth, throat, esophagus, larynx, liver, and breast. Women should have no more than one drink a day. Men should have no more than two drinks a day.
- *Poor diet, lack of physical activity, and being over-weight.* A high-fat diet increases the risk of cancers of the colon, uterus, and prostate. Lack of physical activity and being over-weight increase the risk for cancers of the breast, colon, esophagus, kidney, and uterus.

If detected early, cancer can be treated and controlled (Box 32-1). Treatment depends on the type of tumor, its site and size, and if it has spread. The goal of cancer treatment may be one of the following:
- Cure the cancer
- Control the disease
- Reduce symptoms for as long as possible

Some cancers respond to one type of treatment. Others respond best to two or more types. Cancer treatments also damage healthy cells and tissues. Side effects depend on the type and extent of the treatment.

- Thickening or lump in the breast or any other part of the body
- New mole or an obvious change in an existing mole
- A sore that does not heal
- Hoarseness or cough that does not go away
- Changes in bowel or bladder habits
- Discomfort after eating
- A hard time swallowing
- Weight gain or loss with no known reason
- Unusual bleeding or discharge
- Feeling weak or very tired

From National Cancer Institute: *What you need to know about cancer: an overview*, NIH Publication No. 05-1566, Bethesda, Md, posted October 4, 2006.

- *Surgery.* Surgery removes tumors. It is done to cure or control cancer. It also relieves pain from advanced cancer. The person has some pain after surgery. The pain is controlled with pain-relief drugs. The person may feel weak or tired for a while. Some surgeries are very disfiguring. Self-esteem and body image are affected.
- *Radiation therapy.* Radiation therapy also is called *radiotherapy.* It kills cells. X-ray beams are aimed at the tumor. Sometimes radioactive material is implanted in or near the tumor. Cancer cells and normal cells receive radiation. Both are destroyed. Radiation therapy:
  - Destroys certain tumors
  - Shrinks a tumor before surgery
  - Destroys cancer cells that remain in an area after surgery
  - Controls tumor growth to prevent or relieve pain

  Side effects depend on the body part being treated. Burns, skin breakdown, and hair loss can occur at the treatment site. The doctor may order special skin care measures. Fatigue is common. Extra rest is needed. Discomfort, nausea and vomiting, diarrhea, and loss of appetite are other side effects.
- *Chemotherapy.* Chemotherapy involves drugs that kill cells. It is used to:
  - Shrink a tumor before surgery.
  - Kill cells that break off the tumor. The goal is to prevent metastasis.
  - Relieve symptoms caused by the cancer.

  Cancer cells and normal cells are affected. Side effects depend on the drug used:
  - Hair loss **(alopecia).**
  - Gastro-intestinal irritation. Poor appetite, nausea, vomiting, and diarrhea can occur. **Stomatitis,** an inflammation *(itis)* of the mouth *(stomat),* may occur.

- Bone marrow depression (decreased production of blood cells). Bleeding and infection are risks. The person may feel weak and tired.
- *Hormone therapy.* Hormone therapy prevents cancer cells from getting or using hormones needed for their growth. Drugs are given that prevent the production of certain hormones. Organs or glands that produce a certain hormone are removed. For example, a breast cancer might need estrogen for growth. Then the ovaries are removed. A prostate cancer may need testosterone for growth. Then the testicles may be removed. Side effects of hormone therapy include fatigue, fluid retention, weight gain, hot flashes, nausea and vomiting, appetite changes, and blood clots. Fertility is affected in men and women. Men also may experience impotence and loss of sexual desire.
- *Biological therapy.* Biological therapy *(immuno-therapy)* helps the immune system fight the cancer. It also protects the body from the side effects of cancer treatments. Side effects include flu-like symptoms— chills, fever, muscle aches, weakness, loss of appetite, nausea, vomiting, and diarrhea. Bleeding, bruising, and swelling may occur. So can skin rashes.

DRUG THERAPY FOR CANCER

Chemotherapy is most effective when the tumor is small and when cells divide rapidly. The agent used depends on the type of tumor cells, rate of growth, and tumor size.

Approaches to cancer treatment are changing rapidly. Therefore specific agents and dosages are not discussed. See Table 32-1 on pp. 390-396.

See *Delegation Guidelines: Drugs Used in the Treatment of Cancer.*

DELEGATION GUIDELINES
Drugs Used in the Treatment of Cancer

Some drugs used to treat cancer are given parenterally— by subcutaneous, intramuscular, or intravenous injection. You do not give parenteral dose forms. Should a nurse delegate the administration of such to you, you must:

- Remember that parenteral dosages are often very different from dosages for other routes.
- Refuse the delegation. Make sure you explain why. Do not just ignore the request. Make sure the nurse knows that you cannot give the drug and why.

Your state and agency may allow you to give some oral dose forms. Make sure you receive the necessary education about any chemotherapy agents that you will give.

TABLE 32-1	Cancer Chemotherapeutic Agents			

GENERIC NAME	BRAND NAME	TOXICITY		MAJOR INDICATIONS
		ACUTE	DELAYED	
ALKYLATING AGENTS				
busulfan	Myleran	None	Bone marrow depression	Chronic myelogenous leukemia
carboplatin	Paraplatin	Nausea, vomiting	Bone marrow suppression, anemia, nephro–toxicity	Ovarian carcinoma
carmustine	BCNU	Nausea and vomiting; pain along vein of intravenous infusion	Granulocyte and platelet suppression Hepatic, pulmonary, and renal toxicity	Brain, Hodgkin's disease, lympho-sarcoma, myeloma, malignant melanoma
chlorambucil	Leukeran	None	Bone marrow depression (anemia, leukopenia, thrombocytopenia) can be severe with excessive dosage	Chronic lymphocytic leukemia, Hodgkin's disease, non-Hodgkin's lymphoma, trophoblastic neoplasms
cisplatin	Platinol-AQ	Nausea, vomiting	Nephro–toxicity, otoxicity, blurred vision, changes in color perception	Testicular and ovarian cancers; bladder cancer
cyclophosphamide	Cytoxan	Nausea and vomiting	Bone marrow depression, alopecia, cystitis	Hodgkin's disease and other lymphomas, multiple myeloma, lymphocytic leukemia, many solid cancers
ifosfamide	Ifex	Nausea, vomiting, diarrhea	Hematuria, alopecia, confusion, coma	Testicular, lung, breast, ovarian, pancreatic, gastric cancer
lomustine	CCNU, CeeNU	Severe nausea and vomiting; anorexia	Thrombocytopenia, leukopenia, alopecia, confusion, lethargy, ataxia	Brain, Hodgkin's disease
mechlorethamine	Nitrogen mustard; Mustargen	Nausea and vomiting	Moderate depression of peripheral blood count	Hodgkin's disease and other lymphomas, bronchogenic carcinoma
melphalan	Alkeran	Nausea, vomiting, diarrhea	Bone marrow depression	Multiple myeloma, ovarian carcinoma, testicular seminoma

TABLE 32-1 | Cancer Chemotherapeutic Agents—cont'd

GENERIC NAME	BRAND NAME	ACUTE	DELAYED	MAJOR INDICATIONS
ALKYLATING AGENTS—cont'd				
streptozocin	Zanosar	Hypoglycemia, severe nausea, and vomiting	Moderate but transient renal and hepatic toxicity, hypoglycemia, mild anemia, leukopenia	Pancreatic islet cell carcinoma
temozolomide	Temodar	Headache, nausea, vomiting, constipation	Bone marrow depression, seizures	Glioblastoma, astrocytoma
thiotepa	Thioplex	Dizziness, headache, anorexia	Bone marrow depression	Hodgkin's disease, ovary and breast carcinomas, bladder cancer
ANTI-METABOLITES				
capecitabine	Xeloda	Nausea and vomiting, diarrhea, constipation, fatigue	Bone marrow depression, dermatitis, hand-and-foot syndrome, lymphopenia	Breast cancer, colorectal cancer
cladribine	Leustatin	Headache, dizziness, rash, nausea	Bone marrow depression, purpura	Hairy cell leukemia, lymphomas
clofarabine	Clolar	Flushing, hypotension, hypertension, headache, nausea, vomiting	Bone marrow depression, dermatitis	Acute lymphocytic leukemia
cytarabine hydrochloride	Cytosar	Nausea and vomiting, anorexia, oral ulceration	Bone marrow depression, megaloblastosis	Acute leukemias
fludarabine	Fludara	Nausea, vomiting, diarrhea, anorexia, myalgia	Edema, rash, weakness, cough, dyspnea, hemolytic anemia	Chronic lymphocytic leukemia, other leukemias
fluorouracil	5-FU, FU	Nausea	Oral and GI ulceration, stomatitis and diarrhea, bone marrow depression	Breast, large bowel, ovarian, pancreatic, stomach carcinoma
gemcitabine	Gemzar	Nausea, vomiting	Bone marrow suppression, rashes, edema	Pancreatic, breast, lung cancer

Continued

TABLE 32-1	Cancer Chemotherapeutic Agents—cont'd			
		TOXICITY		
GENERIC NAME	**BRAND NAME**	**ACUTE**	**DELAYED**	**MAJOR INDICATIONS**
ANTI-METABOLITES—cont'd				
mercaptopurine	6-MP, Purinethol	Occasional nausea and vomiting, usually well tolerated	Bone marrow depression, occasional hepatic damage	Acute lymphocytic and granulocytic leukemia
methotrexate	MTX	Occasional diarrhea, hepatic necrosis	Oral and GI ulceration, bone marrow depression (anemia, leukopenia, thrombocytopenia), cirrhosis	Acute lymphocytic leukemia, choriocarcinoma, carcinoma of cervix and head and neck area, mycosis fungoides, solid cancers
pemetrexed	Alimta	Nausea, vomiting, diarrhea	Bone marrow depression, renal dysfunction	Malignant pleural mesothelioma, non-small cell lung cancer
pentostatin	Nipent	Nausea, vomiting, muscle pain, headache, bloating, constipation, diarrhea	Bone marrow depression, renal dysfunction	Hairy cell leukemia, lymphomas
thioguanine	TG, Tabloid	Occasional nausea and vomiting, usually well tolerated	Bone marrow depression	Acute non-lymphocytic leukemia
NATURAL PRODUCTS				
etoposide	VePesid, Toposar	Nausea, vomiting, stomatitis, diarrhea	Leukopenia, thrombocytopenia, alopecia	Testicular tumors, small cell carcinoma of the lung, Hodgkin's disease and non-Hodgkin's lymphoma, acute non-lymphocytic leukemia, ovarian carcinoma, Kaposi's sarcoma
docetaxel	Taxotere	Nausea, vomiting, diarrhea	Bone marrow suppression, rashes, hypersensitivity	Breast cancer, prostate cancer
paclitaxel	Taxol	Nausea, vomiting, hypotension, diarrhea	Bone marrow suppression, mucositis, peripheral neuropathy	Ovarian carcinoma, breast carcinoma, AIDS-related Kaposi's sarcoma, lung cancer
vinblastine sulfate	Velban	Nausea and vomiting, local irritant	Alopecia, stomatitis, bone marrow depression, loss of reflexes	Hodgkin's disease and other lymphomas, solid cancers
vincristine sulfate	Oncovin	Local irritant	Areflexia, peripheral neuritis, paralytic ileus, mild bone marrow depression	Acute lymphocytic leukemia, Hodgkin's disease and other lymphomas, solid cancers

TABLE 32-1 | Cancer Chemotherapeutic Agents—cont'd

GENERIC NAME	BRAND NAME	TOXICITY		MAJOR INDICATIONS
		ACUTE	DELAYED	
NATURAL PRODUCTS—cont'd				
vinorelbine	Navelbine	Nausea, vomiting, constipation, diarrhea	Bone marrow suppression, hepatotoxicity, bronchospasm	Non-small cell lung cancer, breast cancer, cervical carcinoma, Kaposi's sarcoma
ANTIBIOTICS				
bleomycin	Blenoxane	Nausea and vomiting, fever, very toxic	Edema of hands, pulmonary fibrosis, stomatitis, alopecia	Hodgkin's disease, non-Hodgkin's lymphoma, squamous cell carcinoma of head and neck, testicular carcinoma
dactinomycin	Actinomycin D; Cosmegen	Nausea and vomiting, local irritant	Stomatitis, oral ulcers, diarrhea, alopecia, mental depression, bone marrow depression	Testicular carcinoma, Wilms' tumor, rhabdomyosarcoma, Ewing's and osteogenic sarcoma, and other solid tumors
daunorubicin	Cerubidine	Nausea, vomiting, diarrhea, fever, chills	Bone marrow suppression, reversible alopecia	Acute non-lymphocytic leukemia in adults; acute lymphocytic leukemia in children and adults
doxorubicin	Adriamycin	Nausea, red urine (not hematuria)	Bone marrow depression, cardiotoxicity, alopecia, stomatitis	Soft tissue, osteogenic and miscellaneous sarcomas, Hodgkin's disease, non-Hodgkin's lymphoma, bronchogenic and breast carcinoma, thyroid cancer, leukemias
epirubicin	Ellence	Nausea, vomiting, red urine (not hematuria), rash, diarrhea	Bone marrow depression, cardiotoxicity, alopecia, stomatitis	Breast cancer
idarubicin	Idamycin	Nausea, vomiting, diarrhea	Bone marrow suppression, cardiotoxicity, mucositis, hemorrhage	Acute myelocytic leukemia
mitomycin C	Mutamycin	Nausea and vomiting, flu-like syndrome	Bone marrow depression, skin toxicity; pulmonary, renal, CNS effects	Cancer of the cervix, stomach, pancreas, and bladder
mitoxantrone	Novantrone	Nausea, vomiting, diarrhea	Heart failure; GI bleeding; cough, dyspnea	Acute non-lymphocytic leukemia, prostate cancer
valrubicin	Valstar	Bladder spasm, hematuria, abdominal pain	Rash	Carcinoma-in-situ of the urinary bladder

Continued

TABLE 32-1	Cancer Chemotherapeutic Agents—cont'd			
		TOXICITY		
GENERIC NAME	BRAND NAME	ACUTE	DELAYED	MAJOR INDICATIONS
OTHER SYNTHETIC AGENTS				
aldesleukin	Proleukin	Confusion, dyspnea, nausea, diarrhea	Bone marrow depression, liver dysfunction	Melanoma, renal cell carcinoma, T-cell lymphoma
altretamine	Hexalen	Nausea, vomiting	Anemia, leukopenia, thrombocytopenia, peripheral neuropathy	Ovarian cancer
dacarbazine	DTIC-Dome; DIC	Nausea and vomiting, flu-like syndrome	Bone marrow depression (rare)	Metastatic malignant melanoma, Hodgkin's disease
hydroxyurea	Hydrea	Mild nausea and vomiting	Bone marrow depression	Chronic granulocytic leukemia, ovarian cancer, melanoma
interferon alfa-2a	Roferon-a	Flu-like syndrome	Bone marrow depression	Hairy cell leukemia, Kaposi's sarcoma
interferon alfa-2b	Intron a	Flu-like syndrome	Bone marrow depression	Hairy cell leukemia, Kaposi's sarcoma, malignant melanoma
levamisole	Ergamisol	Nausea, diarrhea	Dermatitis, alopecia, leukopenia	Colon cancer
leuprolide acetate	Lupron	Hot flashes; initial exacerbation of symptoms	Dysrhythmias, edema	Prostatic carcinoma, breast carcinoma
mitotane	Lysodren	Nausea and vomiting	Dermatitis, diarrhea, mental depression	Adrenal cortical carcinoma
procarbazine hydrochloride	Matulane	Nausea and vomiting	Bone marrow depression, CNS depression	Hodgkin's disease, non-Hodgkin's lymphoma, lung cancer, melanoma
HORMONES				
abarelix	Plenaxis	Sleep disturbance, headache	Gyneco-mastia, hot flashes	Prostate cancer
anastrozole	Arimidex	Nausea, vomiting, headache	Hot flashes, diarrhea, constipation, pelvic pain, edema	Breast cancer in post-menopausal women with disease progression following tamoxifen therapy

TABLE 32-1	Cancer Chemotherapeutic Agents—cont'd			
		TOXICITY		
GENERIC NAME	BRAND NAME	ACUTE	DELAYED	MAJOR INDICATIONS
HORMONES—cont'd				
bicalutamide	Casodex	Nausea, constipation, peripheral edema, diarrhea	Hepatitis, gyneco-mastia, dyspnea	Prostate cancer
estramustine	Emcyt	Nausea, diarrhea	Thrombosis, hypergly-cemia, hepatic dys-function, breast tenderness	Prostate cancer
Ethinyl estradiol		None	Fluid retention, hyper-calcemia, feminiza-tion, uterine bleeding	Breast and prostate carcinomas
exemestane	Aromasin	Nausea, fatigue, insomnia	Depression, anxiety, hot flashes, dyspnea	Breast cancer in post-menopausal women with disease progression follow-ing tamoxifen therapy
fluoxymesterone		None	Fluid retention, mas-culinization, choles-tatic jaundice	Breast carcinoma
flutamide	Eulexin	Nausea, vomiting	Hot flashes, loss of libido, impotence, gyneco-mastia, hepato–toxicity	Metastatic prostatic carcinoma
fulvestrant	Faslodex	Nausea, headache, constipation	Dyspnea, rash	Breast cancer
goserelin	Zoladex	Anorexia, dizziness, pain	Hot flashes, sexual dysfunction	Prostate and breast cancer
histrelin	Vantas	Insertion site reaction	Hot flashes, gyneco-mastia, fatigue	Prostate cancer
letrozole	Femara	Nausea, vomiting, headache	Muscle aches, hot flashes, constipa-tion, diarrhea, fatigue	Breast cancer in post-menopausal women with disease progression follow-ing anti-estrogen therapy
medroxyprogesterone acetate		None	None	Endometrial carci-noma, renal cell, breast cancer
nilutamide	Nilandron	Insomnia, headache, nausea, constipation	Hot flashes, impaired adaptation to dark	Prostate cancer

Continued

TABLE 32-1   Cancer Chemotherapeutic Agents—cont'd

| GENERIC NAME | BRAND NAME | TOXICITY | | MAJOR INDICATIONS |
		ACUTE	DELAYED	
HORMONES—cont'd				
tamoxifen	Nolvadex	Nausea, vomiting, hot flashes	Increased bone and tumor pain, thrombocytopenia, leukopenia, edema, hypercalcemia	Breast cancer (estrogen sensitive)
testolactone	Teslac	None	Fluid retention, masculinization	Breast carcinoma
testosterone enanthate	Delatestryl	None	Fluid retention, masculinization	Breast carcinoma
toremifene	Fareston	Nausea, vomiting	Hot flashes, sweating, vaginal discharge	Metastatic breast cancer in postmenopausal women with estrogen positive tumors
triptorelin	Trelstar	Vomiting, fatigue	Hot flashes, impotence, insomnia	Prostate cancer
DNA TOPOISOMERASE INHIBITORS				
irinotecan	Camptosar	Nausea, vomiting, anorexia, diarrhea, constipation, shortness of breath	Diarrhea, bone marrow suppression, alopecia	Carcinoma of the colon and rectum
topotecan	Hycamtin	Nausea, vomiting, diarrhea, shortness of breath	Alopecia, bone marrow depression, stomatitis	Ovarian cancer, small cell lung cancer

REVIEW QUESTIONS

Circle the BEST answer.

1 A person has cancer. You know that
   a the tumor will not threaten life
   b the tumor can spread to other body parts
   c the tumor is benign
   d the person's mouth is inflamed

2 Which is *not* a warning sign of cancer?
   a painful, swollen joints
   b a sore that does not heal
   c unusual bleeding or discharge
   d discomfort after eating

3 A person had surgery for cancer. The person's care will likely include
   a pain-relief measures
   b mouth care for stomatitis
   c skin care for burns at the treatment site
   d measures to prevent hair loss

4 Chemotherapy is most effective
   a when the tumor is first diagnosed
   b after surgery
   c after radiation therapy
   d when the tumor is small

5 A person receiving chemotherapy will likely experience
   a diarrhea
   b burns
   c skin breakdown
   d weight gain

Circle T if the statement is true. Circle F if the statement is false.

6 T F   Nausea and vomiting are common side effects from chemotherapy.

7 T F   Hormones are used to treat some cancers.

8 T F   Some antibiotics are used in the treatment of cancer.

Answers to these questions are on p. 447.

33

Drugs Affecting Muscles and Joints

OBJECTIVES

- Define the key terms and key abbreviations used in this chapter.
- Describe the goals of therapy when muscle relaxants are given.
- Describe the different types of muscle relaxants.
- Explain how to assist with the nursing process when giving muscle relaxants.
- Describe gout.
- Describe the drugs used to treat gout.
- Explain how to assist with the nursing process when giving drugs to treat gout.

KEY TERMS

clonus Rapidly alternating involuntary contraction and relaxation of skeletal muscles

hyper-reflexia Increased reflex actions

spasm An involuntary muscle contraction of sudden onset

KEY ABBREVIATIONS

CNS Central nervous system
g Gram
GI Gastro-intestinal
mg Milligram
PO Per os (orally)

Musculoskeletal disorders may produce varying degrees of pain and immobility. Nervous system disorders often affect the muscles. The person's ability to perform activities of daily living is affected. The person may need drug therapy to relax the muscles. See Box 33-1 for structure and function of the muscles.

Arthritis is a common joint disease. It is treated with non-steroidal anti-inflammatory agents (Chapter 17) and cortico-steroids (Chapter 28). Gout is a very painful form of arthritis (p. 401).

See *Delegation Guidelines: Drugs Affecting Muscles and Joints.*

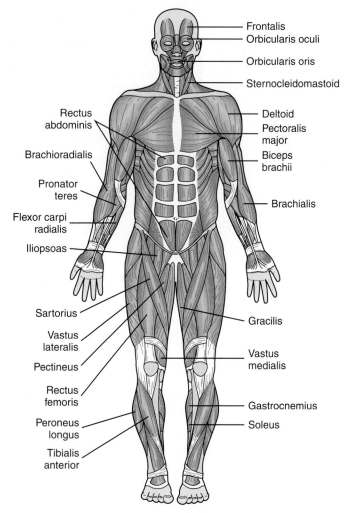

Fig. 33-1 Anterior view of the muscles of the body.

BOX 33-1 Muscles: Structure and Function

The human body has more than 500 *muscles* (Figs. 33-1 and 33-2). Some are voluntary. Others are involuntary.

- *Voluntary muscles* can be consciously controlled. Muscles attached to bones *(skeletal muscles)* are voluntary. Arm muscles do not work unless you move your arm; likewise for leg muscles. Skeletal muscles are *striated*. That is, they look striped or streaked.
- *Involuntary muscles* work automatically. You cannot control them. They control the action of the stomach, intestines, blood vessels, and other body organs. Involuntary muscles also are called *smooth muscles*. They look smooth, not streaked or striped.
- *Cardiac muscle* is in the heart. It is an involuntary muscle. However, it appears striated like skeletal muscle.

Muscles have three functions:
- Movement of body parts
- Maintenance of posture
- Production of body heat

Strong, tough connective tissues called *tendons* connect muscles to bones. When muscles contract (shorten), tendons at each end of the muscle cause the bone to move. The body has many tendons. See the Achilles tendon in Figure 33-2. Some muscles constantly contract to maintain the body's posture. When muscles contract, they burn food for energy. Heat is produced. The more muscle activity, the greater the amount of heat produced. Shivering is how the body produces heat when exposed to cold. Shivering is from rapid, general muscle contractions.

DELEGATION GUIDELINES
Drugs Affecting Muscles and Joints

Some drugs affecting muscles and joints are given parenterally—by intramuscular or intravenous injection. Some are injected into the spinal column. Because you do not give such dose forms, they are not included in this chapter. Should a nurse delegate the administration of such to you, you must:

- Remember that parenteral dosages are often very different from dosages for other routes.
- Refuse the delegation. Make sure you explain why. Do not just ignore the request. Make sure the nurse knows that you cannot give the drug and why.

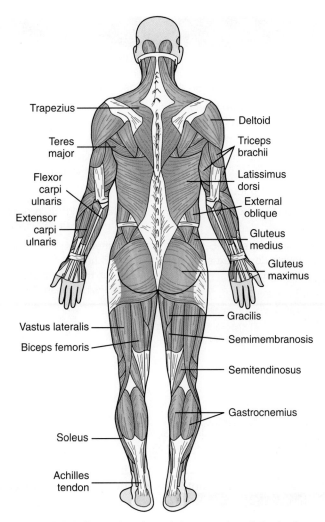

Fig. 33-2 Posterior view of the muscles of the body.

DRUG CLASS: Centrally Acting Skeletal Muscle Relaxants

Centrally acting skeletal muscle relaxants are used to relieve acute muscle spasm. A spasm is an involuntary muscle contraction of sudden onset. Muscle spasms are often painful. Drugs in this class depress the central nervous system (CNS). They do not have a direct effect on muscles or nerve conduction. All drugs in this class cause some degree of sedation.

The drugs listed in Table 33-1 on p. 400 are used with physical therapy, rest, and analgesics. The goal of therapy is relief of muscle spasm.

Assisting With the Nursing Process

When giving centrally acting skeletal muscle relaxants, you assist the nurse with the nursing process.

ASSESSMENT
- Measure vital signs.
- Observe level of alertness.

PLANNING
See Table 33-1 for "Adult Dosage."

IMPLEMENTATION
See Table 33-1 for "Comments."

EVALUATION
Report and record:
- *Sedation, weakness, lethargy, gastro-intestinal (GI) complaints.* These are usually mild and tend to resolve with continued therapy. Provide for safety. Remind the person to avoid driving or using machines.
- *Dizziness.* Provide for safety.
- *Sore throat, fever, jaundice, weakness.* These may signal changes in red blood cells and white blood cells.
- *Anorexia, nausea, vomiting, jaundice.* These may signal liver toxicity.

TABLE 33-1	Centrally Acting Muscle Relaxants		
GENERIC NAME	**BRAND NAME**	**ADULT DOSAGE**	**COMMENTS**
carisoprodol	Soma	PO: 350 mg four times daily	Onset of action: 30 minutes; duration: 4 to 6 hours
cyclobenzaprine	Flexeril	PO: 10 mg three times daily; do not exceed 30 mg	Recommended only for short-term treatment (2-3 weeks) of painful musculo-skeletal conditions; very sedating
metaxalone	Skelaxin	PO: 800 mg three or four times daily	Use with caution in persons with liver disease; causes false-positive Clinitest reaction
methocarbamol	Robaxin	PO: 1-1.5 g four times daily	
orphenadrine citrate	Norflex	PO: 100 mg two times daily	Also has analgesic properties; do not use in persons with glaucoma or prostatic hyperplasia
tizanidine	Zanaflex	PO: 4-8 mg every 6 to 8 hours; do not exceed 36 mg daily	Peak effects at 1 to 2 hours and dissipates between 3 to 6 hours Used for management of increased muscle tone associated with spasticity

DRUG CLASS: Direct-Acting Skeletal Muscle Relaxant

The following is a direct-acting skeletal muscle relaxant:

- dantrolene (dan' tro leen); Dantrium (dan tree' um)

This drug acts directly on skeletal muscle. It produces mild weakness of skeletal muscles. It decreases the force of reflex muscle contractions, muscle stiffness, involuntary muscle movements, and spasticity. It also decreases:

- **Clonus**—rapidly alternating involuntary contraction and relaxation of skeletal muscles
- **Hyper-reflexia**—increased reflex actions

The drug is used to control spasticity of chronic disorders such as cerebral palsy, multiple sclerosis, spinal cord injury, and stroke. The goal of therapy is relief from muscle spasm.

Assisting With the Nursing Process

When giving dantrolene (Dantrium), you assist the nurse with the nursing process.

ASSESSMENT

- Measure vital signs.
- Observe muscle spasms that may be present.

PLANNING

The oral dose forms are 25, 50, and 100 mg capsules.

IMPLEMENTATION

- The initial adult dose is 25 mg daily.
- The dose is increased to 25 mg two, three, or four times daily at 4- to 7-day intervals.
- The dosage is gradually increased up to 100 mg two, three, or four times a day.
- Some persons may require 200 mg four times daily.

EVALUATION

Report and record:

- *Weakness, diarrhea, drowsiness.* These are usually mild and tend to resolve with continued therapy.
- *Dizziness, light-headedness.* Provide for safety.
- *Photo-sensitivity.* This is sensitivity to sunlight and ultra-violet light (sunlamps, tanning beds). The person should avoid exposure to sunlight, sunlamps, and tanning beds. He or she should apply a sunscreen and wear long-sleeved garments, a hat, and sunglasses when outdoors. Sunburn needs medical attention.
- *Anorexia, nausea, vomiting, jaundice.* These may signal liver toxicity.

OTHER MUSCLE RELAXANTS

The following drug relaxes muscles by partially inhibiting reflex activity at the spinal cord:

- baclofen (bak' lo fen); Lioresal (ly or' e sahl)

The drug is used to manage muscle spasticity from multiple sclerosis, spinal cord injury, and other spinal cord diseases. The goal of therapy is relief of muscle spasm.

Assisting With the Nursing Process

When giving baclofen (Lioresal), you assist the nurse with the nursing process.

ASSESSMENT

Observe level of alertness.

PLANNING

The oral dose forms are:
- 10 and 20 mg tablets
- 10 and 20 mg orally disintegrating tablets

IMPLEMENTATION
- The oral adult dose is 5 mg three times a day.
- The dosage may be increased by 5 mg every 3 to 7 days based on the person's response.
- The best effects usually occur with dosages of 40 to 80 mg daily.
- Orally disintegrating tablets provide more rapid onset of action. They are used for persons who have swallowing problems.

EVALUATION

Report and record:
- *Nausea, fatigue, headache, drowsiness.* These are usually mild and tend to resolve with continued therapy.
- *Dizziness.* Provide for safety.

DRUGS USED TO TREAT GOUT

Gout occurs when uric acid builds up in the body. The build-up can lead to kidney stones and sharp uric acid crystal deposits in the joints. Uric acid comes from the breakdown of substances called *purines*. Purines are in all body tissues and in some foods. Liver, dried beans and peas, and anchovies are examples.

Normally uric acid is excreted from the body through urine. It can build up in the blood when:
- The body makes too much uric acid
- The kidneys do not excrete enough uric acid
- A person eats too many foods high in purine

The first gout attack often occurs in the big toe. The toe is very sore, red, warm, and swollen. Gout can also affect the insteps, ankles, heels, knees, wrists, fingers, and elbows (Fig. 33-3). Signs and symptoms include:
- Pain
- Swelling
- Redness
- Heat
- Stiff joints

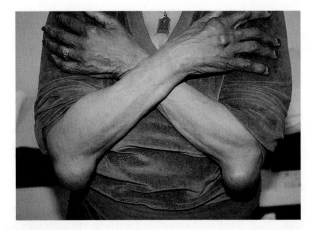

Fig. 33-3 Gout. (From Swartz MH: *Textbook of physical diagnosis, history, and examination*, ed 4, Philadelphia, 2002, Saunders.)

Stress, alcohol, drugs, and other illnesses can lead to gout. The next attack may not occur for months or years.

Drugs used to treat gout are:
- Non-steroidal anti-inflammatory agents (Chapter 17)
- Cortico-steroids (Chapter 28)
- Other agents:
  - allopurinol (al oh pur' in ol); Aloprim (ahl' oh prim) and Zyloprim (zy' lo prim)
  - Colchicine (kol' chi sin)
  - Probenecid (pro ben' eh sid)

allopurinol (Aloprim and Zyloprim)

Allopurinol (Aloprim and Zyloprim) prevents uric acid from forming. The goals of therapy are to:
- Reduce uric acid blood levels
- Reduce the frequency of acute gout attacks

Assisting With the Nursing Process

When giving allopurinol (Aloprim and Zyloprim), you assist the nurse with the nursing process.

ASSESSMENT

Ask about GI complaints.

PLANNING

The oral dose forms are 100 and 300 mg tablets.

IMPLEMENTATION
- The initial adult dose is 100 mg daily.
- The daily dosage is increased by 100 mg per week as needed to lower uric acid blood levels.
- The maximum daily dosage is 800 mg.
- Give the drug with food or milk if gastric irritation occurs.

EVALUATION

Report and record:

- *Anorexia, nausea, vomiting, jaundice.* These may signal liver toxicity.
- *Sore throat, fever, jaundice, weakness.* These may signal changes in red blood cells and white blood cells.
- *Fever, itching, rash.* These may signal an allergic reaction. Tell the nurse at once. Do not give the next dose unless approved by the nurse.

colchicine

Colchicine is used to prevent or relieve acute gout attacks. Joint pain and swelling begin to subside within 48 to 72 hours after therapy is started.

The goal of therapy is to relieve joint pain caused by an acute gout attack.

Assisting With the Nursing Process

When giving colchicine, you assist the nurse with the nursing process.

ASSESSMENT

- Ask about GI complaints.
- Measure intake and output.

PLANNING

The oral dose forms are 0.5 and 0.6 mg tablets.

IMPLEMENTATION

- The initial adult dose is 0.5 to 1.2 mg.
- The initial dose is followed by 0.6 mg every 1 to 2 hours until pain subsides or nausea, vomiting, and diarrhea develop.
- A total dose of 4 to 10 mg may be required.
- After the acute attack, 0.5 to 0.6 mg should be given every 6 hours for a few days to prevent a relapse.
- To prevent re-current gout, the dose is 0.5 to 0.6 mg every 1 to 3 days.
- The person should drink 8 to 12 eight-ounce glasses of fluid daily.

EVALUATION

Report and record:

- *Nausea, vomiting, diarrhea.* Drug therapy is discontinued when these develop.
- *Red blood in vomitus, "coffee ground" vomitus, dark tarry stools.* These signal GI bleeding.
- *Sore throat, fever, jaundice, weakness.* These may signal changes in red blood cells and white blood cells.

probenecid

Probenecid promotes the excretion of uric acid through the urine. It prevents the kidneys from re-absorbing urate. This results in reduced uric acid in the blood.

The goal of therapy is to prevent acute attacks of gouty arthritis.

Assisting With the Nursing Process

When giving probenecid, you assist the nurse with the nursing process.

ASSESSMENT

Ask about GI complaints.

PLANNING

The oral dose form is 500 mg tablets.

IMPLEMENTATION

- The initial adult dose is 250 mg twice a day for 1 week. Then it is increased to 500 mg twice a day.
- The dosage may be increased by 500 mg every few weeks.
- The maximum daily dosage is 2 to 3 g daily.
- Give the drug with food or milk to prevent gastric irritation.
- The person should drink 8 to 12 eight-ounce glasses of fluid daily.

EVALUATION

Report and record:

- *Sign and symptoms of acute gout attacks* (p. 401). These may increase for the first few months of therapy.
- *Nausea, anorexia, vomiting.* These may signal peptic ulcer disease.
- *Red blood in vomitus, "coffee ground" vomitus, dark tarry stools.* These signal GI bleeding.
- *Hives, itching, rash.* These may signal an allergic reaction. Tell the nurse at once. Do not give the next dose unless approved by the nurse.

REVIEW QUESTIONS

Circle the **BEST** answer.

1 An involuntary muscle contraction of sudden onset is called
a clonus
b hyper-reflexia
c a spasm
d a jerk

2 The rapidly alternating involuntary contraction and relaxation of skeletal muscles is called
a clonus
b hyper-reflexia
c a spasm
d jerking

3 Centrally acting skeletal muscle relaxants act
a directly on the muscle
b by depressing the CNS
c by inhibiting reflex activity at the spinal cord
d by blocking nerve impulses

4 All centrally acting skeletal muscle relaxants cause some degree of
a confusion
b orthostatic hypotension
c sedation
d spasticity

5 The goal of therapy for centrally acting muscle relaxants is relief of
a clonus
b hyper-reflexia
c muscle spasm
d jerking

6 Which has a dose form of orally disintegrating tablets?
a dantrolene (Dantrium)
b baclofen (Lioresal)
c carisoprodol (Soma)
d tizanidine (Zanaflex)

7 Which is *not* a centrally acting muscle relaxant?
a dantrolene (Dantrium)
b cyclobenzaprine (Flexeril)
c methocarbamol (Robaxin)
d carisoprodol (Soma)

8 Direct-acting skeletal muscle relaxants decrease
a clonus, hyper-reflexia, and muscle spasm
b cerebral palsy and multiple sclerosis
c spinal cord injury and stroke
d photo-sensitivity, sedation, and drowsiness

9 Which is a direct-acting skeletal muscle relaxant?
a dantrolene (Dantrium)
b baclofen (Lioresal)
c metaxalone (Skelaxin)
d orphenadrine citrate (Norflex)

10 Baclofen (Lioresal) is used in the management of
a clonus, hyper-reflexia, and muscle spasm
b cerebral palsy and stroke
c spinal cord injury and multiple sclerosis
d photo-sensitivity, sedation, and drowsiness

11 Allopurinol (Aloprim) is given for gout. The initial adult dose is
a 100 mg daily
b 200 mg daily
c 300 mg daily
d 400 mg daily

12 Allopurinol (Zyloprim) is given
a before meals
b on an empty stomach
c with food or milk
d at bedtime

13 After therapy is started, a person receiving colchicine should begin to see symptom relief within
a 12 to 24 hours
b 1 to 2 days
c 2 to 3 days
d 1 week

14 Persons receiving colchicine or probenecid should drink
a 4 to 8 eight-ounce glasses of fluid daily
b 8 to 12 eight-ounce glasses of fluid daily
c milk with every meal
d milk at bedtime

15 Persons receiving drug therapy for gout should be observed for
a dysrhythmias
b tremors
c GI symptoms
d confusion

Answers to these questions are on p. 447.

34

Drugs Used to Treat Infections

OBJECTIVES

- Define the key terms and key abbreviations used in this chapter.
- Identify the signs and symptoms of an infection.
- Describe healthcare-associated infections and how to prevent them.
- Identify the pathogens destroyed by anti-microbial agents.
- Identify the safety measures needed when giving anti-microbial agents.
- Identify the signs of an allergic reaction to anti-microbial agents.

KEY TERMS

aerobe A microbe that lives and grows in the presence of oxygen *(aer)*

anaerobe A microbe that lives and grows in the absence *(an)* of oxygen *(aer)*

antibiotics Anti-microbials derived from living microorganisms

anti-microbial agents Chemicals that eliminate pathogens

bacteria One-celled plant life that multiply rapidly and can cause an infection in any body system; germs

carrier A human or animal that is a reservoir for microbes but does not have the signs and symptoms of infection

fungi Plants that live on other plants or animals

germs See "bacteria"

healthcare-associated infection (HAI) An infection that develops in a person cared for in any setting where health care is given; the infection is related to receiving health care

infection A disease state resulting from the invasion and growth of microbes in the body

microbe See "microorganism"

microorganism A small *(micro)* living plant or animal *(organism)* seen only with a microscope; a microbe

non-pathogen A microbe that does not usually cause an infection

Continued

normal flora Microbes that live and grow in a certain area

opportunistic infection An infection caused by non-pathogens in a person with a weakened immune system

pathogen A microbe that is harmful and can cause an infection

protozoa One-celled animals that can infect the blood, brain, intestines, and other body areas

secondary infection An infection caused by a microbe that follows the first infection caused by a different microbe

viruses Microbes that grow in living cells

KEY ABBREVIATIONS

AIDS Acquired immunodeficiency syndrome
CDC Centers for Disease Control and Prevention
g Gram
GI Gastro-intestinal
HAI Healthcare-associated infection
HBV Hepatitis B virus
HIV Human immunodeficiency virus
IM Intramuscular
IV Intravenous
kg Kilogram
mg Milligram
mL Milliliter
STD Sexually transmitted disease
TB Tuberculosis
UTI Urinary tract infection

A **microorganism (microbe)** is a small *(micro)* living plant or animal *(organism)*. It is seen only with a microscope. Microbes are everywhere—in the mouth, nose, respiratory tract, stomach, and intestines. They are on the skin and in the air, soil, water, and food. They are on animals, clothing, and furniture.

Some microbes are harmful and can cause infections. They are called **pathogens. Non-pathogens** are microbes that do not usually cause an infection.

Normal flora are microbes that live and grow in a certain area. Certain microbes are in the respiratory tract, in the intestines, and on the skin. They are non-pathogens when in or on a natural reservoir. When a non-pathogen is transmitted from its natural site to another site or host, it becomes a pathogen. *Escherichia coli (E. coli)* is found in the colon. If it enters the urinary system, it can cause an infection.

INFECTION

The immune system protects the body from disease and infection (Box 34-1). An **infection** is a disease state resulting from the invasion and growth of microbes in the body. A *local infection* is in a body part. A *systemic infection* involves the whole body. (*Systemic* means *entire.*) The person has some or all of the signs and symptoms listed in Box 34-2 on p. 406. See Box 34-3 on p. 406 for common infections.

See *Focus on Older Persons: Infection* on p. 408.

Text continued on p. 408

BOX 34-1 **The Immune System: Structure and Function**

The immune system protects the body from disease and infection. Abnormal body cells can grow into tumors. Sometimes the body produces substances that cause the body to attack itself. Microbes (bacteria, viruses, and other germs) can cause an infection. The immune system defends against threats inside and outside the body.

The immune system gives the body *immunity*. Immunity means that a person has protection against a disease or condition. The person will not get or be affected by the disease:

- *Specific immunity* is the body's reaction to a certain threat.
- *Non-specific immunity* is the body's reaction to anything it does not recognize as a normal body substance.

Special cells and substances function to produce immunity:

- *Antibodies*—normal body substances that recognize abnormal or unwanted substances. They attack and destroy such substances.
- *Antigens*—abnormal or unwanted substances. An antigen causes the body to produce antibodies. The antibodies attack and destroy the antigens.
- *Phagocytes*—white blood cells that digest and destroy microbes and other unwanted substances (Fig. 34-1, p. 406).
- *Lymphocytes*—white blood cells that produce antibodies. Lymphocyte production increases as the body responds to an infection.
- *B lymphocytes (B cells)*—cause the production of antibodies that circulate in the plasma. The antibodies react to specific antigens.
- *T lymphocytes (T cells)*—cells that destroy invading cells. *Killer T cells* produce poisons near the invading cells. Some T cells attract other cells. The other cells destroy the invaders.

When the body senses an antigen (an unwanted substance), the immune system acts. Phagocyte and lymphocyte production increases. Phagocytes destroy the invaders through digestion. The lymphocytes produce antibodies that attack and destroy the unwanted substances.

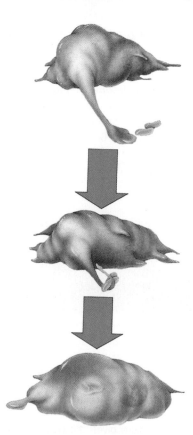

Fig. 34-1 A phagocyte digests and destroys a microorganism. (From Thibodeau GA, Patton KT: *Structure and function of the body*, ed 11, St Louis, 2000, Mosby.)

BOX 34-3 **Common Infections—cont'd**

You may care for persons with AIDS or those who are HIV carriers. You may have contact with the person's blood or body fluids. Protect yourself and others from the virus. Follow Standard Precautions and the Bloodborne Pathogen Standard (Appendix C). A person may have the HIV virus but no symptoms. In some persons, HIV or AIDS is not yet diagnosed.

Persons age 45 years and older are at risk. The Centers for Disease Control and Prevention (CDC) reported that from the beginning of the epidemic through 2005, there were over 220,900 cases of AIDS in persons age 45 years and older.

- Ages 45 to 49—over 102,700 cases
- Ages 50 to 54—over 56,900 cases
- Ages 55 to 59—over 30,400 cases
- Ages 60 to 64—over 16,400 cases
- Ages 65 and older—over 14,500 cases

Older persons get and spread HIV through sexual contact and IV drug use. However, many do not consider themselves to be at risk. Older persons tend to be less informed about the disease. And they tend not to practice safe sex. A blood transfusion between 1978 and 1985 increases the risk of HIV.

Aging and some diseases can mask the signs and symptoms of AIDS. Older persons are less likely to be tested for HIV/AIDS. Often the person dies without the disease being diagnosed. You must follow Standard Precautions and the Bloodborne Pathogen Standard.

HEALTHCARE-ASSOCIATED INFECTION

A healthcare-associated infection (HAI) is an infection that develops in a person cared for in any setting where health care is given. The infection is related to receiving health care. Hospitals, nursing centers, clinics, and home care settings are examples. HAIs also are called *nosocomial infections.* (*Nosocomial* comes from the Greek word for hospital.) HAIs are caused by normal flora. Or they are caused by microbes transmitted to the person from other sources.

For example, *E. coli* is normally in the colon. Feces contain *E. coli.* Poor wiping after bowel movements can cause *E. coli* to enter the urinary system. The hands can transmit *E. coli* to other body areas. If hand washing is poor, *E. coli* spreads to any body part or anything the hands touch. It also can be transmitted to other people.

Microbes can enter the body through equipment used in treatments, therapies, and tests. Such items must be free of microbes. Staff can transfer microbes from one person to another and from themselves to others. Common sites for HAIs are:

- The urinary system
- The respiratory system
- Wounds
- The bloodstream

Patients and residents are weak from disease or injury. Some have wounds or open skin areas. Infants and older persons have a hard time fighting infections. The health team must prevent the spread of infection. HAIs are prevented by:

- Medical asepsis (This includes hand hygiene.)
- Surgical asepsis
- Standard Precautions
- Transmission-Based Precautions
- The Bloodborne Pathogen Standard (Appendix C)

HEPATITIS B

Hepatitis B is caused by the hepatitis B virus (HBV). It is present in the blood and body fluids (saliva, semen, vaginal secretions) of infected persons. It is spread by:

- IV drug use and sharing needles
- Accidental needle sticks
- Sex without a condom, especially anal sex
- Contaminated tools used for tattoos or body piercings
- Sharing a toothbrush, razor, or nail clippers with an infected person

HEPATITIS C

Hepatitis C is spread by blood contaminated with the virus. A person may have the virus but no symptoms. Serious liver disease and damage may show up years later. Even without symptoms, the person can transmit the disease. Hepatitis C is treated with drugs. The virus is spread by:

- Blood contaminated with the virus
- IV drug use and sharing needles
- Inhaling cocaine through contaminated straws
- Contaminated tools used for tattoos or body piercings
- High-risk sexual activity—sex with an infected person, multiple sex partners
- Sharing a toothbrush, razor, or nail clippers with an infected person

HERPES ZOSTER (SHINGLES)

This is caused by the same virus that causes chickenpox. The virus lies dormant in nerve tissue. (*Dormant* means to be *inactive.*) The virus can become active years later. The person has a rash or blisters on the skin. At first the person has a burning or tingling pain, numbness, or itching. This occurs in an area on one side of the body or one side of the face. After a few days or a week, a rash with fluid-filled blisters appears (Fig. 34-2, p. 408). The person has mild to intense pain. Itching is a common complaint. The doctor orders anti-viral drugs and drugs for pain relief.

TUBERCULOSIS

Tuberculosis (TB) is a bacterial infection in the lungs. It also can occur in the kidneys, bones, joints, nervous system (including the spine), muscles, and other parts of the body. If TB is not treated, the person can die.

TB is spread by airborne droplets with coughing, sneezing, speaking, singing, or laughing. Nearby persons can inhale the bacteria. Those who have close, frequent contact with an infected person are at risk.

TB can be present in the body but not cause signs and symptoms. An active infection may not occur for many years. Only persons with an active infection can spread the disease to others.

- Appetite: loss of
- Cough
- Depression
- Diarrhea lasting more than a week
- Energy: lack of
- Fever
- Headache
- Memory loss, confusion, and forgetfulness
- Mouth or tongue:
  - Brown, red, pink, or purple spots or blotches
  - Sores or white patches
- Night sweats
- Pneumonia
- Shortness of breath
- Skin:
  - Rashes or flaky skin
  - Brown, red, pink, or purple spots or blotches on the skin, eyelids, or nose
- Swallowing: painful or difficult
- Swollen glands: neck, underarms, and groin
- Tiredness: may be extreme
- Vision loss
- Weight loss

FOCUS ON OLDER PERSONS

Infection

Like other body systems, changes occur in the immune system with aging. When an older person has an infection, he or she may not show the signs and symptoms listed in Box 34-2. The person may have only a slight fever or no fever at all. Redness and swelling may be very slight. The person may not complain of pain. Confusion and delirium may occur.

An infection can become life-threatening before the older person has obvious signs and symptoms. You must be alert to the most minor changes in the person's behavior or condition. Report any concerns to the nurse at once.

Older persons are at risk for infection. Healing takes longer than in younger persons. Therefore rehabilitation can take longer. The person's independence and quality of life are affected.

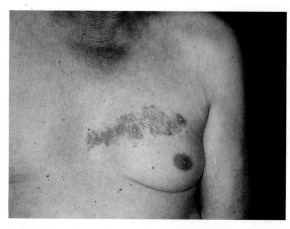

Fig. 34-2 Shingles. (Courtesy Department of Dermatology, School of Medicine, University of Utah. In McCance KL, Huether SE: *Pathophysiology: the biologic basis for disease in adults and children*, ed 5, 2006, St Louis.)

ANTI-MICROBIAL AGENTS

Anti-microbial agents are chemicals that eliminate pathogens. **Antibiotics** are anti-microbials derived from living microorganisms. For example, penicillin was first derived from a mold. Most antibiotics are harvested from large colonies of microbes. The microbes are purified and chemically modified into semi-synthetic anti-microbial agents.

Anti-microbials are first classified according to the type of pathogen to be destroyed:

- Bacteria—anti-bacterial agents. **Bacteria** are one-celled plant life that multiply rapidly. They are often called **germs.** They can cause an infection in any body system. A staining method is used to classify bacteria. (This method is named after Hans Gram. He was the Danish doctor who developed the staining method.)
  - Gram-negative bacteria—have a pink color when stained.
  - Gram-positive bacteria—have a violet color when stained.
- Fungi—anti-fungal agents. **Fungi** are plants that live on other plants or animals. Mushrooms, yeasts, and molds are common fungi. Fungi can infect the mouth, vagina, skin, feet, and other body areas.
- Viruses—anti-viral agents. **Viruses** are microbes that grow in living cells. They cause many diseases. The common cold, herpes, acquired immunodeficiency syndrome (AIDS), and hepatitis are examples.

Anti-bacterials are further classified into drug classes. Penicillins and tetracyclines are examples. The anti-bacterial ordered depends on the pathogen present.

The goal of anti-microbial therapy is to eliminate the infection. Sometimes secondary infections develop. A **secondary infection** is an infection caused by a microbe that follows the first infection. The first infection was caused by a different microbe.

See *Delegation Guidelines: Anti-Microbial Agents.*

See *Promoting Safety and Comfort: Anti-Microbial Agents.*

DELEGATION GUIDELINES
Anti-Microbial Agents

Some drugs used to treat infections are given parenterally—by intramuscular (IM) or intravenous (IV) injection. Because you do not give parenteral dose forms, they are not included in this chapter. Should a nurse delegate the administration of such to you, you must:

- Remember that parenteral dosages are often very different from dosages for other routes.
- Refuse the delegation. Make sure you explain why. Do not just ignore the request. Make sure the nurse knows that you cannot give the drug and why.

PROMOTING SAFETY AND COMFORT
Anti-Microbial Agents

SAFETY

Always check for allergies any time you give an anti-microbial. Closely observe all persons for allergic reactions to anti-microbials. Persons with histories of allergies, asthma, or rhinitis are at risk. So are persons taking many drugs.

Everyone should be observed carefully for at least the first 20 to 30 minutes after the drug is given. However, some drug reactions may not occur for several days. Should a reaction occur, tell the nurse at once. Do not give the next dose until the nurse directs you to do so.

A serious allergic reaction may occur with the first dose. Repeated exposures can be life-threatening. Tell the nurse at once if the person shows any sign of an allergic reaction:

- Swelling, redness, or pain at an injection site
- Hives
- Rash
- Itching
- Nasal congestion and discharge
- Wheezing
- Dyspnea
- Severe respiratory distress
- Nausea
- Vomiting
- Diarrhea
- Fever
- Malaise
  Follow the nurse's directions. You may be asked to:
- Activate the agency's rapid response team.
- Bring the emergency cart (crash cart) to the person's bedside.
- Provide cardio-pulmonary resuscitation.

COMFORT

Anti-microbials are usually given at regular intervals to maintain blood levels of the drug. For example, an antibiotic is given every 6 hours. You may need to awaken the person.

DRUG CLASS: **Amino-Glycosides**

Amino-glycosides are antibiotics that kill bacteria by inhibiting protein synthesis. They are used against gram-negative microbes that cause gram-negative infections including:

- Urinary tract infections (UTIs)—Chapter 30.
- Meningitis—an infection or inflammation of the membranes covering the brain and spinal cord.
- Wound infections.
- Septicemia—a systemic infection in which pathogens are present in the blood. It can be caused by the spread of an infection from any body part.

Most drugs in this class are given IM or IV. The following is given orally:

- neomycin (nee oh mye' sin); Neo-Fradin (nee oh frae din)

Assisting With the Nursing Process

When giving neomycin (Neo-Fradin), you assist the nurse with the nursing process.

ASSESSMENT

- Ask about the person's signs and symptoms.
- Measure vital signs.
- Measure intake and output.
- Observe for hearing loss.

PLANNING

The oral dose forms are:

- 500 mg tablets
- 125 mg/5 mL in 480 mL bottle

IMPLEMENTATION

The usual adult oral dose is 4 to 12 g daily in 4 divided doses.

EVALUATION

Report and record:

- *Dizziness, tinnitus (ringing in the ears), signs of hearing loss.* The drug can cause hearing damage.
- *Decreasing urinary output, bloody or smoky-colored urine.* These signal kidney toxicity.
- See *Promoting Safety and Comfort: Anti-Microbial Agents.*

DRUG CLASS: **Cephalo-Sporins**

Cephalo-sporins inhibit cell wall synthesis in bacteria. These drugs are related to the penicillins. They may be used for persons allergic to penicillins.

Cephalo-sporins are used for:

- UTIs
- Respiratory tract infections
- Abdominal infections
- Bacteremia (the presence of bacteria in the blood)
- Meningitis
- Osteo-myelitis (an infection of the bone and bone marrow)

TABLE 34-1	Cephalo-Sporins		
GENERIC NAME	**BRAND NAME**	**ORAL DOSE FORMS**	**ADULT DOSAGE RANGE**
cefaclor	Ceclor	250, 500 mg capsules 375, 500 mg extended-release tablets 125, 187, 250, 375 mg chewable tablets 125, 187, 250, 375 mg/5 mL suspension	250-500 mg every 8 hours; do not exceed 4 g/day
cefadroxil	Duricef	500 mg capsules 1000 mg tablets 125, 250, 500 mg/5 mL suspension	1-2 g daily in 1-2 doses daily
cefdinir	Omnicef	300 mg capsules 125 mg/5 mL suspension 250 mg/5 mL suspension	300-600 mg every 12 hours
cefixime	Suprax	100 mg/5 mL suspension	200 mg every 12 hours or 400 mg once daily
cefpodoxime	Vantin	100, 200 mg tablets 50, 100 mg/5 mL suspension	200 mg every 12 hours for 7-14 days
cefprozil	Cefzil	250, 500 mg tablets 125, 250 mg/5 mL suspension	250-500 mg every 12 hours for 10 days
ceftibuten	Cedax	400 mg capsules 90 mg/5 mL suspension	400 mg once daily 2 hours before or 1 hour after meals for 10 days
cefuroxime	Zinacef, Ceftin	125, 250, 500 mg tablets 125, 250 mg/5 mL suspension	250-500 mg every 12 hours
cephalexin	Keflex	250, 500 mg capsules, tablets 125, 250 mg/5 mL suspension	250-1000 mg every 6 hours
cephradine	Velosef	250, 500 mg capsules 125, 250 mg/5 mL suspension	250-500 mg every 6 hours; do not exceed 8 g/day

Assisting With the Nursing Process

When giving cephalo-sporins, you assist the nurse with the nursing process.

ASSESSMENT
- Ask about the person's signs and symptoms.
- Measure vital signs.
- Measure intake and output.

PLANNING
See Table 34-1 for "Oral Dose Forms."

IMPLEMENTATION
See Table 34-1 for "Adult Dosage Range."

EVALUATION
Report and record:
- *Diarrhea.* The normal flora of the gastro-intestinal (GI) tract is altered. Observe for signs and symptoms of dehydration if diarrhea is severe or does not resolve.
- *Genital and anal itching, vaginal discharge, thrush (a fungal infection of the mouth).* These signal secondary infections. Remind the person of the need for good oral and perineal hygiene.
- *Bleeding, easy bruising, bleeding gums, nosebleeds.* These signal changes in platelets.
- *Changes in alertness and orientation to person, time, and place; confusion; muscle cramps; nausea.* These may signal electrolyte imbalance (potassium, sodium, and chloride).
- See *Promoting Safety and Comfort: Anti-Microbial Agents,* p. 409.

TABLE 34-2 Macrolides			
GENERIC NAME	**BRAND NAME**	**ORAL DOSE FORMS**	**ADULT DOSAGE RANGE**
azithromycin	Zithromax	250, 500, 600 mg tablets 100, 167, 200, 1000 mg/5 mL suspension	500 mg as a single dose on day 1, followed by 250 mg once daily on days 2-5 for a total dose of 1.5 g
clarithromycin	Biaxin Biaxin XL	250, 500 mg tablets 125, 250 mg/5 mL suspension 500 and 1000 mg extended-release tablets	250-500 mg every 12 hours for 7-14 days
erythromycin	Eryc, Ilosone, E-Mycin, many others	333, 500 mg enteric-coated tablets 250, 500 mg chewable tablets 250, 500 mg film-coated tablets 333, 500 mg enteric-coated pellets in capsules 125, 200, 250, 400 mg/5 mL suspension 100 mg/mL and 100 mg/2.5 mL drops	250 mg four times daily for 10-14 days

DRUG CLASS: **Ketolides**

The following drug is a ketolide:
- telithromycin (tel ith roh my' sin); Ketek (kee' tec)

This drug prevents bacteria from synthesizing new proteins. It is used to treat:
- Acute bacterial sinusitis
- Bronchitis
- Pneumonia

Assisting With the Nursing Process

When giving telithromycin (Ketek), you assist the nurse with the nursing process.

ASSESSMENT
- Ask about the person's signs and symptoms.
- Measure vital signs.
- Measure intake and output.
- Ask about GI symptoms.
- Ask about vision problems.

PLANNING

The oral dose forms are 300 and 400 mg tablets.

IMPLEMENTATION
- The usual dose is 800 mg daily for 5, 7, or 10 days.
- The length of therapy depends on the infection. Sinusitis and bronchitis are usually treated for 5 days. Pneumonia is treated for 7 to 10 days.

EVALUATION

Report and record:
- *Diarrhea, nausea, and vomiting.* These are the most common side effects from this drug. They are usually mild and tend to resolve with continued therapy.

- *Dizziness.* This tends to resolve. Provide for safety. Remind the person not to drive or perform dangerous tasks.
- *Blurred vision, difficulty focusing, double vision.* These may occur after the first or second dose and last for several hours. Provide for safety. Remind the person not to drive or perform dangerous tasks.
- See *Promoting Safety and Comfort: Anti-Microbial Agents*, p. 409.

DRUG CLASS: **Macrolides**

Macrolides inhibit protein synthesis in susceptible bacteria. They kill bacteria or prevent bacteria from multiplying.

Drugs in this class are often used when other classes of drugs cannot be used. They are used for:
- Respiratory infections
- GI infections
- Skin infections
- Soft tissue infections
- Sexually transmitted diseases (STDs)

Assisting With the Nursing Process

When giving macrolides, you assist the nurse with the nursing process.

ASSESSMENT
- Ask about the person's signs and symptoms.
- Measure vital signs.
- Measure intake and output.
- Ask about GI symptoms.

PLANNING

See Table 34-2 for "Oral Dose Forms."

IMPLEMENTATION

See Table 34-2, p. 411, for "Adult Dosage Range."

EVALUATION

Report and record:

- *Diarrhea, nausea, vomiting, abnormal taste.* These are the most common side effects from this drug. They are usually mild and tend to resolve with continued therapy.
- See *Promoting Safety and Comfort: Anti-Microbial Agents,* p. 409.

DRUG CLASS: Penicillins

Penicillins were the first true antibiotics. They remain one of the most widely used classes of antibiotics.

Penicillins interfere with bacterial cell wall synthesis. The resulting cell wall is weak because of a defective structure. Bacteria are destroyed.

Penicillins are most effective against bacteria that multiply rapidly. Many bacteria that are sensitive to penicillin develop a protective mechanism against the drug. They can resist penicillin therapy. Some penicillin drugs have been modified to prevent this problem.

Penicillins are used to treat:

- Middle ear infections (otitis media)
- Pneumonia
- Meningitis
- UTIs
- Syphilis

Penicillins also are ordered for some persons before surgery and before dental procedures. The goal is to prevent infection in persons with a history of rheumatic fever. *Rheumatic fever* is a systemic inflammatory disease that may develop as a delayed reaction to a poorly treated upper respiratory infection. It usually occurs in young school-age children. Rheumatic fever may affect the brain, heart, joints, skin, or subcutaneous tissues.

Assisting With the Nursing Process

When giving penicillins, you assist the nurse with the nursing process.

ASSESSMENT

- Ask about the person's signs and symptoms.
- Measure vital signs.
- Measure intake and output.

PLANNING

See Table 34-3 for "Oral Dose Forms."

IMPLEMENTATION

See Table 34-3 for "Adult Dosage Range."

EVALUATION

Report and record:

- *Diarrhea.* Penicillins alter the normal flora of the GI tract. Observe for signs and symptoms of dehydration if diarrhea is severe or does not resolve.
- *Changes in alertness and orientation to person, time, and place; confusion; muscle cramps; nausea.* These may signal electrolyte imbalance (potassium, sodium, and chloride).
- See *Promoting Safety and Comfort: Anti-Microbial Agents,* p. 409.

TABLE 34-3 Penicillins			
GENERIC NAME	**BRAND NAME**	**ORAL DOSE FORMS**	**ADULT DOSAGE RANGE**
amoxicillin	Amoxil, Trimox	500, 875 mg tablets 125, 200, 250, 400 mg chewable tablets 250, 500 mg capsules 50 mg/mL and 125, 200, 250, 400 mg/ 5 mL suspension 200, 400 mg tablets for suspension	250-500 mg/8 hours
ampicillin	Principen	250, 500 mg capsules	250-500 mg/6 hours
carbenicillin	Geocillin	382 mg tablets	382-764 mg four times daily
dicloxacillin	Dicloxacillin	250, 500 mg capsules 62.5 mg/5 mL suspension	250-500 mg/6 hours
oxacillin	Oxacillin	250 mg/5 mL suspension	250-500 mg/4-6 hours
penicillin V potassium	Penicillin VK, Veetids	250, 500 mg tablets 125, 250 mg/5 mL suspension	250-500 mg/6 hours
COMBINATION PRODUCTS			
amoxicillin and potassium clavulanate (co-amoxiclav)	Augmentin	125, 200, 250, 400 mg chewable tablets 250, 500, 875 mg tablets 1000 mg extended-release tablets 125, 200, 250, 400, 600 mg/5 mL suspension	250-600 mg/8 hours

DRUG CLASS: Quinolones

Quinolone antibiotics prevent bacteria from reproducing. They are effective in treating initial and re-current UTIs.

A new sub-class—the fluoro-quinolones—inhibit the activity of an enzyme needed for bacteria to multiply. Drugs in this sub-class show great promise against many gram-positive and gram-negative bacteria. This includes some anaerobes—microbes that live and grow in the absence *(an)* of oxygen *(aer)*. Aerobes are microbes that live and grow in the presence of oxygen *(aer)*.

Assisting With the Nursing Process

When giving quinolones, you assist the nurse with the nursing process.

ASSESSMENT

- Ask about the person's signs and symptoms.
- Measure vital signs.
- Measure intake and output.
- Ask about GI symptoms.

PLANNING

See Table 34-4 for "Oral Dose Forms."

IMPLEMENTATION

See Table 34-4 for "Adult Dosage Range."

EVALUATION

Report and record:

- *Nausea, vomiting, diarrhea, GI discomfort.* These are usually mild and tend to resolve with continued therapy.
- *Dizziness, light-headedness.* These tend to be self-limiting. Remind the person not to drive or do dangerous tasks. Provide for safety.
- *Photo-sensitivity.* This is sensitivity to sunlight and ultra-violet light (sunlamps, tanning beds). The person should avoid exposure to sunlight, sunlamps, and tanning beds. He or she should apply a sunscreen and wear long-sleeved garments, a hat, and sunglasses when outdoors. Sunburn needs medical attention.
- *Tinnitus (ringing in the ears), headache, dizziness, depression, drowsiness, confusion.* These are nervous system effects. Provide for safety.
- See *Promoting Safety and Comfort: Anti-Microbial Agents*, p. 409.

TABLE 34-4 Quinolones			
GENERIC NAME	**BRAND NAME**	**ORAL DOSE FORMS**	**ADULT DOSAGE RANGE**
ciprofloxacin	Cipro	Tablets: 100, 250, 500, 750 mg Tablets, extended-release: 500, 1000 mg Suspension: 250, 500 mg/5 mL	0.5-1.5 g daily in two divided doses 2 hours after meals.
gemifloxacin	Factive	Tablets: 320 mg	320 mg once daily. It may be taken without regard to meals.
levofloxacin	Levaquin	Tablets: 250, 500, 750 mg Suspension: 25 mg/mL	500 mg once daily.
lomefloxacin	Maxaquin	Tablets: 400 mg	400 mg once daily. It may be taken without regard to meals.
moxifloxacin	Avelox	Tablets: 400 mg	400 mg once daily. It may be taken without regard to meals.
nalidixic acid	NegGram	Tablets: 250, 500, 1000 mg	1 g four times daily for 7-14 days. Take with meals.
norfloxacin	Noroxin	Tablets: 400 mg	400 mg twice daily for 7-10 days. Take 1 hour before or 2 hours after meals with a large glass of fluid. Do not exceed 800 mg daily.
ofloxacin	Floxin	Tablets: 200, 300, 400 mg	600-800 mg daily in two divided doses every 12 hours, 1 hour before or 2 hours after meals, with a large glass of fluid.

GENERIC NAME	BRAND NAME	ORAL DOSE FORMS	ADULT DOSAGE RANGE
sulfadiazine	Sulfadiazine	500 mg tablets	Initial dose: 2-4 g, then 4-8 g/24 hours in divided doses
sulfasalazine	Azulfidine	500 mg tablets 500 mg delayed-release tablets	Initial therapy: 3-4 g daily in divided doses; maintenance dosage is 2 g daily
sulfisoxazole	Sulfisoxazole, Gantrisin	500 mg tablets 500 mg/5 mL suspension	Initial dose: 2-4 g; maintenance dose is 4-8 g/24 hours divided into three to six doses
co-trimoxazole	Bactrim, Septra, Bactrim DS, Septra DS	Tablets, suspension	Two to four tablets daily, depending on strength and the disease being treated
erythromycin-sulfisoxazole	Pediazole, Eryzole	Suspension	2.5-10 mL every 6 hours, depending on the person's weight

TABLE 34-5 Sulfonamides

DRUG CLASS: Sulfonamides

Sulfonamides are highly effective anti-bacterial agents. They inhibit bacteria from making folic acid, causing bacterial death. Folic acid is needed for cell growth and reproduction.

Drugs in this class are used to treat UTIs and otitis media. They may be used to treat other infections in persons allergic to penicillin.

Assisting With the Nursing Process

When giving sulfonamides, you assist the nurse with the nursing process.

ASSESSMENT
- Ask about the person's signs and symptoms.
- Measure vital signs.
- Measure intake and output.
- Ask about GI symptoms.

PLANNING
See Table 34-5 for "Oral Dose Forms."

IMPLEMENTATION
- See Table 34-5 for "Adult Dosage Range."
- The person should drink water several times a day.

EVALUATION
Report and record:
- *Nausea, vomiting, diarrhea, GI discomfort.* These are usually mild and tend to resolve with continued therapy.
- *Photo-sensitivity.* This is sensitivity to sunlight and ultra-violet light (sunlamps, tanning beds). The person should avoid exposure to sunlight, sunlamps, and tanning beds. He or she should apply a sunscreen and wear long-sleeved garments, a hat, and sunglasses when outdoors. Sunburn needs medical attention.

- *Sore throat, fever, jaundice, weakness.* These may signal changes in red blood cells and white blood cells.
- *Tinnitus (ringing in the ears), headache, dizziness, depression, drowsiness, confusion.* These are nervous system effects. Provide for safety.
- See *Promoting Safety and Comfort: Anti-Microbial Agents*, p. 409.

DRUG CLASS: Tetracyclines

Tetracyclines are effective against gram-negative and gram-positive bacteria. They inhibit bacteria cells from making protein.

These drugs are often used in persons allergic to penicillin to treat:
- Certain STDs
- UTIs
- Upper respiratory infections
- Pneumonia
- Meningitis
- Acne

Tetracyclines may stain the teeth if taken during tooth development—last half of pregnancy through 8 years of age. These drugs are secreted in breast milk. Nursing mothers should feed infants formula or cow's milk.

Assisting With the Nursing Process

When giving tetracyclines, you assist the nurse with the nursing process.

ASSESSMENT
- Ask about the person's signs and symptoms.
- Measure vital signs.
- Measure intake and output.
- Ask about GI symptoms.

TABLE 34-6	Tetracyclines		
GENERIC NAME	**BRAND NAME**	**ORAL DOSE FORMS**	**ADULT DOSAGE RANGE**
demeclocycline	Declomycin	150, 300 mg tablets	150 mg four times daily or 300 mg twice daily
doxycycline	Vibramycin	50, 100 mg tablets 50, 100 mg capsules 25, 50 mg/5 mL syrup	200 mg on day 1, then 100 mg divided in two doses
minocycline	Minocin	50, 75, 100 mg capsules 50, 75, 100 mg tablets 50 mg/5 mL suspension	200 mg, followed by 100 mg/12 hours
tetracycline	Sumycin	250, 500 mg capsules and tablets 125 mg/5 mL suspension and syrup	250-500 mg four times daily

PLANNING

See Table 34-6 for "Oral Dose Forms."

IMPLEMENTATION

- See Table 34-6 for "Adult Dosage Range."
- Give the drug 1 hour before or 2 hours after the person ingests antacids, milk or other dairy products, or products containing calcium, aluminum, magnesium, or iron. (Note: Food and milk interfere with the absorption of demeclocycline.)

EVALUATION

Report and record:

- *Nausea, vomiting, diarrhea, GI discomfort.* These are usually mild and tend to resolve with continued therapy.
- *Photo-sensitivity.* This is sensitivity to sunlight and ultra-violet light (sunlamps, tanning beds). The person should avoid exposure to sunlight, sunlamps, and tanning beds. He or she should apply a sunscreen and wear long-sleeved garments, a hat, and sunglasses when outdoors. Sunburn needs medical attention.
- See *Promoting Safety and Comfort: Anti-Microbial Agents*, p. 409.

DRUG CLASS: **Anti-Tubercular Agents**

Tuberculosis (TB) is described in Box 34-3. These drugs are used in the treatment of TB:

- ethambutol (e tham' bu tol); Myambutol (my am' bu tol)
- isoniazid (i so ny' ah zid); INH
- rifampin (rif am' pin); Rifadin (rif' ah din)

ethambutol (Myambutol)

This drug inhibits bacterial growth. It is used with other anti-tubercular agents to prevent the development of resistant organisms. The goal of therapy is to eliminate the TB.

Assisting With the Nursing Process

When giving ethambutol (Myambutol), you assist the nurse with the nursing process.

ASSESSMENT

- Ask about the person's signs and symptoms.
- Measure vital signs.
- Measure intake and output.
- Ask about GI symptoms.
- Observe level of alertness and orientation to person, time, and place.

PLANNING

The oral dose forms are 100 and 400 mg tablets.

IMPLEMENTATION

- The dosage is based on the person's body weight.
- The drug is given once a day with food or milk.

EVALUATION

Report and record:

- *Nausea, vomiting, diarrhea, abdominal cramps.* These are usually mild and tend to resolve with continued therapy. Give the drug with food to lessen nausea and vomiting.
- *Confusion, hallucinations.* Provide for safety.
- *Blurred vision, red-green vision changes.* Provide for safety during blurred vision.
- See *Promoting Safety and Comfort: Anti-Microbial Agents*, p. 409.

isoniazid (INH)

This drug appears to disrupt the bacteria's cell wall and inhibits the cell from multiplying.

The drug is used to prevent and treat TB. If TB is active, it is used with other anti-tubercular agents. The goals of therapy are to:

- Prevent TB in persons who test positive for the disease.
- Eliminate TB in persons with active TB.

Assisting With the Nursing Process

When giving isoniazid (INH), you assist the nurse with the nursing process.

ASSESSMENT

- Ask about the person's signs and symptoms.
- Measure vital signs.
- Measure intake and output.
- Ask about GI symptoms.

PLANNING

The oral dose forms are:

- 50, 100, and 300 mg tablets
- 50 mg/5 mL syrup

IMPLEMENTATION

- The dosage is based on the person's body weight.
- The dosage is usually a single daily dose. It may be given in divided doses.
- Give the drug on an empty stomach.

EVALUATION

Report and record:

- *Tingling and numbness of the hands and feet.* These are common and are dose related. Observe for signs of skin breakdown. Test water temperature to prevent burns.
- *Nausea, vomiting.* These are common and are dose related.
- *Dizziness, ataxia (staggering gait, imbalance, poor coordination).* Provide for safety during ambulation.
- *Anorexia, nausea, vomiting, jaundice.* These may signal liver toxicity.
- See *Promoting Safety and Comfort: Anti-Microbial Agents,* p. 409.

rifampin (Rifadin)

This drug blocks key pathways needed for cells to grow and multiply. It is used with other drugs to treat TB.

Rifampin (Rifadin) also is used to eliminate certain bacteria in the naso-pharynx of carriers showing no symptoms. A **carrier** is a human or animal that is a reservoir for microbes but does not have the signs and symptoms of infection. Such bacteria are:

- *N. meningitidis*—it may cause septicemia or meningitis.
- *H. influenzae* type B (Hib disease)—it may cause meningitis, pneumonia, joint or bone infections, and throat inflammations. Hib disease mainly affects children in the first 5 years of life.

Assisting With the Nursing Process

When giving rifampin (Rifadin), you assist the nurse with the nursing process.

ASSESSMENT

- Ask about the person's signs and symptoms.
- Measure vital signs.
- Measure intake and output.
- Ask about GI symptoms.

PLANNING

The oral dose forms are 150 and 300 mg capsules.

IMPLEMENTATION

- The usual adult dose is 600 mg once daily.
- The drug is given 1 hour before or 2 hours after a meal.

EVALUATION

Report and record:

- *Reddish-orange secretions.* Urine, feces, saliva, sputum, sweat, and tears may be tinged reddish-orange. This is harmless and resolves with continued therapy.
- *Nausea, vomiting.* These are usually mild and tend to resolve with continued therapy.
- *Nausea, vomiting, fever, chills, muscle or bone pain, bruising, yellowish color of the skin or eyes.* The person needs further medical attention.
- See *Promoting Safety and Comfort: Anti-Microbial Agents,* p. 409.

DRUG CLASS: **Other Antibiotics**

Other antibiotics used to treat infections are:

- clindamycin (klin dah my' sin); Cleocin (klee o' sin)
- metronidazole (met row nyd' a zol); Flagyl (fla' jil)
- tinidazole (tin id' a zol); Tindamax (tin dah' max)
- vancomycin (van ko my' sin); Vancocin (van ko' sin)

clindamycin (Cleocin)

This drug inhibits the bacteria from making protein. It is used against:

- Gram-negative aerobes
- Gram-positive anaerobes
- Gram-negative anaerobes

Assisting With the Nursing Process

When giving clindamycin (Cleocin), you assist the nurse with the nursing process.

ASSESSMENT

- Ask about the person's signs and symptoms.
- Measure vital signs.
- Measure intake and output.
- Ask about bowel elimination patterns.

PLANNING

The oral dose forms are:

- 75, 150, and 300 mg capsules
- 75 mg/5 mL suspension

IMPLEMENTATION

- The usual adult oral dose is 150 to 450 mg every 6 hours.
- Do not refrigerate the suspension. It is stable at room temperature for 14 days.

EVALUATION

Report and record:

- *Diarrhea.* This is usually mild and tends to resolve with continued therapy.
- *Severe diarrhea.* This is signaled by 5 or more stools per day.
- *Blood or mucus in the stool.* The person needs further medical attention.
- See *Promoting Safety and Comfort: Anti-Microbial Agents,* p. 409.

metronidazole (Flagyl)

This drug kills bacteria and some protozoa. **Protozoa** are one-celled animals. They can infect the blood, brain, intestines, and other body areas. The drug is used to treat:

* Trichomoniasis—a vaginal infection.
* Giardiasis—diarrhea usually caused by water contaminated with feces. It also is called *traveler's diarrhea.*
* Amebic dysentery—an inflammation of the intestine. The person has frequent loose stools with flecks of blood and mucus. The liver may be involved—amebic liver abscess.
* Anaerobic bacterial infections.

Assisting With the Nursing Process

When giving metronidazole (Flagyl), you assist the nurse with the nursing process.

ASSESSMENT

* Ask about the person's signs and symptoms.
* Measure vital signs.
* Measure intake and output.
* Ask about GI symptoms.
* Observe level of alertness and orientation to person, time, and place.

PLANNING

The oral dose forms are:

* 250 and 500 mg tablets
* 375 and 500 mg capsules
* 750 mg extended-release tablets

IMPLEMENTATION

* The dosage depends on the infection needing treatment.
* The person should avoid alcoholic beverages and drugs containing alcohol (cough medications, mouthwashes).

EVALUATION

Report and record:

* *Nausea, vomiting, diarrhea.* These are usually mild and tend to resolve with continued therapy.
* *Dizziness.* Provide for safety.
* *Confusion, seizures.* Provide for safety. Follow the care plan for seizure precautions.
* See *Promoting Safety and Comfort: Anti-Microbial Agents,* p. 409.

tinidazole (Tindamax)

This drug is similar to metronidazole (Flagyl). It is used to treat:

* Trichomoniasis in men and women
* Giardiasis
* Amebic dysentery
* Amebic liver abscess

Assisting With the Nursing Process

When giving tinidazole (Tindamax), you assist the nurse with the nursing process.

ASSESSMENT

* Ask about the person's signs and symptoms.
* Measure vital signs.
* Measure intake and output.
* Ask about GI symptoms.
* Observe level of alertness and orientation to person, time, and place.

PLANNING

The oral dose forms are 250 and 500 mg tablets.

IMPLEMENTATION

* The dosage depends on the infection needing treatment.
* The person should avoid alcoholic beverages and drugs containing alcohol (cough medications, mouthwashes).

EVALUATION

Report and record:

* *Nausea, vomiting, diarrhea.* These are usually mild and tend to resolve with continued therapy.
* *Dizziness.* Provide for safety.
* *Confusion, seizures.* Provide for safety. Follow the care plan for seizure precautions.
* See *Promoting Safety and Comfort: Anti-Microbial Agents,* p. 409.

vancomycin (Vancocin)

This drug prevents cell walls from forming. It is effective against gram-positive bacteria. The drug has severe adverse effects. Therefore it is reserved for persons with potentially life-threatening infections who cannot be treated with penicillins or cephalo-sporins.

Assisting With the Nursing Process

When giving vancomycin (Vancocin), you assist the nurse with the nursing process.

ASSESSMENT

* Ask about the person's signs and symptoms.
* Measure vital signs.
* Measure intake and output.
* Observe for hearing loss.

PLANNING

The oral dose forms are 125 and 250 mg capsules.

IMPLEMENTATION

The usual adult dose is 500 mg every 6 hours or 1 g every 12 hours.

EVALUATION

Report and record:

* *Dizziness, tinnitus (ringing in the ears), signs of hearing loss.* The drug can cause hearing damage.
* *Decreasing urinary output, bloody or smoky-colored urine.* These signal kidney toxicity.
* *Genital and anal itching, vaginal discharge, thrush (a fungal infection of the mouth).* These signal secondary infections. Remind the person of the need for good oral and perineal hygiene.
* See *Promoting Safety and Comfort: Anti-Microbial Agents,* p. 409.

DRUG CLASS: **Topical Anti-Fungal Agents**

Anti-fungal agents change cell membranes. Proteins and electrolytes can leak from cells. Cells cannot take in the nutrients needed for their growth.

Topical agents are used to treat:

- Athlete's foot
- Jock itch
- Ringworm
- Thrush
- Diaper rash
- Vaginal yeast infection

Assisting With the Nursing Process

When applying topical anti-fungal agents, you assist the nurse with the nursing process.

ASSESSMENT

Ask about the person's signs and symptoms.

PLANNING

See Table 34-7 for "Topical Dose Forms."

IMPLEMENTATION

- See Table 34-7 for "Adult Dosage Range."
- See Chapter 11 for applying topical agents. Wear gloves.
- For athlete's foot: the person should wear cotton socks. They should be changed 2 or 3 times a day.
- For jock itch or ringworm: the person should wear clothing that fits well, is not constrictive, and is well-ventilated.
- Eye contact: eye contact with the drug should be avoided. Wash eyes at once if contact occurs.

EVALUATION

Report and record:

- *Vaginal applications: vaginal or perineal burning, itching, discharge, soreness, swelling.* These are usually mild and tend to resolve with continued therapy.
- *Redness, swelling, blistering, oozing.* These may signal an allergic reaction.
- See *Promoting Safety and Comfort: Anti-Microbial Agents*, p. 409.

TABLE 34-7	Topical Anti-Fungal Agents		
GENERIC NAME	**BRAND NAME**	**TOPICAL DOSE FORMS**	**ADULT DOSAGE RANGE**
butenafine	Lotrimin Ultra, Mentax	Cream: 1%	For ringworm, jock itch, athlete's foot: Apply topically to affected area once or twice daily for 1-4 weeks
butoconazole	Gynazole-1 Mycelex-3	Vaginal cream: 2%	For vaginal candidiasis: Gynazole-1: One full applicator intra-vaginally at bedtime once Mycelex-3: One full applicator intra-vaginally at bedtime for 3 days; may be extended to 6 days, if needed
ciclopirox	Loprox	Cream: 0.77% Lotion: 0.77% Shampoo: 1% Solution for nails: 8%	For ringworm, jock itch, athlete's foot, cutaneous candidiasis, and tinea versicolor: Massage cream or lotion into affected skin twice daily for at least 4 weeks Shampoo: Twice weekly for 4 weeks
clotrimazole	Gyne-Lotrimin Mycelex-7 Desenex Lotrimin AF Mycelex	Vaginal tablets: 200 mg Vaginal cream: 1% Cream: 1% Solution: 1% Oral lozenges: 10 mg (troches)*	For vaginal candidiasis: Tablets: Insert one 200 mg tablet intra-vaginally at bedtime for 3-7 nights Cream: One full applicator at bedtime for 3-7 nights For ringworm, jock itch, athlete's foot: Apply topically to affected skin morning and evening; gently rub in For oral candidiasis: Allow one lozenge to dissolve slowly in mouth five times daily for 14 consecutive days
econazole	Spectazole	Cream: 1%	For ringworm, jock itch, athlete's foot, tinea versicolor: Apply over affected area once daily For cutaneous candidiasis: Apply twice daily, morning and evening
ketoconazole	Nizoral	Cream: 2%	For ringworm, jock itch, athlete's foot, cutaneous candidiasis, and tinea versicolor: Massage in cream to affected and surrounding tissue once daily; may require 2-4 weeks of treatment

*This is an oral dose form.

TABLE 34-7 Topical Anti-Fungal Agents—cont'd

GENERIC NAME	BRAND NAME	TOPICAL DOSE FORMS	ADULT DOSAGE RANGE
ketoconazole—cont'd	Nizoral—cont'd	Cream: 2%—cont'd	For seborrheic dermatitis: Massage in cream to affected area twice daily for 4 weeks
		Shampoo: 2%	For dandruff: Moisten hair and scalp with water; apply shampoo and lather gently for 1 minute; rinse and reapply, leaving lather on scalp for 3 minutes; rinse thoroughly and dry hair; apply shampoo twice weekly for 4 weeks with at least 3 days between shampooing
miconazole	Monistat 3	Vaginal suppositories: 200 mg	For vaginal candidiasis: Monistat 3: Insert one suppository intra-vaginally at bedtime for 3 days
	Monistat 7	Vaginal suppositories: 100 mg Vaginal cream: 2%	Monistat 7: Insert one full applicator or one suppository intra-vaginally at bedtime for 3-7 days
	Micatin	Cream: 2% Powder: 2% Spray: 2%	For ringworm, jock itch, athlete's foot, cutaneous candidiasis, and tinea versicolor: Cover affected areas twice daily, morning and evening; treatment may require 2-4 weeks

naftifine	Naftin	Cream: 1%
		Gel: 1%
			For ringworm, jock itch, athlete's foot:
			   Cream: Massage into affected area once daily
			   Gel: Massage into affected area twice daily

nystatin	Mycostatin	Vaginal tablets: 100,000 units	For vaginal candidiasis: One tablet intra-vaginally daily for 2 weeks
	Mycostatin, Nilstat	Oral suspension: 100,000 units/mL*	For oral candidiasis: 4-6 mL four times daily; retain in mouth as long as possible before swallowing
	Mycostatin pastilles	Oral lozenges: 200,000 units (troches)*	One or two tablets four or five times daily; do not chew or swallow
	Mycostatin, Nilstat	Cream, ointment, powder	For cutaneous candidiasis: Apply to affected area two or three times daily
oxiconazole nitrate	Oxistat	Cream: 1% Lotion: 1%	For ringworm, jock itch, athlete's foot: Massage into affected areas once daily at bedtime
sertaconazole	Ertaczo	Cream: 2%	For athlete's foot: Apply twice daily for 4 weeks
sulconazole	Exelderm	Cream: 1% Solution: 1%	For ringworm, jock itch, athlete's foot: Massage into affected area twice daily
terbinafine	Lamisil AT	Cream: 1% Spray: 1%	Massage into affected area twice daily; treatment may require 2-4 weeks

terconazole	Terazol 7
	Terazol 3
		Vaginal cream: 0.4%
		Vaginal cream: 0.8%
		
		Vaginal suppository: 80 mg
			For vaginal candidiasis:
			   Insert one full applicator intra-vaginally daily at bedtime for 3 (Terazol 3) or 7 (Terazol 7) consecutive days
			   Insert one suppository intra-vaginally once daily at bedtime for 3 consecutive days

tioconazole	Vagistat-1 Monistat-1	Vaginal ointment: 6.5%	For vaginal candidiasis: Insert one full applicator intra-vaginally at bedtime once
tolnaftate	Tinactin	Cream: 1% Solution: 1% Gel: 1% Spray: 1% Powder: 1%	For ringworm, jock itch, athlete's foot, cutaneous candidiasis, and tinea versicolor: Cover affected areas twice daily, morning and evening; treatment may require 2-4 weeks

*This is an oral dose form.

DRUG CLASS: Systemic Anti-Fungal Agents

The following systemic anti-fungal agents are given orally:

- fluconazole (flu kon' a zol); Diflucan (dye' flu can)
- flucytosine (flu sy' toe seen); Ancobon (on' ko bon)
- griseofulvin (griz ee o ful' vin); Fulvicin (ful' vi sin) and Grifulvin (gri ful' vin)
- itraconazole (it rah kon' a zol); Sporanox (spor' ahn ox)
- ketoconazole (key toe kon' a zol); Nizoral (nis' or ral)
- terbinafine (ter bin' ah feen); Lamisil (lahm' ih sil)

fluconazole (Diflucan)

The drug interferes with cell wall formation. The drug is used:

- For fungal infections affecting:
  - The meninges
  - Mouth and pharynx
  - Esophagus
  - Vagina
- To prevent fungal infections in:
  - Bone marrow transplant patients who are receiving radiation or chemotherapy
  - Persons with HIV
  - Persons with weakened immune systems

Assisting With the Nursing Process

When giving fluconazole (Diflucan), you assist the nurse with the nursing process.

ASSESSMENT

- Ask about the person's signs and symptoms.
- Measure vital signs.
- Measure intake and output.
- Ask about GI symptoms.

PLANNING

The oral dose forms are:

- 50, 100, 150, and 200 mg tablets
- 10 and 40 mg/mL

IMPLEMENTATION

- The usual adult dose is 100 to 400 mg daily.
- The dosage depends on the infection being treated.

EVALUATION

Report and record:

- *Nausea, vomiting, and diarrhea.* These are usually mild and tend to resolve with continued therapy.
- *Anorexia, nausea, vomiting, jaundice.* These may signal liver toxicity.
- See *Promoting Safety and Comfort: Anti-Microbial Agents,* p. 409.

flucytosine (Ancobon)

This drug is thought to prevent the cell from making protein. It is used to treat fungal infections affecting:

- The blood
- Heart
- Urinary tract
- Meninges
- Lungs

Assisting With the Nursing Process

When giving flucytosine (Ancobon), you assist the nurse with the nursing process.

ASSESSMENT

- Ask about the person's signs and symptoms.
- Measure vital signs.
- Measure intake and output.
- Ask about GI symptoms.
- Observe level of alertness and orientation to person, time, and place.

PLANNING

The oral dose forms are 125 and 250 mg capsules.

IMPLEMENTATION

- The dose depends on body weight.
- The drug is given every 6 hours.

EVALUATION

Report and record:

- *Nausea, vomiting, and diarrhea.* These are usually mild and tend to resolve with continued therapy.
- *Rash, sore throat, fever, jaundice, weakness.* These may signal changes in red blood cells and white blood cells.
- *Decreasing urinary output, bloody or smoky-colored urine.* These signal kidney toxicity.
- *Anorexia, nausea, vomiting, jaundice.* These may signal liver toxicity.
- See *Promoting Safety and Comfort: Anti-Microbial Agents,* p. 409.

griseofulvin (Fulvicin and Grifulvin)

These drugs stop cell division and new cell growth. They are used to treat ringworm of the scalp, body, nails, and feet.

Assisting With the Nursing Process

When giving griseofulvin (Fulvicin and Grifulvin), you assist the nurse with the nursing process.

ASSESSMENT

- Ask about the person's signs and symptoms.
- Measure vital signs.
- Measure intake and output.
- Ask about GI symptoms.

PLANNING

The oral dose forms are:

- 125, 250, and 500 mg tablets
- 125 mg/5 mL oral suspension

IMPLEMENTATION

- Dosage depends on the microbe and location of the infection—usually 500 mg to 1 g in one dose or in divided doses daily.
- A high-fat meal may increase drug absorption.

EVALUATION

Report and record:

- *Nausea, vomiting, anorexia, abdominal cramps.* These are usually mild and tend to resolve with continued therapy.
- *Confusion.* Provide for safety.
- *Dizziness.* Provide for safety.
- *Genital and anal itching, vaginal discharge, thrush (a fungal infection of the mouth).* These signal secondary infections. Remind the person of the need for good oral and perineal hygiene.
- *Photo-sensitivity.* This is sensitivity to sunlight and ultra-violet light (sunlamps, tanning beds). The person should avoid exposure to sunlight, sunlamps, and tanning beds. He or she should apply a sunscreen and wear long-sleeved garments, a hat, and sunglasses when outdoors. Sunburn needs medical attention.
- *Sore throat, fever, jaundice, weakness.* These may signal changes in red blood cells and white blood cells.
- *Decreasing urinary output, bloody or smoky-colored urine.* These signal kidney toxicity.
- *Anorexia, nausea, vomiting, jaundice.* These may signal liver toxicity.
- See *Promoting Safety and Comfort: Anti-Microbial Agents,* p. 409.

itraconazole (Sporanox)

This drug interferes with the cell wall. Cell contents leak out of the cell. The drug is used to treat a variety of fungal infections.

Assisting With the Nursing Process

When giving itraconazole (Sporanox), you assist the nurse with the nursing process.

ASSESSMENT

- Ask about the person's signs and symptoms.
- Measure vital signs.
- Measure intake and output.
- Ask about GI symptoms.
- Observe for signs and symptoms of heart failure (Chapter 21).

PLANNING

The oral dose forms are:

- 100 mg capsules
- 10 mg/mL oral solution in 150 mL containers

IMPLEMENTATION

- The usual adult dose is 100 to 400 mg daily.
- Doses greater than 200 mg are given in 2 divided doses.
- Give the drug with a full meal.

EVALUATION

Report and record:

- *Nausea, vomiting.* These are usually mild and tend to resolve with continued therapy.
- *Anorexia, nausea, vomiting, jaundice.* These may signal liver toxicity.
- *Dyspnea, chest pain, fatigue, edema, syncope (fainting), palpitations.* These are signs of heart failure.
- See *Promoting Safety and Comfort: Anti-Microbial Agents,* p. 409.

ketoconazole (Nizoral)

This drug interferes with the cell wall. Cell contents leak out of the cell. The drug is used to treat a variety of fungal infections.

Assisting With the Nursing Process

When giving ketoconazole (Nizoral), you assist the nurse with the nursing process.

ASSESSMENT

- Ask about the person's signs and symptoms.
- Measure vital signs.
- Measure intake and output.
- Ask about GI symptoms.

PLANNING

The oral dose form is 200 mg tablets.

IMPLEMENTATION

- The usual adult dose is 200 to 400 mg once daily.
- Give the drug at least 2 hours before giving drugs that reduce stomach acidity.
- Give the drug with food.
- The person should avoid alcoholic beverages and drugs containing alcohol (cough medications, mouthwashes).

EVALUATION

Report and record:

- *Nausea, vomiting.* These are usually mild and tend to resolve with continued therapy.
- *Anorexia, nausea, vomiting, jaundice.* These may signal liver toxicity.
- See *Promoting Safety and Comfort: Anti-Microbial Agents,* p. 409.

terbinafine (Lamisil)

The drug affects enzymes that cells need to live. The drug is used to treat fungal infections affecting toenails and fingernails.

Assisting With the Nursing Process

When giving terbinafine (Lamisil), you assist the nurse with the nursing process.

ASSESSMENT

- Ask about the person's signs and symptoms.
- Measure vital signs.
- Measure intake and output.
- Ask about GI symptoms.

PLANNING

The oral dose form is 250 mg tablets.

IMPLEMENTATION

- Fingernail infections: 250 mg daily for 6 weeks
- Toenail infections: 250 mg daily for 12 weeks

EVALUATION

Report and record:

- *Decreasing urinary output, bloody or smoky-colored urine.* These signal kidney toxicity.
- *Anorexia, nausea, vomiting, jaundice.* These may signal liver toxicity.
- See *Promoting Safety and Comfort: Anti-Microbial Agents*, p. 409.

DRUG CLASS: **Anti-Viral Agents**

The following are anti-viral agents:

- acyclovir (a sy' klo veer); Zovirax (zoh' ve rahx)
- famciclovir (pham sik' lo veer); Famvir (pham' veer)
- valacyclovir (vahl ah syk' lo veer); Valtrex (vahl' trex)
- abacavir (ah bak' ah veer); Ziagen (ziy' ah jen)
- atazanavir (at ah zan' ah veer); Reyataz (ray' ah taz)
- didanosine (die dahn' oh seen); Videx (vye' dex)
- efavirenz (ef ahv' er enz); Sustiva (sus tee' vha)
- emtricitabine (em tree sit' a bean); Emtriva (em tree' vah)
- lamivudine (lahm ih' vu deen); Epiver and Epivir-HBV (ep' i vihr)
- stavudine (stav' u deen); Zerit (zair' it) and Zerit XR
- zidovudine (zid ohv' u deen); Retrovir (ret' roh veer)
- amantadine hydrochloride (ah man' tah deen); Symmetrel (sim' eh trel)
- oseltamivir (oh sel tahm' ah veer); Tamiflu (tahm' ih fluh)
- zanamivir (zahn am' ah veer); Relenza (rehl en' zah)
- ribavirin (ribe ah vi' rihn); Virazole (vi' rah zohl) and Rebetol (rehb et' ohl)

acyclovir (Zovirax)

This drug prevents viral cells from multiplying. It is used to treat genital herpes infections (Chapter 29).

Assisting With the Nursing Process

When giving acyclovir (Zovirax), you assist the nurse with the nursing process.

ASSESSMENT

- Ask about the person's signs and symptoms.
- Measure vital signs.
- Measure intake and output.
- Observe level of alertness and orientation to person, time, and place.

PLANNING

The dose forms are:

- Topical: 5% ointment and cream
- Oral:
  - 200 mg capsules
  - 400 and 800 mg tablets
  - 200 mg/5 mL suspension

IMPLEMENTATION

- Topical: apply to each lesion every 3 hours six times a day for 7 days. Wear gloves and practice hand hygiene.
- Oral:
  - Initial treatment: The usual adult dosage is 200 mg every 4 hours while awake. The total daily dosage is 1000 mg for 10 days.
  - Suppressive therapy: 400 mg two to five times a day for up to 12 months.
  - Intermittent therapy: 200 mg every 4 hours while awake. The total daily dosage is 1000 mg for 5 days. The drug is started at the earliest sign of symptoms.

EVALUATION

Report and record:

- *Sweating.* Follow the care plan for fluid intake.
- *Decreasing urinary output, bloody or smoky-colored urine.* These signal kidney toxicity.
- *Hypotension.* Blood pressure is measured in the supine and standing positions. Provide for safety. Remind the person to rise slowly from a supine or sitting position. Have the person sit or lie down if he or she feels faint.
- *Confusion.* Provide for safety.
- See *Promoting Safety and Comfort: Anti-Microbial Agents*, p. 409.

famciclovir (Famvir)

This drug prevents the virus cell from multiplying. It is used to treat:

- Recurrent genital herpes
- Herpes zoster (shingles)

Assisting With the Nursing Process

When giving famciclovir (Famvir), you assist the nurse with the nursing process.

ASSESSMENT

- Ask about the person's signs and symptoms.
- Measure vital signs.
- Measure intake and output.
- Ask about GI symptoms.
- Observe level of alertness and orientation to person, time, and place.

PLANNING

The oral dose forms are 125, 250, and 500 mg tablets.

IMPLEMENTATION

- For genital herpes: 125 mg two times a day for 5 days. Therapy should be started within 6 hours of the first sign or symptom.
- For herpes zoster (shingles): 500 mg every 8 hours for 7 days. Therapy should be started within 72 hours of symptom onset.

EVALUATION

Report and record:

- *Nausea, vomiting, headache.* These are usually mild and resolve with continued therapy.
- *Confusion.* Provide for safety.
- See *Promoting Safety and Comfort: Anti-Microbial Agents,* p. 409.

valacyclovir (Valtrex)

This drug inhibits the viral cell from multiplying. It is used to treat herpes zoster (shingles). The drug also is used to treat or suppress genital herpes.

Assisting With the Nursing Process

When giving valacyclovir (Valtrex), you assist the nurse with the nursing process.

ASSESSMENT

- Ask about the person's signs and symptoms.
- Measure vital signs.
- Measure intake and output.

PLANNING

The oral dose forms are 500 mg and 1 g caplets.

IMPLEMENTATION

- For herpes zoster: 1 g three times a day for 7 days
- For genital herpes: 500 mg two times a day for 7 days

EVALUATION

See acyclovir (Zovirax).

abacavir (Ziagen)

This drug prevents viral growth. It is used with other anti-viral agents to:

- Slow the progression of HIV.
- Reduce the frequency of opportunistic infections. An **opportunistic infection** is caused by non-pathogens in a person with a weakened immune system. Risk factors include diabetes, HIV infection, cancer, and urinary catheterization.

Assisting With the Nursing Process

When giving abacavir (Ziagen), you assist the nurse with the nursing process.

ASSESSMENT

- Ask about the person's signs and symptoms.
- Measure vital signs.
- Measure intake and output.
- Ask about GI symptoms.

PLANNING

The oral dose forms are:

- 300 mg tablets
- 20 mg/mL oral solution in 240 mL bottles

IMPLEMENTATION

The usual adult dose is 300 mg twice a day. It is given with other anti-viral agents.

EVALUATION

Report and record:

- *Anorexia, nausea, vomiting, jaundice.* These may signal liver toxicity.
- See *Promoting Safety and Comfort: Anti-Microbial Agents,* p. 409.

atazanavir (Reyataz)

This drug prevents virus cells from maturing. Immature virus cells are not infectious. The drug is used with other anti-viral agents to:

- Slow the progression of HIV
- Reduce the frequency of opportunistic infections

Assisting With the Nursing Process

When giving atazanavir (Reyataz), you assist the nurse with the nursing process.

ASSESSMENT

- Ask about the person's signs and symptoms.
- Measure vital signs.
- Measure intake and output.

PLANNING

The oral dose forms are 100, 150, 200, and 300 mg capsules.

IMPLEMENTATION

The usual adult dose is 400 mg once daily with food.

EVALUATION

Report and record:

- *Jaundice.* This reverses when the drug is discontinued.
- *Rash.* This usually resolves within 1 to 2 weeks.
- *Severe rash, blisters, fever.* The person needs medical attention.
- *Signs and symptoms of hyperglycemia.* See Chapter 27.
- *Anorexia, nausea, vomiting, jaundice.* These may signal liver toxicity.
- See *Promoting Safety and Comfort: Anti-Microbial Agents,* p. 409.

didanosine (Videx)

This drug prevents cells from multiplying. The drug is used to:

- Slow the progression of HIV
- Reduce the frequency of opportunistic infections

Assisting With the Nursing Process

When giving didanosine (Videx), you assist the nurse with the nursing process.

ASSESSMENT

- Ask about the person's signs and symptoms.
- Measure vital signs.
- Measure intake and output.
- Ask about GI symptoms.

PLANNING

The adult oral dose forms are:

- 25, 50, 100, 150, and 200 mg chewable tablets
- 125, 200, 250, and 400 mg delayed-release capsules
- 10 mg/mL powder for oral solution after reconstitution

IMPLEMENTATION

- Chewable tablets:
  - 125 mg every 12 hours for persons weighing less than 132 pounds (60 kg)
  - 200 mg every 12 hours for persons weighing more than 132 pounds (60 kg)
  - Tablets must be thoroughly chewed. Crushed tablets should be well dispersed in at lease 1 ounce of water.
- Delayed-release capsules:
  - 250 mg once a day for persons weighing less than 132 pounds (60 kg)
  - 400 mg once a day for persons weighing more than 132 pounds (60 kg)
- Powder:
  - 167 mg every 12 hours for persons weighing less than 132 pounds (60 kg)
  - 250 mg every 12 hours for persons weighing more than 132 pounds (60 kg)

- The powder form is prepared by a pharmacist. The person should drink the ordered dose immediately. Do not mix the powder with fruit juice or other liquids containing acid.
- Give all drug forms on an empty stomach. The dose is given 1 hour before or 2 hours after meals.

EVALUATION

Report and record:

- *Diarrhea.* This is more common with the powder form.
- *Abdominal pain, nausea, vomiting.* These may signal pancreatitis.
- *Numbness, tingling, pain in the feet and hands.* These signal nervous system involvement.
- See *Promoting Safety and Comfort: Anti-Microbial Agents,* p. 409.

efavirenz (Sustiva)

This drug inhibits HIV from multiplying. It is used with other agents to:

- Slow the progression of HIV
- Reduce the frequency of opportunistic infections

Assisting With the Nursing Process

When giving efavirenz (Sustiva), you assist the nurse with the nursing process.

ASSESSMENT

- Ask about the person's signs and symptoms.
- Measure vital signs.
- Measure intake and output.
- Ask about GI symptoms.

PLANNING

The oral dose forms are:

- 50, 100, and 200 mg capsules
- 600 mg tablets

IMPLEMENTATION

- The usual adult dose is 600 mg once a day with other anti-viral agents.
- The drug should be taken on an empty stomach at bedtime. Food increases absorption and the risk of toxic effects.
- Women who are or may become pregnant should not take this drug. Fetal deaths are associated with the drug.

EVALUATION

Report and record:

- *Drowsiness, dizziness, impaired concentration, vivid dreams, depression, delusions.* These may improve after 2 to 4 weeks of therapy.
- *Rash.* This usually resolves within 1 month of therapy.
- *Severe rash, blisters, fever.* The person needs medical attention.

- *Anorexia, nausea, vomiting, jaundice.* These may signal liver toxicity.
- See *Promoting Safety and Comfort: Anti-Microbial Agents*, p. 409.

emtricitabine (Emtriva)

This drug inhibits HIV from multiplying. It is used with other agents to:
- Slow the progression of HIV
- Reduce the frequency of opportunistic infections

Assisting With the Nursing Process

When giving emtricitabine (Emtriva), you assist the nurse with the nursing process.

ASSESSMENT
- Ask about the person's signs and symptoms.
- Measure vital signs.
- Measure intake and output.
- Ask about GI symptoms.

PLANNING
The oral dose forms are:
- 200 mg capsules
- 10 mg/mL solution

IMPLEMENTATION
- The usual adult doses are:
  - 200 mg capsule once a day
  - 240 mg oral solution once a day
- The dosage is reduced for persons with impaired kidney function.

EVALUATION
Report and record:
- *Anorexia, nausea, vomiting, jaundice.* These may signal liver toxicity.
- *Malaise, muscle pains, respiratory distress, hypotension.* These signal a build up of lactic acid in the blood (lactic acidosis). See Chapter 27.
- *Changes in skin color.* This may occur on the palms and soles of the feet.
- *Diarrhea, nausea, rhinitis, rash, weakness, cough, headache.*
- See *Promoting Safety and Comfort: Anti-Microbial Agents*, p. 409.

lamivudine (Epiver and Epivir-HBV)

This drug prevents the HIV and the hepatitis B virus (HBV) from multiplying. It is used to:
- Slow the progression of HIV infection when used with zidovudine (Retrovir)
- Slow the progression of HBV infection
- Reduce the frequency of opportunistic infections

Assisting With the Nursing Process

When giving lamivudine (Epiver and Epivir-HBV), you assist the nurse with the nursing process.

ASSESSMENT
- Ask about the person's signs and symptoms.
- Measure vital signs.
- Measure intake and output.
- Ask about GI symptoms.
- Ask about numbness, tingling, and pain in the hands and feet.

PLANNING
The oral dose forms are:
- 100, 150, and 300 mg tablets
- 5 and 10 mg/mL oral solution in 240 mL bottles

IMPLEMENTATION
- For HIV infection: 150 mg two times a day with zidovudine (Retrovir)
- For HBV infection: 100 mg once a day

EVALUATION
Report and record:
- *Anorexia, nausea, vomiting, jaundice.* These may signal liver toxicity.
- *Malaise, muscle pains, respiratory distress, hypotension.* These signal a build up of lactic acid in the blood (lactic acidosis). See Chapter 27.
- *Abdominal pain, nausea, vomiting.* These may signal pancreatitis.
- *Numbness, tingling, pain in the feet and hands.* These signal nervous system involvement.
- See *Promoting Safety and Comfort: Anti-Microbial Agents*, p. 409.

stavudine (Zerit and Zerit XR)

These drugs are used with other anti-viral agents in the treatment of HIV infection. The goals of therapy are to:
- Slow the progression of HIV infection
- Reduce the frequency of opportunistic infections

Assisting With the Nursing Process

When giving stavudine (Zerit and Zerit XR), you assist the nurse with the nursing process.

ASSESSMENT
- Ask about the person's signs and symptoms.
- Measure vital signs.
- Measure intake and output.
- Ask about GI symptoms.
- Ask about numbness, tingling, and pain in the hands and feet.

PLANNING
The oral dose forms are:
- 15, 20, 30, and 40 mg capsules
- 37.5, 50, 75, and 100 mg extended-release capsules
- 1 mg/mL powder for oral solution

IMPLEMENTATION
- Capsules:
  - For persons weighing less than 132 pounds (60 kg): 30 mg every 12 hours
  - For persons weighing more than 132 pounds (60 kg): 40 mg every 12 hours
- Extended-release capsules:
  - For persons weighing less than 132 pounds (60 kg): 75 mg once a day
  - For persons weighing more than 132 pounds (60 kg): 100 mg once a day

EVALUATION
Report and record:
- *Anorexia, nausea, vomiting, jaundice.* These may signal liver toxicity.
- *Malaise, muscle pains, respiratory distress, hypotension.* These signal a build up of lactic acid in the blood (lactic acidosis). See Chapter 27.
- *Abdominal pain, nausea, vomiting.* These may signal pancreatitis.
- *Numbness, tingling, pain in the feet and hands.* These signal nervous system involvement.
- See *Promoting Safety and Comfort: Anti-Microbial Agents,* p. 409.

zidovudine (Retrovir)

This drug prevents HIV from multiplying. It is used to:
- Slow the progression of HIV infection
- Reduce the frequency of opportunistic infections

Assisting With the Nursing Process
When giving zidovudine (Retrovir), you assist the nurse with the nursing process.
ASSESSMENT
- Ask about the person's signs and symptoms.
- Measure vital signs.
- Measure intake and output.
- Ask about numbness, tingling, and pain in the hands and feet.

PLANNING
The oral dose forms are:
- 100 mg capsules
- 300 mg tablets
- 50 mg/5 mL syrup

IMPLEMENTATION
- Persons without symptoms of HIV infection: 100 mg every 4 hours while awake. Total dosage is 500 mg/day.
- Persons with symptoms of HIV infection: 200 mg every 4 hours. After 1 month the dosage is reduced to 100 mg every 4 hours.

EVALUATION
Report and record:
- *Fatigue, dizziness, headache, pallor, dyspnea on exertion.* These may signal changes in red blood cell production.
- *Numbness, tingling, pain in the feet and hands.* These signal nervous system involvement.
- See *Promoting Safety and Comfort: Anti-Microbial Agents,* p. 409.

amantadine hydrochloride (Symmetrel)

This drug acts against the influenza A virus. It is also used to treat Parkinson's disease. The drug is discussed in Chapter 14.

oseltamivir (Tamiflu)

This drug inhibits an enzyme on the viral cell coat. The enzyme is needed for cell reproduction and the spread of viral cell particles. The drug is used to reduce flu symptoms—nasal congestion, sore throat, cough, muscle aches, fatigue, headache, chills, sweats.

Assisting With the Nursing Process
When giving oseltamivir (Tamiflu), you assist the nurse with the nursing process.
ASSESSMENT
- Ask about the person's signs and symptoms.
- Measure vital signs.
- Measure intake and output.
- Ask about GI symptoms.

PLANNING
The oral dose forms are:
- 75 mg capsules
- 12 mg/mL oral suspension

IMPLEMENTATION
- The usual adult dosage is 75 mg two times a day for 5 days.
- Treatment should begin within 2 days of flu symptom onset.
- Give the drug with food or milk.

EVALUATION
Report and record:
- *Nausea, vomiting.* Give the drug with food or milk to lessen nausea and vomiting.
- *Cough, yellow or green sputum, sore throat, fever, continuing symptoms.* The person needs further medical attention.
- See *Promoting Safety and Comfort: Anti-Microbial Agents,* p. 409.

zanamivir (Relenza)

This drug inhibits an enzyme on the viral cell coat. The enzyme is needed for cell reproduction and the spread of viral cell particles. The drug is used to reduce flu symptoms—nasal congestion, sore throat, cough, muscle aches, fatigue, headache, chills, sweats. The drug may prevent the secondary infection of pneumonia.

Assisting With the Nursing Process

When giving zanamivir (Relenza), you assist the nurse with the nursing process.

ASSESSMENT

- Ask about the person's signs and symptoms.
- Measure vital signs.
- Measure intake and output.

PLANNING

The dose form is 5 mg blisters of powder for inhalation.

IMPLEMENTATION

The usual adult dosage is:

- 2 inhalations (one 5 mg blister per inhalation for a total of 10 mg) every 12 hours for 5 days.
- Treatment should begin within 2 days of flu symptom onset.
- Inhaled broncho-dilators should be taken before this drug.

EVALUATION

Report and record:

- *Asthma, broncho-spasm, shortness of breath, chest soreness.* The person must stop taking the drug and seek medical attention.
- *Cough, yellow or green sputum, sore throat, fever, continuing symptoms.* The person needs further medical attention.
- See *Promoting Safety and Comfort: Anti-Microbial Agents,* p. 409.

ribavirin (Rebetol)

This drug inhibits viral activity. For adults, it is used with other drugs in the treatment of hepatitis C. See Box 34-3.

Assisting With the Nursing Process

When giving ribavirin (Rebetol), you assist the nurse with the nursing process.

ASSESSMENT

- Ask about the person's signs and symptoms.
- Measure vital signs.
- Measure intake and output.
- Ask about GI symptoms.

PLANNING

The oral dose form is 200 mg capsules.

IMPLEMENTATION

- For persons weighing less than 165 pounds (75 kg):
  - 400 mg in the morning
  - 600 mg in the evening
- For persons weighing more than 165 pounds (75 kg):
  - 600 mg in the morning
  - 600 mg in the evening

EVALUATION

Report and record:

- *Fatigue, dizziness, headache, pallor, dyspnea on exertion.* These may signal changes in red blood cell production.
- See *Promoting Safety and Comfort: Anti-Microbial Agents,* p. 409.

REVIEW QUESTIONS

Circle the **BEST** answer.

1 Microbes that grow in living cells are called
   a bacteria   c germs
   b fungi   d viruses

2 Plants that live on other plants or animals are called
   a bacteria   c germs
   b fungi   d viruses

3 Chemicals that eliminate pathogens are called
   a antibiotics   c anti-virals
   b anti-microbials   d non-pathogens

4 A person with a weakened immune system develops an infection. It is caused by a non-pathogen. The person has
   a a bacterial infection
   b a healthcare-associated infection
   c an opportunistic infection
   d a secondary infection

5 A person is being treated for an infection. Another infection develops. This is called
   a a bacterial infection
   b a healthcare-associated infection
   c an opportunistic infection
   d a secondary infection

Continued

REVIEW QUESTIONS—cont'd

6 Before giving any anti-microbial, you must first
   a check for allergies
   b observe for an allergic reaction
   c put on gloves
   d observe the person for 20 to 30 minutes

7 The following signal an allergic reaction *except*
   a bleeding   c hives
   b dyspnea   d nasal congestion

8 To maintain blood levels of the drug, anti-microbials are usually given
   a at regular intervals
   b at the same time every day
   c every 6 hours
   d every 12 hours

9 Neo-Fradin is an amino-glycoside. It can cause
   a diabetes   c meningitis
   b hearing loss   d septicemia

10 Which drug class can cause staining of the teeth?
   a cephalo-sporins   c sulfonamides
   b penicillins   d tetracyclines

11 Cephalo-sporins and ketolides are given to treat infections caused by
   a bacteria   c penicillins
   b fungi   d viruses

12 Which is *not* a cephalo-sporin?
   a co-amoxiclav (Augmentin)
   b cefaclor (Ceclor)
   c cephalexin (Keflex)
   d cefixime (Suprax)

13 Which is *not* an anti-tubercular agent?
   a metronidazole (Flagyl)   c ethambutol (Myambutol)
   b isoniazid (INH)   d rifampin (Rifadin)

14 Which is *not* a penicillin?
   a Amoxil   c Principen
   b Cipro   d Trimox

15 A common side effect from penicillin is
   a diarrhea   c photo-toxicity
   b hearing loss   d tingling

16 Doxycycline (Vibramycin) is a
   a cephalo-sporin   c sulfonamide
   b penicillin   d tetracycline

17 Fluoro-quinolones are effective against many of the following *except*
   a gram-positive bacteria   c gram-negative bacteria
   b anaerobic bacteria   d fungi and viruses

18 Isoniazid (INH) is given
   a on an empty stomach   c 30 minutes before a meal
   b with food or milk   d 30 minutes after a meal

19 Anti-tubercular agents are usually given
   a in a single daily dose   c every 4 hours
   b in divided doses   d every 6 hours

20 Which antibiotic has the most severe adverse effects?
   a clindamycin (Cleocin)   c tinidazole (Tindamax)
   b metronidazole (Flagyl)   d vancomycin (Vancocin)

21 Which is similar to metronidazole (Flagyl)?
   a clindamycin (Cleocin)   c terbinafine (Lamisil)
   b tinidazole (Tindamax)   d vancomycin (Vancocin)

22 Which is a systemic anti-fungal agent?
   a fluconazole (Diflucan)   c tioconazole (Monistat-1)
   b butenafine (Lotrimin)   d nystatin (Mycostatin)

23 Which anti-fungal agent is used to treat fungal infections affecting the blood and lungs?
   a flucytosine (Ancobon)   c griseofulvin (Fulvicin)
   b fluconazole (Diflucan)   d terbinafine (Lamisil)

24 The following are used to treat genital herpes *except*
   a famciclovir (Famvir)   c valacyclovir (Valtrex)
   b zidovudine (Retrovir)   d acyclovir (Zovirax)

25 Anti-viral drugs used to treat HIV also are used to reduce the frequency of
   a hepatitis B   c opportunistic infections
   b hepatitis C   d secondary infections

26 Which has a powder oral dose form?
   a valacyclovir (Valtrex)   c efavirenz (Sustiva)
   b atazanavir (Reyataz)   d didanosine (Videx)

27 Which drug is inhaled?
   a ribavirin (Rebetol)   c zidovudine (Retrovir)
   b zanamivir (Relenza)   d oseltamivir (Tamiflu)

28 Which is used to treat hepatitis C?
   a ribavirin (Rebetol)   c zidovudine (Retrovir)
   b zanamivir (Relenza)   d oseltamivir (Tamiflu)

Circle T if the statement is true. Circle F if the statement is false.

29 T F Aerobic microbes live and grow in the presence of oxygen.

30 T F Sulfonamides are used to treat HIV and opportunistic infections.

31 T F Tetracyclines are given with dairy products to promote drug absorption.

32 T F Clindamycin (Cleocin) suspension should be refrigerated.

33 T F Metronidazole (Flagyl) is applied topically.

34 T F Famciclovir (Famvir) and valacyclovir (Valtrex) are used to treat shingles.

Answers to these questions are on p. 448.

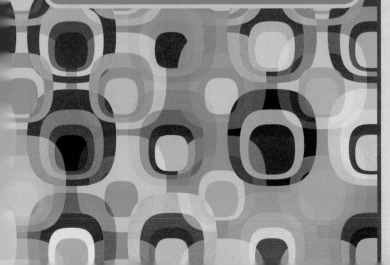

Nutrition and Herbal and Dietary Supplement Therapy

OBJECTIVES

- Define the key terms and key abbreviations used in this chapter.
- Explain the purpose and use of the MyPyramid Food Guidance System.
- Explain how to use the Dietary Guidelines for Americans.
- Describe the functions and sources of vitamins and minerals.
- Describe the therapies for malnutrition.
- Explain how you assist the nurse with therapies for malnutrition.
- Identify common herbs and dietary supplements.

KEY TERMS

aspiration Breathing fluid, food, vomitus, or an object into the lungs

calorie The amount of energy produced when the body burns food

enteral nutrition Giving nutrients into the gastro-intestinal (GI) tract *(enteral)* through a feeding tube

gastrostomy tube A tube inserted through a surgically created opening *(stomy)* in the stomach *(gastro)*; stomach tube

jejunostomy tube A feeding tube inserted into a surgically created opening *(stomy)* in the *jejunum* of the small intestine

malnutrition Any disorder of nutrition; *mal* means *bad*

naso-duodenal tube A feeding tube inserted through the nose *(naso)* into the *duodenum* of the small intestine

naso-gastric (NG) tube A feeding tube inserted through the nose *(naso)* into the stomach *(gastro)*

naso-intestinal tube A feeding tube inserted through the nose *(naso)* into the small intestine *(intestinal)*

naso-jejunal tube A feeding tube inserted through the nose *(naso)* into the *jejunum* of the small intestine

Continued

KEY TERMS—cont'd

nutrient A substance that is ingested, digested, absorbed, and used by the body

nutrition The processes involved in the ingestion, digestion, absorption, and use of foods and fluids by the body

parenteral nutrition Giving nutrients through a catheter inserted into a vein; *para* means *beyond*; *enteral* relates to the *bowel*

percutaneous endoscopic gastrostomy (PEG) tube A feeding tube inserted into the stomach (*gastro*) through a small incision (*stomy*) made through (*per*) the skin (*cutaneous*); a lighted instrument (*scope*) allows the doctor to see inside a body cavity or organ (*endo*)

regurgitation The backward flow of stomach contents into the mouth

KEY ABBREVIATIONS

AIDS Acquired immunodeficiency syndrome
BPH Benign prostatic hyperplasia
CNS Central nervous system
GI Gastro-intestinal
IV Intravenous
MAR Medication administration record
mg Milligram
mL Milliliter
NG Naso-gastric
PEG Percutaneous endoscopic gastrostomy
TPN Total parenteral nutrition

The body needs a regular source of energy to support and maintain its functions. Such functions include respiration, nerve transmission, circulation, physical work, and maintaining body temperature. For some people, the daily diet provides needed energy sources. Other people use herbs and dietary supplements to enhance the daily diet.

NUTRITION

Nutrition is the processes involved in the ingestion, digestion, absorption, and use of foods and fluids by the body. Good nutrition is needed for growth, healing, and body functions. A well-balanced diet and correct calorie intake are needed. A high-fat and high-calorie diet causes weight gain and obesity. Weight loss occurs with a low-calorie diet.

Foods and fluids contain nutrients. A **nutrient** is a substance that is ingested, digested, absorbed, and used by the body. Nutrients are grouped into fats, proteins, carbohydrates, vitamins, minerals, and water.

Fats, proteins, and carbohydrates give the body fuel for energy. The amount of energy provided by a nutrient is measured in calories. A **calorie** is the amount of energy produced when the body burns food:

- 1 gram of fat—9 calories
- 1 gram of protein—4 calories
- 1 gram of carbohydrate—4 calories

Dietary Guidelines

The *Dietary Guidelines for Americans 2005* are for persons 2 years of age and older (Box 35-1). Through diet and physical activity, the guidelines serve to:

- Promote health
- Reduce the risk of chronic diseases

Certain diseases are linked to poor diet and the lack of physical activity. They include cardiovascular diseases, hypertension (high blood pressure), diabetes, being over-weight, obesity, osteoporosis, and some cancers.

MyPyramid

The *MyPyramid Food Guidance System* (Fig. 35-1, p. 433) is based on the *Dietary Guidelines for Americans 2005.* Smart and healthy food choices and daily activity are encouraged.

The MyPyramid symbol shows the "Steps to a Healthier You."

- *The kind and amounts of food to eat daily.* This depends on the person's age, gender (male or female), and activity level.
- *Gradual improvement.* People can take small steps each day to improve their diet and life-style.
- *Physical activity.* This is shown by the steps and the person climbing them. They are a reminder of the importance of physical activity. For health benefits, at least 30 minutes of physical activity are needed on most days of the week. It is best to do so every day. Activity should be moderate or vigorous. The activity can be done in one 30-minute period. Or it can be done in 2 or 3 parts as long as the total time is at least 30 minutes a day.
- *Variety.* The six color bands stand for the 5 food groups and oils. Foods from the 5 groups are needed each day for good health.
- *Moderation.* This means to avoid extremes. The bands narrow as they go from the bottom to the top of the pyramid. Foods near the base have the most nutritional value and the fewest calories. They have little or no solid fats, added sugars, or caloric sweeteners. Foods lower in the band should be chosen more often than those higher in the band.
- *The right amount from each food group band.* The bands differ in width. The widths suggest how much food to choose from each group. The wider the band, the more foods the person should choose from that group.

BOX 35-1 Dietary Guidelines for Americans 2005

CONSUME AN ADEQUATE AMOUNT OF NUTRIENTS WITHIN YOUR DAILY CALORIE NEEDS

- Consume a variety of nutrient-dense foods and beverages from the basic food groups. Nutrient-dense foods have little or no solid fats or added sugar.
  - Limit the intake of fats, cholesterol, added sugars, salt, and alcohol.
- Use the MyPyramid Food Guidance System or the DASH Eating Plan (Dietary Approaches to Stop Hypertension). Use the plans to determine energy needs (calories needed) for your gender (male or female), age, and activity level.

WEIGHT MANAGEMENT

- To maintain a healthy body weight—balance your calorie intake with the calories used for energy.
- To prevent gradual weight gain over time—make small decreases in calorie intake and increase physical activity.

PHYSICAL ACTIVITY

- Engage in regular physical activity to promote health, mental well-being, and a healthy body weight. Avoid a sedentary life-style. *Sedentary* means a life-style with little or no physical activity.
  - To reduce the risk of chronic disease in adulthood—engage in at least 30 minutes of moderate to vigorous activity on most days of the week. This activity is in addition to your usual activity at work or at home.
  - For greater health benefits—engage in physical activity that is more vigorous or longer in duration.
  - To manage body weight and prevent gradual, unhealthy weight gain—engage in up to 60 minutes of moderate to vigorous activity on most days of the week. Do not exceed calorie needs.
  - To maintain weight loss in adulthood—engage in 60 to 90 minutes of moderate activity daily. Do not exceed calorie needs.
- To achieve physical fitness include the following physical activities:
  - Cardiovascular conditioning
  - Stretching exercises for flexibility
  - Resistance exercise or calisthenics for muscle strength and endurance

FOOD GROUPS TO ENCOURAGE

- Eat enough fruits and vegetables but stay within energy (calorie) needs.
  - For a daily intake of 2000 calories—2 cups of fruit and 2½ cups of vegetables are recommended.
  - For a daily intake of more than 2000 calories—more than 2 cups of fruit and 2½ cups of vegetables are recommended.

- For daily intake of less than 2000 calories—less than 2 cups of fruit and 2½ cups of vegetables are recommended.
- Choose a variety of fruits and vegetables each day. Select from all five vegetable subgroups—dark green, orange, legumes, starchy vegetables, and others. Do so several times a week.
- Eat at least 3 ounces of whole-grain products a day. An ounce-equivalent of whole grain is the amount of whole grain that equals a 1-ounce slice of bread.
- At least half of the daily grain requirement should come from whole grains. Examples include brown rice, buckwheat, bulgur, oatmeal, and wild rice. Whole wheat bran, crackers, pasta, and tortillas are other examples.
- The rest of the daily grain requirement comes from enriched or whole-grain products.
- Consume 3 cups per day of fat-free or low-fat milk or equivalent milk products:
  - 1 cup yogurt = 1 cup of fat-free or low-fat milk
  - 1½ ounces natural cheese = 1 cup of fat-free or low-fat milk
  - 2 ounces processed cheese = 1 cup of fat-free or low-fat milk

FATS

- Limit intake of fats and oils high in:
  - Saturated fats—fat from animal products such as meat and dairy products (milk, cheese). Many of these fats are solid at room temperature—butter, lard, and shortening.
  - *Trans* fats—fats found in shortening and commercially prepared baked goods, snack foods, fried foods, and margarine. Trans fats also are found in dairy products, beef, and lamb.
  - Cholesterol—a fat-related substance that is found in all animal foods. It is not found in plants. Main sources are egg yolks and organ meats (liver, kidneys). Other sources include meat, poultry, fish, and shellfish.
- Keep total fat intake between 20% and 30% of calories. Most fat should come from fish, nuts, and vegetable oils.
- Select and prepare meat, poultry, dry beans, milk, and milk products that are lean, low-fat, or fat-free.

CARBOHYDRATES

- Choose fiber-rich fruits, vegetables, and whole grains often.
- Choose and prepare foods and beverages with little added sugars or caloric sweeteners.
- Consume sugar- and starch-containing foods and beverages less frequently. Along with good oral hygiene, this helps prevents dental caries (cavities).

Modified from *Dietary Guidelines for Americans 2005* and *Finding Your Way to a Healthier You: Based on the Dietary Guidelines for Americans,* U.S. Department of Health and Human Services and U.S. Department of Agriculture. *Continued*

BOX 35-1   Dietary Guidelines for Americans 2005—cont'd

SODIUM AND POTASSIUM
- Consume less than 2300 mg (about 2 teaspoons of salt) of sodium per day.
- Choose and prepare foods with little salt.
- Consume potassium-rich foods. Fruits and vegetables are examples.

ALCOHOLIC BEVERAGES
- Persons who drink alcohol should do so sensibly and in moderation. Moderation means 12 ounces of regular beer, 5 ounces of wine, or 1½ ounces of 80-proof distilled spirits.
  - Women—up to 1 drink per day
  - Men—up to 2 drinks per day
- Alcohol should not be consumed by:
  - Persons who cannot restrict their alcohol intake
  - Women of child-bearing age who may become pregnant
  - Pregnant and breast-feeding women
  - Children and adolescents
  - Persons taking drugs that interact with alcohol
  - Persons with certain medical conditions
- Alcohol should not be consumed by persons who engage in activities that require attention, skill, or coordination. Driving and operating machinery are examples.

FOOD SAFETY
- To avoid food-borne illnesses:
  - Wash your hands.
  - Clean food contact surfaces.
  - Clean fruits and vegetables.
  - Do not wash or rinse meat and poultry.
  - Separate raw, cooked, and ready-to-eat foods while shopping, preparing, or storing foods.
  - Cook foods to a safe temperature to kill microbes.
  - Chill perishable foods promptly.
  - Defrost foods properly.
  - Avoid the following foods:
    - Raw (unpasteurized) milk or any products made from unpasteurized milk
    - Raw or partially cooked eggs or food containing raw eggs
    - Raw or undercooked meat and poultry
    - Unpasteurized juices
    - Raw sprouts

Nutrients

No food or food group has every essential nutrient. A well-balanced diet ensures an adequate intake of essential nutrients.

- *Protein*—is the most important nutrient. It is needed for tissue growth and repair. Sources include meat, fish, poultry, eggs, milk and milk products, cereals, beans, peas, and nuts.
- *Carbohydrates*—provide energy and fiber for bowel elimination. They are found in fruits, vegetables, breads, cereals, and sugar. Carbohydrates break down into sugars during digestion. The sugars are absorbed into the bloodstream. Fiber is not digested. It provides the bulky part of chyme for elimination.
- *Fats*—provide energy. They add flavor to food and help the body use certain vitamins. Sources include meats, lard, butter, shortening, oils, milk, cheese, egg yolks, and nuts. Dietary fat not needed by the body is stored as body fat (*adipose tissue*).
- *Vitamins*—are needed for certain body functions. They do not provide calories. The body stores vitamins A, D, E, and K. Vitamin C and the B complex vitamins are not stored. They must be ingested daily. The lack of a certain vitamin results in signs and symptoms of an illness. Table 35-1 on p. 434 lists the sources and major functions of common vitamins.
- *Minerals*—are used for many body processes. They are needed for bone and tooth formation, nerve and muscle function, fluid balance, and other body processes. Table 35-2 on p. 434 lists the major functions and dietary sources of common minerals.
- *Water*—is needed for all body processes. Death can result from too much or too little water. Water is ingested through fluids and foods. Water is lost through urine, feces, and vomit. It is also lost through the skin (perspiration) and the lungs (expiration). An adult needs 1500 mL of water daily to survive. About 2000 to 2500 mL of fluid per day are needed for normal fluid balance. The water requirement increases with hot weather, exercise, fever, illness, and excess fluid losses.

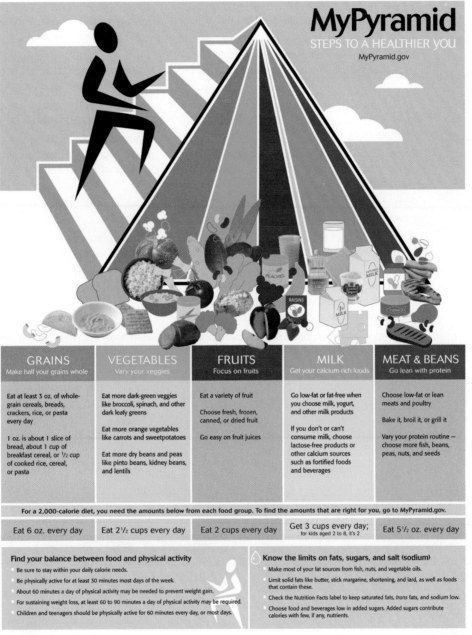

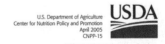

Fig. 35-1 MyPyramid: Steps to a Healthier You. (Courtesy U.S. Department of Agriculture, Center for Nutrition and Policy Promotion, April 2005, CNPP-15.)

TABLE 35-1   Functions and Sources of Common Vitamins

VITAMIN	MAJOR FUNCTIONS	SOURCES
Vitamin A	Growth; vision; healthy hair, skin, and mucous membranes; resistance to infection	Liver, spinach, green leafy and yellow vegetables, yellow fruits, fish liver oils, egg yolks, butter, cream, whole milk
Vitamin B_1 (thiamin)	Muscle tone, nerve function, digestion, appetite, normal elimination, carbohydrate use	Pork, fish, poultry, eggs, liver, breads, pastas, cereals, oatmeal, potatoes, peas, beans, soybeans, peanuts
Vitamin B_2 (riboflavin)	Growth, healthy eyes, protein and carbohydrate metabolism, healthy skin and mucous membranes	Milk and milk products, liver, green leafy vegetables, eggs, breads, cereals
Vitamin B_3 (niacin)	Protein, fat, and carbohydrate metabolism; nervous system function; appetite; digestive system function	Meat, pork, liver, fish, peanuts, breads and cereals, green vegetables, dairy products
Vitamin B_{12}	Formation of red blood cells, protein metabolism, nervous system function	Liver, meats, poultry, fish, eggs, milk, cheese
Folate (folic acid)	Formation of red blood cells, intestinal function, protein metabolism	Liver, meats, fish, poultry, green leafy vegetables, whole grains
Vitamin C (ascorbic acid)	Formation of substances that hold tissues together; healthy blood vessels, skin, gums, bones, and teeth; wound healing; prevention of bleeding; resistance to infection	Citrus fruits, tomatoes, potatoes, cabbage, strawberries, green vegetables, melons
Vitamin D	Absorption and metabolism of calcium and phosphorus, healthy bones	Fish liver oils, milk, butter, liver, exposure to sunlight
Vitamin E	Normal reproduction, formation of red blood cells, muscle function	Vegetable oils, milk, eggs, meats, cereals, green leafy vegetables
Vitamin K	Blood clotting	Liver, green leafy vegetables, egg yolks, cheese

TABLE 35-2   Functions and Sources of Common Minerals

MINERAL	MAJOR FUNCTIONS	SOURCES
Calcium	Formation of teeth and bones, blood clotting, muscle contraction, heart function, nerve function	Milk and milk products, green leafy vegetables, whole grains, egg yolks, dried peas and beans, nuts
Phosphorus	Formation of bones and teeth; use of proteins, fats, and carbohydrates; nerve and muscle function	Meat, fish, poultry, milk and milk products, nuts, egg yolks, dried peas and beans
Iron	Allows red blood cells to carry oxygen	Liver, meat, eggs, green leafy vegetables, breads and cereals, dried peas and beans, nuts
Iodine	Thyroid gland function, growth, metabolism	Iodized salt, seafood, shellfish
Sodium	Fluid balance, nerve and muscle function	Almost all foods
Potassium	Nerve function, muscle contraction, heart function	Fruits, vegetables, cereals, meats, dried peas and beans

Malnutrition

Nutrition plays a vital role in the recovery from illness, surgery, and injury. Adequate nutrient intake is needed to restore normal body processes and to rebuild and repair tissue. If nutritional needs are not met, malnutrition results. **Malnutrition** is any disorder of nutrition. *(Mal means bad.)*

Persons who are malnourished are at risk for infections and organ failure. Complications, other diseases, and death may occur. Malnutrition usually results from:

- Inadequate intake of protein and calories
- A deficiency of one or more vitamins and minerals

Therapy for Malnutrition. Therapy for malnutrition involves partial or full supplementation. To *supplement* means to complete or add to. The diet can be supplemented by:

- *Oral supplements.* The person drinks one of the oral formulas listed in Table 35-3.
- *Enteral nutrition.* **Enteral nutrition** is giving nutrients into the gastro-intestinal (GI) tract *(enteral)* through a feeding tube. The doctor orders the type of formula, the amount to give, and when to give tube feedings. Most formulas contain proteins, carbohydrates, fats, vitamins, and minerals. Tube feedings are given at certain times (scheduled feedings). Or they are given over a 24-hour period (continuous feedings). These feeding tubes are common:
  - **Naso-gastric (NG) tube.** A feeding tube is inserted through the nose *(naso)* into the stomach *(gastro).* See Figure 35-2.
  - **Naso-intestinal tube.** A feeding tube is inserted through the nose *(naso)* into the small intestine *(intestinal).* A **naso-duodenal tube** is inserted into the *duodenum.* A **naso-jejunal tube** is inserted into the *jejunum.* See Figure 35-3.

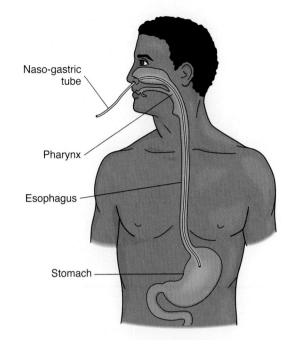

Fig. 35-2 A naso-gastric tube inserted through the nose and esophagus and into the stomach.

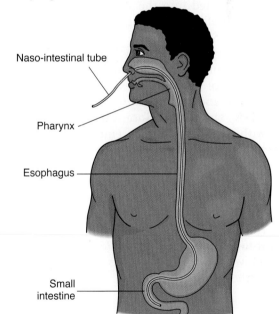

Fig. 35-3 A naso-intestinal tube is inserted through the nose and into the duodenum or jejunum of the small intestine.

TABLE 35-3	**Oral Nutritional Supplements**	
FORMULA TYPE	**BRAND NAMES**	**COMMENTS**
Oral supplements	Ensure Liquid Ensure Plus HN Ensure Plus ProSure Boost	These products are dietary supplements and are available in a variety of flavors for oral use. Requires full digestive capability by gut. At recommended dosages, these formulas provide 100% of the recommended dietary allowance for vitamins and minerals.

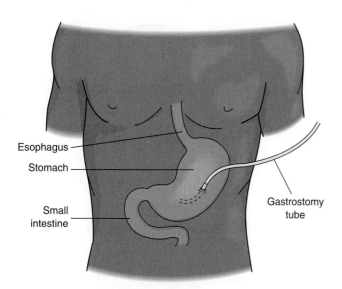

Fig. 35-4 A gastrostomy tube.

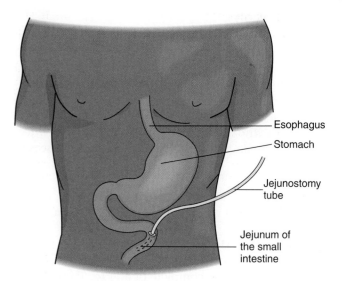

Fig. 35-5 A jejunostomy tube.

- **Gastrostomy tube.** Also called a *stomach tube,* it is inserted into the stomach. A doctor surgically creates an opening *(stomy)* in the stomach *(gastro).* See Figure 35-4.
- **Jejunostomy tube.** A feeding tube inserted into a surgically created opening *(stomy)* in the *jejunum* of the small intestine. See Figure 35-5.
- **Percutaneous endoscopic gastrostomy (PEG) tube.** The doctor inserts the feeding tube with an endoscope. An endoscope is a lighted instrument *(scope)* used to see inside a body cavity or organ *(endo).* The tube is inserted through the mouth and esophagus and into the stomach. The doctor makes a small incision *(stomy)* through *(per)* the skin *(cutaneous)* and into the stomach *(gastro).* A tube is inserted into the stomach through the incision (Fig. 35-6). The endoscope allows the doctor to see correct tube placement in the stomach.

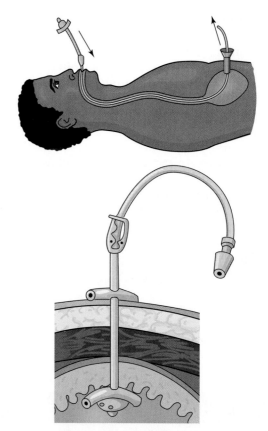

Fig. 35-6 A percutaneous endoscopic gastrostomy (PEG) tube.

• *Parenteral nutrition.* **Parenteral nutrition** is giving nutrients through a catheter inserted into a vein (Fig. 35-7). (*Para* means *beyond; enteral* relates to the *bowel*). A nutrient solution is given directly into the bloodstream. Nutrients do not enter the GI tract for absorption. Parenteral nutrition is often called *total parenteral nutrition (TPN)* or *hyperalimentation. (Hyper* means *high* or *excessive. Alimentation* means *nourishment.)* The nutrient solution contains water, proteins, carbohydrates, vitamins, and minerals. The solution drips through a catheter inserted into a large vein. This method is used when the person cannot receive oral feedings or enteral feedings. Or it is used when oral or enteral feedings are not enough to meet the person needs.

See *Delegation Guidelines: Therapy for Malnutrition.*

See *Promoting Safety and Comfort: Therapy for Malnutrition,* p. 438.

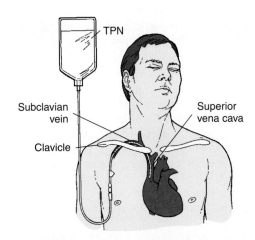

Fig. 35-7 Parenteral nutrition. (*Mosby's dictionary of medicine, nursing, and health professions,* ed 7, St Louis, 2006, Mosby.)

DELEGATION GUIDELINES
Therapy for Malnutrition

The nurse is responsible for all aspects of TPN. You assist the nurse by carefully observing the person.

You assist the nurse with tube feedings. In some states and agencies, you are allowed to give tube feedings. *Remember, you are never responsible for inserting feeding tubes or checking their placement.* This is the RN's responsibility.

Before giving tube feedings, make sure that:
• Your state allows you to perform the procedure
• The procedure is in your job description
• You have had the necessary education and training
• You know how to use the agency's equipment and supplies
• You review the procedure in the agency's procedure manual
• You review the procedure with the nurse
• A nurse is available to answer questions and to supervise you
• An RN has identified and labeled all other tubes, catheters, and needles
• An RN checks tube placement

If the above conditions are met, you need this information from the nurse, the MAR, and the care plan:
• The type of tube—NG, naso-intestinal, PEG, or jejunostomy
• What feeding method to use—syringe, feeding bag, or feeding pump
• What size syringe to use—usually 30 or 60 mL for an adult
• How to position the person for the feeding—Fowler's or semi-Fowler's
• How to position the person after the feeding and for how long—Fowler's or semi-Fowler's

• What formula to use
• How much formula to give
• How high to raise the syringe or hang the feeding bag—usually 18 inches above the stomach or intestines
• The amount of flushing solution to use—usually 30 to 60 mL (1 to 2 ounces) of water for an adult
• How fast to give the feeding if using a syringe—usually over 30 minutes
• The flow rate if a feeding bag is used (Flow rate is the number of drops per minute.)
• The flow rate if a feeding pump is used
• If ice is kept around the bag for a continuous feeding
• What observations to report and record:
  • Nausea
  • Discomfort during the feeding
  • Vomiting
  • Distended (enlarged and swollen) abdomen
  • Coughing
  • Complaints of indigestion or heartburn
  • Redness, swelling, drainage, odor, or pain at the ostomy site
  • Fever
  • Signs and symptoms of respiratory distress
  • Increased pulse rate
  • Complaints of flatulence
  • Diarrhea
• When to report observations
• What specific patient or resident concerns to report at once

PROMOTING SAFETY AND COMFORT
Therapy for Malnutrition

SAFETY

The person may have an intravenous (IV) line, a breathing tube (tracheostomy or endo-tracheal tube), and drainage tubes. You must know the purpose of each tube. Ask the nurse to label each tube to identify its purpose. Formula must enter only the feeding tube. Otherwise, the person can die.

Before giving a tube feeding always:

- Turn on the light if the room is dark. Do so even if the person is sleeping.
- Check and inspect the feeding tube and label with the nurse.
- Make sure an RN checks for tube placement.
- Make sure every tube, catheter, and needle is labeled.
- Trace the feeding tube back to the insertion site. Start at the end of the tube into which you will give the feeding. Trace the tube backward. For example, if the person has an NG tube, you will end at the nose. If the person has a gastrostomy tube, you will end at the abdomen. If you do not end at the correct place, do not give the tube feeding. Call for the nurse.

Aspiration is a major risk that can occur from tube feedings. Aspiration is breathing fluid, food, vomitus, or an object into the lungs. It can cause pneumonia and death. Aspiration can occur:

- *During insertion.* NG tubes and naso-intestinal tubes are passed through the esophagus and then into the stomach or small intestine. The tube can slip into the airway. An x-ray is taken after insertion to check tube placement.
- *From tube movement out of place.* Coughing, sneezing, vomiting, suctioning, and poor positioning are common causes. A tube can move from the stomach or intestines into the esophagus and then into the airway. The RN checks tube placement before every scheduled tube feeding. With continuous feedings, the RN checks tube placement every 4 hours. To do so, the RN attaches a syringe to the tube. Gastro-intestinal secretions are withdrawn through the syringe. Then the pH of the secretions is measured. *You are never responsible for checking feeding tube placement.*

- *From regurgitation.* Regurgitation is the backward flow of stomach contents into the mouth. Delayed stomach emptying and over-feeding are common causes.

To assist the nurse in preventing regurgitation and aspiration:

- Position the person in Fowler's or semi-Fowler's position before the feeding. Follow the care plan and the nurse's directions.
- Maintain Fowler's or semi-Fowler's position after the feeding. The position may be required for 1 to 2 hours after the feeding or at all times. The position allows formula to move through the GI tract. Follow the care plan and the nurse's directions.
- Avoid the left side-lying position. When the person lies on the left side, the stomach cannot empty into the small intestine.

Persons with NG or gastrostomy tubes are at great risk for regurgitation. The risk is less with intestinal tubes. Formula passes directly into the small intestine. Also, formula is given at a slow rate. During digestion, food slowly passes from the stomach into the small intestine. The stomach handles larger amounts of food at one time than does the small intestine.

Nasal secretions may contain blood or microbes. So can drainage at an ostomy site. Wear gloves. Follow Standard Precautions and the Bloodborne Pathogen Standard (Appendix C).

Remind visitors to call for a nurse if any tube becomes disconnected or needs to be reconnected. They could connect the wrong tubes together.

HERBAL AND DIETARY SUPPLEMENTS

Many people use herbs and dietary supplements to promote and maintain health. Hundreds of herbal medicines and dietary supplements are marketed in the United States. The vast majority of health benefit claims made for herbal and dietary supplements are not proven. See Table 35-4 for some commonly used herbs. See Table 35-5 on p. 441 for some common dietary supplements.

TABLE 35-4	Herbal Therapy			
COMMON NAME	**OTHER NAMES**	**USES**	**DOSE FORMS**	**SIDE EFFECTS**

aloe	aloe vera
	salvia
	burn plant
		Arthritis
		Colitis
		Common cold
		Ulcers
		Hemorrhoids
		Seizures
		Glaucoma
		Pain
		Inflammation
		Itching
		Sunburn
		Skin ulcers
		Psoriasis
		Frostbite
			Aloe gel:
			  Moisturizing lotion
			  Shampoo
			  Hair conditioner
			  Gels
			  Toothpaste
			  Aloe juice for topical
			    application
			  Capsules and tinc-
			    tures for oral use
			Aloe latex:
			  Juice drinks
			  Juice
				Oral forms may
				  cause diarrhea

black cohosh	squawroot black snakeroot bugbane bugwort	Pre-menstrual syndrome Menstrual cramps Menopause	Elixirs Tablets Capsules	Upset stomach is a rare side effect
echinacea	purple coneflower coneflower black sampson	Common cold Flu Urinary tract infection Wounds	Dried roots Teas Tinctures Powder	Allergic reactions can occur but are rare
feverfew	featherfoil flirtwort bachelor's buttons	Migraine headache Rheumatoid arthritis	Leaf powder for tea Tablets	Mouth ulcers Lip swelling Allergic reactions

garlic		Reduce cholesterol and
		  triglycerides
		Lower blood pressure
		Anti-platelet activity
			Cloves
			Oil
			Enteric-coated tablets
			Capsules
			Elixirs
				Taste
				Odor
				Commercial prepara-
				  tions may cause
				  nausea, vomiting,
				  and burning of the
				  mouth and stomach

ginger	African ginger Jamaica ginger race ginger	Nausea and vomiting Rheumatoid arthritis Osteoarthritis Muscle discomfort	Powdered ginger-root Tea from ginger-root	Heartburn Diarrhea Mouth and throat irritation

ginkgo	maidenhair tree	Short-term memory loss
		Headache
		Dizziness
		Tinnitus
		Emotional instability
		Anxiety
		Alzheimer's disease
		Improve walking
		  distance
		Erectile dysfunction
		Improve peripheral blood
		  flow in diabetes
		Hearing
			Liquid
			Tablets
			Capsules
				Restlessness
				Diarrhea
				Nausea
				Vomiting
				Dizziness

Continued

TABLE 35-4	Herbal Therapy—cont'd			
COMMON NAME	**OTHER NAMES**	**USES**	**DOSE FORMS**	**SIDE EFFECTS**
ginseng	aralia cinquefoil five fingers tartar root red berry	Health maintenance Stress Vitality	Teas Powders Capsules Tablets Liquids	Insomnia Diarrhea Skin eruptions
goldenseal	yellow root Indian dye Indian paint jaundice root	Canker sores Sore mouth Cracked and bleeding lips	Powder for tea Tincture Fluid extract Freeze-dried root	High doses may cause: Nausea Vomiting Diarrhea CNS stimulation
green tea	Chinese tea teagreen	CNS stimulation Increased blood pressure and heart rate Diuretic Diarrhea Lower cholesterol and triglycerides Reduce the risk of bladder, esophageal, and pancreatic cancers	Tea bags	Anxiety Nervousness Headache Diuresis Insomnia Tremors Irritability Palpitations Dysrhythmias Dependence
saw palmetto	palmetto scrub sabal American dwarf palm tree cabbage palm	Benign prostatic hyperplasia (BPH) Reduce risks from urinary retention Lessen the need for BPH surgery	Dietary supplement	Upset stomach Diarrhea
St. John's wort	klamath weed hardhay amber	Depression Heal wounds	Powder Tablets Capsules Liquid Semi-solids for topical use	Photo-sensitivity Serotonin syndrome (from taking two or more drugs that affect serotonin levels): Confusion Agitation Shivering Fever Sweating Nausea Diarrhea Muscle spasms Tremors Coma
valerian	amantilla setwall heliotrope vandal root	Restlessness Sleep	Tea Tincture Extract Tablets Capsules	Excitability Uneasiness Headache

TABLE 35-5 Dietary Supplements

COMMON NAME	OTHER NAMES	USES	DOSE FORMS	SIDE EFFECTS
coenzyme Q$_{10}$	CoQ$_{10}$ ubiquinone	Heart failure Angina Hypertension Dysrhythmias Heart valve replacement Cancers of the breast, lung, prostate, pancreas, colon Muscular dystrophy Periodontal disease AIDS	Powder-filled capsules Tablets Liquid-filled gel capsules Chewable wafers Intra-oral spray	Insomnia
creatine	creatine monohydrate	Muscle performance	Powder Candy Gum Liquid	Weight gain from water retention
lycopene		May reduce the risk of prostate cancer and possibly lung, colon, and breast cancer Lower cholesterol Protect against heart attack and stroke Cataracts Macular degeneration	Tomato powder Tomato extract	None reported
melatonin	sleep hormone MEL MLT	Jet lag Anti-aging	Tablets Liquid	Drowsiness Sedation Lethargy Agitation Insomnia
policosanal	polycosanol N-octacosanol	Lower cholesterol Inhibit platelets	Tablets	Nervousness Headache Diarrhea Insomnia Weight loss Excess urination
S-adenosylmethionine (SAM-e)	Sammy SAM ademetionine	Depression Osteoarthritis Fibromyalgia	Tablets Capsules	Mild stomach distress

REVIEW QUESTIONS

Circle the **BEST** answer.

1 Nutrition is
   a fats, proteins, carbohydrates, vitamins, and minerals
   b the many processes involved in the ingestion, digestion, absorption, and use of foods and fluids by the body
   c the MyPyramid Food Guidance System
   d the balance between calories taken in and used by the body

2 The MyPyramid Food Guidance System encourages the following *except*
   a the same diet for everyone
   b smart food choices
   c physical activity
   d small steps to improve diet and life-style

3 Vitamin A is needed for
   a vision
   b muscle tone
   c formation of red blood cells
   d healthy bones

4 Vitamin B_{12} is needed for
   a nervous system function
   b growth
   c healthy eyes
   d digestive system function

5 Vitamin K is needed for
   a blood clotting
   b resistance to infection
   c healthy bones
   d protein metabolism

6 Sodium is needed for
   a blood clotting
   b bone and teeth formation
   c thyroid gland function
   d fluid balance

7 Which is needed for nerve and heart function?
   a phosphorus
   b iron
   c iodine
   d potassium

8 Enteral nutrition
   a requires an NG tube
   b is given into a central venous site
   c is given into the GI tract
   d requires an IV

9 For a tube feeding, the person is positioned in
   a Fowler's or semi-Fowler's position
   b the left side-lying position
   c the right side-lying position
   d the supine position

10 The nurse checks feeding tube placement to prevent
   a aspiration
   b regurgitation
   c over-feeding
   d cramping

11 Which position is used to prevent regurgitation after a tube feeding?
   a Fowler's or semi-Fowler's position
   b the supine position
   c the left or right side-lying position
   d the prone position

12 A nurse asks you to give a tube feeding. The procedure is not in your job description. What should you do?
   a Refuse to perform the task.
   b Give the tube feeding.
   c Tell the director of nursing.
   d Ask another nurse what you should do.

13 Which is an oral nutritional supplement?
   a Ensure
   b aloe
   c green tea
   d St. John's wort

14 Herbs and dietary supplements have proven nutritional value.
   a True
   b False

15 Which is an herb?
   a folic acid
   b ginger
   c iodine
   d thiamin

Answers to these questions are on p. 448.

Review Question Answers

Chapter 1
The Medication Assistant

1 d
2 a
3 a
4 b
5 d
6 d
7 b
8 b
9 d
10 a
11 c
12 c
13 a
14 b
15 a
16 T
17 F
18 F
19 F
20 F

Chapter 2
Delegation

1 c
2 b
3 a
4 a
5 b
6 c
7 b
8 b
9 c
10 d

Chapter 3
Ethics and Laws

1 b
2 c

3 a
4 d
5 c
6 a
7 b
8 a
9 c
10 c
11 a
12 d
13 c
14 b
15 a
16 d
17 d
18 a
19 b
20 a
21 c
22 b
23 c
24 c

Chapter 4
Assisting With the Nursing Process

1 a
2 d
3 b
4 c
5 d
6 b
7 a
8 c
9 c
10 b
11 d
12 c
13 a
14 b

15 c
16 d
17 c
18 b
19 b
20 d
21 c
22 a
23 d
24 b
25 T
26 T
27 F
28 F
29 T
30 F

Chapter 5
Body Structure and Function

1 a
2 b
3 d
4 c
5 c
6 a
7 b
8 c
9 d
10 d
11 b
12 a
13 b
14 b
15 b
16 c
17 d
18 a
19 d
20 a
21 b

Chapter 6
Basic Pharmacology

1 a
2 c
3 b
4 a
5 c
6 d
7 b
8 d
9 d
10 d
11 d
12 a
13 d
14 a
15 c

Chapter 7
Life Span Considerations

1 b
2 a
3 a
4 d
5 a
6 a
7 a
8 b
9 c
10 a
11 d
12 a
13 d
14 a
15 b
16 d
17 b
18 c

Chapter 8
Drug Orders and
Prescriptions

1 c
2 a
3 b
4 c
5 a
6 d
7 c
8 a
9 c
10 b
11 b
12 a
13 b
14 b
15 b
16 d

17 b
18 a
19 F
20 T
21 T
22 T
23 F
24 F
25 T
26 F
27 F
28 F
29 F
30 T

Chapter 9
Medication Safety

1 b
2 c
3 b
4 a
5 d
6 a
7 c
8 a
9 b
10 a
11 b
12 c
13 a
14 d
15 a
16 a
17 d
18 a
19 b
20 a
21 a
22 b
23 a
24 b
25 b
26 a
27 c
28 b
29 c
30 d
31 F
32 F
33 F
34 T
35 T
36 T
37 T
38 T
39 F
40 T
41 F
42 F

Chapter 10
Oral, Sublingual, and Buccal
Drugs

1 c
2 a
3 d
4 b
5 c
6 d
7 c
8 c
9 d
10 a
11 c
12 d
13 a
14 c
15 d
16 b
17 F
18 F
19 T
20 F
21 T
22 T
23 F
24 T
25 F

Chapter 11
Topical Drugs

1 a
2 d
3 b
4 b
5 a
6 b
7 a
8 a
9 b
10 b
11 c
12 T
13 F
14 T
15 T
16 T
17 F
18 F

Chapter 12
Eye, Ear, Nose, and Inhaled
Drugs

1 b
2 a
3 c
4 b
5 d
6 d
7 a

8   c
9   b
10   a
11   d
12   c
13   c
14   d
15   b
16   c
17   b
18   b
19   b
20   d
21   c
22   F
23   T
24   T
25   F
26   F

Chapter 13
Vaginal and Rectal Drugs

1   d
2   d
3   a
4   a
5   d
6   b
7   a
8   b
9   b
10   a
11   a
12   T
13   T
14   T
15   F

Chapter 14
Drugs Affecting the Nervous System

1   d
2   a
3   a
4   b
5   a
6   c
7   c
8   d
9   a
10   a
11   d
12   a
13   a
14   d
15   c
16   b
17   c
18   b
19   T

20   T
21   T
22   T
23   F
24   T
25   F
26   T

Chapter 15
Drugs Used for Mental Health Disorders

1   d
2   a
3   a
4   d
5   b
6   a
7   b
8   a
9   c
10   a
11   d
12   b
13   c
14   a
15   c
16   a
17   b
18   c
19   a
20   c
21   a
22   a
23   T
24   T
25   F
26   T
27   F
28   F

Chapter 16
Drugs Used for Seizure Disorders

1   b
2   c
3   a
4   a
5   b
6   c
7   a
8   c
9   b
10   b
11   a
12   c
13   a
14   d
15   T
16   T
17   F

18   F
19   F
20   F

Chapter 17
Drugs Used to Manage Pain

1   b
2   c
3   b
4   c
5   a
6   b
7   b
8   a
9   c
10   d
11   d
12   a
13   a
14   d
15   a
16   T
17   F
18   F
19   T
20   F
21   T
22   F

Chapter 18
Drugs Used to Lower Lipids

1   d
2   b
3   a
4   c
5   c
6   b
7   a
8   b
9   b
10   c
11   a
12   b
13   T
14   T
15   F

Chapter 19
Drugs Used to Treat Hypertension

1   b
2   a
3   d
4   d
5   a
6   a
7   b
8   c
9   a
10   b
11   a

12 a
13 a
14 d
15 d
16 c
17 c
18 c
19 a
20 a
21 a
22 a
23 d
24 b
25 F
26 T
27 F
28 T

Chapter 20
Drugs Used to Treat Dysrhythmias

1 b
2 c
3 c
4 d
5 d
6 d
7 a
8 d
9 b
10 d
11 b
12 b
13 b
14 b
15 c
16 d
17 c
18 b
19 c
20 T
21 T
22 F

Chapter 21
Drugs Used to Treat Angina, Peripheral Vascular Disease, and Heart Failure

1 a
2 d
3 a
4 b
5 a
6 a
7 b
8 c
9 d
10 c

11 b
12 b
13 b
14 a
15 a
16 a
17 b
18 c
19 a
20 a
21 b
22 T
23 F
24 T
25 T
26 T
27 T
28 F
29 T
30 T

Chapter 22
Drugs Used for Diuresis

1 a
2 b
3 a
4 d
5 d
6 d
7 b
8 c
9 b
10 a
11 d
12 a

Chapter 23
Drugs Used to Treat Thrombo-Embolic Diseases

1 d
2 b
3 a
4 d
5 b
6 c
7 b
8 a
9 a
10 a
11 c
12 b
13 T
14 T
15 T
16 T
17 F
18 F
19 T
20 T

Chapter 24
Drugs Used to Treat Respiratory Diseases

1 a
2 b
3 b
4 c
5 a
6 d
7 a
8 c
9 d
10 d
11 c
12 a
13 b
14 d
15 d
16 b
17 d
18 b
19 d
20 c
21 b
22 b
23 c
24 F
25 F
26 T
27 F
28 T
29 T
30 T
31 T
32 F

Chapter 25
Drugs Used to Treat Gastro-Esophageal Reflux and Peptic Ulcer Diseases

1 d
2 d
3 a
4 a
5 a
6 a
7 a
8 d
9 c
10 a
11 a
12 c
13 a
14 d
15 a
16 b
17 a
18 c

Chapter 26
Drugs Used to Treat Nausea, Vomiting, Constipation, and Diarrhea

1 d
2 c
3 a
4 d
5 b
6 a
7 d
8 c
9 d
10 c
11 c
12 T
13 F
14 F
15 F

Chapter 27
Drugs Used to Treat Diabetes and Thyroid Diseases

1 b
2 b
3 d
4 b
5 d
6 b
7 a
8 b
9 b
10 c
11 d
12 c
13 a
14 d
15 d
16 d
17 c
18 T
19 F
20 F

Chapter 28
Corico-Steroids and Gonadal Hormones

1 d
2 c
3 d
4 d
5 a
6 b
7 c
8 a
9 a
10 a
11 d
12 a
13 b
14 c
15 F
16 T
17 T
18 T

Chapter 29
Drugs Used in Men's and Women's Health

1 a
2 c
3 d
4 b
5 d
6 b
7 a
8 d
9 b
10 b
11 c
12 F
13 F
14 T

Chapter 30
Drugs Used to Treat Urinary System Disorders

1 a
2 d
3 c
4 d
5 a
6 c
7 d
8 c
9 c
10 T
11 F
12 F

Chapter 31
Drugs Used to Treat Eye Disorders

1 a
2 b
3 b
4 a
5 b
6 b
7 c
8 c
9 a
10 a
11 c
12 a
13 c
14 d
15 d
16 d
17 a
18 d
19 F
20 T
21 T
22 T

Chapter 32
Drugs Used in the Treatment of Cancer

1 b
2 a
3 a
4 d
5 a
6 T
7 T
8 T

Chapter 33
Drugs Affecting Muscles and Joints

1 c
2 a
3 b
4 c
5 c
6 b
7 a
8 a
9 a
10 c
11 a
12 c
13 c
14 b
15 c

Chapter 34
Drugs Used to Treat
Infections

1 d
2 b
3 b
4 c
5 d
6 a
7 a
8 a
9 b
10 d
11 a
12 a
13 a
14 b
15 a
16 d
17 d
18 a
19 a
20 d
21 b
22 a
23 a
24 b
25 c
26 d
27 b
28 a
29 T
30 F
31 F
32 F
33 F
34 T

Chapter 35
Nutrition and Herbal and
Dietary Supplement Therapy

1 b
2 a
3 a
4 a
5 a
6 d
7 d
8 c
9 a
10 a
11 a
12 a
13 a
14 b
15 b

A Review of Arithmetic

APPENDIX **A**

ROMAN NUMERALS

OBJECTIVE

- Read and write selected numerical values using Roman numerals.

Roman numerals are occasionally used by the health care provider in prescribing drugs. Key symbols are as follows:

I = 1	V = 5	X = 10	L = 50
C = 100	D = 500	M = 1000	

Whenever a Roman numeral is repeated or a smaller numeral follows, the numerals are added.

EXAMPLES:

I = 1	II = 2	III = 3	VI = 6
1 + 0 = 1	1 + 1 = 2	1 + 1 + 1 = 3	5 + 1 = 6

VII = 7	XI = 11	XII = 12
5 + 1 + 1 = 7	10 + 1 = 11	10 + 1 + 1 = 12

Whenever a smaller Roman numeral appears *before* a larger Roman numeral, subtract the smaller numeral.

EXAMPLES:

IV = 4	IX = 9	XC = 90
5 − 1 = 4	10 − 1 = 9	100 − 10 = 90

Whenever a smaller Roman numeral appears between two larger Roman numerals, subtract the smaller number from the numeral following it.

EXAMPLES:

XIX = 19	XIV = 14	XCIX = 99
10 + 10 − 1 = 19	10 + 5 − 1 = 14	100 − 10 + 10 − 1 = 99

The most common Roman numerals associated with drug administration are:

ss = ½, i = 1, ii = 2, iii = 3, iv = 4, v = 5, vi = 6, vii = 7, viiss = 7½, viii = 8, ix = 9, x = 10, and xv = 15

FRACTIONS

OBJECTIVE

- Demonstrate proficiency in mathematic problems using addition, subtraction, multiplication, and division of fractions.

Fractions are one or more of the separate parts of a whole number or amount.

EXAMPLE:

$$1 - ½ = ½$$

Common Fractions

A common fraction is part of a whole number. The numerator (dividend) is the number above the line. The denominator (divisor) is the number below the line.

The line separating the numerator and denominator tells us to divide.

Numerator (names how many parts are used)

Denominator (tells how many pieces into which the whole is divided)

EXAMPLES:

The denominator represents the number of parts or pieces the whole is divided into.

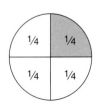

Adapted from Clayton BD, Stock YN, Harroun RD: *Basic pharmacology for nurses,* ed 14, St. Louis, 2007, Mosby.

¼ means graphically that the whole circle is divided into four (4) parts; one (1) of the parts is being used.

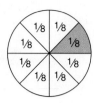

⅛ means graphically that the whole circle is divided into eight (8) parts; one (1) of the parts is being used.

From these two examples, ¼ and ⅛, you can see that the *larger* the *denominator* number, the *smaller* the *portion* is. In the example above, each section in the ⅛ circle is smaller than each section in the ¼ circle.

Common fractions are an important concept to understand when calculating drug doses. For example, the medicine ordered may be ¼ g and the drug source available is ½ g tablet. Before proceeding to do any formal calculations, you should first decide if the dose you need to give is smaller or larger than the drug source available.

EXAMPLES:

Visualize:

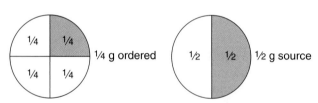

¼ g ordered   ½ g source

Decision: "Is what I need to give a larger or smaller portion than the drug available?"

Answer: ¼ g is smaller. Therefore, it would be less than one tablet.

Try a second example: ⅛ g is ordered. The drug source is ½ g.

Visualize:

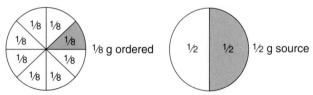

⅛ g ordered   ½ g source

Decision: "Is what I need to give a larger or smaller portion than the drug available?"

Answer: ⅛ g is smaller than the drug source. Therefore, it would be less than one tablet.

Types of Common Fractions

Common fractions are expressed in various formats:
1. *Simple:* Contains *one* numerator and *one* denominator: ¼, ¹⁄₂₀, ¹⁄₆₀, ¹⁄₁₀₀

2. *Complex:* May have a simple fraction in the numerator or denominator:

$$\frac{1}{2} \text{ over } 4 = \frac{\frac{1}{2}}{4}$$

$$\text{or}$$

$$\frac{1}{2} \div 4 =$$

$$\frac{1}{2} \div \frac{4}{1} =$$

$$\frac{1}{2} \times \frac{1}{4} = \frac{1}{8}$$

3. *Proper:* Numerator is smaller than denominator: ⅛, ⅖, ¹⁄₁₀₀

4. *Improper:* Numerator is larger than denominator: ⁴⁄₃, ⁶⁄₄, ¹⁰⁰⁄₁₀

5. *Mixed number:* A whole number and a fraction: 4⅝, 6⅔, 1⁵⁄₁₀₀

6. *Decimal:* Fractions written on the basis of a multiple of 10: 0.5 = ⁵⁄₁₀, 0.05 = ⁵⁄₁₀₀, 0.005 = ⁵⁄₁₀₀₀

7. *Equivalent:* Fractions that have the same value: ⅓ and ²⁄₆

Working With Fractions
Reducing to Lowest Terms
Divide the numerator and the denominator by a number that will divide into both evenly (a common denominator).

EXAMPLE:

$$\frac{25}{125} \div \frac{25}{25} = \frac{1}{5}$$

Finding the lowest common denominator of a series of fractions is not always easy. Remember:
- If the numerator and denominator are even numbers, 2 will work as a common denominator but it may not be the smallest one.
- If the numerator and denominator end with 0 or 5, 5 will work as a common denominator but it may not be the smallest one.
- Check to see if the numerator divides evenly into the denominator. This will be the smallest term. When all else fails, use the prime number method to find the lowest common denominator. A prime number is a whole number, greater than 1, that can be divided only by itself and 1 (2, 3, 5, 7, 11, 19, 23, etc.).

Addition
Adding Common Fractions. When denominators are the same figure, add the numerators.

EXAMPLE:

$$\frac{1}{4} + \frac{2}{4} + \frac{3}{4} = \frac{6}{4} = 1\frac{1}{2}$$

Add the following:

$$\frac{2}{6} + \frac{3}{6} + \frac{4}{6} = \frac{9}{6} = 1\frac{1}{2}$$

$$\frac{1}{100} + \frac{3}{100} + \frac{5}{100} = \frac{9}{100}$$

When the denominators are unlike, change the fractions to equivalent fractions. Do so by finding the lowest common denominator.

EXAMPLE:

$$\frac{2}{5} + \frac{3}{10} + \frac{1}{2} = \underline{\hspace{1cm}}$$

1. Determine the lowest common denominator. In this example, 10 is the lowest common denominator.
2. Divide the denominator of the fraction being changed into the common denominator. Multiply the product (answer) by the numerator.

$\dfrac{2}{5} = \dfrac{4}{10}$ Divide 5 into 10. Multiply the answer [2] by 2.

$\dfrac{3}{10} = \dfrac{3}{10}$ Divide 10 into 10. Multiply the answer [1] by 3.

$\dfrac{1}{2} = \dfrac{5}{10}$ Divide 2 into 10. Multiply the answer [5] by 1.

$\dfrac{12}{10} = 1\dfrac{1}{5}$ Add the numerators and place the total over the denominator [10]. Convert the improper fraction to a mixed number and reduce to lowest terms.

Add the following:

a. $\dfrac{2}{8} = \dfrac{}{64}$

   $+\dfrac{4}{64} = \dfrac{}{64}$

   $+\dfrac{5}{16} = \dfrac{}{64}$

      $\dfrac{}{64}$ *Answer:* $\dfrac{5}{8}$

b. $\dfrac{3}{7} = \dfrac{}{28}$

   $+\dfrac{9}{14} = \dfrac{}{28}$

   $+\dfrac{1}{28} = \dfrac{}{28}$

      $\dfrac{}{28}$ *Answer:* $1\dfrac{3}{28}$

Adding Mixed Numbers. Add the fractions first. Then add the whole numbers.

EXAMPLE:

$$2\frac{3}{4} + 2\frac{1}{2} + 3\frac{3}{8} = \underline{\hspace{1cm}}$$

1. Determine the lowest common denominator. In this example, 8 is the common denominator.

2. Divide the denominator of the fraction being changed into the common denominator. Multiply the product (answer) by the numerator.

$2\dfrac{3}{4} = 2\dfrac{6}{8}$ Divide 4 into 8. Multiply the answer [2] by 3.

$2\dfrac{1}{2} = 2\dfrac{4}{8}$ Divide 2 into 8. Multiply the answer [4] by 1.

$+3\dfrac{3}{8} = 3\dfrac{3}{8}$ Divide 8 into 8. Multiply the answer [1] by 3.

$\dfrac{13}{8}$ Add the numerators. Place the total over the denominator [8].

Convert the improper fraction $\left[\dfrac{13}{8}\right]$ to a mixed number $\left[1\dfrac{5}{8}\right]$. Add it to the whole numbers.

$$7 + \frac{13}{8} = 7 + 1\frac{5}{8} = 8\frac{5}{8}$$

Add the following:

a. $\dfrac{1}{4}$

   $+\dfrac{3}{4}$

   $\dfrac{}{4}$ *Answer:* $\dfrac{4}{4} = 1$

b. $\dfrac{1}{2} = \dfrac{}{6}$

   $+\dfrac{1}{3} = \dfrac{}{6}$

   $+\dfrac{1}{6} = \dfrac{}{6}$

   $= \dfrac{}{6}$ *Answer:* $\dfrac{6}{6} = 1$

c. $\dfrac{3}{5} = \dfrac{}{50}$

   $+\dfrac{4}{50} = \dfrac{}{50}$ *Answer:* $\dfrac{34}{50} = \dfrac{17}{25}$

   $= \dfrac{}{50}$ (Reduced to lowest term)

Subtraction

Subtracting Fractions. When the denominators are unlike, change the fractions to an equivalent fraction. Do so by finding the lowest common denominator.

EXAMPLE:

$$\frac{1}{4} - \frac{3}{16} = \underline{\hspace{1cm}}$$

1. Determine the lowest common denominator. In this example, 16 is the lowest common denominator.

2. Divide the denominator of the fraction being changed into the common denominator. Multiply the product (answer) by the numerator.

$$\frac{1}{4} = \frac{4}{16}$$ Divide 4 into 16. Multiply the answer [4] by 1.

$$-\frac{3}{16} = \frac{3}{16}$$

$$\frac{1}{16}$$ Subtract the numerators. Place the total [1] over the denominator [16].

Subtract the following:

a. $\dfrac{3}{8}$

   $-\dfrac{2}{8}$

     $\dfrac{1}{8}$ *Answer:* $\dfrac{1}{8}$

b. $\dfrac{1}{100} = \dfrac{}{300}$

   $-\dfrac{1}{150} = \dfrac{}{300}$

     $\dfrac{}{300}$ *Answer:* $\dfrac{1}{300}$

Subtracting Mixed Numbers. Subtract the fractions first. Then subtract the whole numbers.

EXAMPLE:

$$4\frac{1}{4} - 1\frac{3}{4} = \underline{\hspace{2cm}}$$

$$4\frac{1}{4} = 3\frac{5}{4}$$ You cannot subtract $\frac{3}{4}$ from $\frac{1}{4}$.

$$-1\frac{3}{4} = 1\frac{3}{4}$$ Therefore borrow 1 (which equals $\frac{4}{4}$) from the whole numbers. Then add

$$3\frac{5}{4} - 1\frac{3}{4} = 2\frac{2}{4} \quad \frac{4}{4} + \frac{1}{4} = \frac{5}{4}.$$

$$2\frac{2}{4} = 2\frac{1}{2}$$ Subtract the numerators. Place answer over the denominator (4). Reduce to lowest terms. Subtract the whole numbers.

When the denominators are unlike, change the fractions to equivalent fractions by finding the lowest common denominator.

EXAMPLE:

$$2\frac{5}{8} - 1\frac{1}{4} = \underline{\hspace{2cm}}$$

1. Determine the lowest common denominator. In this example, 8 is the common denominator.

2. Divide the denominator of the fraction being changed into the common denominator. Multiply the product (answer) by the numerator.

$$2\frac{5}{8} = 2\frac{5}{8}$$ Divide 8 into 8. Multiply the answer (1) by 5.

$$-1\frac{1}{4} = 1\frac{2}{8}$$ Divide 4 into 8. Multiply the answer (2) by 1.

$$2\frac{5}{8} - 1\frac{2}{8} = 1\frac{3}{8}$$ Subtract the numerators. Place the total (3) over the denominator (8) and reduce to lowest terms. Subtract the whole numbers.

Subtract the following:

a. $\dfrac{7}{8} = \dfrac{}{24}$

   $-\dfrac{3}{6} = \dfrac{}{24}$

     $\dfrac{}{24}$ *Answer:* $\dfrac{9}{24} = \dfrac{3}{8}$

b. $6\dfrac{7}{8} = \dfrac{}{16}$

   $-3\dfrac{1}{16} = \dfrac{}{16}$

     $\dfrac{}{16}$ *Answer:* $3\dfrac{13}{16}$

Multiplication
Multiplying a Whole Number by a Fraction

EXAMPLE:

$$3 \times \frac{5}{8} = \underline{\hspace{2cm}}$$

1. Place the whole number over 1 ($\frac{3}{1}$).
2. Multiply the numerators (top numbers) and denominators (bottom numbers).

$$\frac{3}{1} \times \frac{5}{8} = \frac{15}{8}$$

3. Change the improper fraction to a mixed number.

$$\frac{15}{8} = 1\frac{7}{8}$$

Multiply the following:

a. $2 \times \dfrac{3}{4} = \underline{\hspace{1.5cm}}$ *Answer:* $\dfrac{3}{2} = 1\dfrac{1}{2}$

b. $15 \times \dfrac{3}{5} = \underline{\hspace{1.5cm}}$ *Answer:* $\dfrac{9}{1} = 9$

Multiplying Two Fractions

EXAMPLE:

$$\frac{1}{4} \times \frac{2}{3} = \underline{\hspace{1cm}}$$

1. Use cancellation to speed the process.

$$\frac{1}{\overset{}{\underset{2}{\cancel{4}}}} \times \frac{\overset{1}{\cancel{2}}}{3} = \frac{1}{6}$$

2. Multiply the numerators and denominators.

$$\frac{1}{2} \times \frac{1}{3} = \frac{1}{6}$$

Multiplying Mixed Numbers

EXAMPLE:

$$3\frac{1}{2} \times 2\frac{1}{5} = \underline{\hspace{1cm}}$$

1. Change the mixed numbers (a whole number and a fraction) to an improper fraction (numerator is larger than denominator).

$$3\frac{1}{2} \times 2\frac{1}{5} = \underline{\hspace{1cm}}$$

Multiply the denominator times the whole number and add the numerator.

$$\frac{7}{2} \times \frac{11}{5} = \underline{\hspace{1cm}}$$

2. Multiply the numerators and denominators.

$$\frac{7}{2} \times \frac{11}{5} = \frac{77}{10}$$

3. Change the product (answer), an improper fraction, to a mixed number. Divide the denominator into the numerator and reduce to lowest terms.

$$\frac{7}{2} \times \frac{11}{5} = \frac{77}{10} = 7\frac{7}{10}$$

Multiply the following:

a. $1\frac{2}{3} \times \frac{3}{6} = \underline{\hspace{1cm}}$ *Answer:* $\frac{5}{6}$

b. $1\frac{7}{8} \times 1\frac{1}{4} = \underline{\hspace{1cm}}$ *Answer:* $\frac{75}{32} = 2\frac{11}{32}$

Division

Dividing Fractions

EXAMPLE:

$$4 \div \frac{1}{2} = \underline{\hspace{1cm}}$$

1. Change the division sign to a multiplication sign.
2. Invert the divisor (the number after the division sign).
3. Reduce the fractions using cancellation.

4. Multiply the numerators and denominators.

$$4 \div \frac{1}{2} = \frac{4}{1} \times \frac{2}{1} = \frac{8}{1} = 8$$

Dividing with a Mixed Number

1. Change the mixed number to an improper fraction.
2. Change the division sign to a multiplication sign.
3. Invert the divisor.
4. Reduce whenever possible.

EXAMPLES:

$$4\frac{1}{2} \div \frac{3}{4} = \frac{9}{2} \div \frac{3}{4} = \frac{\overset{3}{\cancel{9}}}{\underset{1}{\cancel{2}}} \times \frac{\overset{2}{\cancel{4}}}{\underset{1}{\cancel{3}}} = \frac{6}{1} \text{ or } 6$$

$$6\frac{1}{4} \div 1\frac{1}{4} = \frac{25}{4} \div \frac{5}{4} = \frac{\overset{5}{\cancel{25}}}{\underset{1}{\cancel{4}}} \times \frac{\overset{1}{\cancel{4}}}{\underset{1}{\cancel{5}}} = \frac{5}{1} \text{ or } 5$$

Fractions as Decimals

Fractions can be changed to a decimal form by dividing the numerator by the denominator.

EXAMPLE:

$$\frac{1}{2} = 2\overline{)1.0}^{\,0.5}$$

Change the following fractions to decimals:

$\frac{1}{100} = \underline{\hspace{1cm}}$ *Answer:* 0.01

$\frac{5}{8} = \underline{\hspace{1cm}}$ *Answer:* 0.625

$\frac{1}{2} = \underline{\hspace{1cm}}$ *Answer:* 0.5

Using Cancellation to Speed Your Work

1. Determine a number that will divide evenly into both the numerator and denominator.
2. Continue the process of dividing both the numerator and denominator by the same number until all numbers are reduced to the lowest terms.
3. Complete the multiplication of the problem.

EXAMPLE:

$$\frac{\overset{1}{\cancel{5}}}{\underset{2}{\cancel{6}}} \times \frac{\overset{3}{\cancel{9}}}{\underset{2}{\cancel{10}}} = \underline{\hspace{1cm}}$$

$$\frac{1}{2} \times \frac{3}{2} = \frac{3}{4}$$

4. Complete the division of the problem.

EXAMPLE:

$$\frac{6}{9} \div \frac{5}{8} = \underline{\hspace{1cm}}$$

Change the division sign to a multiplication sign and invert the number after the division sign. Reduce and complete the multiplication of the problem.

$$\frac{2}{3} \times \frac{8}{5} = \frac{16}{15} = 1\frac{1}{15}$$

DECIMAL FRACTIONS

OBJECTIVES

- Calculate problems using addition, subtraction, multiplication, and division of decimals.
- Convert decimals to fractions and fractions to decimals.

When fractions are written to decimal form, the denominators are not written. Decimal means "10."

When reading decimals, the numbers to the left of the decimal point are whole numbers. It helps to think of them as whole dollars. Numbers to the right of the decimal are fractions of the whole number. Think of them as "cents."

EXAMPLES:

    1.0 = one
    11.0 = eleven
    111.0 = one hundred eleven
    1111.0 = one thousand one hundred eleven

Numbers to the right of the decimal point are read as follows:

EXAMPLES:

Decimal(s):	Fraction(s):
0.1 = one tenth	1/10
0.01 = one hundredth	1/100
0.465 = four hundred sixty-five thousandths	465/1000
0.0007 = seven ten thousandths	7/10,000

Here is another way to view reading decimals:

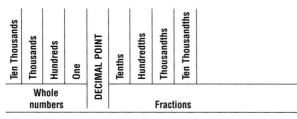

Ten Thousands	Thousands	Hundreds	One	DECIMAL POINT	Tenths	Hundredths	Thousandths	Ten Thousandths
	Whole numbers					Fractions		

			.	1	equals one-tenth (1/10)
			.	2 2	equals twenty-two hundredths (22/100)
			.	1 1 2	equals one hundred twelve thousandths (112/1000)
			.	0 1 1 2	equals one hundred twelve ten thousandths (112/10,000)

1 .	equals number one
1 0 .	equals number ten
1 0 0 .	equals number one hundred
1 0 0 0 .	equals number one thousand

On prescriptions another way of expressing the decimal is by using a slanted line.

EXAMPLES:

1 mg	= 0.001 g	= 0/001 g
0.1 mg	= 0.0001g	= 0/0001 g
30 mg	= 0.030 g	= 0/030 g
100 mg	= 0.100 g	= 0/100 g
1000 mg	= 1.000 g	= 1 g

Note: Often the decimal point is not recognized and very large doses have been accidentally administered. *The rule is: Do not use trailing 0s to the right of decimal points.*

$$250 \text{ mg} = 0.250 \text{ g} = 0/250 \text{ g}$$

Multiplying Decimals

Multiplying Whole Numbers and Decimals

1. The multiplicand is the top number.
2. The multiplier is the bottom number with the × (multiplication sign) before it.
3. Count as many places in the answer, starting from the right, as there are places in the decimal involved in the multiplication.

EXAMPLES:

```
    500            1000           1000
  × 0.02         × 0.04         × 0.009
  10.00 (10)     40.00 (40)     9.000 (9)

                   7.25           500
                 ×    4         × 0.009
                 29.00 (29)     4.500 (or 4.5)
```

Multiplying a Decimal by a Decimal

1. Multiply the problem as if the numbers were both whole numbers.
2. Count decimal places in the answer, starting from the right, as many decimal places as there are in both of the numbers that were multiplied.

EXAMPLE:

```
    3.75
  ×  0.5
  1.875
```

There are two decimal places in 3.75 and one decimal place in 0.5, making three decimal places. Count three decimal places from the right.

Multiplying Numbers With Zero

EXAMPLES:

1. Multiply 223 by 40.
   a. Multiply 223 by 0. Write the answer, 0, in the unit column of the answer.
   b. Then multiply 223 by 4. Write this answer in front of the 0 in the product.

```
     223
   ×  40
     000
     892
    8920
```

2. Multiply 124 by 304.
   a. First multiply 124 by 4. The answer is 496.
   b. Now multiply 124 by 0. Write the answer, 0, under the 9 in 496.
   c. Multiply 124 by 3. Write this answer in front of the 0 in the product.

$$
\begin{array}{r}
124 \\
\times\ 304 \\
\hline
496 \\
000 \\
372 \\
\hline
37{,}696
\end{array}
$$

Dividing Decimals

1. If the divisor (number by which you divide) is a decimal, make it a whole number. Do so by moving the decimal point to the right of the last number.
2. Move the decimal point in the dividend (the number inside the bracket) as many places to the right as you move the decimal point in the divisor.
3. Place the decimal point for the quotient (answer) directly above the new decimal point of the dividend and divide dividend by the divisor.

EXAMPLES:

$$0.25\overline{)10} = 25\overline{)1000.}\ \ \ \ 0.3\overline{)99.3} = 3\overline{)993.}$$

$$0.4\overline{)1.68} = 4\overline{)16.8}$$

Changing Decimals to Common Fractions

1. Remove the decimal point.
2. Place the appropriate denominator under the number.
3. Reduce to lowest terms.

EXAMPLES:

$$0.2 = \frac{2}{10} = \frac{1}{5} \qquad 0.2 = \frac{20}{100} = \frac{1}{5}$$

Changing Common Fractions to Decimal Fractions

Divide the numerator of the fraction by the denominator.

EXAMPLE:

$$\frac{1}{4} \text{ means } 1 \div 4 \text{ or } 4\overline{)1.00}\ \ (0.25)$$

PERCENTS

OBJECTIVES

- Calculate problems using percentages.
- Convert percents to fractions, percents to decimals, decimal fractions to percents, and common fractions to percents.

Determining the Percent of One Number Relative to Another

1. Divide the smaller number by the larger number.
2. Multiply the quotient by 100. Add the percent sign.

EXAMPLE:

A certain 1000-part solution is 10 parts drug. What percent of the solution is drug?

$$1000\overline{)10.00}\ \ (0.01)$$

$$0.01 \times 100 = 1.\text{ or }1\%$$

Changing Percents to Fractions

1. Omit the percent sign to form the numerator.
2. Use 100 for the denominator.
3. Reduce the fraction.

EXAMPLES:

$$5\% = \frac{5}{100} = \frac{1}{20} \qquad 75\% = \frac{75}{100} = \frac{3}{4}$$

Changing Percents to Decimal Fractions

1. Omit the percent signs.
2. Insert a decimal point *two places to the left* of the last number; or express decimally as hundredths.

EXAMPLES:
$$5\% = 0.05 \qquad 15\% = 0.15$$

Numbers that are already expressed in hundredths, such as 10%, 15%, 25%, 50%, merely need to have the decimal point placed in front of the first numbers. That is because they are already expressed in hundredths. Whereas 1%, 2%, 4%, 5% needed to have a zero placed in front of the number to express them as hundredths.

If the percent is a mixed number, it should have the fraction expressed as a decimal. Then change the percent to a decimal. Do so by moving the decimal point two places to the left.

EXAMPLES:

$$12\frac{1}{2}\% = 12.5\% \text{ or } 0.125 \qquad \frac{1}{4}\% = 0.25\% \text{ or } 0.0025$$

Changing Common Fractions to Percents

1. Divide the numerator by the denominator.
2. Multiply the quotient by 100. Then add the percent sign.

   EXAMPLE:

   $$\frac{1}{50} = 50\overline{)1.00}^{\,0.02} = 0.02 \times 100 = 2\%$$

   Change the following:

   $\frac{1}{400} = $ ____   Answer = 0.25%

   $\frac{1}{8} = $ ____   Answer = 12.5%

Changing Decimal Fractions to Percents

1. Move the decimal point two places to the right.
2. Omit the decimal point if a whole numbers results.
3. Add the percent signs. This is the same as multiplying the decimal fraction by 100 and adding the percent sign.

   EXAMPLE:

   $0.01 = 1.00 = 1\%$ (or $\frac{1}{100}$)

Points to Remember in Reading Decimals

1. 1. is the whole number 1. When it is written 1.0, it is still one or 1.
2. The whole number is usually written like this: 1 or 2 or 3 or 4, and so on. Remember, do not use trailing 0s.
3. Can you read 0.1? This is one tenth. There is one number after the decimal point.
4. Can you read .1? This is also one tenth. The zero in front of the decimal point does not change its value. One tenth can be written in two ways: 0.1 and .1. The leading 0 to the left of the decimal should be used to help prevent errors.

SYSTEMS OF WEIGHTS AND MEASURES

OBJECTIVES

- Know the basic equivalents of the household and metric systems.

- Convert drug problems using the household and metric systems.

Two systems of measurement are used during the calculation, preparation, and administration of medicines: Household and Metric

Household Measurements

Household measurements are often the way drugs are given at home. However, they are the least accurate. Household measurements include drops, teaspoons, tablespoons, teacups, cups, glasses, pints, quarts, and gallons. The first three measurements—drops, teaspoons, and tablespoons—are used for drugs depending on the amount prescribed.

COMMON HOUSEHOLD EQUIVALENTS

1 quart = 4 cups
1 pint = 2 cups
1 cup = 8 ounces
1 teacup = 6 ounces
1 tablespoon = 3 teaspoons
1 teaspoon = approximately 5 mL

The metric system uses the **meter** as the standard unit of length. The **liter** is the standard unit of volume. The **gram** is the standard unit of weight.

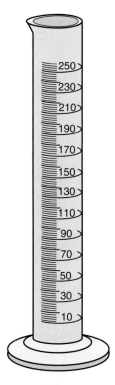

UNITS OF LENGTH (METER)

1 millimeter = 0.001	meaning 1/1000
1 centimeter = 0.01	meaning 1/100
1 decimeter = 0.1	meaning 1/10
1 meter = 1	meter

UNITS OF VOLUME (LITER)

1 milliliter = 0.001	meaning 1/1000
1 centiliter = 0.01	meaning 1/100
1 deciliter = 0.1	meaning 1/10
1 liter = 1	liter

UNITS OF WEIGHT (GRAM)

1 microgram = 0.000001	meaning 1/1,000,000
1 milligram = 0.001	meaning 1/1000
1 centigram = 0.01	meaning 1/100
1 decigram = 0.1	meaning 1/10
1 gram = 1	gram

Other Prefixes

Deca means ten or 10 times as much. *Hecto* means one hundred or 100 times as much. *Kilo* means one thousand or 1000 times as much. These three prefixes can be combined with the words *meter, gram, or liter.*

EXAMPLES:
   1 decaliter = 10 liters
   1 hectometer = 100 meters
   1 kilogram = 1000 grams

Arabic numbers are used to write metric doses.

EXAMPLES:

500 milligrams, 5 grams, 15 milliliters

Prefixes added to the units (meter, liter, or gram) indicate smaller or larger units. All units are derived by dividing or multiplying by 10, 100, or 1000.

COMMON METRIC EQUIVALENTS

1000 milliliters (mL)	= 1 liter (L)
1000 milligrams (mg)	= 1 gram (g)
1000 micrograms (mcg)	= 1 milligram (mg)
1,000,000 micrograms (mcg)	= 1 gram (g)
1000 grams (g)	= 1 kilogram (kg)

Differentiate among metric weight and metric volume. Mark each of the following MW for metric weight or MV for metric volume.

1. microgram = _____   Answer: MW
2. liter = _____   Answer: MV
3. gram = _____   Answer: MW

Conversion of Metric Units

The first step in calculating the drug dosage is to make sure that the drug ordered and the drug source on hand are *both* in the same *system of measurement* (preferably in the metric system) and in the *same unit of weight* (for example, both **milligrams** or **grams**).

Converting Milligrams to Grams
(1000 mg = 1 g)

Divide the number of milligrams by 1000 or move the decimal point of the milligrams three places to the left.

EXAMPLES:
   200 mg = 0.2 g
   0.6 mg = 0.0006 g

In the following example, both the doctor's order and the drug available are in the metric system. They are *not* both in the *same unit of weight* within the metric system.

EXAMPLE:

The doctor orders 0.25 g of a drug. The label on the drug bottle says 250 mg. This means that each capsule contains 250 mg of the drug.

To change the gram dose into milligrams, multiply 0.25 by 1000. Move the decimal point three places to the right (a milligram is one thousandth of a gram). 0.250 g = 250 mg. You would give one tablet of this drug.

TRY THIS ONE: The doctor orders 0.1 g of a drug. The bottle label states that the strength of the drug is 100 mg/capsule.

To change the gram dose into milligrams, move the decimal point three places to the right: 0.1 g = 100 mg. That is exactly what the bottle label strength states.

Solid Dosage for Oral Administration

If the dosage on hand and dosage ordered are both in the same system and in the same unit of weight, calculate the dosage using one of these methods.

EXAMPLE:

The doctor orders 1 g of ampicillin. The ampicillin bottle states that each tablet in the bottle contains 0.5 g.

PROBLEM:

You do not have the 1 g as ordered. How many tablets will you give? Notice that the amount ordered and the amount available are in the same system of measurement (metric) and the same unit of weight (grams).

SOLUTION:

$$\frac{Dose\ desired}{Dose\ on\ hand} = \frac{1\ g}{0.5\ g} = 2$$

You will give two 0.5 g capsules for the 1.0 g ordered.

The dosage on hand and dosage ordered are both in the same system of measurement, but they are *not* in the same unit of weight within the system. The units of weight must first be converted.

EXAMPLE:

The doctor orders 1000 milligrams (metric) of ampicillin. On hand: 0.25 gram (metric) per tablet.

Rule: Converting grams (metric) to milligrams (metric) (1 g = 1000 mg)

Multiply the number of grams by 1000. Move the decimal point of the grams three places to the right. 0.25 g = 250 mg

SOLUTION:

$$\frac{Dose\ desired}{Dose\ on\ hand} = \frac{1000\ mg}{250\ mg} = 4 \quad \text{Give four 0.25 g tablets.}$$

Conversion Problems

Some students understand problems in tablet or capsule dosage for oral administration if presented with their fractional equivalents as follows:

1. The doctor orders 2 g of a drug in oral tablet form. The medicine bottle label states that the strength on hand is 0.5 g. This means each tablet in the bottle is the strength 0.5 g.

   How many tablets should you give? 1, 2, 3, 4, or 5?
   Answer: 4

   What strength is ordered? 2 g

   What strength is on the bottle label? 0.5 g

   What is the fractional equivalent of 0.5 g? ½ g

   How many ½ g (0.5 g) tablets would equal 2 g? 4

   $$2 \div \frac{1}{2} = \frac{2}{1} \times \frac{2}{1} = 4 \text{ tablets}$$

2. The doctor orders 0.2 mg of a drug in oral tablet form. The medicine bottle label states that the strength on hand is 0.1 mg. This means each tablet in the bottle is the strength 0.1 mg.

   How many tablets should you give? 1, 2, 3, or 4?
   Answer: 2 tablets

   What strength is ordered? 0.2 mg

   What is the fractional equivalent of 0.2 mg? ²⁄₁₀

   What strength is on the bottle label? 0.1 mg

   What is the fractional equivalent of 0.1 mg? ¹⁄₁₀

   How many ¹⁄₁₀ mg (0.1 mg) tablets would equal ²⁄₁₀ mg (0.2 mg)? 2

   $$\begin{array}{l} 0.1 \text{ mg} = \text{¹⁄₁₀ mg or 1 tablet} \\ +0.1 \text{ mg} = \text{¹⁄₁₀ mg or 1 tablet} \\ \hline 0.2 \text{ mg} = \text{²⁄₁₀ mg or 2 tablets} \end{array}$$

   Dosage desired ÷ dosage on hand =

   $$or \ \frac{2}{10} \div \frac{1}{10} = \frac{2}{\overset{}{\underset{1}{10}}} \times \frac{\overset{1}{10}}{1} = 2 \text{ tablets}$$

3. The doctor orders 0.5 mg of a drug in oral capsule form. The medicine bottle label states that the strength on hand is 0.25 mg. This means each capsule in the bottle is the strength 0.25 mg.

   How many tablets should you give? 1, 2, 3, 4, or 5?
   Answer: 2 tablets

   What strength is ordered? 0.5 mg

   What fractional equivalent equals 0.5 mg? ½ mg

   What strength is on the bottle label? 0.25 mg

   What fractional equivalent equals the strength on hand? ¼ mg

   How many ¼ mg (0.25 mg) tablets would equal ½ mg (0.5 mg)? 2

   $$\begin{array}{l} 0.25 \text{ mg} = \text{¼ mg or 1 tablet} \\ +0.25 \text{ mg} = \text{¼ mg or 1 tablet} \\ \hline 0.50 \text{ mg} = \text{½ mg or 2 tablets} \end{array}$$

Dosage desired ÷ dosage on hand =

$$or \ \frac{1}{2} \div \frac{1}{4} = \frac{1}{2} \times \frac{4}{1} = 2 \text{ tablets}$$

4. The doctor orders 0.25 mg of a drug in oral capsule form. The medicine bottle label states that the strength on hand is 0.5 mg. This means that every capsule in the bottle is the strength 0.5 mg.

   How many tablets should you give? ½, 1, 1½, 2, 2½, 3, 4, or 5? *Answer:* ½ tablet

   What strength did the doctor order? 0.25 mg

   What is the fractional equivalent of the strength the ordered? ¼ mg

   What strength is on the bottle label? 0.5 mg

   What is the fractional equivalent of the strength on the bottle label? ½ mg

   Which is less: 0.5 mg (½ mg) or 0.25 mg (¼ mg)?
   Answer: 0.25 mg (¼ mg)

   Was the amount ordered less than the strength on hand or more? *Answer:* Less

   $$0.5 \text{ mg} = \frac{1}{2} \text{ mg or 1 tablet}$$

   $$0.25 \text{ mg} = \frac{1}{4} \text{ mg or half as much or } \frac{1}{2} \text{ tablet}$$

   $$or \ \frac{1}{4} \div \frac{1}{2} = \frac{1}{4} \times \frac{2}{1} = \frac{1}{2} \text{ tablet}$$

   Note: If the drug is available in 0.25 mg tablets, request this size from the pharmacy. A tablet should be divided only when scored. Even then, the practice is not advised because the tablet often fragments into unequal pieces.

ARITHMETIC EXERCISES— ON YOUR OWN

Roman Numerals

Express the following numbers in Roman numerals.

1. 3 _____
2. 20 _____
3. 101 _____
4. 9 _____
5. 18 _____
6. 499 _____
7. 10 _____
8. 49 _____
9. 1979 _____

Express the following Roman numerals in Arabic numbers.

10. iv _____
11. xxxix _____
12. xix _____
13. vi _____
14. ix _____
15. xv _____

Working with Fractions

Reduce the following fractions to lowest terms.

16. 5/100 = _____
17. 3/21 = _____
18. 6/36 = _____
19. 12/44 = _____
20. 2/4 = _____

Changing Decimals to Common Fractions

Convert the following decimals to common fractions.

21. 0.3 = _____
22. 0.25 = _____
23. 0.4 = _____
24. 0.50 = _____
25. 0.5 = _____
26. 0.75 = _____
27. 0.05 = _____
28. 0.002 = _____

Changing Common Fractions to Decimal Fractions

Convert the following common fractions to decimal fractions.

29. ½ = _____
30. ¾ = _____
31. 1/6 = _____
32. 1/50 = _____
33. 2/3 = _____

Changing Percents to Fractions

Convert the following percentages to fractions.

34. 25% = 25/100 = _____
35. 2% = 2/100 = _____
36. 15% = 15/100 = _____
37. 12 1/2% = 12.5/100 = _____
38. 10% = 10/100 = _____
39. ¼% = 1/4/100 = _____
40. 20% = 20/100 = _____
41. 150% = 150/100 = _____
42. 50% = 50/100 = _____
43. 4% = 4/100 = _____

Changing Percents to Decimal Fractions

Convert the following percents to decimal fractions.

44. 4% = _____
45. 25% = _____
46. 1% = _____
47. 50% = _____
48. 2% = _____
49. 10% = _____

Changing Decimal Fractions to Percents

Convert the following decimal fractions to percentages.

50. 0.05 = _____
51. 0.25 = _____
52. 0.15 = _____
53. 0.125 = _____
54. 0.0025 = _____

Converting Milligrams to Grams

Convert the following milligrams (mg) to grams (g).

55. 0.4 mg = _____g
56. 0.12 mg = _____g
57. 0.2 mg = _____g
58. 0.1 mg = _____g
59. 500 mg = _____g
60. 125 mg = _____g
61. 100 mg = _____g
62. 200 mg = _____g
63. 50 mg = _____g
64. 400 mg = _____g

Convert the following grams (g) to milligrams (mg)

65. 0.2 g = _____mg
66. 0.250 g = _____mg
67. 0.125 g = _____mg
68. 0.006 g = _____mg
69. 0.004 g = _____mg
70. 2.5 g = _____mg

Answers:

1. III 2. XX 3. CI 4. IX 5. XVIII 6. ID
7. X 8. IL 9. MXMCXXIX 10. 4 11. 39
12. 19 13. 6 14. 9 15. 15 16. 1/20
17. 1/7 18. 1/6 19. 3/11 20. ½ 21. 3/10
22. ¼ 23. 2/5 24. ½ 25. ½ 26. ¾
27. 1/20 28. 1/500 29. 0.5 30. 0.75
31. 0.1666 32. 0.02 33. 0.66 34. ¼ 35. 1/50
36. 3/20 37. 1/8 38. 1/10 39. 1/400 40. 1/5
41. 3/2 or 1 1/2 42. ½ 43. 1/25 44. 0.04
45. 0.25 46. 0.01 47. 0.5 48. 0.02 49. 0.1
50. 5% 51. 25% 52. 15% 53. 12.5%
54. 0.25% 55. 0.0004 g 56. 0.00012 g
57. 0.0002 g 58. 0.0001 g 59. 0.5 g 60. 0.125 g
61. 0.1 g 62. 0.2 g 63. 0.05 g 64. 0.4 g
65. 200 mg 66. 250 mg 67. 125 mg 68. 0.6 g
69. 4 mg 70. 2500 mg

Transmission-Based Precautions

CONTACT PRECAUTIONS

- Used for persons with known or suspected infections or conditions that increase the risk of contact transmission.
- Patient or resident placement:
  - A single room is preferred.
  - Do the following if a room is shared with another person who is not infected with the same agent:
    - Keep the privacy curtain between the beds closed.
    - Change personal protective equipment (PPE) and perform hand hygiene between contact with persons in the same room. Do so regardless of whether one or both persons are on Contact Precautions.
- Gloves:
  - Don gloves upon entering the person's room or care setting.
  - Wear gloves whenever touching the person's intact skin.
  - Wear gloves whenever touching surfaces or items near the person.
- Gowns:
  - Wear a gown whenever clothing may have direct contact with the person.
  - Wear a gown whenever contact is likely with surfaces or equipment near the person.
  - Don the gown upon entering the person's room or care setting.

Modified from Siegel JD, Rhinehart E, Jackson M, Chiarello L, and the Healthcare Infection Control Practices Advisory Committee: *Guideline for Isolation Precautions: Preventing Transmission of Infectious Agents in Healthcare Settings 2007,* Centers for Disease Control and Prevention, June 2007.

- Remove the gown and perform hand hygiene before leaving the person's room or care setting.
- After removing the gown, make sure your clothing and skin do not touch potentially contaminated surfaces.
- Patient or resident transport:
  - Limit transport and movement of the person outside of the room to medically necessary purposes.
  - Cover the area of the person's body that is infected.
  - Remove and discard contaminated PPE and perform hand hygiene before transporting the person.
  - Don clean PPE to handle the person at the transport destination.
- Care equipment:
  - Follow Standard Precautions.
  - Use disposable equipment when possible. If possible, leave non-disposable equipment in the person's room.
  - Clean and disinfect non-disposable and multiple-use equipment before use on another person.
  - For home care settings:
    - Limit the amount of non-disposable care items brought into the home. Leave them in the home as long as they are needed.
    - Clean and disinfect items that cannot be left in the home. Stethoscopes and blood pressure cuffs are examples. Clean and disinfect care items before taking them from the home. Or place them in a plastic bag for transport for later cleaning and disinfection.

DROPLET PRECAUTIONS

- Used for persons known or suspected to be infected with pathogens transmitted by respiratory droplets. Such droplets are generated by a person who is coughing, sneezing, or talking.

- Patient or resident placement:
  - A single room is preferred.
  - Do the following if a room is shared with another person who is not infected with the same agent:
    - Keep the privacy curtain between the beds closed.
    - Change PPE and perform hand hygiene between contact with persons in the same room. Do so regardless of whether one or both persons are on Droplet Precautions.
- Personal protective equipment:
  - Don a mask upon entering the person's room or care setting.
- Patient or resident transport:
  - Limit transport and movement of the person outside of the room to medically necessary purposes.
  - Have the person wear a mask.
  - Instruct the person to follow Respiratory Hygiene/Cough Etiquette (see "Standard Precautions" in Chapter 9).
  - No mask is required for health team members transporting the person.

AIRBORNE PRECAUTIONS

- Used for persons known or suspected to be infected with pathogens transmitted by person-to-person by the airborne route. Tuberculosis, measles, chickenpox, smallpox, and severe acute respiratory syndrome (SARS) are examples.

- The patient or resident is placed in an airborne infection isolation room (AIIR). If one is not available, the person is transferred to an agency with an AIIR.
- Health team members susceptible to the infection are restricted from entering the room. This is if immune staff members are available.
- Personal protective equipment:
  - An approved respirator is worn upon entering the room or home of a person with tuberculosis.
  - Respiratory protection is recommended for all health team members when caring for persons with smallpox.
- Patient or resident transport:
  - Limit transport and movement of the person outside of the room to medically necessary purposes.
  - Have the person wear a surgical mask.
  - Instruct the person to follow Respiratory Hygiene/Cough Etiquette (see "Standard Precautions").
  - Cover skin lesions infected with the microbe.
  - No mask or respirator is required for health team members transporting the person if:
    - The person is wearing a mask or respirator
    - Skin lesions are covered

Bloodborne Pathogen Standard

The human immunodeficiency virus (HIV) and the hepatitis B virus (HBV) are major health concerns. The health team is at risk for exposure to these viruses. The Bloodborne Pathogen Standard is intended to protect them from exposure. It is a regulation of the Occupational Safety and Health Administration (OSHA).

HIV and HBV are found in the blood. They are bloodborne pathogens. They exit the body through blood. They are spread to others by blood. Other potentially infectious materials (OPIM) also spread the viruses:

- Human body fluids—semen, vaginal secretions, cerebrospinal fluid, synovial fluid, pleural fluid, pericardial fluid, peritoneal fluid, amniotic fluid, saliva in dental procedures, any body fluid that is visibly contaminated with blood, and all body fluids when it is difficult or impossible to differentiate between them
- Any tissue or organ (other than intact skin) from a human (living or dead)
- HIV-containing cell or tissue cultures, organ cultures, and HIV- or HBV-containing culture medium or other solutions; blood, organs, or other tissues from experimental animals infected with HIV or HBV

EXPOSURE CONTROL PLAN

The agency must have an exposure control plan. It identifies staff at risk for exposure to blood or OPIM. All caregivers and the laundry, central supply, and housekeeping staffs are at risk. The plan includes actions to take for an exposure incident.

Staff at risk receive free training. Training occurs upon employment and yearly. Training is also required for new or changed tasks involving exposure to bloodborne pathogens. Training must include:

- An explanation of the standard and where to get a copy
- The causes, signs, and symptoms of bloodborne diseases
- How bloodborne pathogens are spread
- An explanation of the exposure control plan and where to get a copy
- How to know which tasks might cause exposure
- The use and limits of safe work practices, engineering controls, and personal protective equipment
- Information about the hepatitis B vaccination
- Who to contact and what to do in an emergency
- Information on reporting an exposure incident, post-exposure evaluation, and follow-up
- Information on warning labels and color-coding

PREVENTIVE MEASURES

Preventive measures reduce the risk of exposure. Such measures follow.

Hepatitis B Vaccination

Hepatitis B is a liver disease. It is caused by the hepatitis B virus (HBV). HBV is spread by blood and sexual contact.

The hepatitis B vaccine produces immunity against hepatitis B. *Immunity* means protection against a certain disease. He or she will not get the disease.

A *vaccination* involves giving a vaccine to produce immunity against an infectious disease. A *vaccine* is a preparation containing dead or weakened microbes. The hepatitis B vaccination involves 3 injections. The second injection is given 1 month after the first. The third injection is given 6 months after the second one. The vaccination can be given before or after exposure to HBV.

You can receive the hepatitis B vaccination within 10 working days of being hired. The agency pays for it. You can refuse the vaccination. If so, you must sign a statement refusing the vaccine. You can have the vaccination at a later date.

Engineering and Work Practice Controls

Engineering controls reduce employee exposure in the workplace. Special containers for contaminated sharps (needles, broken glass) and specimens remove and isolate the hazard from staff. Containers are puncture-resistant, leak-proof, and color-coded in red. They have the *BIOHAZARD* symbol.

Work practice controls also reduce exposure risks. All tasks involving blood or OPIM are done in ways to limit splatters, splashes, and sprays. Producing droplets also is avoided. OSHA requires these work practice controls:

- Do not eat, drink, smoke, apply cosmetics or lip balm, or handle contact lenses in areas of occupational exposure.
- Do not store food or drinks where blood or OPIM are kept.
- Practice hand hygiene after removing gloves.
- Wash hands as soon as possible after skin contact with blood or OPIM.
- Never recap, bend, or remove needles by hand. When recapping, bending, or removing contaminated needles is required, use mechanical means (forceps) or a one-handed method.
- Never shear or break contaminated needles.
- Discard contaminated needles and sharp instruments (such as razors) in containers that are closable, puncture-resistant, and leak-proof. Containers are color-coded in red and have the *BIOHAZARD* symbol. Containers must be upright and not allowed to over-fill.

Personal Protective Equipment (PPE)

This includes gloves, goggles, face shields, masks, laboratory coats, gowns, shoe covers, and surgical caps. Blood or OPIM must not pass through them. They protect your clothes, undergarments, skin, eyes, mouth, and hair.

PPE is free to employees. Correct sizes are available. The agency makes sure that PPE is cleaned, laundered, repaired, replaced, or discarded. OSHA requires these measures for the safe handling and use of PPE.

- Remove PPE before leaving the work area.
- Remove PPE when a garment becomes contaminated.
- Place used PPE in marked areas or containers when being stored, washed, decontaminated, or discarded.

- Wear gloves when you expect contact with blood or OPIM.
- Wear gloves when handling or touching contaminated items or surfaces.
- Replace worn, punctured, or contaminated gloves.
- Never wash or decontaminate disposable gloves for re-use.
- Discard utility gloves that show signs of cracking, peeling, tearing, or puncturing. Utility gloves are decontaminated for re-use if the process will not ruin them.

Equipment

Contaminated equipment is cleaned and decontaminated. Decontaminate work surfaces with a proper disinfectant:

- Upon completing tasks
- At once when there is obvious contamination
- After any spill of blood or OPIM
- At the end of the work shift when surfaces became contaminated since the last cleaning

Use a brush and dustpan or tongs to clean up broken glass. Never pick up broken glass with your hands, not even with gloves. Discard broken glass into a puncture-resistant container.

Waste

Special measures are required when discarding regulated waste:

- Liquid or semi-liquid blood or OPIM
- Items contaminated with blood or OPIM
- Items caked with blood or OPIM
- Contaminated sharps

Closable, puncture-resistant, and leak-proof containers are used. Containers are color-coded in red. They have the *BIOHAZARD* symbol.

Housekeeping

The agency must be kept clean and sanitary. A cleaning schedule is required. It includes decontamination methods and the tasks and procedures to be done.

Laundry

OSHA requires these measures for contaminated laundry:

- Handle it as little as possible.
- Wear gloves or other needed PPE.
- Bag contaminated laundry where it is used.
- Mark laundry bags or containers with the *BIOHAZARD* symbol for laundry sent off-site.
- Place wet, contaminated laundry in leak-proof containers before transport. The containers are color-coded in red or have the *BIOHAZARD* symbol.

EXPOSURE INCIDENTS

An *exposure incident* is any eye, mouth, other mucous membrane, non-intact skin, or parenteral contact with blood or OPIM. *Parenteral* means piercing the mucous membranes or the skin barrier. Piercing occurs through needle sticks, human bites, cuts, and abrasions.

Report exposure incidents at once. Medical evaluation, follow-up, and required tests are free. Your blood is tested for HIV and HBV. If you refuse testing, the blood sample is kept for at least 90 days. Testing is done later if you change your mind.

Confidentiality is important. You are told of the evaluation results. You also are told of any medical conditions that may need treatment. You receive a written opinion of the medical evaluation within 15 days after its completion.

The *source individual* is the person whose blood or body fluids are the source of an exposure incident. His or her blood is tested for HIV or HBV. State laws vary about releasing the results. The agency informs you about laws affecting the source's identity and test results.

Selected Illustrations, Boxes, and Tables
from *Basic Pharmacology for Nurses*

Illustrations, boxes, and tables originally published in Clayton BD, Stock YN, Harroun RD: Basic pharmacology for nurses, ed 14, St Louis, 2007, Mosby.

Glossary

absorption The process by which a drug is transferred from its site of body entry to circulating body fluids (blood, lymph) for distribution

abuse The intentional mistreatment or harm of another person

accountable Being responsible for one's actions and the actions of others who performed the delegated tasks; answering questions about and explaining one's actions and the actions of others

adrenergic blocking agent A drug that inhibits adrenergic effects

adrenergic fibers Nerve endings that release norepinephrine (a neurotransmitter)

advance directive A document stating a person's wishes about health care when that person cannot make his or her own decisions

adverse drug reaction (ADR) An unintended effect on the body from using a legal drug, illegal drug, or two or more drugs; drug reaction

aerobe A microbe that lives and grows in the presence of oxygen *(aer)*

agonist A drug that acts on a certain type of cell to produce a predictable response

aldosterone A substance that causes the kidneys to retain sodium

allergic reaction An unfavorable response to a substance that causes a hyper-sensitivity reaction

alopecia Hair loss

anaerobe A microbe that lives and grows in the absence *(an)* of oxygen *(aer)*

analgesic A drug that relieves pain; *an* means *without*, *algesic* means *pain*

anaphylactic reaction See "anaphylaxis"

anaphylaxis A severe, life-threatening sensitivity to an antigen; anaphylactic reaction

androgens Steroid hormones that produce masculine effects

angiotensin A substance that causes vaso-constriction, increased blood pressure, and the release of aldosterone

antacids Drugs that buffer, neutralize, or absorb hydrochloric acid in the stomach; *ant* means *against, acid* means *sour*

antagonist A drug that exerts an opposite action to that of another; or it competes for the same receptor sites

anti-anxiety drugs Drugs used to treat anxiety

antibiotics Anti-microbials derived from living microorganisms

anti-cholinergic agent A drug that blocks or inhibits cholinergic activity

anti-coagulants Drugs that prevent arterial and venous thrombi; "blood thinners"

anti-convulsants Drugs used to prevent or reduce seizures

anti-depressants Several classes of drugs used to treat mood disorders

anti-diabetic agents Drugs used to prevent or relieve the symptoms of diabetes

anti-diarrheals Drugs that relieve the symptoms of diarrhea

anti-dysrhythmic agents Drugs used to prevent or correct abnormal heart rhythms

anti-emetics Drugs used to treat nausea and vomiting

antihistamines Drugs that compete with released histamine for receptor sites in the arterioles, capillaries, and glands in mucous membranes

anti-hypertensive agents Drugs that reduce blood pressure

anti-microbial agents Chemicals that eliminate pathogens

anti-platelet agents See "platelet inhibitors"

anti-spasmodic agents Drugs that have an anti-cholinergic action and prevent acetylcholine from attaching to cholinergic receptors in the GI tract

anti-thyroid agents Drugs used to suppress the production of thyroid hormones

antitussives Drugs that suppress the cough center in the brain; cough suppressants

anxiety A vague, uneasy feeling in response to stress

arrhythmia Without (*a*) a rhythm (*rhythmia*); dysrhythmia

artery A blood vessel that carries blood away from the heart

ascites The abnormal accumulation of fluid in the peritoneal cavity

aspiration Breathing fluid, food, vomitus, or an object into the lungs

assault Intentionally attempting or threatening to touch a person's body without the person's consent

assessment Collecting information about the person; a step in the nursing process

bacteria One-celled plant life that multiply rapidly and can cause an infection in any body system; germs

barbiturate A drug that depresses the central nervous system, respirations, blood pressure, and temperature

battery Touching a person's body without his or her consent

benign tumor A tumor that does not spread to other body parts; it can grow to a large size

blood pressure The amount of force exerted against the walls of an artery by the blood

boundary crossing A brief act or behavior outside of the helpful zone

boundary signs Acts, behaviors, or thoughts that warn of a boundary crossing or violation

boundary violation An act or behavior that meets your needs, not the person's

broncho-dilators Drugs that relax the smooth muscles of the tracheo-bronchial tree

buccal Inside the cheek (*bucco*)

calorie The amount of energy produced when the body burns food

cancer Malignant tumor

capillary A tiny blood vessel; food, oxygen, and other substances pass from the capillaries to the cells

capsule A gelatin container that holds a drug in a dry powder or liquid form

cardiac output The amount of blood pumped with each heartbeat

carrier A human or animal that is a reservoir for microbes but does not have the signs and symptoms of infection

cell The basic unit of body structure

cerumen Ear wax

chart See "medical record"

cholesterol A waxy, fat-like substance found in all body cells

cholinergic fibers Nerve endings that release acetylcholine (a neurotransmitter)

cilia Small hair-like structures that project outward from the surfaces of some cells

civil law Laws concerned with relationships between people

clinical record See "medical record"

clonus Rapidly alternating involuntary contraction and relaxation of skeletal muscles

coating agents Drugs that form a substance that adheres to the crater of an ulcer

constipation The passage of a hard, dry stool

contraception The processes or methods used to prevent (*contra*) pregnancy

cortico-steroids Hormones secreted by the adrenal cortex of the adrenal glands

cough suppressants See "antitussives"

cream A semi-solid emulsion containing a drug

cretinism Congenital hypothyroidism

crime An act that violates a criminal law

criminal law Laws concerned with offenses against the public and society in general

cystitis Inflammation (*itis*) of the bladder (*cyst*)

debride To remove

decongestants Drugs that cause vaso-constriction of the nasal mucosa

defamation Injuring a person's name and reputation by making false statements to a third person

delegate To authorize another person to perform a nursing task in a certain situation

desired action Expected response

diabetes A disorder in which the body cannot produce or use insulin properly

diarrhea The frequent passage of liquid stools

digestion The process of physically and chemically breaking down food so that it can be absorbed for use by the cells

digitalization Giving a larger dose of digoxin for the first 24 hours, then giving the person a daily dose

dilute To add the correct amount of water or other liquid

distribution The ways drugs are transported by circulating body fluids to the sites of action (receptors) and to the sites of metabolism and excretion

diuresis The increased formation and excretion of urine; *dia* means *through, ur* means *urine*

diuretic A drug that promotes the formation and excretion of urine; *dia* means *through, ur* means *urine*

dose The amount of drug to give

drug A chemical substance that has an effect on a living organism

drug blood level The amount of a drug present in the blood

drug diversion Taking a person's drugs for your own use

drug interaction When the action of one drug is altered by the action of another drug

drug order An order for a drug written on the agency's (hospital, nursing center) physician's order form for a patient or resident; medication order

drug reaction See "adverse drug reaction"

dyslipidemia An abnormality of one or more of the blood fats (lipids)

dysrhythmia An abnormal *(dys)* rhythm *(rhythmia)*; arrhythmia

elixir A clear liquid made up of a drug dissolved in alcohol and water

embolus A small part of a thrombus that breaks off and travels through the vascular system until it lodges in a blood vessel

emesis Vomiting, vomitus

emulsion An oral dose form containing small droplets of water-in-oil or oil-in-water

endometriosis A condition *(osis)* in which the tissue that lines *(endo)* the inside of the uterus *(metri)* grows outside the uterus

enteral nutrition Giving nutrients into the gastro-intestinal (GI) tract *(enteral)* through a feeding tube

enteral route Drugs are given directly into the gastro-intestinal (GI) tract; *enteral* means *bowel*

enzymes Substances produced by body cells; using oxygen, enzymes break down glucose and other nutrients to release energy for cellular work

epilepsy A brain disorder in which clusters of nerve cells sometimes signal abnormally

erectile dysfunction (ED) The inability of the male to have an erection; impotence

estrogen The female hormone

ethics Knowledge of what is right conduct and wrong conduct

eunuchism A condition in which the male lacks male hormones

euphoria An exaggerated feeling or state of physical or mental well-being

evaluation To measure if goals in the planning step were met; a step in the nursing process

excretion The elimination of a drug from the body

expectorants Drugs that liquify mucus to promote the ejection of mucus from the lungs and tracheo-bronchial tree

false imprisonment Unlawful restraint or restriction of a person's freedom of movement

fatty oxidase enzyme inhibitor A drug that reduces the oxygen needed by myocardial cells to cause muscle contractions

fecal impaction The prolonged retention and build-up of feces in the rectum

fraud Saying or doing something to trick, fool, or deceive a person

fungi Plants that live on other plants or animals

gastro-intestinal prostaglandins Drugs that inhibit gastric acid secretion

gastrostomy tube A tube inserted through a surgically created opening *(stomy)* in the stomach *(gastro)*; stomach tube

generic name The drug's common name

germs See "bacteria"

gluco-corticoids Hormones that regulate carbohydrate, protein, and fat metabolism; they have anti-inflammatory, anti-allergenic, and immuno-suppressant activity

gonads The reproductive glands

griping Severe and spasm-like pain in the abdomen caused by an intestinal disorder; gripping

gynecologic Pertains to diseases of the female reproductive organs and breasts

healthcare-associated infection (HAI) An infection that develops in a person cared for in any setting where health care is given; the infection is related to receiving health care

hemoglobin The substance in red blood cells that carries oxygen and gives blood its color

hemorrheologic agent A drug that prevents the clumping of red blood cells and platelets: hemorrheologic relates to the science *(logic)* of blood *(hemo)* flow *(rrheo)*

histamine A substance released in response to allergic reactions and tissue damage from trauma or infection

histamine (H_2)-receptor antagonists Drugs that block the action of histamine; histamine blockers

hives See "urticaria"

homeostasis A constant internal environment

hormone A chemical substance secreted by the endocrine glands into the bloodstream

hyperglycemia High *(hyper)* sugar *(glyc)* in the blood *(emia)*

hyperlipidemia Excess *(hyper)* lipids *(fats)* in the blood *(emia)*

hyper-reflexia Increased reflex actions

hypertension The systolic pressure is 140 mm Hg or higher *(hyper)*, or the diastolic pressure is 90 mm Hg or higher; high blood pressure

hyperthyroidism The disease that occurs from the excess *(hyper)* production of the thyroid hormones

hypnotic A drug that produces sleep

hypoglycemia Low *(hypo)* sugar *(glyc)* in the blood *(emia)*

hypo-glycemic agents Drugs that lower *(hypo)* the blood *(emic)* glucose *(glyc)* level

hypogonadism A condition in which the body does not produce enough *(hypo)* testosterone

hypothyroidism The disease that results from inadequate *(hypo)* thyroid hormone production

idiosyncratic reaction Something unusual or abnormal that happens when a drug is first given

immunity Protection against a disease or condition; the person will not get or be affected by the disease

implementation To perform or carry out nursing measures in the care plan; a step in the nursing process

impotence See "erectile dysfunction"

infarction A local area of tissue death

infection A disease state resulting from the invasion and growth of microbes in the body

inhibitor A drug that prevents or restricts a certain action

inotropic agents Drugs that stimulate the heart to increase the force of contractions

insomnia A chronic condition in which the person cannot sleep or stay asleep all night

instill To enter drop by drop

insulin A hormone produced by the pancreas; it is needed for glucose to enter skeletal muscles, heart muscle, and fat

intermittent claudication A pain pattern usually described as aching, cramping, tightness, or weakness in the calves usually during walking; it is relieved with rest

intramuscular (IM) Within *(intra)* a muscle *(muscular)*

intra-nasal Within *(intra)* the nose *(nasal)*

intravenous (IV) Within *(intra)* a vein *(venous)*

invasion of privacy Violating a person's right not to have his or her name, photo, or private affairs exposed or made public without giving consent

ischemia A decreased supply of oxygenated blood to a body part

jejunostomy tube A feeding tube inserted into a surgically created opening *(stomy)* in the jejunum of the small intestine

lactic acid A product of glucose metabolism

lactic acidosis A build up of lactic acid in the blood

lavage Washing out the stomach

law A rule of conduct made by a government body

laxatives Substances that cause evacuation of the bowel; *laxare* means *to loosen*

leukorrhea An abnormal whitish *(leuko)* vaginal discharge *(rrhea)*

libel Making false statements in print, writing, or through pictures or drawings

lipids Fats

lotion A watery preparation containing suspended particles

lozenge A flat disk containing a medicinal agent with a flavored base; troche

malignant tumor A tumor that invades and destroys nearby tissue and can spread to other body parts; cancer

malnutrition Any disorder of nutrition; *mal* means *bad*

malpractice Negligence by a professional person

medical record The written account of a person's condition and response to treatment and care; chart or clinical record

medication A drug used to prevent and treat disease; medicine

medication assistant-certified (MA-C) Nursing assistive personnel who are allowed by state law to give drugs

medication order See "drug order"

medication reminder Reminding the person to take drugs, observing them being taken as prescribed, and charting that they were taken

medicine See "medication"

medicine cup A plastic container with measurement scales

medicine dropper A small glass or plastic tube with a hollow rubber ball at one end

menstruation The process in which the lining of the uterus breaks up and is discharged from the body through the vagina

metabolism The burning of food for heat and energy by the cells; the process by which the body in-activates drugs

metabolite A product of drug metabolism

metastasis The spread of cancer to other body parts

microbe See "microorganism"

microorganism A small *(micro)* living plant or animal *(organism)* seen only with a microscope; a microbe

mineralo-corticoids Hormones that maintain fluid and electrolyte balance

miosis Narrowing of the pupil

mucolytic agents Drugs that reduce the stickiness and thickness of pulmonary secretions

mydriasis Dilation of the pupil

myxedema Hypothyroidism that occurs during adult life

nasal Nose

naso-duodenal tube A feeding tube inserted through the nose *(naso)* into the duodenum of the small intestine

naso-gastric (NG) tube A feeding tube inserted through the nose *(naso)* into the stomach *(gastro)*

naso-intestinal tube A feeding tube inserted through the nose *(naso)* into the small intestine *(intestinal)*

naso-jejunal tube A feeding tube inserted through the nose *(naso)* into the *jejunum* of the small intestine

nausea The sensation of abdominal discomfort that may lead to the urge or need to vomit

neglect Failure to provide the person with the goods or services needed to avoid physical harm, mental anguish, or mental illness

negligence An unintentional wrong in which a person did not act in a reasonable and careful manner and a person or the person's property was harmed

neuron The basic nerve cell of the nervous system

neurotransmitter A chemical substance that transmits nerve impulses

non-pathogen A microbe that does not usually cause an infection

normal flora Microbes that live and grow in a certain area

nurse practice act The law that regulates nursing practice in a state

nursing assistive personnel Individuals employed to give direct hands-on care and perform delegated nursing care tasks under the supervision of a licensed nurse

nursing care plan A written guide about the person's care; care plan

nursing diagnosis Describes a health problem that can be treated by nursing measures; a step in the nursing process

nursing intervention An action or measure taken by the nursing team to help the person reach a goal

nursing process The method nurses use to plan and deliver nursing care; its five steps are assessment, nursing diagnosis, planning, implementation, and evaluation

nursing task Nursing care or a nursing function, procedure, activity, or work that does not require an RN's professional knowledge or judgment

nutrient A substance that is ingested, digested, absorbed, and used by the body

nutrition The processes involved in the ingestion, digestion, absorption, and use of foods and fluids by the body

objective data Information that is seen, heard, felt, or smelled by an observer; signs

observation Using the senses of sight, hearing, touch, and smell to collect information

ocular Pertains to the eye

ointment A semi-solid preparation containing a drug in an oily base

ophthalmic Pertains to the eye

opiate A drug that contains opium, is derived from opium, or has opium-like activity

opium The milky substance from unripe poppy seed pods; *opion* means poppy juice

opportunistic infection An infection caused by non-pathogens in a person with a weakened immune system

oral contraceptives Birth control pills

organ Groups of tissues with the same function

osmotic agents Drugs that cause fluid to be drawn from outside of the vascular system into the blood

otic Pertains to the ear

over-active bladder (OAB) A syndrome characterized by urinary frequency, urgency, and incontinence; urge syndrome or urgency/frequency syndrome

pain To ache, hurt, or be sore; discomfort

parenteral nutrition Giving nutrients through a catheter inserted into a vein; *para* means *beyond*; *enteral* relates to the bowel

parenteral route Drugs bypass the GI tract (*para* means *beyond*; *enteral* means *bowel*)

pathogen A microbe that is harmful and can cause an infection

peptic Pertains to digestion or the enzymes and secretions needed for digestion

peptic ulcer An ulcer in the stomach, duodenum, or other part of the GI system exposed to gastric juices

percutaneous endoscopic gastrostomy (PEG) tube A feeding tube inserted into the stomach *(gastro)* through a small incision *(stomy)* made through *(per)* the skin *(cutaneous)*; a lighted instrument *(scope)* allows the doctor to see inside a body cavity or organ *(endo)*

percutaneous route Drugs are given through *(per)* the skin *(cutaneous)* or a mucous membrane

peristalsis Involuntary muscle contractions in the digestive system that move food down the esophagus through the alimentary canal

pharmacology The study of drugs and their actions on living organisms

placebo A drug dosage form that has no active ingredients

planning Setting priorities and goals; a step in the nursing process

platelet aggregation inhibitor A drug that prevents platelets from clumping together and causes vaso-dilation

platelet inhibitors Drugs that prevent platelet aggregation (clumping); anti-platelet agents

powder A finely ground drug in a talc base

pre-hypertension When the systolic pressure is between 120 and 139 mm Hg or the diastolic pressure is between 80 and 89 mm Hg

prescription A drug order written for a person leaving the hospital or nursing center or for a person seen in a clinic or doctor's office; it is written on a prescription pad or it is called in, faxed, or emailed to the pharmacy by the doctor

priapism A prolonged or constant erection

PRN order The nurse decides when to give the drug based on the person's needs

professional boundaries That which separates helpful behaviors from behaviors that are not helpful

professional sexual misconduct An act, behavior, or comment that is sexual in nature and occurs within the scope of employment

progesterone The hormone associated with body changes that favor pregnancy and lactation

prokinetic agents Drugs that stimulate movement or motility

prostatitis Inflammation (*itis*) of the prostate (*prostat*)

protected health information Identifying information and information about the person's health care that is maintained or sent in any form (paper, electronic, oral)

proton pump inhibitors Drugs that inhibit the gastric acid pump of the parietal cells

protozoa One-celled animals that can infect the blood, brain, intestines, and other body areas

psychosis A state of severe mental impairment; the person does not view the real or unreal correctly

pyelonephritis Inflammation (*itis*) of the kidney (*nephr*) pelvis (*pyelo*)

reconstitute To add water or other liquid to a powder or solid form of a drug

regurgitation The backward flow of stomach contents into the mouth

renin An enzyme that affects blood pressure

respiration The process of supplying the cells with oxygen and removing carbon dioxide from them

retching The involuntary, labored, spasmodic contractions of the abdominal and respiratory muscles without vomitus; "dry heaves"

rhinitis medicamentosa Drug-induced congestion

rhinorrhea Nasal discharge (*rhino* means *nose*; *rrhea* means *discharge*); runny nose

route How and where the drug enters the body

secondary infection An infection caused by a microbe that follows the first infection caused by a different microbe

sedative A drug that quiets the person; it gives a feeling of relaxation and rest

seizure Violent and sudden contractions or tremors of muscle groups; convulsion

semi-synthetic A natural substance that has been partially altered by chemicals

side effect An unintended reaction to a drug given in a normal dosage

signs See "objective data"

single order A drug is to be given at a certain time and only one time

slander Making false statements orally

souffle cup A small paper or plastic cup used for solid drug forms

spasm An involuntary muscle contraction of sudden onset

standard of care Refers to the skills, care, and judgment required by nursing assistive personnel under similar conditions

standing order A drug is to be given for a certain number of doses or for a certain number of days

STAT order The drug is to be given at once and only one time

stomatitis Inflammation (*itis*) of the mouth (*stomat*)

subcutaneous Beneath (*sub*) the skin (*cutaneous*)

subjective data Things a person tells you about that you cannot observe through your senses; symptoms

sublingual Under (*sub*) the tongue (*lingual*)

suppository A cone-shaped, solid drug that is inserted into a body opening; it melts at body temperature

suspension A liquid containing solid drug particles

symptoms See "subjective data"

synapse The junction between one neuron and the next

synthetic A substance that is made rather than naturally occurring

syringe A plastic measuring device with three parts—tip, barrel, and plunger

syrup An oral dose form containing a drug dissolved in sugar

system Organs that work together to perform special functions

tablet A dried, powdered drug compressed into a small disk

testosterone The male hormone

therapeutic drug monitoring The measurement of a drug's concentration in body fluids

thrombo-embolic diseases Diseases associated with abnormal clotting within blood vessels

thrombosis The process of clot formation

thrombus A blood clot

thyroid replacement hormones Drugs that replace thyroid hormones in the treatment of hypothyroidism

tissue A group of cells with similar functions

topical Refers to a surface of a part of the body

topical medication A drug applied to the skin

tort A wrong committed against a person or the person's property

toxicity Exposure to large amounts of a substance that should not cause problems in smaller amounts; the reaction when side effects are severe

tracheo-bronchial tree The trachea, bronchi, and bronchioles

trademark The brand name or trade name of the drug

tranquilizers Anti-anxiety drugs

transdermal Through *(trans)* the skin *(dermal)*

triglycerides Fatty compounds that come from animal and vegetable fats

troche See "lozenge"

tumor A new growth of abnormal cells; tumors are benign or malignant

ulcer A shallow or deep crater-like sore of a mucous membrane

urethritis Inflammation *(itis)* of the urethra *(urethr)*

urinary anti-microbial agents Substances that have an antiseptic effect on urine and the urinary tract

urticaria Raised, irregularly shaped patches on the skin and severe itching; hives

vaso-dilators Drugs that widen blood vessels to increase blood flow

vaso-spasm A sudden contraction of a blood vessel causing vaso-constriction

vein A blood vessel that returns blood back to the heart

viruses Microbes that grow in living cells

vital signs Temperature, pulse, respirations, blood pressure, and pain

vomiting Expelling stomach contents through the mouth; emesis

vomitus The food and fluids expelled from the stomach through the mouth; emesis

vulnerable adult A person 18 years old or older who has a disability or condition that makes him or her at risk to be wounded, attacked, or damaged

Key Abbreviations

ACE Angiotensin-converting enzyme

ACTH Adrenocorticotropic hormone

AD Alzheimer's disease

ADE Adverse drug event

ADH Antidiuretic hormone

ADME Absorption, distribution, metabolism, excretion

ADR Adverse drug reaction

AHA American Hospital Association

AIDS Acquired immunodeficiency syndrome

ALR Assisted living residence

ARB Angiotensin II receptor blocker

AV bundle Atrio-ventricular bundle

AV node Atrio-ventricular node

BPH Benign prostatic hyperplasia

C Celsius; centigrade

CAD Coronary artery disease

CDC Centers for Disease Control and Prevention

CHF Congestive heart failure

CNA Certified nursing assistant

CNS Central nervous system

CO$_2$ Carbon dioxide

COMT Catechol O-methyltransferase

COPD Chronic obstructive pulmonary disease

DEA Drug Enforcement Administration

DNR Do not resuscitate

ECG Electrocardiogram

ED Erectile dysfunction

EMT Emergency medical technician

F Fahrenheit

FDA Food and Drug Administration

g Gram

GED General education diploma

GERD Gastro-esophageal reflux disease

GH Growth hormone

GI Gastro-intestinal

h Hour

HAI Healthcare-associated infection

HBV Hepatitis B virus

HDL High-density lipo-protein

Hg Mercury

HIPAA Health Insurance Portability and Accountability Act of 1996

HIV Human immunodeficiency virus

ID Identification

IM Intramuscular

IOP Intra-ocular pressure

ISMP Institute for Safe Medication Practices

IV Intravenous; intravenously

kg Kilogram

LDL Low-density lipo-protein

LNA Licensed nursing assistant

LPN Licensed practical nurse

LVN Licensed vocational nurse

MA-C Medication assistant-certified

MAOI Monoamine oxidase inhibitor

MAR Medication administration record

mcg Microgram

MDI Metered-dose inhaler

MDS Minimum Data Set

mg Milligram

MI Myocardial infarction

mL Milliliter

mm Millimeter

mm Hg Millimeters of Mercury

NANDA-I North American Nursing Diagnosis Association International

NCSBN National Council of State Boards of Nursing

NDC National Drug Code

NG Naso-gastric

NSAID Non-steroidal anti-inflammatory drug

O$_2$ Oxygen

OAB Over-active bladder

OBRA Omnibus Budget Reconciliation Act of 1987

OCD Obsessive-compulsive disorder
ODT Orally disintegrating tablet
OPIM Other potentially infectious materials
OSHA Occupational Safety and Health Administration
OTC Over-the-counter

PAC Premature atrial contraction
PAT Paroxysmal atrial tachycardia
PDR Physicians' Desk Reference
PEG Percutaneous endoscopic gastrostomy
PG Prostaglandin
PO By mouth (per os); per os (orally)
PPE Personal protective equipment
PPI Proton pump inhibitor
PRN, prn As needed, when necessary, when needed
PTSD Post-traumatic stress disorder

PUD Peptic ulcer disease
PVC Premature ventricular contraction
PVD Peripheral vascular disease

q Every

RBC Red blood cell
RN Registered nurse
RNA Registered nurse aide

SA node Sino-atrial node
SSRI Selective serotonin re-uptake inhibitor
STAT Immediately; at once
STD Sexually transmitted disease
subcut Subcutaneous; subcutaneously

T$_3$ Tri-iodothyronine
T$_4$ Thyroxine
TB Tuberculosis
TCA Tri-cyclic anti-depressant
TDD Transdermal drug delivery

TED hose Thrombo-embolic disease hose
TH Thyroid hormone; thyroxine
TIA Transient ischemic attack
TLC Therapeutic Lifestyle Changes
TO Telephone order
TPN Total parenteral nutrition
TSH Thyroid-stimulating hormone
TURP Trans-urethral resection of the prostate
TZD Thiazolidinedione

UTI Urinary tract infection

VC Vomiting center
VF Ventricular fibrillation
V fib Ventricular fibrillation
VO Verbal order
VT Ventricular tachycardia

WBC White blood cell

Index

Page numbers followed by *f* indicate figures; *t*, tables; *b*, boxes.